Effective
Dental
Assisting

Effective Dental Assisting

SHIRLEY PRATT SCHWARZROCK, PH.D.

Clinical Assistant Professor
Faculty of the School of Dentistry
University of Minnesota

JAMES R. JENSEN, D.D.S.

Associate Dean
School of Dentistry
University of Minnesota

Wm. C. Brown Company Publishers
Dubuque, Iowa

Copyright © 1954, 1959 by L.H. Schwarzrock and S.P. Schwarzrock

Copyright © 1967, 1973 by Wm. C. Brown Company Publishers

Library of Congress Catalog Card Number: 72—92850

ISBN 0—697—05705—4

Third Printing, 1975

Printed in the United States of America

CONTENTS

PREFACE FOR THE DENTAL ASSISTANT

A career as a dental assistant can be a most rewarding way of life. You assist people to be more comfortable. You are part of a service profession which improves the health and welfare of people. Dental assistants are intelligent, effective, and personable health professionals.

The profession requires the learning of a vast amount of detail about dentistry and people. This text attempts to start you on your career with a mastery of fundamentals. The Workbook, which accompanies the text, has a "Preface for the Prospective Dental Assistant" which will help you learn how to study, accomplish your goals, take examinations, and be interviewed by a prospective employer. It will also help you organize your study habits and use of time.

Today oral health care is being provided more frequently by a team of health professionals directed by the dentist. The dental assistant is an effective team member in this important health profession. Notice the Frontispiece. It shows an excellent dental assistant serving her dentist. Wouldn't you like to be working as she is? You can.

Shirley Schwarzrock
James R. Jensen

PREFACE FOR THE DENTIST

The team concept of oral health care delivery has drastically altered the practice of dentistry. Four-handed, sit-down dentistry is now common. Dental assisting is a necessity. Preferably, more than one assistant can and should be utilized.

Effective Dental Assisting, the *Workbook for Effective Dental Assisting,* and the *Manual for the Workbook* have been written to aid in training (1) dental assistants in formal training courses and (2) dental assistants in the office of the individual dentist who is faced with the problems of training a new employee. Even the dentist who hires a certified dental assistant will find *Effective Dental Assisting* helpful for purposes of review and clarification of office routine, provided he has organized his office in the manner suggested.

The 1973 edition of *Effective Dental Assisting* attempts to provide an opportunity for familiarity with the old as well as the new, inasmuch as the dental assistants will find themselves confronted with many ages of armamentarium. It has been our goal, however, to illustrate as many techniques of assisting with materials and processes as possible.

As in the previous editions, the authors have attempted to provide specific and detailed routines commonly used in a dental office. Insofar as the space limitation imposed by one volume permits, the illustrations present typical samples of each item with which a dental assistant should be familiar. The manufacturer may vary, the form may be slightly different, but the illustrations, including instruments, equipment, and business records, are intended to help the student learn by recognition from photographs when actual specimens are not available.

It is recognized that routines differ in various dental offices, but it is also recognized that learning a basic routine and being familiar with instrumentation and key processes hasten adaptation to the individual office when the student becomes an employed assistant.

Your new assistant will appreciate an orderly approach to her training for the new job. The time and effort required to teach her to work in the manner which you prefer for your office can be reduced, and your production level raised.

You, the dentist, should be familiar with the complete text. Wherever necessary, adapt the instructions to your particular methods of operating and administering your office. It is recommended that you indicate the order in which you wish your assistant to learn the various procedures and duties. The new assistant should then be expected to know only those sections or procedures which she has been assigned until she has mastered all the techniques which you require.

Use of the Workbook will aid materially in helping her understand the textbook. You, the dentist, can ask your new assistant to answer the questions in the Workbook for the section which you have assigned her in the text.

The *Manual to the Workbook* is a publication designed for the dentist or teacher. Part one contains suggestions about effective teaching procedures. Part two states each Workbook question with the correct answer and the page number of *Effective Dental Assisting* where the correct answer will be found.

Now, why have an assistant?

Dentistry is a self-limiting profession. With the exception of the dental hygienist's work and that performed by a laboratory technician, every operation for which the dentist receives remuneration is one he must perform with his two hands during the number of hours he feels he must— or can—spend in the dental office. The use of dental assistants to perform all tasks which are interruptions of the dentist's chair time and to increase production through chairside assisting is the best solution to a difficult problem in economics and personal health.

Any task which a dental assistant can be taught to do for the dentist should be delegated to an assistant. The degree to which this delegation of tasks is successfully carried in various dental offices often accounts for the variation in production and, as a direct result, in the amount of time the dentist must work.

There are a number of sources of lost productive time that apply to any office, regardless of the fact that not all dentists are capable of producing at the same rate. One important cause of lost productive time is disorganization of the dentist's work habits at the chair. In order to produce efficiently, the dentist's operative procedures must always be the same in sequence of procedure and instrumentation for each type of operation. The use of diamond and/or carbide instruments for operative procedures at the higher operating speeds *requires* a systematic procedure, together with the use of a well-trained assistant, to achieve maximum benefits.

Any dentist who has worked alone is thoroughly aware of production-disturbing factors in the dental office. Answering the telephone, making appointments, collecting fees, processing X rays, purchasing supplies, talking with salesmen, cleaning up after operative work, sterilizing instruments—these are but a few of the production-disturbing factors. Hiring an assistant to take over these duties, when the patient load warrants, creates an increase in services rendered which is very apparent. The dentist's output of energy and the degree of strain become less when he secures the many benefits of good office efficiency.

The dental assistant's *primary* job is to keep the dentist at the chair providing dental care which *no one* else in the office can provide. This means that she is to control or eliminate production-disturbing factors while serving the public graciously; she is also to assist in the production of dentistry at the chair.

If the dental assistant is to succeed, she must be trained to exercise control of the office by the best means possible. The dentist must be cooperative in her exercise of such control.

Dental assisting is a complex job. It requires a high level of intelligence, social adjustment, emotional stability, speech ability, manual dexterity, and personal drive to be a success, together with good health and the personal habits of good grooming which make up a pleasing individual. With these tangible and intangible qualifications, a girl has an excellent chance of becoming a good assistant if her training is well organized.

Through long practice, the dentist has become familiar with his office procedures; the details are a simple matter of routine. To a new employee these are a thousand-and-one *confusing* details. Responsibility for but one new idea at a time gives the new assistant an orderly approach to these details. She will be a better assistant in less time if allowed to pursue this training program.

In order to facilitate the use of this text in his office, the dentist should take time to accomplish the following:

1. Organize his own instrumentation and sequence in all dental operations.
2. Make the necessary changes or additions in the text, especially in the operative section, to suit his own pattern of work.
3. Indicate to the assistant the order in which she is to be held responsible for learning the various duties and operations. Carefully verify her answers in the Workbook and be sure that she understands the material she has studied.
4. Make a list of the time required for typical operations, from the average number of surfaces of amalgam restorations per hour to the time required for denture work and its associated laboratory requirements —for all routine procedures performed in your practice—to be typed and mounted inside the back cover of the appointment book or placed in a permanent location at the desk where appointments are made.
5. Turn to page 594 and fill in the exposure time for X rays as used in your office.

6. Be cooperative in delegating authority to your dental assistant as she grows in ability. Any indication of lack of confidence on the part of an employer can seriously impair the self-confidence and performance of an employee.

The procedures outlined in this text are not assumed to apply to all dental offices, nor to include all dental procedures. They are presented with the sole purpose of providing a starting point in training for the neophyte. If no outline of procedure for a specific duty were used, only generalities would remain. The dental assistant, regardless of her training or experience, *must always learn the procedures as used in the office in which she is employed.*

Shirley Schwarzrock
James R. Jensen

ACKNOWLEDGMENTS

The most remarkable factor in the production of this fourth edition of *Effective Dental Assisting* is the great kindness and generosity of many people. My gratitude to them is beyond expression. With revision impending, generous offers of assistance came from all parts of the United States. For these offers I am deeply grateful.

The selection of Dean James R. Jensen to coauthor and supervise the dental technology is fortunate. He was a close friend of Doctor Rocky. His areas of concern in dentistry and his teaching efforts in Minnesota's dental auxiliary utilization program prior to his appointment as Assistant Dean have given him insights which are invaluable in the revision of this text.

It is with deep gratitude for the long hours devoted to my education and for the contributions to our joint effort that I welcome Jim as coauthor.

Shirley Schwarzrock

Others have been very helpful, and we wish to acknowledge their contributions:

Doctor Rocky looked on Hugh Silkenson, D.D.S., M.S.D., as an adopted son; and Hugh contributed the revision materials for History, Anatomy, and Microbiology and Sterilization. We wish to thank Hugh.

Donald Hauptfeuhrer of the Department of Radiology of the University of Illinois College of Dentistry has been a gracious guide in radiography for several years. With this revision Don offered invaluable editorial assistance.

Fred Hayes, D.D.S., member of the American Society of Oral Surgeons, former Mayo Clinic Fellow, another of Doctor Rocky's close friends, added new materials for oral surgery.

Dorothy Carbonaro, Readers Services Librarian, Bureau of Library Services, American Dental Association, contributed to the necessary research, suggesting materials to read and verifying bibliography.

Fritz Schöen, Prof. Dr. med., Dr. med. dent., and Brigitte Gierl, dental assistant, for permission to use the washed-field technique.

Members of the University of Minnesota Dental School Staff deserve a special thanks:

Helen Tuchner, C.D.A., B.S., Director, Dental Assistants' Training Program,

Leroy Christianson, R.B.P., Senior Medical Photographer, Director of the Dental Illustration Laboratory, and his staff including: Art Work —Mrs. Susan Ball and Mrs. Joan Dako,

Anna Hampel, D.D.S., M.S.D., Director Admissions, Treatment Planning, and Comprehensive Care,

Carl Bandt, D.D.S., M.S.D., Director of Clinics,

Allan D. Petersen, D.D.S., Associate Professor of Prosthodontics, and Norman O. Holte, D.D.S., M.S., Professor of Oral Surgery.

Robert Silha, D.D.S., of Eastman Kodak, assisted with illustrations from Eastman Kodak.

The educational directors Andrew Nagy, of Siemens, and Ron Newman, of S. S. White, were most helpful, as was Charles Stevenson, President of Rinn Corporation, and M. M. Bennett and his staff at General Electric.

Our continued appreciation to these individuals for their contributions to the several editions:

Sumter S. Arnim, D.D.S., Ph.D., Professor of Dentistry, University of Texas, Houston, Texas.

Bruce Fenchell, D.D.S., Cedar Rapids, Iowa.

Andrew Froehlich, C.P.A., Minneapolis, Minnesota.

James Kershaw, D.D.S., West Warwick, Rhode Island.

Harry Lykins, Regional Manager, Healthco, Columbus, Ohio.

John Marcus, Marcus Dental Supply Co., Minneapolis, Minnesota.

Lawrence W. McIver, D.D.S., American Association of Orthodontists, National Angle Society, Minneapolis, Minnesota.

Roscoe Miller, M.D., Professor of Radiology, Indiana University Medical Center, Indianapolis, Indiana.

Albert G. Richards, D.D.S., Professor of Dentistry, University of Michigan, Ann Arbor, Michigan.

A. T. Thorson, D.D.S., Fellow, ICD. Former Director of the Dental Assistants' Training Program at the University of Minnesota, Minneapolis, Minnesota.

Edward T. Wentworth, D.D.S., Rochester, New York.

To the many dental firms who supplied illustrations and legend material we are grateful.

Shirley Schwarzrock
James R. Jensen

PART ONE | DENTISTRY AND PEOPLE

*A dental office is
centered around relationships among people
and is a place where
people meet to give and receive service.*

Some patients are apprehensive, some are relaxed, some are joyous, and some are withdrawn, fearful, or belligerent. The gamut of emotions are expressed by patients.

The attitudes of the personnel who dispense service for these patients can and do affect the attitudes of patients, and vice versa. Those who provide the service ought to remain pleasant and cheerful even when attitudes encountered in patients cause *frustrations* (defeats to one's attempts to do something; discouragements). The dental office personnel should be able to accept the problems as part of a day's work.

The chapters in part one are written to help the dental assistant gain perspective for her work as a member of the oral health care delivery team. They will provide her with techniques in the areas of communication and human relations, so essential for her work with her dentist and his patients.

1 The Profession of Dentistry... A Team Approach

Service to the Public

Good health—including a healthy mouth—is becoming the right of every person in today's world. More people are comprehending that good *oral health* (mouth health) is essential to good general health.

"The beginning of preventive medicine is care of the mouth" is a widely quoted statement by one of the famed Mayo brothers, founders of the Mayo Clinic in Rochester, Minnesota. The relationship of good oral health to good general health was recognized very early. According to one translator, in 668-626 B.C. an Assyrian court physician recommended the removal of a patient's teeth because the physician felt they were the cause of the patient's systemic difficulties.

The need for dental services has accompanied the existence of a civilized society from early history to the present. Prinz reports that the earliest written information concerning dentistry appeared on one of several clay tablets, probably made about 7,000 years ago, which were found in the valley of the Euphrates river (Iraq).[1] This reference consisted of a treatment for painful teeth.

1. Herman Prinz, *Dental Chronology*, p. 15.

In the 1930s, Dr. Weston A. Price conducted investigations of dental deformities and dental decay among various racial groups all over the world. His report on the South Sea Islanders was typical of his reports on other groups studied: When the Islanders retained their primitive ways of life and existed on native foods, they did not develop dental deformities nor dental decay; yet such deformities and decay were common among the Islanders who lived on imported foods.[2] *Dental deformities* and *dental decay* are therefore often called *diseases of civilization.*

Today the dental profession is making a most important contribution to society through its services to individuals. Dentistry can provide the care which helps the individual maintain good oral health, good personal appearance, and the ability to *masticate* (chew) food properly. It can also prevent pain by preventive care and provide relief from pain when pain is already present. The relationship of these services to the general physical and mental health of the individual cannot be overemphasized.

Pain is one of the basic reasons, or motivating forces, for seeking dental treatment. Also, with the general improvement in the quality of dental treatment and in the public's appreciation of that treatment, the *prevention* of pain has become a strong motivating force for seeking professional care regularly.

The maintenance of personal appearance is dependent to a high degree upon the maintenance of oral health. People who have teeth missing present a ridiculous appearance—consider the circus clowns who blacken several teeth to produce laughs. Personal appearance, therefore, provides a third motivating force for seeking dental treatment. In fact, *in the mind of the average patient, personal appear-*

2. W. A. Price, *Nutrition and Physical Degeneration,* pp. 116-128.

ance ranks well ahead of most reasons for seeking dental care.

The oral cavity is the portal through which all nourishment enters the body. The first step in the digestion of food occurs in the mouth with the action of ptyalin in the saliva beginning the conversion of starches to sugars. The teeth are used to break up the larger food particles by a grinding action, making it easier for the ptyalin to begin its work, and also to prepare the food for swallowing. The ability to properly masticate food taken into the mouth is therefore important for the entire process of digestion as well as for pleasure in eating.

Oral health and general health are very closely related. Many systemic diseases have oral manifestations; a high percentage of cancer originates in the mouth area. Thus, maintaining oral health is one of the basic functions of the dental profession.

The purpose of dentistry, then, is to serve the public by:

1. helping to maintain good oral health,
2. helping to maintain the ability to masticate food for as long as one lives,
3. helping to maintain or to improve personal appearance,
4. preventing oral diseases and pain by practicing preventive dentistry, and
5. providing relief from oral pain.

Oral Health Care Delivery

A study of literature about dentistry reveals many statements (supported by statistics) which indicate an impending shortage of dentists.

There never has been doubt about the *need* for dental care. Dental caries infects ninety-eight percent of our population. Periodontal disease and malocclusions are nearly as rampant. There is an almost universal need for dental treatment of some kind for all individuals.

The *demand* for oral health care services unfortunately does not even closely approach the need. Today four out of five potential dental patients do not receive the care they need. Why? Some people cannot afford to pay for the services, some areas of the country are without enough dentists to adequately care for the demand for services, some people fear dentistry, and some people are ignorant of dentistry's contribution to comfort, appearance, and improved ability to masticate food. (Some are ignorant of the importance to general health of one's ability to masticate food.) These are all reasons potential patients fail to seek the care they need.

However, there is more demand for dental care today than there was twenty-five years ago. During World War II, many men who had not experienced dental care as civilians learned the meaning of good dentistry as members of the armed services. As they established homes on their release from service, they resolved to provide dental care for their families; and the demand for good care grew. The population explosion following the war further increased the demand for services.

It is also true that health care, including oral health care, is receiving more attention by local, state, and federal legislators searching for means to broaden health-coverage benefits for all citizens.

A statement made by Aristotle in 384-322 B.C. seems to be guiding public sentiment today. He said:

Health of mind and body is so fundamental to the good life that if we believe that men have any personal rights at all as human beings, then they have an absolute moral right to such a measure of good health as society and society alone is able to give.

Currently, many segments of society are provided health care benefits through governmental programs, private insurance carriers, union contracts, employers' fringe benefits, and dental service plans. Third-party payment plans are rapidly eliminating the economic barrier which prevents many segments of the population from seeking adequate health care. (Third-party payment means that someone who does not receive the service pays for it—such as government agencies, unions, employers, or insurance carriers.)

Consequently, people who formerly were unable or unwilling to pay for dentistry are now seeking dental care, thus increasing the number of patients to be treated. In some areas a critical shortage of dentists already exists, and the shortage is likely to worsen generally. Dental leaders in government, organized dentistry, and dental education recognize that the increased demand for dental services has created the necessity for new approaches to the problem of providing adequate care for new patients.

A logical solution is the establishment of the dental health team. The dentist is responsible for the diagnosis and care plan for each patient. He employs a staff of assistants who have been trained in the services they provide. He directs the delivery of service to his patients, while he performs only the treatments needing his skills and judgment. As the various dental auxiliaries are created and as the expanded duty training programs develop, the dentist of the future may do less routine dentistry, delegating the repetitive phases of dental treatment to well-trained and certified assistants.

Thus, the dental health team is of growing significance. A dentist is likely to staff his office with several assistants who have experienced different training programs and therefore will make varying contributions to the oral health care delivery team.

It is also true that the day of the individual solo practice seems to be waning. Dentists are discovering the advantages of group practice whereby it is easier for emergencies to be met and for hours to be regulated, with more consideration for the health and well-being of the dentist while maintaining excellent service for the patients.

Laws are being changed so that dentists may incorporate and thus provide fringe benefits for their employees and receive the same tax benefits which businessmen achieve by incorporation.

Thus we find that more assistants will be working in a group practice and on a team which consists of more than two or three persons.

The Role of the Dentist

The dentist is a well-educated individual. Educationally, dentistry today requires a minimum of two years of training in cultural and scientific studies before entry into the dental school. Most people do not realize that in the beginning years of professional training, dental students and medical students may be in the same classes. If the courses are offered separately, they are similar in content, differing only in emphasis relating to each profession. The dental student's studies are not confined to the oral cavity, nor, indeed, to the head. His studies in anatomy, for example, range through *gross anatomy* (the study of the complete body and its various parts), *embryology* (the study of the growth and development of the body before birth), *comparative anatomy* (the comparison of human anatomy with that of other animals), *histology* (the study of microscopic anatomy of normal tissues), and *dental anatomy* (the study of the form of individual teeth and their usual shape, and their relationship to each other in the dental arch).

The dental student's studies in other fields are equally thorough. For the most part, the public as a whole is not aware of the type and thoroughness of training the dentist receives in the field of medical sciences nor of the complexity of his training in the dental sciences. Today, dentists are frequently becoming members of hospital health care delivery teams, taking their rightful place next to the physician.

The dentist is a highly trained specialist. This, in turn, points up another consideration in dental practice: a highly trained specialist should devote his time and ability to that work for which he is specifically trained and which only he is capable of performing. In order to achieve the objective of providing more and better service to more people, the dentist needs to employ assistants to take over the duties in the dental office which do not require his professional training. (Dental educators now agree that many of the routine details which a dentist performs do not require as high a degree of skill as he must perform in other operations. Thus many areas can be delegated to other persons who are not as highly skilled as the dentist, provided they have been educated in the performance of these skills.)

Most dentists are engaged in the general practice of dentistry; that is, the dental procedures which they accomplish for their patients may be in any field of dentistry. In rural or isolated areas, the dentist is more likely to engage in most of the types of work which comprise the total dental field. In metropolitan areas, where specialists are more readily available, the "general" dentist is more likely to refer patients with particularly difficult problems to specialists for treatments requiring a high degree of skill in a limited dental field.

Dental Specialties

Increase in knowledge in various fields in dentistry, as in medicine, which require advanced training and special skills has created the need for specialists. The growth of urban centers of population and the development of transportation facilities have provided the opportunity for specialists to serve.

A *specialist* in dentistry is a dentist who limits his practice to one type of work, in contrast to the *general* dentist who practices in more than one field of dentistry. In dentistry there are eight specialties recognized as such at this time by the American Dental Association.[3] Each specialty has qualifications and examinations to be met before a dentist can announce himself a specialist. These eight specialties are as follows:

1. *Oral surgery* is restricted to the diagnosis of diseases, injuries, and defects of the human jaws and associated structures and the treatment by surgical techniques.
2. *Orthodontics* is restricted to correcting dental anomalies, which usually means improving the appearance and the ability to masticate of patients whose dental arches and/or jaws are malformed. The public generally refers to this process as "straightening teeth," but a much more complicated process is involved. This specialist must be skillful in understanding functions and aesthetics of teeth within the jaws and in correcting the relationships of upper and lower arches to create a pleasing outward appearance while providing ability to masticate food effectively.
3. *Pedodontics* is restricted to dentistry for children. "It includes training the child to accept dentistry, restoring and maintaining the primary, mixed, and permanent dentitions, applying preventive measures for dental caries and periodontal disease, and preventing, intercepting, and correcting various problems of occlusion."[4]

4. *Periodontics* is restricted to the diagnosis, treatment, and prevention of diseases of the supporting structures of the teeth, including deviations from normal anatomy and physiology. The public commonly refers to all these diseases and problems under one misleading word, "pyorrhea."
5. *Prosthodontics* is restricted to the restoration and maintenance of oral function by the replacement of missing teeth and structures by artificial devices. It includes "providing suitable substitutes [called prosthetic replacements] for the coronal portions of teeth or for one or more lost or missing natural teeth and their associated parts in order that impaired function, appearance, comfort, and health of the patient may be restored."[5] Some of the devices are referred to as "fixed" because they are cemented permanently to existing teeth, but some replacements are removable. A full denture is the replacement for all the teeth in one arch; it restores aesthetics and function. The prosthetic replacement of part of the teeth in one arch is called a partial denture. An improper term for a denture is "plate."
6. *Oral pathology* is restricted to the study of oral diseases, their diagnosis or identification, their causes, how they proceed, and what effect they produce, as well as their relationships to the rest of the body.
7. *Dental public health* is confined to working with public education in dental health, prevention, and treatment programs for any department of health, whether it is supported by federal, state, county, or local governments.
8. *Endodontics* is restricted to working with the etiology (causative factors), diagnosis, prevention, and treatment of diseases of

---

3. "Specialties and Announcement of Practice Limitation," *ADA Journal* 69 (August 1964): 193.
4. Carl O. Boucher, *Current Clinical Dental Terminology*, p. 271.

5. *Ibid.*, p. 297.

the dental pulp and with the aftereffects of these diseases on the various structures which compose the pulp and periapical tissues.

The dentist in general practice may refer patients to a specialist in the aforementioned fields, may ask for consultation with him regarding a particular case, or may ask for assistance from a specialist in a particular field in the normal conduct of his dental practice.

Types of Practice

Whether they are general practitioners or specialists, dentists may have a private practice or a practice with several other dentists in what is called group practice.

In private practice, as the name implies, a dentist works by himself in his own office. He may rent the space or own his building, but he alone is responsible for the dentistry performed in his office. He may even share a reception room with another dentist or a physician, but his practice is private—his own.

A group practice consists of several men working together under some plan on which they have agreed. It may be a group of specialists and generalists or it may be a group of general practitioners. Any agreement which is satisfactory to them is acceptable. They may share their reception room, office expenses, employees, a working code, and even their office space and/or income. In this situation one of the dentists may even employ other dentists.

Group practice may also apply to a dental practice in association with members of other health professions who have formally agreed on certain central arrangements designed to advance the economical and efficient conduct of their practices in order to render an improved health service to the patient. Such groups may also contract with unions or employers to perform service for a group of workers—another form of private practitioners ar-

ranging to care for a group of patients rather than accepting these patients on an individual basis.

Principles of Ethics

Dentists have a very high ethical standard by which they practice. It may help you to understand the high level of your own profession if you understand what the dental profession as a whole expects of each individual who has been licensed to practice dentistry.

Here, then, are quoted the important points of the Principles of Ethics of the American Dental Association as revised in 1971:

The practice of dentistry first achieved the stature of a profession in the United States where, through the heritage bestowed by the efforts of many generations of dentists, it acquired the three unfailing characteristics of a profession: education beyond the usual level, the primary duty of service to the public and the right to self-government.

The maintenance and enrichment of this heritage of professional status place on everyone who practices dentistry an obligation which should be willingly accepted and willingly fulfilled. This obligation cannot be reduced to a changeless series of urgings and prohibitions for, while the basic obligation is constant, its fulfillment may vary with the changing needs of a society composed of the human beings that a profession is dedicated to serve. The spirit and not the letter of the obligation, therefore, must be the guide of conduct for the professional man. In its essence, this obligation has been summarized for all time and for all men in the golden rule which asks only that "whatsoever ye would that men should do to you, do ye even so to them."

The following statements constitute the *Principles of Ethics* of the American Dental Association. The constituent and component societies are urged to adopt additional provisions or interpretations not in conflict with these *Principles of Ethics* which would enable them to serve more faithfully the traditions, customs and desires of the members of these societies.

Section 1

Education Beyond the Usual Level. The right of a dentist to professional status rests in the knowledge, skill and experience with which he serves his patients and society. Every dentist has the obligation of keeping his knowledge and skill freshened by continuing education through all of his professional life.

Section 2

Service to the Public. The dentist's primary duty of serving the public is discharged by giving the highest type of service of which he is capable and by avoiding any conduct which leads to a lowering of esteem of the profession of which he is a member.

In serving the public, a dentist may exercise reasonable discretion in selecting patients for his practice. However, a dentist may not refuse to accept a patient into his practice or deny dental service to a patient solely because of the patient's race, creed, color or national origin.

Section 3

Government of a Profession. Every profession receives from society the right to regulate itself, to determine and judge its own members. Such regulation is achieved largely through the influence of the professional societies, and every dentist has the dual obligation of making himself a part of a professional society and of observing its rules of ethics.

Section 4

Leadership. The dentist has the obligation of providing freely of his skills, knowledge and experience to society in those fields in which his qualifications entitle him to speak with professional competence. The dentist should be a leader in his community, including all efforts leading to the improvement of the dental health of the public.

Section 5

Emergency Service. The dentist has an obligation when consulted in an emergency by the patient of another dentist to attend to the conditions leading to the emergency and to refer the patient to his regular dentist who should be informed of the conditions found and treated.

Section 6

Use of Auxiliary Personnel. The dentist has an obligation to protect the health of his patient by not delegating to a person less qualified any service or operation which requires the professional competence of a dentist. The dentist has a further obligation of prescribing and supervising the work of all auxiliary personnel in the interests of rendering the best service to the patient.

Section 7

Consultation. The dentist has the obligation of seeking consultation whenever the welfare of the patient will be safeguarded or advanced by having recourse to those who have special skills, knowledge and experience. A consultant will hold the details of a consultation in confidence and will not undertake treatment without the consent of the attending practitioner.

Section 8

Unjust Criticism and Expert Testimony. The dentist has the obligation of not referring disparagingly, orally or in writing, to the services of another dentist to a member of the public. A lack of knowledge of conditions under which the services were afforded may lead to unjust criticism and to a lessening of the public's confidence in the dental profession. If there is indisputable evidence of faulty treatment, the welfare of the patient demands that corrective treatment be instituted at once and in such a way as to avoid reflection on the previous dentist or on the dental profession. The dentist also has the obligation of cooperating with appropriate public officials on request by providing expert testimony.

Section 9

Rebates and Split Fees. The dentist may not accept or tender "rebates" or "split fees."

Section 10

Secret Agents and Exclusive Methods. The dentist has an obligation not to prescribe, dispense or promote the use of drugs or other agents whose complete formulae are not available to the dental profession. He also has the obligation not to prescribe or dispense, except for limited investigative purposes, any therapeutic agent, the value of which is not supported by scientific evidence. The dentist has the further obligation of not holding out as exclusive, any agent, method or technic.

Section 11

Patents and Copyrights. The dentist has the obligation of making the fruits of his discoveries and labors available to all when they are useful in safeguarding or promoting the health of the public.

Patents and copyrights may be secured by a dentist provided that they and the remuneration derived from them are not used to restrict research, practice or the benefits of the patented or copyrighted material.

Section 12

Advertising. Advertising reflects adversely on the dentist who employs it and lowers the public esteem of the dental profession. The dentist has the obligation of advancing his reputation for fidelity, judgment and skill solely through his professional services to his patients and to society. The use of advertising in any form to solicit patients is inconsistent with this obligation.

Section 13

Cards, Letterheads and Announcements. A dentist may properly utilize professional cards, announcement cards, recall notices to patients of record and letterheads when the style and text are consistent with the dignity of the profession and with the custom of other dentists in the community.

Announcement cards may be sent when there is a change in location or an alteration in the character of practice, but only to other dentists, to members of other health professions and to patients of record.

Section 14

Office Door Lettering and Signs. A dentist may properly utilize office door lettering and signs provided that their style and text are consistent with the dignity of the profession and with the custom of other dentists in the community.

Section 15

Use of Professional Titles and Degrees. A dentist may use the titles or degrees, Doctor, Dentist, D.D.S. or D.M.D., in connection with the name on cards, letterheads, office door signs and announcements. A dentist who also possesses a medical degree may use this degree in connection with his name on cards, letterheads, office door signs and announcements. A dentist who has been certified by a national certifying board for one of the specialties approved by the American Dental Association may use the title "diplomate" in connection with his specialty on his cards, letterheads and announcements if such usage is consistent with the custom of dentists in the community. A

dentist may not use his title or degree in connection with the promotion of any commercial endeavor.*

The use of eponyms in connection with drugs, agents, instruments or appliances is generally to be discouraged.

Section 16

Health Education of the Public. A dentist may properly participate in a program of health education of the public involving such media as the press, radio, television and lecture, provided that such programs are in keeping with the dignity of the profession and the custom of the dental profession of the community.

Section 17

Contract Practice. A dentist may enter into an agreement with individuals and organizations to provide dental health care provided that the agreement does not permit or compel practices which are in violation of these *Principles of Ethics.*

Section 18

Announcement of Limitation of Practice. Only a dentist who limits his practice exclusively to one of the special areas approved by the American Dental Association for limited practice may include a statement of his limitation in announcements, cards, letterheads and directory listings (consistent with the custom of dentists of the community), provided at the time of the announcement, he has met the existing educational requirements and standards set by the American Dental Association for members wishing to announce limitation of practice.

In accord with the established ethical ruling that dentists should not claim or imply superiority, use of the phrases "Specialist in ...." or "Specialist on ...." in announcements, cards, letterheads or directory listings should be discouraged. The use of the phrase "Practice limited to ...." is preferable.

*The resolution adopted by the 1970 House of Delegates inadvertently referred to "the last sentence" of Section 15 rather than "the last sentence of the first paragraph" of Section 15. At its January, 1971 meeting the Judicial Council voted that the intent was obviously "the last sentence of the first paragraph." This matter will be brought to the attention of the 1971 House of Delegates.

A dentist who uses his eligibility to announce himself as a specialist to make the public believe that specialty services rendered in his dental office are being rendered by ethically qualified specialists when such is not the case, is engaged in unethical conduct. The burden is on the specialist to avoid any inference that general practitioners who are associated with him are ethically qualified to announce themselves as specialists.

Section 19

Directories. A dentist may permit the listing of his name in a directory provided that all dentists in similar circumstances have access to a similar listing and provided that such listing is consistent in style and text with the custom of the dentists in the community.

Section 20

Name of Practice. A dentist may practice in a partnership, or as a solo practitioner, professional corporation or professional association. The use of practice names other than the names of participating dentists is unethical, except that corporate designations may be used if required by state law. Designations such as "Professional Corporation," "Inc.," "Group," "Clinic," or similar designations, may not be used as a part of the name of a practice on cards, letterheads, signs, directories and announcements, unless required by state law.

Note. The following policy was approved by the 1970 House of Delegates: Resolved, that dentists using assumed names for their dental practices prior to June 1, 1970 be allowed to continue to use ethically such assumed names until not later than January 1, 1972.

Section 21

Judicial Procedure. Problems involving questions of ethics should be solved at the local level within the broad boundaries established in these *Principles of Ethics* and within the interpretation of the code of ethics of the component society. If a satisfactory decision cannot be reached, the question should be referred, on appeal, to the constituent society and the Judicial Council of the American Dental Association, as provided in Chapter XI of the *Bylaws* of the American Dental Association.

Abiding by the principles of ethics which have been evolved by the national and local dental organizations, the dentist practices in any number of ways, depending on his mode of operation and choice of specialty. He will maintain an office and hire personnel to complete his team which he selects with consideration for his needs for assistance.

Formation of a Team

A team means a number of persons working together. The critical words are *working together.* A team means cooperation, getting a job done. In the dental office it is also necessary to perform this job harmoniously—with each team member carrying his or her responsibilities effectively so other team members can accomplish their parts of the joint effort.

The oral health team attempts to provide excellent care for each patient who enters the office. It is to be expected that a practicing dentist will have his team well organized, and as a new assistant enters the team relationship, she should be made aware of her place within the group. Perhaps nothing will be said about the "team," but it is hoped that the new assistant will feel the team spirit of these oral health delivery team professionals.

What positions exist on the dental health team? How can one move from one position to another? The dentist is the captain of the team. He determines which work he wishes to have accomplished by others and then hires the assistants to fulfill these needs. The important factor is that *a dentist is privileged to decide just what he believes his needs to be and forms his team around those needs.*

Soon, if not now, most dental offices may have an office administrator who oversees the coordination of the efforts of all employees. Other employees may include the chairside assistant, hygienist, expanded duties assistants, laboratory technicians, and certain business office employees whose titles will vary from office to office. The most common titles in that group will be receptionist, bookkeeper, and patient educator. The office administrator may be the person whose responsibilities are reception of patients and/or bookkeeping and/or patient education. In some offices the office administrator will have separate responsibilities, and all or some of these functions will be performed by other staff members. For purposes of clarifying specific tasks, we will consider the separate responsibilities of reception, bookkeeping, and patient education.

As a patient enters a dental office, he may encounter members of the oral health care delivery team in this order: receptionist, bookkeeper, hygienist, patient educator, dental assistant or chairside assistant, floater, laboratory assistant, expanded duties personnel, and laboratory technician.

The *receptionist* is a most important team member. She plans the appointments, scheduling patients carefully so that time is not wasted. She is responsible for the telephone—one of the most important instruments in the office since it is often the first contact a patient has with the office and thereby creates his first impression. From this first contact, he forms an opinion about the dental office. He may confuse quality of dental care with the degree of friendliness he experiences in his telephone contact. Through the use of the telephone, patients can be lost or gained, service can be rendered or people turned away in frustration and anger.

The receptionist also greets patients and cares for anyone who enters the reception room, including salesmen and professional colleagues of the dentist. Her job requires the use of excellent communication techniques so performed that patients enjoy coming to this particular office. She may also be responsible for making the financial arrangements during case presentations.

The *bookkeeper* may be the receptionist or a full-time bookkeeper with no other responsibilities; or a bookkeeping service may be utilized by the dentist.

The *hygienist* is a certified and licensed employee of the dentist, permitted by state law to perform certain specific tasks under the direction of the dentist. Prophylaxis, taking dental X rays, and patient education are tasks which a hygienist may perform under the supervision of the dentist-employer. A minimum two-year course of study is necessary prior to certification or licensing.

The *patient educator* teaches home oral hygiene—preventive care of the mouth. Her responsibility is to see that patients learn to care for their mouths, to keep them clean and well exercised at home, so that the excellent restorations which are placed by the dentist receive proper maintenance between recalls.

Although treatment of disease is necessary, prevention is the first consideration for all diseases affecting the human body. Oral diseases are no exception. If a disease can be prevented, treatment will not be necessary. If a disease is treated, the patient should be told how to avoid a recurrence. Oral health needs far exceed the ability of the dental profession to provide adequate treatment. It is the goal of the dental profession, therefore, not only to provide the necessary corrective treatment, but to prevent occurrence and recurrence by teaching good preventive dental care. Such preventive educational programs need professional guidance, a responsibility usually assigned to the auxiliaries on the team: the dental assistant, the dental hygienist, or, in many offices, the patient educator.

The *dental assistant* or *chairside assistant* sits beside the patient and is the dentist's second pair of hands—thus the common term "four-handed dentistry." She makes it possible for him to keep his eyes concentrated on his work, without the need to reach for instruments and materials, and to keep his hands close to the area of operation in the patient's mouth. This assistant will anticipate the dentist's needs and be ready to supply the materials as he indicates he has finished with the previous step. She will know his routines as well as he does. Usually the dentist and his chair assistant develop a private communication system utilizing the turn of the hand, movement of the head, or even a short word such as "Now" to indicate the change in instrumentation or procedure. Watching an efficient dentist-chairside assistant team can be fascinating.

The *floater*, another trained chairside assistant, is an additional pair of hands to serve the assistant who serves the dentist. She, too, learns to recognize the routines so well that she anticipates the materials needed by the chair assistant, who never leaves the patient. The floater is expected to supply anything not already at the chair. These two assistants in conjunction with the dentist provide what is known as six-handed dentistry.

The *laboratory assistant* may spend her time in the dental laboratory preparing impressions, waxing restorations, pouring models—doing any of the many tasks which are necessary to complete restorations the dentist is designing for his patients.

New team members are being added as recognition of the need for their services develops. The new team members are referred to as assistants who perform expanded duties, or *expanded duties personnel*. These duties have not as yet been entirely delineated. However, many of the repetitive treatments which the dentist has been performing will be delegated to these expanded duties assistants who have been trained in specific tasks and then certified as able to perform them in the dental office. Currently, some state boards permit certified expanded duties personnel to perform some intraoral processes. (Minnesota students graduating from courses in intraoral processes permitted by the State Board of

Dentistry are called *Registered Assistants.*) In the future, more duties will be added to this list, and new functions and training will follow.

The number of intraoral duties performed by auxiliary personnel may increase as time goes on. Formerly, an assistant was not permitted to work inside the mouth. Now the assistant is being trained in many intraoral procedures to further expand the production capabilities of the dental team. There will be several levels of expanded duties, and it is conceivable that a good dental assistant can return to school from time to time to develop more skills. Given the capacity and determination and by continuing to acquire education, such an assistant could continue to study until she becomes a dentist.

The *laboratory technician* may or may not be a part of the office staff. If the dentist employs him and provides space in the office for his work, then he is a member of the team. If the dentist prefers to utilize the services of a commercial laboratory, the team relationship may not be as evident, but nevertheless, cooperation and goodwill must exist.

The dental laboratory technician at this time is neither registered nor licensed by law. However, in 1957 a program for certification was formally endorsed by the American Dental Association and the National Association of Dental Laboratories. By July 1963 more than 5,000 dental technicians had been certified.[6] On June 8, 1964, the Joint Committee of the American Dental Association and the National Association of Dental Laboratories launched a nationwide program of accreditation for existing laboratories.[7]

The technician is trained to perform laboratory operations primarily concerned with the

6. National Board for Certification, Roster of Certified Dental Technicians, Washington, D. C., July 1963.
7. American Dental Association, *ADA Journal* 69, no. 2 (August 1964): 202.

fabrication of appliances such as fixed and removable prostheses.

The oral health care delivery team of the future may consist of the office administrator, the hygienist, the chair assistant, the floater, expanded duties personnel, receptionist, bookkeeper, and laboratory technician—all directed by the dentist.

Role of the Dental Assistant

Dental assistants most certainly play an important role on the team with ever-increasing responsibilities. This book is written for the *beginning* dental assistant who must experience training either in the office or in a school. How does one decide whether personal satisfaction exists in this profession?

Some girls look for a job when they finish school—something to occupy them until they find a husband to support them. Other girls look for a career—a career to pursue for a lifetime—in spite of marriage, in addition to marriage, or in place of marriage. The philosophy a person develops in a career approach to the world of work is vastly different from that developed by a girl who is just marking time until Mr. Right comes along. A career can be a stimulating, challenging experience, with one's outlook broadened considerably and opportunities for advancement and for interesting experiences greatly increased. In addition, no woman is safe to assume that she will marry and never have to seek employment again. Every woman needs a career—to give her stimulus in living, to give her a way of adding to the family income if necessary, and to support herself and her children should she be widowed.

How does one acquire this career outlook? Every woman should discover her vocational interests by taking a test most high schools give to determine these interests, such as the Strong's Interest Inventory.[8] With some understanding of her interests and high-school grades, it is possible for a woman to find a career opportunity which will be a challenge and a lifelong interest.

The individual whose interests indicate that a career in dental assisting would be desirable is likely to find dental assisting a career of intense personal satisfaction.

Let us look at the role of the beginning dental assistant.

A dental assistant is usually a fine young woman with a constitution of steel, a good sense of humor, a pleasant personality, and a sense of enjoyment in serving people.

Do you feel happy when you help someone with a problem which he cannot solve by himself? When another human being looks at you, smiles, and says, "Thanks! That was a big help to me!" do you feel personal satisfaction?

That's the way a good dental assistant can feel about her job *every day,* because she is helping people to be more comfortable and healthier even though they may not always smile their appreciation.

Work Opportunities

Where can you find a position as a dental assistant? You will readily think of working for a dentist in either private practice or group practice, but there are at least two other fields for your consideration: a job with a federal agency or one with the armed services. Federal agency jobs are found in either the U. S. Public Health Department or the Veterans' Administration. Both have clinics and hospitals where dental assistants are employed. These employees are under Civil Service. The armed services have a special classification for

8. This type of test must be administered by a competent Certified Psychologist or Counselor. If a high school does not offer such a counseling program, most colleges test and counsel individuals for a nominal fee.

dental assistants. They sometimes use civilian personnel for these jobs, but usually the assistants are members of the services. All services —army, navy, air force, and marines—use dental assistants.

Regardless of *where* you choose to work— for a private practitioner, a group practitioner, Civil Service, or the armed forces—you will find that your dentist has spent many years learning his profession and will never be through with learning. This same opportunity is yours; learn all you possibly can about the job you are performing and about the profession of dentistry. Borrow books from your dentist. If you have access to a dental library, read other books which will help to give you a background in dentistry. The library of the American Dental Association provides such services. This library is one of the finest in the nation, and books are regularly loaned through mail services. It is not possible to exhaust your opportunities to know more about your work.

One way to improve yourself professionally is to become a member of the American Dental Assistants Association. This organization, formed in 1924, has established educational requirements whereby a dental assistant can become a *Certified Dental Assistant.* The rise in status of the dental assistant can be largely attributed to the dedicated individuals who have worked diligently as members of the American Dental Assistants Association. In 1960 the goal of certification and educational requirements for the dental assistant were established by action of the American Dental Association.[9]

The Dental Assistant, the journal of the American Dental Assistants Association, is a most helpful publication which you can read regularly. When you have become eligible for

9. Lois Kryger, "A.D.A.A. Guideposts," *The Dental Assistant,* American Dental Assistants Association, July-August 1962, p. 35.

membership and actually join the American Dental Assistants Association, you receive this periodical. *Reading* the journal, attending meetings, and continuing to study—all help one improve professional skills.

Duties

What can you expect as duties? The dental assistant may be the only employee in the office, in which case she assists at the chair, receives patients, and is the office secretary. In an office where there is more than one employee, she may be a chair assistant, helping only with dentistry at the chair and perhaps doing some laboratory work. If there are two or more assistants, the second assistant may be a receptionist and office administrator, caring for the business routines of the office.

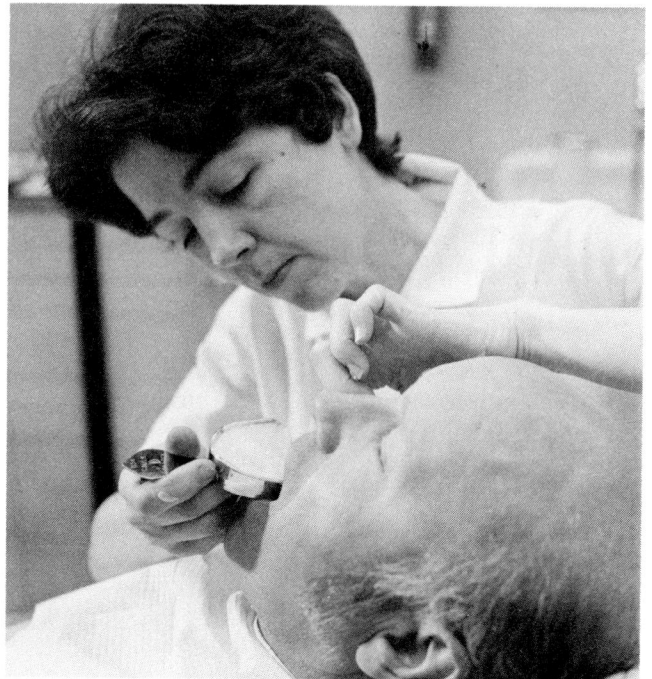

Fig. 1.1. The dental assistant takes an impression for a study model.

It will become obvious that the practice of dentistry involves a great many subjects in addition to those of a technical nature. It is the purpose of this text to help you *begin* your association with the duties which are yours in the dental office and to serve as a reference.

The job of the dental assistant is primarily to *save the dentist's time:* to do for the dentist those things which do not require his technical training and would interrupt his actual production of dental work for patients; secondarily, to aid directly in the production of dental services at the chair. There are literally hundreds of duties, operations, techniques, instruments, medications, and other details to learn. No single operation is an exact replication of another; no two patients are just alike in their reactions or needs. Remember that, in spite of its complexity, learning this work can become confusing only if you let it become so.

Your job will be easier to learn if you will take *one* operation at a time and learn thoroughly what is required for it and what it is meant to accomplish. Then, and only then, learn a new operation. Aim for the ability to anticipate the needs of the dentist in your preparations in the office. Learn to work in close harmony with him. If you first understand just what a particular job is meant to accomplish, you will approach your part of it with more confidence and understanding. Consequently, you will be able to assist more successfully.

While no single dental service is an exact repetition when performed for different patients, there are certain basic points which will be repeated time and again. You can learn these basic points for any given operation. Experience will teach you how to take care of the variable elements of all operations. That phase of the work will come with time and *intelligent observation* on your part. Always prepare everything which is normally required for an operation. Be prepared to handle the unusual

quickly on request, or, if possible, before such request—upon observing its need.

The outlines of routine dental operations in the text are given as examples to aid in breaking down your particular office routine. It is not possible to write outlines of procedure which will satisfy all dentists. Nearly all dental offices have differences in procedure to some extent: in the way patients are treated, in the way an inlay preparation or an amalgam preparation is made, or in the manner the practice is conducted. It is your duty to *fit into* an office, not to revolutionize it—unless you are specifically invited to reorganize some phase. There are many paths to the same goal —there are many ways, for example, to construct full upper and lower dentures. Adapt yourself to the routines *your* dentist desires in his office.

Memorize one basic routine at a time. Learn *by name* the instruments, materials, or medications required for that routine; learn the sequence of their use and where each belongs in the cabinet or laboratory before proceeding to another routine. Ask all the questions you feel are necessary, but cultivate the note-taking habit so that you will not find it necessary to ask the same question twice.

To repeat: The object in having a dental assistant in the first place is to save *time*. The more *time* you save your dentist, the better assistant you are. You are there to help the dentist; the more quickly you learn the various routines and the more rapidly you perform each one, the better you are doing your job. Whatever your work of the moment, *learn to do it rapidly and thoroughly.*

Make it your objective to know your work to the last detail, to maintain a constant interest in the patient as an individual, to do each job quietly and efficiently, and to be part of a smooth-running organization. Join your Dental Assistants Association and take an active part in its programs and functions. Cultivate a feeling of enthusiasm about your work and about the dental profession.

Know that you have an important part in providing a very necessary service to humanity.

Standard of Conduct

Regardless of the size of the office staff with which you work, there are certain principles of behavior which are necessary for work in the office. A standard of professional conduct in keeping with the high principles of dental ethics is necessary.

The American Dental Assistants Association has formulated this Code of Ethics:

The spirit of the Golden Rule should be the guiding principle of conduct for the dental assistant. In all her contacts with the dental profession and society she should maintain honesty, loyalty, and a desire to serve to the best of her ability her employer and his patients.

The dental assistant should give to her employer the cooperation he needs to serve his patients capably and efficiently. She will hold in confidence the details of professional services rendered by her employer. She should refrain from performing any service for patients which requires the professional competence of the dentist, or which may be prohibited by the dental practice act of the state in which she is employed.

She should avoid making any disparaging remarks about the conduct of the profession she serves, or of her employer's treatment of his patients.

The dental assistant has the obligation of increasing her skill and efficiency by availing herself of the educational opportunities provided by the Association and its component societies. She should take part in the efforts of these groups to improve the educational status of the dental assistant and should support this Code of Ethics.

In providing a service to the public, as in the dental office, it is inevitable that you will come into contact with much information which is to be treated with the strictest confidence. The personal records which the office keeps of the dental work, physical history, and details of the patient are the property of the dentist, not of the patient. This does not imply freedom to use such information for any purpose other than that for which it is intended. There is no justification *ever* for reporting outside the office the slightest bit of information you have learned while in that office. It is confidential information. Treat it as such.

Records should not be left where a patient might see and (with a natural curiosity) read them, whether they are those of the patient himself or of another patient. Always place them in such a position as to make it inconvenient for the patient to see the records, even though he should make a deliberate effort to do so.

Recently one of the nationally syndicated columnists published a letter in which the writer expressed anger. She was employed in the downtown area of a city. At lunch the dental assistants, lawyers' secretaries, medical assistants, a minister's secretary, and nurses with whom she ate were always discussing over the luncheon table the personal business of patients and clients. She was angry because she felt that there was nowhere she could go for care of her personal health problems, religious problems, or legal problems and feel that the matter would be treated confidentially. From the points of view of the dentist who is pledged to confidential care and the patient who is at the mercy of the dentist and his staff, this accusation could not be more serious. Be certain that you do not fall into this category of thoughtless assistants. Remember, *What you see here, what you hear here, stays here.*

In the dental office you are in a "service" profession. A service profession assumes certain obligations to the public it serves. It must honor the confidentiality of personal information above any consideration, perform its services in the best interests of the patients, and strive to achieve the highest standards of service and cleanliness (moral, mental, and physical). Being a dental assistant is somewhat like being an ambassador in a foreign country. An ambassador attempts to create an excellent impression so that people who meet him will think highly of his country. Ask yourself, What kind of impression am I creating for my dentist? What kind of impression am I creating for my profession of dentistry?

Before your dentist can practice his profession, he must have a patient. What brings that patient to your dentist's office? What keeps him as a patient?

Dentists cannot advertise in the usual sense of the word. You, yourself, become one of the personal advertisements of the office for which you work. In your contacts outside that office, you can do much to bring patients into it; your conduct inside the office can do much to keep those patients who do come. Psychology applied to working with people is of prime importance in all walks of life; under the conditions of the dental office it cannot be overemphasized. In chapter two you will find practical guides for your work with patients.

The dental assistant will learn much about the dentist for whom she works. Every phase of his personal life eventually becomes known to her to some degree—from how well he gets along with his wife to how he spends his income. It is never wise to indicate that you know any of these details. They are not subjects for comment. The dentist knows that you will learn many of these details, but he also prefers that you let the information "go in one ear and out the other." The dental assistant who lives with her family sometimes finds it difficult to resist the family's curiosity about patients, office details, and the dentist for whom she works. Make it a habit to divulge no information. Again: there is no justification *ever* for reporting outside the office the slightest bit of information you have learned while in that office. It is confidential information. Treat it as such. Do not gossip!

The dentist and his dental assistant are necessarily in a closely interdependent relationship for a considerable part of each day. This in itself tends to produce frictions, the severity of which is governed by the adjustment of the personalities involved. It would be unusual to have every day, week after week, month after month, year after year, go by without occasional irritation. If all office relationships are maintained on a plane of harmony and teamwork to perform office routines, with as little interjection of personal elements as is possible, the dentist-assistant team has the best opportunity for continuous harmonious association. Should it become evident that the personalities of the dentist and his assistant are not compatible, it is far preferable to terminate the association than to continue to work under conditions which are not pleasant. Moreover, any such friction in the office is very soon evident to patients.

Familiarity can breed contempt. It is best to apply the same principle to the relationship of dentist and assistant. For example, the dentist's wife should always remain "Mrs. Smith" to the dental assistant unless there is an extremely strong reason for the relationship to reach the familiarity of first names.

However familiar the office staff may be with each other when by themselves, the dentist should be addressed as "Doctor" when in the presence of patients. "This material is ready, Doctor." When speaking about the dentist, refer to him as "Doctor Smith." "Doctor Smith will see you at three o'clock, Mrs. Jones." It is best to retain this terminology at all times in the office.

When a dentist's wife acts as his dental assistant, it is even more important that addressing each other in a professional manner be remembered. Not all patients who enter the office may be familiar with the fact that the dentist and his assistant are man and wife. Terms of endearment, unconsciously applied, may offend. The use of a familiar manner is too easily carried over into the presence of patients, and in a professional office this is decidedly unbecoming.

The patient's impression of the dentist often begins with his contact with the dental assistant—first on the telephone, later in the reception room. If the telephone contact is effective, the patient looks forward to seeing the office. The condition of the reception room affects his impression, but the *attitude* of the dental assistant can reinforce or obliterate that impression. Therefore, the standard of conduct of the dental assistant should be that which is expected in a professional office: dignified, efficient, tactful—but friendly.

Personal Impression Created by the Dental Assistant

The impression which we create on others is determined by our personal appearance and our ability to express ourselves—bodily and vocally. A good dental assistant creates a favorable impression on the people who enter the office.

In order to create this impression, there are certain matters which must be given careful attention.

Grooming

To create a good impression on patients, the most scrupulous personal grooming is an absolute essential in the dental office.

How refreshing it is to greet someone who smells of soap or who is so clean that cleanliness just radiates from her. The sweet smell of a really clean person is a satisfaction to all who come near.

In dental assisting this type of cleanliness is important. You are in very close contact with humans all day long. A thoroughly clean body to begin the day will help keep you refreshing in your contacts. It would be advisable for every dental assistant to have a soapy shower or tub bath each morning prior to leaving for work. (This, incidentally, is a delightful habit. It is refreshing and leaves one's body feeling wonderful—a luxury we all ought to enjoy.) With the soaps available today, most of the body odor is controlled for a twenty-four-hour period. If your problem is especially difficult, using a good deodorant immediately after your bath ought to keep you pleasant to be near for the entire time you are at the office.

If you have any special problems with body odors, such as especially strong menstruation odor, be sure to take extra precautions with special deodorants and frequent changes of pads during those periods when you are having difficulty. Perfume never completely masks such odors. To some people it makes them only more nauseating.

Of course, a clean body should be put into all clean clothing. It takes such a few minutes to suds out your personal underthings at night—and keeps them fresh and clean without harsh scrubbing. Liquid soaps make the task easy. There is no excuse for a dental assistant to appear at the office any way but scrupulously clean.

It is also important to shampoo your hair at least weekly. Some young women find it necessary to shampoo every other day if they have problems with excessive oil. Our world today is full of smog and dirt; therefore, a weekly shampoo is a must. Needless to say, tidy hair is important. A simple hairstyle is probably most acceptable in the dental office—nothing high-style which interferes with good assisting. It is a little difficult to be touching your hair to keep it coiffed and to assist at the chair at the same time. Hair and mouths simply do not go together!

In recapitulation, then, the dental assistant must be scrupulously neat about her person. Her work brings her into close contact with patients throughout the day, always under critical observation. Here are an even dozen reminders:

1. Uniform. Color is being used more frequently for dental uniforms. The traditional white uniform for the dental assistant is still preferred by many dentists, but in a number of offices dentists are substituting color. The psychological reason lies in part in children's association between white and the nurse or physician who has given them a "shot" which has caused pain. It is also possible that some adult patients may subconsciously feel this discomfort with white.

   The design of uniforms has improved. They are more attractive and comfortable, whether they are dresses or the very popular uniform pants suit. Regardless of the color of the uniform which your office requires, cleanliness is of utmost importance. An extra uniform at the office is a necessity in case there should be an accident which makes it desirable to change during the day.

2. If your uniform is white, your slip should be white also, since colored slips under white uniforms are unattractive. Of course it must be of the correct length, ending in the hemline of the uniform so that it does not show above the hem nor hang below the uniform.

3. Hose should be of a light color. White hose, if preferred, are deductible from income tax as a professional expense. One pair per week is allowed.

4. Shoes. If your uniform is white, white shoes, kept white and in good repair, are in order. Whatever color the shoes required in your office, they ought to be of a conservative type, properly groomed. If you have two pair for use on alternate days, they last longer and give your feet a much needed rest. White shoes are deductible from your income tax as a professional expense.

5. Neat hair. If a cap is not part of the uniform, a hairnet should be worn if there is any question of loose strands.

6. Fingernails should be scrupulously clean, neatly trimmed, and not an excessive length. Use only clear or natural polish. Hands should be kept clean throughout the day. Wash before assisting at the chair and before handling instruments which are to be used.

7. Cosmetics should be used sparingly and in good taste. Remember that the dental assistant receives very close scrutiny. Makeup which might be acceptable when viewed from some distance may not look very attractive when seen twelve or fifteen inches away.

8. Perfume, if any, should be very mild. Be certain that the deodorant which you use is effective. Perfume is not a substitute for baths and a good deodorant.

9. Jewelry, except for a wristwatch (preferably with a sweep-second hand), should not be worn. Mercury, used in most dental offices, is extremely detrimental to gold. Many dental assistants who are married wish to wear their wedding rings in the office. It would be wise to wear an inexpensive substitute during office hours.

10. Avoid chewing gum. It is offensive to many patients.

11. Wear an apron for the initial daily office dusting.

12. Give yourself a double check on your appearance before receiving the first morning patient. The dental assistant should be able to finish her office-opening duties and check herself before the first patient arrives.

Inadvertent Communication

In addition to grooming, our ability to express ourselves—bodily and vocally—determines the impression we make on others. The way we walk, hold our heads, use our hands, our eyes, and our shoulders gives those we meet emotional impressions that may speak louder than our voices. The tone with which we greet people often implies more than the words we say. It indicates our mental attitude and provokes a similar response from the person we address. It helps to look directly into the patient's eyes as you speak. If you speak pleasantly, people are inclined to respond pleasantly.

Watch several strangers walk down the street. Some have good posture and carry their bodies easily; some slouch forward, eyes on the ground, glance occasionally and restively around; some stride forward, shoulders back, fists clenched, chin out. Each suggests something about his mental attitude—from timidity and fear to aggressive belligerence.

Good posture, maintained with an appearance of ease, is the foundation for all good public impression. It suggests self-confidence.

The appearance of lightness on the feet may be attained by practicing this one exercise: Imagine that a wire is attached to your sternum (breastbone), lifting you until the soles of your shoes barely touch the floor. Walk around feeling this sense of "lift." Practice several times daily until it becomes automatic.

If properly done, the result will be excellent posture, maintained with ease. Add a cheery smile and a friendly eye contact. You express self-confidence and such radiance that people will enjoy being near you. This manner is the basis for pleasant office and patient relationships. Remember, those who listen to us speak learn what kind of persons we are from the tone we use, the formation of our words, the rapidity with which we speak, and our choice of words. Study the chapter on communications to improve your speaking and listening abilities.

From the foregoing discussions of the role of the dental assistant, we can list these ideas as a guide for her conduct until such time as she has studied enough to have her code of conduct become a matter of routine behavior.

1. The office assistant should be dignified but not pompous nor belittling of patients.
2. She should be clean and neat.
3. She should behave in a manner befitting the principles laid down in Dental Ethics.
4. She must be accurate in the performance of any services requested of her.
5. She should maintain dignified, courteous relationships with all patients and with her dentist and other staff members.
6. A dental assistant has a responsibility to the community because she is thought to be more of an authority on dentistry than someone who does not work in a dental office. People are apt to ask her questions of a dental nature and believe her answers. She therefore must remember her legal limitations in diagnosis and prescription, consider her responsibilities to the community, and conduct herself accordingly.
7. She never criticizes her dentist to a patient.
8. She remembers: *What you see here, what you hear here, stays here.* Any information which a dental assistant sees or hears at the office is confidential information and should *never* be divulged or commented upon anywhere.

The Desirable Team Member

Whenever people work together, it is necessary to observe some courtesies in order to make it possible for each individual to experience the personal satisfactions which make life enjoyable.

In the dental office, one is often forced to be physically close to other team members and to patients. Such closeness can cause irritation because people need a certain amount of space between themselves and others. This "space bubble" varies with the country in which a person has been raised. For example, in Arabian countries it is customary for people to be very close. In the northern half of the Western Hemisphere more distance between people is customary. If someone moves closer than eighteen inches to a North American, usually the person whose "space bubble" has been invaded finds himself feeling some irritation. Members of the dental health team need to recognize this characteristic of our society and make allowance for it when working with patients and with each other. Space invaded slowly is less offensive than abrupt encroachment. (The study of the space needs of people is called *proxemics.*)

It is also desirable for a team member to be alert to signals from other team members. Sometimes the turn of a hand can mean it is time for a new instrument to be placed in the dentist's hand. Sensitivity to these signals makes for effective teamwork.

Fitting In with the Team That Works with the Patient

The dental health team has a job to do for the patient. The very reason for the existence of the team is that patient . . . that *human* being. It is necessary to remember this fact instead of considering the patients as so many cases, numbers, or inanimate objects to be pushed hither and yon.

In a well-planned and well-run dental office, each staff member will have explicit instructions about his or her particular duties. It is important to have each team member willing

to fit into the pattern of the whole and to work with each other instead of against each other. There must, of necessity, be some flexibility in schedules. There are emergencies which need to be properly handled; there are delays which prevent a dentist from remaining on time; there are patients in pain for whom no time was reserved in the original schedule. It takes good teamwork to handle these upsets in the daily routine, otherwise one member of the team will be unduly burdened or unpleasant frictions will occur. One of the best ways to handle the team effort is to have a written schedule for the team as a whole. This schedule or office administration plan will be discussed later in specific detail.

The comfort and security of the patient are to be uppermost in the minds of the office personnel as they receive, care for, and dismiss patients. An atmosphere of harmony will greatly add to the patient's contentment. There are ten suggestions for a team member to remember about his teammates and how to make the team effort profitable and satisfying. The general ideas behind these ten points will be discussed at greater length in the chapter on psychology; but briefly, here are ten ideas:

1. Emphasize the competence of the person.
2. Feel pride in team accomplishments—and allow each person an opportunity to share your feelings. People react favorably to a smooth-working team. Praise your teamwork whenever you can.
3. Make it easier for each person to accept himself as he is.
4. Make him feel smile-deserving.
5. Encourage him to express his doubts and disagreements about your suggestions. Only by his expression of these doubts and disagreements will you really learn what they are and be able to help remove them.
6. Ask for regularly scheduled staff conferences at which time everyone's satisfac-

tions and discomforts with the working conditions can be discussed calmly. (Even one assistant and one dentist can have a regularly scheduled staff conference.)

7. Be consistent and dependable.
8. Avoid absenteeism.
9. Create a permissive atmosphere—permissive for creative breakthroughs in working out the techniques which will allow you to assist your dentist more effectively.
10. Show and express your appreciation for your teammates.

Summary

Good oral health is essential to good general health, and today good health is considered the right of every person.

The purpose of dentistry is to serve the public by

1. helping to maintain good oral health,
2. helping to maintain throughout life the ability to masticate food,
3. helping to maintain or to improve personal appearance,
4. preventing pain by the practice of preventive dentistry, and
5. providing relief from pain of dental origin.

The oral health care delivery team has become important. The most efficient dental service delivery system seems to be the use of a team composed of the dentist and his auxiliaries: hygienist, chairside assistant, floater, expanded duties personnel, laboratory assistant, office administrator, receptionist, bookkeeper, and patient educator. The dentist organizes the team and decides what auxiliaries he will hire.

There are eight dental specialties at present: oral surgery, orthodontics, pedodontics, periodontics, prosthodontics, oral pathology, dental public health, and endodontics.

The object of having dental assistants is to save time for the dentist by providing assistants to relieve him of tasks which do not require his highly specialized skills.

What you see here, what you hear here, stays here is an important rule for all dental assistants to observe.

Consideration of the fact that patients are human beings is a very important attitude for all dental assistants to possess.

Observing certain standards of conduct and personal habits when in the dental office increases the effectiveness of the service rendered to patients.

Study Questions

1. What can dentistry do for patients?
2. How can patients be served best?
3. Why does a dentist hire assistants?
4. What is a specialist? What are the dental specialties?
5. What are third-party payments?
6. What is an oral health care delivery team? What positions are found on the team?
7. What are the ethics by which a dentist practices?
8. What future is there for dental assistants?
9. What standards of conduct are important for a dental assistant? Why are they important?
10. Why is grooming important?
11. What are the essentials for good grooming in the dental office?
12. What is *inadvertent communication*? Why is it important?
13. What is a desirable team member?
14. How does one help to make a good team?

Bibliography

Boucher, Carl O., ed. *Current Clinical Dental Terminology.* St. Louis, Mo.: C. V. Mosby Co., 1963.

Fast, Julius. *Body Language.* New York: Evans Co., 1970.

Guerini, Vincenzo. *History of Dentistry.* Philadelphia: Lea & Febiger, 1909.

Jensen, James R. "Career Mobility within the Oral Health Care Delivery Team." Paper presented at American Dental Assistants Association Annual Meeting, October 1971. Published in *The Dental Assistant* 41, no. 1 (January 1972): 18-21.

—————. "Dental Manpower and the Responsibilities of the Dental Schools." *American Journal of Public Health* 61, no. 8 (August 1971): 1565-1570; and in *Dental Abstracts of IADR* 17, no. 1 (January 1972): 24-25.

—————, and MESKIN, LAWRENCE H. "A Proposed Format for Auxiliary Education and Utilization." *The Dental Assistant,* the journal of the American Dental Assistants Association, 41, no. 1 (January 1972): 18-21; and *Journal of the American Dental Hygienists Association* 45, no. 3 (May-June 1971): 160-163.

PRICE, W. A. *Nutrition and Physical Degeneration.* New York: P. B. Hoebner, 1939.

PRINZ, HERMAN. *Dental Chronology.* Philadelphia: Lea & Febiger, 1945.

2 | *Fundamental Principles of Human Relations*

Working with People

After the dentist has received his license to practice and has opened his office, he must have patients to treat. What brings patients to him? Why do they continue to come to him instead of finding another dentist?

Obviously, *something* brings the patient to the dentist. It may be pain, poor appearance, or knowledge that regular dental care is desirable, although perhaps not always enjoyable. Patients frequently enter the office apprehensive of the treatment they are about to receive.

What causes a patient to *return* for a second office call? Aside from the area of the country where there is only one dentist for miles around, a patient returns to the dentist because he has confidence in the dentist and likes the way he has been treated in the office. Let's say that again: *He likes the way he has been treated in the office.*

The assistants in the dental office can help create an atmosphere which patients enjoy.

Fundamental Human Needs

In working with people, the dental assistant should recognize that there are fundamental human needs which all people feel and to which they respond. There are many so-called "popular psychology" books in print today which use catchy names for these fundamental needs to help you remember them. Actually, they are not difficult to remember. They include the following:

1. *A feeling of personal worth*—of being important to, or needed by, someone, or contributing to some purpose in life—is basic for all of us.

2. *Self-preservation*—a natural instinct to stay alive, to retard the aging process, and to avoid injury—runs the gamut from protecting oneself from the automobile which is careening around the corner to being concerned with little acts which preserve one's health and youth, such as having a front tooth filled.

3. *A love interest*—a desire to be loved by someone, to belong closely to someone—is present in most humans.

4. *Security* means people must feel safe—protected from whatever real or imagined foes they recognize.

5. *Recognition*—a longing to be noticed or thought worthwhile by other people—is desired by all humans. Some men give large sums of money to a worthwhile movement in order that their names may be kept before the public.

6. *Relief from fear* is sought by all who experience this emotion. Several of our leading psychologists have stated that all people are driven by fear—imaginary or real—to a lesser or a greater degree. Those fears may be created by an actual or an imagined experience. All fears are real to the individual experiencing them, but sometimes he is afraid when there is no reason to be afraid. Some fears—or most fears—stem from experiences in childhood which are no longer consciously remembered, but the emotional memory lingers below the conscious mind and affects behavior. Unfortunately, most children are exposed to gory accounts of some relative's visit to the

dental office, with dramatic descriptions of the accompanying pain. This pain is not actually experienced by the child. The adult has probably exaggerated his own predicament, but the child develops a memory of exaggerated fear of going to the dentist. The child may forget the incident, but he retains the fear of the dental office. Many adults have not been relieved of this feeling about dental offices.

What causes the fear is unimportant. The crucial idea to remember is that people have fears and need to be treated with kindness and reassurance.

Tools for Patient Motivation

These needs, then, are tools with which to work in the office. It is possible to work with people more effectively when you consider their motivational needs.

Learn something about the background of your patients so that you may better understand their moral and socioeconomic problems (the kind of background they have—what kind of income and what type of society they live in). This will help individualize the patient and perhaps explain his needs.

Remember, the most likely motives of these patients for seeking the services of your office are:

Self-preservation—
    People fear the aging of their bodies (losing their teeth), wish to protect themselves (avoid pain), and wish to keep on living;

Love—
    People want love from other humans—love between parents and children, between siblings (brothers and sisters), between other family members, and between friends;

Security—
    People are concerned with their ability to earn money (improved appearance often improves their chance for a better job);

Recognition—

People wish to be recognized as individuals. Perhaps no one wants to be "average" in all respects.

Remember, too, that in addition to the attainment of these goals, patients will also be affected by a desire to experience personal worth, and most patients, consciously or unconsciously, will be experiencing fear.

Your understanding of motivation is important. Actually, the motivation of these basic desires in people may be negatively expressed as *fear that they will not be able to preserve themselves, that they will not be loved, that they will not have the security of a good job, social position, and so forth, and that they will not be recognized as important by other humans.* These feelings are brought into your office, and you must cope with them. Most patients who come to your office will be unaware that they are being controlled by one or all of these basic attitudes toward life.

The oral health care delivery team which can help a patient recognize the dental service as an asset—better appearance, health, or success—has succeeded in eliminating the stage of negation (often expressed as "How large a filling, Doctor?").

The direction of this education of the patient is the business of the dentist, but it is advantageous for each assistant to *understand* the educational process and how the staff is to assist. An assistant's chief responsibility in this area is to develop the patient's confidence in the dentist, the dental office, and the staff.

The dentist tries to educate his patients to the wisdom of sound preventive dentistry and performs services which they actually need, offering them a choice of possible methods if a choice is practical. High-pressure salesmanship by any member of the staff has no place in dentistry. It can mean selling the patient dental services which he may not need and, in some instances, does not want.

From a patient's first contact with the office, whether by telephone or office call, he should be made to feel as much at ease as possible—to form an emotional response of contentment or satisfaction with your office—if he is to remain a long-term patient. The attitude of the entire staff helps set an emotional tone in the office which makes a patient feel comfortable or uncomfortable, depending upon what attitudes the staff holds. The feeling aroused in the patient when he is in your office is known to psychologists and educators as *empathic response.* In the dental office it is most important to arouse a *favorable* empathic response.

You know that a patient's cooperation is necessary to practice dentistry. It is necessary for the patient to open his mouth, sit still, and offer some degree of cooperation if the dentist is to prepare a tooth for an amalgam filling. Learning how to make the patient *like* to cooperate is important to the long-range success of the office.

It is also wise for you to know that income in the office is increased or decreased by the time consumed in producing a given unit of dental service. The income in your office usually affects the salary of the dental assistant. The time consumed by each patient is important. It is unwise to allow any patient to feel "rushed"; neither can you afford to allow a patient to dillydally and consume your dentist's precious time with long conversations. It is therefore necessary for you to learn how to work with people in such a manner that the patient will look forward with a sense of satisfaction to a visit to your office, yet you do not allow any patient to use more of the dentist's time than is necessary.

You should be able to read the behavior of others, to understand why they act as they do, to offer motivation for the kind of behavior you wish from the patients, and to lead them in the office routines which you must maintain if the oral health care delivery team is to perform successfully.

Since everyone possesses a desire to be of value, to fulfill his need for a sense of personal worth, you can utilize this drive effectively in the dental office. If you are able to satisfy the patient's need—to make him feel that in your office he is a very important person whose feelings are considered, whose physical well-being is uppermost in your mind, whose fear you understand, sympathize with, and allay— you will have achieved the objective of making him a long-term patient.

In order to be successful in this task, you must watch for cues from the patient for his emotional tone (the state of emotional excitement he may or may not exhibit). Sometimes the same patient will need to be approached in different ways on different days because his emotional tone may vary from day to day— even hour to hour.

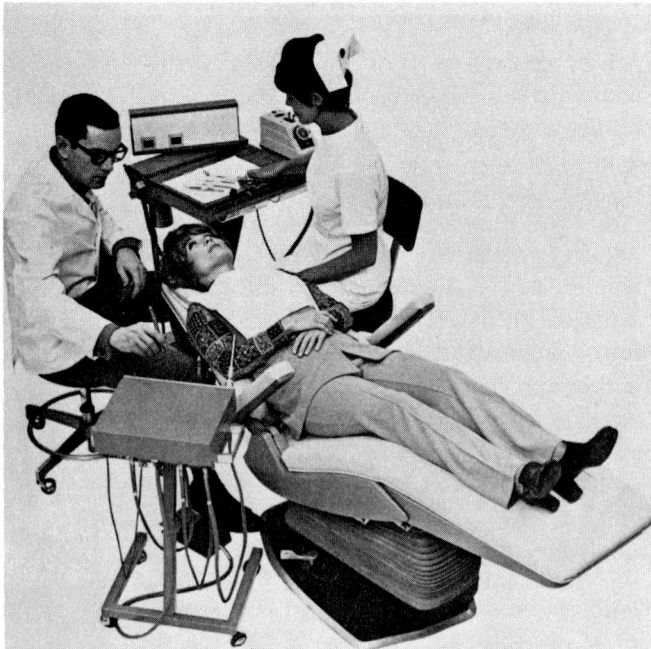

Courtesy Midwest American

Fig. 2.1. Providing every comfort for the patient creates confidence in the dental health team.

It is also necessary to recognize that different ages make differences in the way people react. A person's sense of values varies with his changing age. The three-year-old offers a different reaction to the dental office from that which the six-year-old exhibits. This difference holds true throughout life. Each age group varies. Each individual in the age group may be different from the others in his general group. That is why you must be alert in observing the behavior of every person who enters your office, realizing that his reaction today may differ from his behavior six months ago—or last week.

We will discuss some psychological principles to be applied in working with patients and try to illustrate them with reference to situations in the dental office.

What ought you to know about psychology in the dental office?

Psychology has been called the science of the mind. Psychologists do not agree on any one definition. Modern psychology is a science that studies all the interactions between living organisms and their environment. The ideas (concepts) of emotions, consciousness, instincts, and intelligence are described in relationship to the individual as a whole. The individual is exceedingly complex. Furthermore, the individual changes constantly in some areas of behavior and remains the same in other areas. No two individuals change or behave in the same manner or at the same time.

In more recent psychological studies, human beings are referred to as a "bundle of traits" with varying amounts of abilities for each trait. People and conditions surrounding the individual influence him, and his reactions occur according to the way he feels about these people and conditions.

For example, a five-year-old child who, because of his small stature, is usually called a three-year-old by strangers will react to social situations very differently from the five-year-old who, inches taller than his playmates, is looked upon as being older than five.

It is necessary to understand as thoroughly as possible the development of the individual from the time he was a tiny baby if you are to understand and work with adults. Development does not stop with the end of childhood. The process a person goes through of discovering what he can do as an individual and of trying new skills and ideas ought to continue throughout life. Psychologists have discovered the importance of the *continuing* growth and change of each individual. As research psychologists in the future continue to study, there may be changes in the ideas advanced; but today developmental psychology shows us what appear to be the best ways of approaching people. It is on this philosophy of working with people that our application of psychological principles to various age levels is based.

We will consider some generalizations about behavior of all ages, recognizing that no one person is a specific age. Most people, whether they are five or fifty, show characteristics of several ages. However, one is more likely to see three- to eight-year-old behavior exhibited by a five-year-old. Thus, we have isolated behaviors according to the age at which they are generally exhibited.

Behavior Characteristics of Children

From the developmental psychology research studies, these generalizations regarding behavior from early childhood through adolescence are given because we feel that they have application in working with youngsters in the dental office. They will help you understand a youngster's conduct and will give you an idea of what subjects you can discuss with him or how to help him conform to office routine. (See "Assisting with Children," chap. 44, for other suggestions concerning children.)

General Comments

The child is developing his large muscles and may be engaged in constant activity. He may be a "wiggler" in the dental chair until he is almost eleven. However, with a good, friendly relationship with the dentist, some three-year-olds will sit still and be more cooperative patients than some adults.

Before age six, most children do not have good eye-hand coordination. If you distract the child by asking him to "help" in some fashion, be sure that it is something easy for him to do.

Between ages nine and eleven, control of the small muscles develops, and more physical control is possible.

In early childhood, the only interest the child has in health is when he is ill. Therefore, you cannot expect him to care for his teeth without parental assistance.

Children suffer a serious handicap in their ability to get along in society because their speech development is exceedingly limited. It is years before a child has enough ability to think and express himself so others can understand what he really wants. This ability is called *language facility.*

Language and social development grow together. As the child gains language facility, he gets along better socially.

The child's home life affects speech development. Some parents unintentionally prevent a child from developing speech ability because they answer questions for the child or give him what he wants before he can ask for it, thus sharply cutting his *need* for language development.

Lack of language facility is one of the causes of negativism in the two- to four-year-old. In this negativistic period, children usually respond to any suggestion with a "No, no!" Usually some discipline is needed. Give it pleasantly and firmly to show that this negative attitude is not going to be accepted; that in the dental office cooperation is in order. (Negativism, if not properly treated, may continue into adult life in an otherwise normal individual.)

A three-year-old usually can speak in simple sentences and answer simple questions; however, he cannot tell whether the event happened yesterday or during the morning of the very day you ask the question. He may not remember, he may not be able to frame a sentence, or the sense of time may be too great for him. (Any past event may be said to have happened yesterday—even though it was really six months ago.)

For the three- to six-year-old, laughter is a way of conversing.

Relationships with adults vary with age.

In early years (3-6), adult smiles mean friendliness to the child. Since the child is more interested in being approved by and friends with adults than with children his own age, your friendliness is important in making him like your office. Smile for the *little* youngster!

The young child likes to have you put your arm around him. He enjoys the sense of protection it gives him. By the time a child is eight or nine, however, he may not want you to put your arm around him because now he feels that adults are less necessary in his life. (He is able to do so much for himself.) He still desires adult approval, so be sure to compliment him on the things which he does well. If he shows any signs of desiring physical affection, be sure to give it to him.

Characteristics of Specific Age Groups

The following observations, based on research studies, are useful if you remember that the divisions are not precise according to ages. There is overlapping in either direction in some individuals. At age three, some children will show characteristics of the five-year-old— and perhaps some of the characteristics of the two-year-old, also. The classifications are a guide, however, for your recognition of the type of behavior to expect from the child until you know him personally.

The Twenty-Two-Month- to Twenty-Six-Month-Old Youngster

1. is frightened about being separated from mother at first and may cry;
2. is curious about his surroundings and will usually become interested and stop crying just as soon as the dentist starts doing something for him at the dental chair.

Therefore, you are gentle, slow, ignore his crying, and carry on a process in which he can develop an interest just as soon as possible. Never make fast movements around the youngster of this age.

The Two-Year-Old

1. is negativistic;
2. can be made interested in his surroundings, but must be handled firmly to keep him from becoming so negativistic that it is impossible to work with him;
3. has just succeeded in learning how to manipulate people and will manipulate you as well as his parents unless you are alert.

Therefore, you are firm, gentle, slow, and carry on a process in which he can become interested.

The Three-Year-Old

1. enjoys simple imaginative play. (Join in, in all seriousness, if you want a real thrill. If they feel that you really want to play and understand, you will have little friends who include you in secrets otherwise not divulged.);
2. understands what others do in relationship to his own desires. His language, activities, and life revolve around his own needs and ideas;

3. does not want to share his possessions. Anything he holds in his hands is *his*—anything he wants is *his*. (Watch your choice of words regarding toys and supplies he is using which belong to the dental office.);
4. knows the difference between one, two, and "a lot of";
5. is angry when you interfere with his bodily activity.

The Four-Year-Old

1. wishes to make his own decisions;
2. wishes to understand each problem facing him;
3. has a keen imagination;
4. likes animals and small children;
5. responds to comparisons of his physical size with others. Be careful! Too many people may have commented on how "little" he is;
6. is angry with whoever or whatever upsets him and may attempt to inflict physical punishment on the person or object.

The Five-Year-Old

1. shows off for attention;
2. sometimes is very shy;
3. sulks or becomes destructive when you prevent him from doing what he wants;
4. begins to show interest in everything around him. This interest continues through the seven-year-old period;
5. may embarrass you with the direct way in which he asks you personal questions. Treat the questions casually;
6. may panic with real fear, or just put on a display in order to stop procedures. (Learn to tell the difference.)

The Six-Year-Old

1. begins to be afraid of doctors, blood, a fainting person, dark, and being alone. These five items should be remembered in connection with any six-year-old's visit to your office. Other fears which may appear at this age are fear of ghosts, death, and dead animals. These fears persist through age ten and sometimes last throughout life;
2. is interested in simple factual explanations of everyday life;
3. is angry when you interfere with his plans or possessions, or when you ridicule him or call him names;
4. begins to question *who? what? why?* (with more language facility at his command). He is curious about his environment and eager to experiment by asking questions for more information. You can answer his questions simply, in brief sentences, reducing the language to his level.

The Seven- to Eight-Year-Old

1. compares himself with others his age. He feels superior if he is physically larger or more skillful in any phase of work or play and inferior if he is smaller or less skillful. (Therefore, praise him for his skills.);
2. must dress like his classmates, play as they do, and live by the same code of conduct;
3. is upset by ridicule, loss of prestige, or failure.

The Eight-Year-Old

1. begins to be interested in past cultures. This is good to remember for conversation with the eight-year-old;
2. enjoys imaginative play as pioneers, Indians, pilgrims.

The Eight- to Nine-Year-Old

1. is more interested in his own sex and has as his closest friends members of his own sex.

The Nine- to Eleven-Year-Old

1. gains more satisfaction as he sees his improvement in skills;

2. is interested in factual historical information, but not in political history.

Behavior Characteristics of Adolescents

The eleven- to thirteen-year-olds may be entering adolescence. Many adolescent characteristics begin to show as early as ten.

The Adolescent

1. may be embarrassed by poor posture, awkwardness, pimples (acne), and excessive perspiration;
2. is interested in gang approval rather than adult approval;
3. is learning social graces and tries to be pleasant in his relations, especially with adults;
4. wishes to be treated as an adult when privileges are being considered (driving the car, going to bed, etc.);
5. wishes to remain a child when responsibilities are involved (helping with housework, yard maintenance);
6. wants his adolescent friends to think of him as an adult;
7. is especially anxious to do as his contemporaries do when it comes to dating, dressing, and spending money;
8. has a huge appetite;
9. often has physical coordination and finger dexterity far superior to adults;
10. now feels that being well-groomed and physically attractive is important;
11. behaves in a cocky manner sometimes and may be doing so because he has grown suddenly;
12. grows up mentally, becoming more interested in present environment, ecology, and space programs, and in social, political, and economic life;
13. is interested in good health, in why and how smoking, drinking, and drugs affect

health. The wise adult can do much with the older adolescent on these subjects;
14. may be upset emotionally if his parents have failed in marriage or business—family awareness has developed;
15. may be more interested in one or two hobbies than in any school subject;
16. may steal due to the pressures for items which the family or part-time job cannot provide;
17. often wishes to discuss his personal problems and may ask an adult whom he admires for advice. He is curious about human relationships;
18. may be distressed by a growth spurt which makes him suddenly much bigger than he was a short time ago;
19. in late adolescence wants to be a success in adult terms. He recognizes that he is changing. He even wants to give protection instead of being protected.

An adult, other than the parent, is in a position to help an adolescent to a more responsible use of freedom, since some adolescents revolt against parents who refuse to allow them to make certain decisions. You may find that you are in a position to help an adolescent realize his responsibilities as well as his freedoms.

Behavior of Adults

It has already been stated that all members of the human race have certain fundamental needs or desires—things without which they cannot live. They will go to great lengths to gratify these needs. Most people do not even know that these needs exist. They behave in a certain fashion without knowing why. The need for a sense of personal worth—being important to others—is one of the greatest of these fundamental needs. (That is why you are so happy when you do something for someone else and you know that he values your friendship.)

The need for security is also important. This means that people must feel safe. The patients must develop or have confidence in your office or they won't remain as patients. They must trust your dentist and you to take good care of them—or they do not feel safe or secure. You must satisfy their need for security.

Remembering that it is necessary to make people feel safe and important in your office, let us look at some methods of accomplishing your work each day while making the patients feel safe, important, and like you, your dentist, and your office. These are certain basic ways of approaching people which are more pleasing than others.

Indirect Approach to People

Indirectly presenting ideas is usually a better way of working with people than presenting ideas directly. Some people have developed very negativistically and will not respond to being told directly what to do.

If your attitude is dictatorial or "bossy," the patient may feel that you see him as a puppet or an animal to be pushed around. A patient who feels this way will surely oppose your suggestions and will dislike you intensely. It is wise to avoid the direct approach. The patients will either refuse to do as you command, do so when your back is turned, or walk out on you—except for a few who are very easily influenced or tractable.

Tractable persons will do what you ask without hesitation. Many persons, however, are either passively negativistic (refusing to do what you tell them to do) or actively negativistic (doing the opposite of what you tell them to do).

The indirect presentation of ideas keeps the patient from feeling less important than you, makes him feel his independence, gives him credit for having a good idea of his own, or

makes him afraid that unless he follows through with this good idea which is his, he will lose prestige.

Here are seven indirect approaches to people:

1. *Assume that the patient will do as you wish him to do. (Suggest the behavior if necessary.)*

When you act as if a person knows the correct thing to do and will do so without being told, you are complimenting him most skillfully. You are really saying (without saying it) that this patient is in a very special class. Not all people know the correct thing, and fewer people *do* the correct thing even when they know how they should behave. Because this is true, this patient holds a very high place in your esteem—and in his mind it makes him even more important in your office than other patients who do not know and do not do the correct thing.

Assume that the child will do what is expected without a fuss:

"It's your turn now, Jane," to the seven-year-old when you are ready to lead her to the chair.

"Hop up in the chair now, Bobby. You're so big I can't lift you," to the four-year-old.

"There are some new books on the reading table, Jimmy," to the nine-year-old who must wait a few minutes in the waiting room. You may keep him from rowdy behavior.

Before the adult patient lays his coat on the chair, you say, "You will find the coat rack in the corner, Mr. Jones."

2. *Praise correct behavior when you see it.*

When anyone does what you want him to do, it is a good idea to praise him. He will feel like doing it again.

"I like the way you remembered to put the books back on the shelf, Jimmy."

"Isn't Mrs. Jones a wonderful patient, Dr. Smith? I admire her for the way she takes this today!"

3. *Credit the patient with already knowing what you are about to say.*

It is sometimes necessary to remind patients of office procedures because the long time-lapse between visits allows them to forget routines. It is wise to use great care in approaching the patient, since people often resent being told something they already know—even when they would have forgotten it anyway.

Use such expressions as "There is no need to remind *you* that ...." or "You probably remember ...." or "As you already know ...." *before* you make the statement of what you wish the patient to do.

4. *Show a patient that a certain way of behaving is very desirable.*

Imply that most people do what you are about to suggest to this patient. This is appealing to his sense of desire for social approval.

"The boys and girls who come to see Dr. Smith like to sit on *this* chair made especially for children" (to keep small children from occupying big chairs needed for adult patients).

"Since the usual Coke or 'soda' snack is so unhealthful, a number of high school students are switching to a snack of fruit after school. Maybe you can convince your crowd to do the same." (Since the adolescent feels that he must do as the gang does, you approach him from the idea of being the leader of his gang.)

"It is a good idea to have your teeth checked regularly. Most young adults come for a check-up every six months, but some people find that they need to come every four months."

"Some people have immediate dentures, and their friends hardly know that they have had dentures made."

5. *Disagree tactfully with a patient.*

There are times when it is necessary to disagree with a patient. Be pleasant. Be careful to oppose ideas gently. Listen to the patient carefully and courteously and disagree courteously and quietly—and indirectly, if possible.

A patient may say, "I don't want my teeth cleaned this time. It injures the enamel."

You respond with a question: "Many people feel that way, Mrs. Jones. I wonder whether you know how hard the enamel is on your teeth?"

"No-o-o, I really don't."

"Enamel actually is about the same hardness as steel. The cleaning agent which Dr. Smith uses is only as cleansing as necessary to remove the soft deposits on the surface of that enamel. It is almost always possible to demonstrate the presence of a bacterial plaque—even with the most careful brushing. This plaque is what the dentist removes in cleaning your teeth." (See "Caries" for a discussion of this topic.)

Or you may answer: "Although the cleaning agent is very slightly more abrasive than toothpaste, if a dentist cleaned your teeth twice a year from birth to age eighty, it would only be 160 cleanings—not enough to injure the enamel. Brushing even once a day would be 365 times each year!"

6. *Give the negativistic adult an opportunity to express himself.*

The haughty or domineering person may only be very negative. Sometimes the negation developed between two and four years of age continues throughout life. Sometimes emotional factors in the lives of adults cause them to be very negativistic toward people. You must learn to work well with these persons. Sometimes you can induce these patients to do what is necessary in your office in spite of their negative attitude. Sometimes you find that you must work around the negativism.

Wendell White suggests that a negativistic adult may be approached with any of these wordings before stating the idea you wish to have accepted favorably:

"You may not like this, ..." or "I may have made a mistake, but ...." or "You don't think that ...., do you?"[1]

Any of these approaches gives the patient a chance to disagree and yet agree with you. Negativistic people usually say *no* just out of habit. They can't bring themselves to say *yes*, so you provide the opportunity to allow them to at least partially disagree with you.

If a patient disagrees with your suggestion made after any of the wordings given by Dr. White, drop the idea. If it is a good suggestion, he may bring it up later as his idea. If this happens, let him continue to think that it is his idea. Comment on what an excellent idea he has. Be happy that he does as you wish him to do.

7. *Be pleased with every person who enters the dental office.*

Think in terms of being gracious and kind to everyone—of being pleased with every person who enters the waiting room. No matter what a person does to earn his living, be sure that you express approval of his job. Occasionally a question about some phase of his work may be used as your lead-question when he enters the office. You may learn much from such an approach.

Many patients make a comment, "I can't understand how anyone can be a dentist!"

This is an example of a comment which you must never make about anyone's way of earn-

ing a living. Never even *imply* dislike of any patient's occupation. A comment of interest in the patient's work, such as "Being a baker must be fascinating," is helpful.

Man must find some satisfaction in his work or he is not happy. This applies to you, in your work, as well as to all other people.

Public Relations

Public relations in the dental office is one of the most important phases of assisting! Remember that the patient is constantly appraising you as a person. Are you gentle? Are you cooperative in explaining things? Are you gruff? These intangible, elusive factors make good or bad public relations!

Public relations, as we know it, came into use as a term about 1900. Since that time, much effort has been placed in the promotion of good public relations in every field of human interaction. Briefly, the development of good public relations means the cultivation of goodwill. It is devoted to improving the relations of an organization or individual with the public.

We do not develop good public relations by accident. It is necessary to be constantly aware of the importance of everything we say and do—*how* it is said, *how* it is done—in relationship to the individual with whom we are dealing.

The success with which any one person may "get along" with the public might well be considered on a percentage basis. There will be, under the best circumstances, a small percentage with whom there will be unpleasant relationships. As long as this percentage remains very small, we should feel that our efforts in the field of public relations are successful. If the percentage shows a tendency to rise, the time has come for a close examination of our own personality, our own outlook toward people in general.

1. Wendell White, *Psychology in Living*, p. 20.

In order to work well with people, we must *communicate* with them. However, most people are *preoccupied.* (Preoccupy means complete absorption of the mind or interests; something which causes such absorption; lost in thought.)[2] Preoccupied. Absorbed before. Mind closed. No communication possible. Can't hear you.

Most of the people you meet are preoccupied. Most of what you say is not even heard. What can you do? Let us try to understand preoccupation first, then perhaps we can do something about it.

Preoccupation usually begins in infancy—or is the result of problems from infancy. Powerful emotions which control our lives usually cause preoccupation. The most powerful of these emotions seems to be *fear*, and most people do not even realize that they live with fear.

Children are often treated in ways that produce fear which they must hide. Parents usually do not consciously set out to make their children afraid. However, just the enormity of the size of an adult in the eyes of a child can be fear-inspiring.

One of the authors remembers being towered over by an *immense* first-grade teacher. When the author was age twenty-two, she had occasion to see this teacher again. She "towered" over the teacher who was five feet tall. Even a five-foot-tall adult can seem like a giant to a six-year-old.

A young man, as a high school senior, commented upon seeing the playground of the University Elementary School where he was enrolled through sixth grade, "Why, I used to think it was *immense*. It's small!" He laughed. "You know, I used to wonder how those teachers could bat the ball the *whole*

length of the playground! They were *tremendous*. Why, it's no trick at all. The playground is so *little.*"

We must remember that the adult world viewed through the eyes of a little child is decidedly different from the view of an adult.

If, in addition to seeming like a giant, the adult happens to be stern or angry, the child can be terribly afraid. He is helpless and cannot protect himself effectively from the anger or punishment heaped on him. If his parent is insecure and takes out his hostilities against society on those he can dominate, the child is helpless. He cannot fight effectively, he cannot run away, he cannot even say, "Look, Dad, *I'm* not to blame that you didn't get that promotion."

The human has one more problem. In addition to protecting himself physically, he also must protect his ego—his opinion of himself. The child has to build an image of himself with which he can live the rest of his life. If he is encouraged as a child, he builds a confident image. If he is belittled, not allowed to try certain activities, he soon acquires the idea that he is not very effective. The emotional memory carries into adult life on an unconscious level.

The treatment begins at birth. A child who feels important to his family develops a better picture of himself than the youngster who is constantly belittled. The youngster who is afraid of one of his parents soon becomes anxious. Anxiety keeps him from doing well on tests at school, or anything else which measures his achievement—even making his bed. Anxiety in adult life tends to produce *preoccupation.* The world is full of adults who were ruled by fear when they were children. Emotionally they are confused, ending up as preoccupied, anxiety-ridden adults, unable to admit or even know that they are afraid. They are preoccupied.

2. *Webster's Seventh New Collegiate Dictionary*, p. 671.

The sooner you, the assistant, can recognize a person's problems, the sooner you have conquered the problem of fitting the individual into a smoothly-run office routine. Some patients will present more of a problem than others. We must remember that the problem person is a problem to himself, as well as a problem to others. He sees the situation as his mind allows him to see it, not as other humans see it. He acts on what he sees. No person can do more than that. If you are color-blind and cannot see that the stoplight is red, you will not stop for it. It is your inability to *see* that prevents you from behaving as society thinks you ought to behave. The problem person uses a self-centered approach in every situation. He is preoccupied with his own problems.

A person who continually blunders and creates tension is a person who is never free enough from problems within himself to be interested in the world around him. He is controlled by fear and hostility and creates problems for others because he has no relief from being a problem to himself. This is most commonly illustrated in the dental office by the patient who otherwise may not be a problem person at all. He has an upsetting fear of any dental treatment. He tenses up, squirms, grabs the dentist's arm just as the dentist is about to insert the needle, moans, shoots hostile glances at the assistant; in short, he creates a problem by succumbing to his fear. He is so preoccupied with his fear that he can concentrate on nothing else.

When a person feels that he doesn't amount to much, that he is a cog in a huge factory, an underling, a nobody, he has a hard time living with himself. Sometimes home life can make a person feel this way; sometimes a visit to a dental office can make a person feel unimportant. Giving patients emotional acceptance and approval can raise their opinions of themselves.

You can accept people as they are, deserving of your interest and courtesy. You can give them polite attention even if they are rude. You simply remember that they are being rude to a memory of past treatment by someone else. They are not intentionally being rude to you. Your attitude of the importance of everyone who enters the office will pay off in time. Even the grouches will be less grouchy. This attitude of accepting people as they are, liking them as they are, will help them like themselves, and they will be more pleasant.

For example, in a dental office, recently, a querulous old man came in shouting for the bookkeeper. He waved a letter he had from the dentist. He kept shouting at the receptionist that he wanted the bookkeeper. The waiting room was full of people. Most patients would expect to wait their turn. Not he. He continued shouting. The bookkeeper appeared and said calmly, "I am the bookkeeper."

He began to wave the letter at her. She nodded and invited him to sit by her desk where she disposed of his problem and sent him off in quiet satisfaction that he no longer had a problem.

Many people would have reacted to his antagonism and anger with a hostility which matched his. In some offices he would have been told to sit down and be silent—eventually they would get to him; but the receptionist and bookkeeper were soothing, giving recognition to the seeming urgency of his complaint, commanding his goodwill by providing the environment for him to give goodwill —that which they were giving him. They did not stop and demand his goodwill and courtesy first. The bookkeeper extended the basic courtesy to human nature *as she found it* in a human being, difficult as it might be. You can help people live with their mistakes and shortcomings without being overwhelmed by them. In the final analysis, you must realize that man must be treated as a whole being, and you must recognize the socioeconomic and moral problems he may have, in addition to his dental problems.

Remembering that patients are people and people are preoccupied and fearful, although they don't always know it, you can do some specific things in order to have a smoothly-run office. The next section of this chapter, "Factors Establishing Good Public Relations," is an attempt to give you some specific things to do as you bear in mind that people are preoccupied and fearful. You can overcome these two problems with the right approaches in the office. Breaking the preoccupation barrier will be discussed in chapter three, "Communications."

Factors Establishing Good Public Relations

Consideration of people and their needs indicates that conscious attempts by office personnel can create better public relations. Some of the factors are discusssed in the rest of this chapter. Perhaps you will think of others to be accomplished in the office in which you work.

Create a Friendly Atmosphere in the Office

It is true that the attitudes which you possess are often reflected in those with whom you come into contact. A friendly approach will usually bring a friendly response. A cynical approach will usually bring a response of distrust and dislike. Just what should your attitudes be toward the people you meet in the dental office? Should you be friendly? sympathetic? courteous? sincerely interested? Since it is important for you to help patients like your office, you *must be* friendly, sympathetic, and courteous, no matter what attitude the

patients have. It is up to you to make them feel your friendliness. How good are your self-control and self-discipline?

It is possible to run a very businesslike dental office and yet miss the little touches which build good public relations. Cultivating the habit of letting people know that you appreciate something which they have done for you builds better public relations. It is good practice to close telephone conversations by saying, "Thank you, Mrs. Blank," if you place the call, or "Thank you for calling, Mrs. Blank," if Mrs. Blank telephoned you.

Establishing a friendly atmosphere in the office does not mean that one forgets *why* the dental office exists. Cultivate the habit of thinking in terms of what is to be accomplished in the office. Act accordingly. Guide the patients. Direct conversations into the correct channels to accomplish what you desire to achieve in office administration. Friendly relationships *and* dentistry accomplished on schedule are the ideals to be achieved.

Listen to Patients

Listen carefully and plan your reply carefully. It is helpful to think through the explanations which you must give. They should be phrased so that they are understood correctly and completely. Consider the feelings of others. Try to place yourself in the other person's position in order to consider what that person may be feeling. In short, treat people as they want to be treated and you build good public relations.

Treat the Patient as a VIP

Dentistry is the performance of a personal service for an individual personality. You and the dentist will share the responsibility of making the individual feel that he is the *most important person in your office*. All efforts are made with one point in mind: to serve that patient to the best of your ability. The patient will feel your pride in "your" dentist, your office, and your work. The impression he forms of your dental office is one to which you contribute by your appearance, efficiency, and tact.

We say that an individual is a "human being." Since he is human, he will have his failings or shortcomings. We must accept the fact that each patient will have his peculiarities and his weaknesses. Do we practice looking for the good, the interesting, in each patient —even when his obvious defects are glaringly visible? Someone phrased it this way: There is so much good in the worst of us, and so much bad in the best of us, that it little behooves any of us to speak ill of the rest of us. Or, as Will Rogers put it in his homely philosophy: "I never met a man I didn't like." He did not mean to say that he had never disliked anyone; rather, that when he learned to know a person, the pleasant, interesting, and good part of his character always outweighed the unpleasant characteristics.

The peculiarities and idiosyncrasies of patients should be learned and remembered. The large majority of patients exhibit good common sense and rational behavior with perfectly normal desires to know what is being done for them, how it is to be done, why it is to be done, and for what cost. Maintaining a pleasant professional relationship with this majority is a source of considerable satisfaction to the person who likes people.

Learning to adjust quickly to the individual personality of the patient and exhibiting courtesy and consideration for his interests place "good public relations" in action in the dental office.

Allay His Fear

Fear has been cited as the most important cause of dental neglect. When assisting with a patient, keep in mind that he does not consider dental work a pleasure. When you have

worked for some time in a dental office, you will tend to forget the patient's point of view: that dental work is something of an ordeal. Be sympathetic and reassuring in your comments if the patient expresses his thoughts to you. Use these reactions in a constructive manner by pointing out the ease of regular care at regular intervals. Do not make light of any indication of discomfort or fear with a joking manner or laugh.

One of the best ways to allay fears of the patient with whom you haven't had an opportunity to develop personal ties is to show him an office which runs as smoothly as the proverbial well-oiled machine—one in which each member moves with sureness and certainty to perform an obviously perfected task.

Give the Patient Immediate Attention

A patient who enters the reception room should receive immediate attention. He is being treated most discourteously if he is obliged to wait while an obviously personal conversation is carried on either among the office staff or by a staff member over the telephone. The patient should be made to feel important, that his needs are your first interest, no matter where he may be—in the reception room, operatory, recovery room, or in any other room in your office.

Smile when you first see him enter!

Use the Patient's Name

Learn the patient's name and the names of the members of his family. Use them at every opportunity.

The primary interest of any patient centers in himself. He likes to hear his name. He likes consideration and attention centered completely on his needs and care. Due to this perfectly normal human characteristic, it is wise to listen carefully to the conversation between the patient and the dentist whenever possible. If something is said about the patient's immediate family—a trip to be made, a graduating student, etc.—unobtrusively make a note of the item on the patient's record card in pencil, or clip a note to it, so that either you or the dentist will be reminded to ask or comment about that personal item at the next visit of that patient.

New parents, or about-to-be-parents, are almost always very proud of the fact. Show an interest in their new child, or the expected child, whenever the opportunity presents. A final reminder to the expectant mother to be sure to send the office an announcement will be received with pleasure.

When the announcement comes, immediately send a congratulatory card or a set of miniature dentures (usually available from dental supply houses). In either case, the dentist's personal signature on the card is important. On the outside jacket of both parents' records list the name and date of birth of the new baby. The fact that this is noted allows the dentist an opportunity to say to the patient at the proper time: "I see that Kay will be eighteen months in June, Mrs. Jones. It would be wise to bring her for a training prophylaxis and examination before she is two years of age. Started at this age and recalled every four months, Kay will learn to look forward to dental care instead of fearing it, as you and I do."

In the patient's mind this is far more evidence of interest in the dental care of the family than to ignore the youngster until one of the parents suggests a dental visit.

When you do have occasion to make a remark about a patient in the chair, always do so by naming the patient: "Mrs. Jones certainly is a good patient, Doctor."

Do not use the third person pronouns *he* or *she*.

Explain a Delay to a Waiting Patient

Should an appointment exceed the time reserved, promptly notify the next waiting patient of the delay and the approximate time before he will be taken into the operatory. Specify the approximate time, rather than "a few minutes."

Let your voice show a sincere respect for the fact that Mrs. Jones is one of the two very important people in your office at that moment—the other being the patient still in the operatory. Patients will not develop respect for their appointments with your office unless your office has respect for their time also.

Cope with the Demands of Individual Problems

The occasional unpleasant person, either in the office or on the telephone, is most diplomatically handled with an affirmative type of reply. It is not possible to argue with a *yes*. The person whose voice has risen to an intensity indicating emotional strain is not in a logical frame of mind. He is not ready to hear a reasonable explanation of the situation which concerns him at the moment. It is not, usually, the time to try to give him one. The use of *yes* should include a following short sentence suitable to the situation: "Yes, Mrs. Jones, it *does* look that way" or "Yes, Mr. Jones, I can understand your viewpoint" or "Yes, Mr. Jones, I will check that again."

This reply should be given seriously, not with a smile. You *are* concerned about how to get this individual back to a calm discussion of the situation. It may be possible to do this immediately, but far more frequently it is preferable to defer further discussion until his emotions have had time to return to a normal level, either later the same day (soon after a mealtime is good) or the following day. At that time, be certain that you understand the situation completely, from his viewpoint as well as yours, before discussing it again with the individual concerned. You may discover that the patient has a valid complaint!

Occasionally you will work with a patient whose manner irritates you severely. In such cases, do not allow your feelings to become obvious by the slightest expression of dislike, either facial or verbal. Remain all "sweetness and light" in any and all contacts with those very important people—patients. Again: no matter what occurs in your contacts with patients, remain calm, friendly, poised, and in complete control of your emotions and verbal responses. It is your job to do so.

Another type of person, only rarely encountered, can be quite rude and difficult in routine contacts with the assistant, but becomes most courteous and polite to the dentist himself. Circumstances such as this occur perhaps more frequently on the telephone.

Assume that such a situation arises concerning arrangement for an appointment. If it is your job to make all appointments, then see to it that you do handle the situation diplomatically. If the difficulty concerns some phase of dental practice which is not under your control, do the very best you can to avoid asking the dentist to help you. If you cannot keep the situation under your control, then inform the patient that you will have Dr. Smith call as soon as he is free to do so. Should the patient be present in the office, and the dentist is with another patient at the chair, ask if Dr. Smith can telephone at a specified time. Very often these situations are only an attempt to see the dentist personally without an appointment to do so.

Summary

Patients are *people* who like to be treated as worthwhile human beings, as welcome guests in the office, and as VIPs whose problems are important to the staff.

Motives which lead people to seek dental care include self-preservation, love, security, fear, and recognition. The indirect presentation of ideas, or the power of suggestion, may be used to help patients recognize the value of dental services. It is important for the dental assistant to understand the approaches and purposes of her dentist in working with patients.

The feeling aroused in the patient when he is in your office is known as an *empathic response*. It is desirable to arouse a favorable empathic response in patients—that is, to make them like you and the office. It is wise to learn to read the behavior of others and offer the kind of motivation which results in the conduct and attitudes necessary to a successful dental practice.

Everyone desires to be of value—to feel worthwhile. To make a patient feel that he is a very important person in your dental office is to make him a continuing patient.

Principles of psychology are helpful in working with patients. Generalizations regarding behavior of all humans—children, adolescents, and adults—are an aid in successful dental assisting. Indirect approaches to people which work well in the dental office include the following:

1. assume that the patient will do as you wish him to do,
2. praise the correct behavior when you see it,
3. credit the patient with already knowing what you are about to say,
4. show a patient that a certain way of behaving is very desirable,
5. be tactful when objecting to or disagreeing with a statement,
6. give the negativistic adult an opportunity to express himself, and
7. be pleased with every person who enters the dental office.

The development of good public relations means the cultivation of goodwill.

Factors which contribute to development of good public relations include:

1. establishing a friendly atmosphere in your office,

2. thinking in terms of office accomplishment,
3. cultivating the art of listening to patients,
4. treating the patient as if he were a very important person—he is!

Remember that the patient is a human being and allay his fears; give him immediate attention; use his name when speaking to him or about him, not a third-person pronoun; notify him of a delay if one occurs; and remain calm when working with upset individuals.

The patient is a very important person. Remember to keep him pleased with your office!

Study Questions

1. List four motives which cause patients to seek dental care.
2. What indirect approaches work well in the dental office?
3. Discuss good public relations.
4. List four factors which contribute to attainment of good public relations.
5. What philosophy should you have about patients?

Bibliography

BERNE, ERIC. *Games People Play.* New York: Grove Press, 1964.

BURTON, GENEVIEVE. *Personal, Impersonal, and Interpersonal Relations.* New York: Springer Publishing Co., 1964.

ELLIS, ALBERT, and HARPER, ROBERT A. *A Guide to Rational Living.* North Hollywood, Calif.: Wilshire Book Co., 1971.

FRANCIS, GLORIA M., and MUNJAS, BARBARA. *Promotion of Psychological Comfort.* Dubuque, Ia.: William C. Brown Co. Publishers, 1968.

A Trilogy:

GESELL, ARNOLD, and ILG, FRANCES. *Infant and Child in the Culture of Today.* New York: Harper & Row, 1943.

—————. *The Child from Five to Ten.* New York: Harper & Row, 1943.

—————, and AMES, L. B. *Youth.* New York: Harper & Row, 1956.

JENKINS, GLADYS, et al. *These Are Your Children.* Chicago: Scott, Foresman & Co., 1953.

LAIRD, DONALD A., and LAIRS, ELEANOR C. *The Technique of Handling People.* New York: McGraw-Hill Book Co., 1954.

MASLOW, ABRAHAM H. *Toward a Psychology of Being.* New York: Van Nostrand Reinhold, 1968.

OVERSTREET, BONARO W. *Understanding Fear in Ourselves and Others.* New York: Harper & Row, 1951.

ROGERS, CARL R. *On Becoming a Person.* Boston: Houghton Mifflin Co., 1961.

Webster's Seventh New Collegiate Dictionary. Springfield, Mass.: G. & C. Merriam Co., 1965.

WHITE, WENDELL. *Psychology in Living.* New York: Macmillan Co., 1955.

Pamphlets

The Care of Children's Teeth. American Dental Association, 222 East Superior St., Chicago, Ill., 60611.

How Children Develop. Adventures in Education, University School Series No. 3. Columbus, O.: Ohio State University, 1964.

Your Child from One to Six. Publication #30. Washington, D.C.: U. S. Department of HEW, Children's Bureau, 1962.

Your Child from Six to Twelve. Publication #324. Washington, D.C.: U. S. Department of HEW, Children's Bureau.

3 | Communication Is Public Relations in the Dental Office

Basis for Understanding

How many times this week have you said, "They don't understand" or "I don't understand" or "No, that's not what I meant at all"?

Understanding and being understood are common problems all of us face. Communicating ideas is important because we must work with other people, and to do so necessarily means being able to communicate with them. It would be difficult, indeed, to attempt to perform dentistry if we could not understand and communicate in some form with the patients and our co-workers.

Communication—the accurate transmittal of an idea from one human to another—is affected by many factors. How a person feels as he makes a request may affect the inflection which he uses. In turn, the listener may assume that the speaker meant something else because the listener *interpreted* the inflection according to the way the listener was feeling. The alert, sensitive person will attempt to evaluate the message received and will verify the message with the sender after receiving it. When he is the speaker, this individual will also ask himself, "How can I phrase my request (or statement) to be best understood by my listener?"

The process of transmitting an idea from one person to another (or several others) becomes complicated. Even the way one says "Good morning" differs with circumstances. Consider these instances:

1. The first patient arrives fifteen minutes early. She is an enthusiastic, talkative individual. You are still dusting and have yet to prepare the setups for the operatories. No one else is in the office, the telephone is ringing, and the behavior of this patient in the past indicates that you should give her your undivided attention. Knowing all this, how do you say "Good morning"?

2. An aggressive, overbearing salesman bursts into the office every Tuesday morning at nine, right in the middle of your busy schedule. Your dentist has left instructions that he does not want to see this salesman —ever. Yet your dentist has also instructed you to be courteous to all salesmen but to prevent them from disturbing him. Say "Good morning" to this salesman.

3. The handsome bachelor patient enters. Your dentist has been very clear about professional attitudes toward *all* patients. You like this patient! Say "Good morning."

It is clear that even how one says "Good morning" is influenced by many factors. Consider, then, the problem in transmitting the idea that the X rays have been ruined by some problem with chemicals or that the laboratory has been unable to return the appliance for a difficult patient who is in the office expecting to receive it.

Much communication occurs without the use of words. Our bodies often communicate messages of which we are unaware. For example, the way an individual holds his arms often indicates tension, withdrawal, or openness. Consider Mrs. Doe. She stands before you, arms crossed, body tense, lips set in a firm line, and she says, primly, "I am open to suggestions."

Do you feel certain that she would accept a suggestion? Her body tells you that it would be difficult to find her "open" to anything— yet her words tell you that she is.[1]

Consider the co-worker in your office who takes your arm and says, "I wouldn't dream of intruding." Yet she is standing so close to you that she is touching your shoe with hers, and you find it necesssary to draw back to keep her hair from tickling your nose. She has actually invaded your "space bubble." The study of *proxemics*—space needs of people— will help you understand another way we sometimes receive a double message from an individual.

Often an individual's speech is filled with noises other than words: *uh, er, throat-clearing,* and *nonverbal sounds*. The study of these sounds and their meanings is called *haptics*. They, too, relay messages about the speaker and his true meanings and feeling states.

The important point to remember is that this type of message is one the individual may not be aware he is communicating. (Tests have shown that when a person becomes excited or overjoyed, the pupils of his eyes dilate involuntarily. An inner emotion of elation can be seen if the observer is alert. There seems to be no way an individual can avoid this giveaway of his feeling state.)

Actually, when two people contact each other, there is interaction and communication whether or not the individuals want to communicate or are aware of their communication. When two people interact, there is *some* direct communication. There is some communication which an individual is unaware he is making, there is knowledge he does not communicate for any number of reasons, and there is a large area of unknown information about himself which neither person knows. Two behavioral

1. If you wish to study body language further, there are several books which can be read. Consult the Bibliography.

scientists, Harry Ingham and Joseph Luft, diagramed the expression of this idea and called it the Johari Window (from their first names, Joe and Harry).

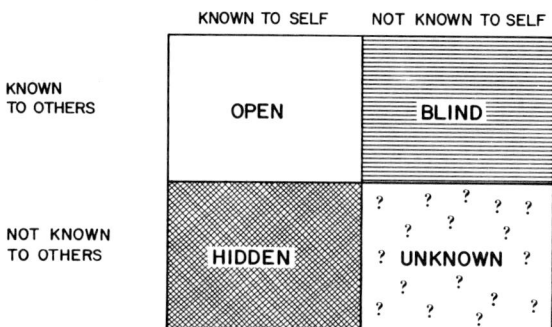

Open area. The individual shares this information knowingly with others.

Blind area. The individual is unaware that he is giving this information to others. Others recognize these feelings but the individual doesn't.

Hidden area. The individual does not share these ideas or feelings with others.

Unknown area. Neither the individual nor his acquaintances are aware of these motivations.[2]

Fig. 3.1. The Johari Window

Dilated pupils of the eyes are an example of communication in the unaware area.

A sensitive individual tries to allow these impressions to help him interpret the entire message he is receiving.

A person who is skilled in techniques of communicating will learn as much as he can about his own message-sending; he will attempt to control his nonverbal communication and make it agree with his verbal communication. (The person who listens and observes carefully while another is speaking to him has a more complete idea of the message given him. He has acquired much data to use in his interpretation of the spoken message.)

2. From Joseph Luft, *Of Human Interaction* (Palo Alto, Calif.: National Press Books, 1969), p. 13.

Transferring a Message

What happens when we try to communicate? Suppose you are a receptionist in a dental office. Your next task is to see that seven-year-old Janie is settled in an operatory and that her mother remains in the reception room.

Step number one is to transfer the idea to Janie that it is now time to go to the operatory. Janie is a somewhat fearful and negative child, rather strongly attached to her mother.

You decide on the sentence which you think will accomplish your goal. The message is "Janie, it's your turn now."

Step number two is to state the message. *How* you say this message will determine, at least in part, her response. If you are nervous, look imploringly at her mother or at the ceiling, hoping that Janie will respond nicely, Janie may refuse to go, cling to her mother, or scream.

You are showing Janie security if you assume a cheerful, positive attitude and demonstrate warmth and love for her. Look directly into her eyes as you smile at her sincerely.

If you express genuine love for a little child and show her by your attitude that she is to receive only kindness and love from you, she is more likely to respond to the security which you offer and come with you.

Notice that you attract her attention *before* you tell her what she is to do. The full impact of your message will be received only when you have her full attention. Further, if you will walk across the reception room and stand near Janie, smile, and hold out your hand, you will be inviting her participation. It would be very hard for her to refuse an offer of such loving attention.

Another approach might be to look through the reception window and say, "Come on, Janie. Doctor's waiting for you," perhaps a little gruffly because you feel distracted. (The other assistant is asking about Mrs. Jones's appointment, and the telephone is ringing.) Under these circumstances Janie is quite likely to cling to Mother, scream, and refuse to go into the operatory (which to her has less than pleasant associations).

If you say, "Do you want to come now?" It is easy for her to say "No!" and then you have a problem in forcing her to come anyway.

Whatever method you use, the message is received by Janie (Step 3). She translates into personal meaning for her all the communication which she receives: your words, your bodily messages, your attitudes, and the atmosphere of the office. She interprets these things in relationship to her past experience: with her parents, her teachers, other "nurses" and "doctors," and whether her previous dental visits have been pleasant. She is also affected by her present emotional state. If she has been fighting with siblings for parental attention and love that morning, or if she has been belittled, she will react differently from the way she may react on a day when she has been praised and loved. If she has been taught to be afraid of life or the assistant or adults, it may show in her reaction. *All* her emotional pressures will affect her answer.

If the sense of love, gentleness, and security she receives from your manner and tone is strong, it will offset negation on her part, and she will respond to your held-out hand by putting her hand in yours and walking with you—perhaps slowly, but neverthelesss trusting you to care for her. The more kindness and interest in *Janie as a person* you can show on (what seems to her) that long walk to the chair, the more secure she will feel.

Briefly, the process of transferring a message from one person to another is this:

1. the need for a message is recognized,
2. the message is formed,
3. the message is given,
4. the message is received,
5. the message is translated or interpreted by the receiver, and
6. the response is given (which becomes a form of feedback).

Note that the message may not be interpreted as the giver intended, but some kind of meaning is received.

Feedback is another way of judging whether your message was received as intended. The reaction of the listener tells the speaker much about the success of his attempt to transmit an idea—*but only if the speaker observes his listener's responses.*

Complexities of Person-to-Person Communication

Obviously there is much more to communication than simply saying a few words. Awareness of the fact that unsuspected problems can occur is important.

The complexities of person-to-person communication can be summarized thus:

1. Sometimes the interpretation which an individual makes when he receives a message may change the meaning of the message the sender thought he was transmitting. Sometimes what the sender fails to say or do affects the receiver as much as or more than what the sender says.
2. Meanings are in people, not in words. Unless the receivers understand the sender as the sender intended, there is communication breakdown.
3. Ability to communicate is determined by how an individual is treated when he communicates. People tend to respond to being treated kindly. Thus, the boss who becomes unconsciously threatening when told something unpleasant is likely to receive only good news because his employees have learned to avoid telling him anything unpleasant.

4. Misunderstanding is bound to occur in communication. Corrections can be made through feedback. (In this usage, feedback means asking the receiver to repeat this message in his own words.)
5. A wise response to trouble is "How can we correct this problem?" not "Whose fault is it?" This technique results in accomplishment of goals instead of ego-crushing.

These are the basic factors about communication. Skill in communication is another area. How does one *effectively* use his speaking mechanism? A brief, practical résumé of the processs of speech and how an individual can apply it for himself follows.

Skillful Use of the Speech Mechanism

Whenever one speaks, the resulting sounds should be pleasing to the audience—whether that audience is one person or a hundred persons. Effective use of the body to produce pleasant speech is something which can be accomplished by anyone who wishes to do so. It is a matter of understanding how good voice control is accomplished and then working with exercises to produce the desired results.

If you need to improve your voice production (and most of us do), perhaps you can take a speech course at your nearby college or night school. If this is impossible, the following discussion, with exercises, will be of help to you.

Good Voice Production

Four sections of the body are involved in good voice production. Based on the work they perform in the speech process, they are referred to as the bellows, the vibrators, the resonators, and the articulators.

The *bellows*: Good speech begins with good breath control. Technically, good breath con-

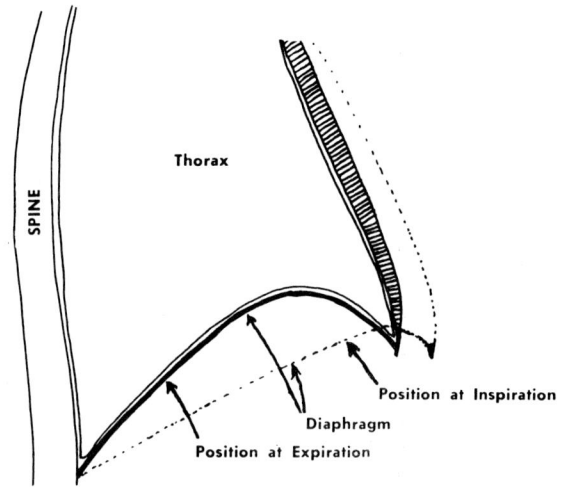

Figure 3.2. Schematic drawing showing action of the diaphragm.

trol is attained by diaphragmatic breathing. The diaphragm is a large muscle which divides the thorax (chest cavity) from the abdomen. When the lungs fill with air in diaphragmatic breathing, the diaphragm is pushed down, thus enlarging the thorax to make room for air.

The other method of breathing—frequently called upper chest breathing—enlarges the thorax by lifting the ribs and sternum. In upper chest breathing there is very little control over the airstream used in speech. The resulting voice is usually referred to as thin, high, weak, or ineffective. If it is necessary to speak for any length of time, the speaker finds his throat aching and tired from the strain.

Diaphragmatic breathing produces a strong, steady stream of air, which in turn produces a good voice tone and leaves the throat relaxed and able to work for hours.

It is important to check on your own method of breathing and to discover diaphragmatic breathing for yourself. (Most women are upper chest breathers.)

It is important for you to use diaphragmatic breathing. If you will lie down, relax, and breathe naturally, you will soon discover that you are breathing diaphragmatically. (The diaphragm area just below the ribs will be rising with each inhalation and falling with each exhalation.) Inhale, and as you exhale, laugh, *ha, ha, ha.* Continue to practice the *feel* of diaphragmatic breathing at intervals until you are using it for your speech. Nothing will make your voice more pleasing than a steady stream of air through a relaxed throat. This can be attained only through diaphragmatic breathing. Practice the following exercises to develop this method of breathing:

1. Work at inhaling and exhaling while standing and while sitting, until you can breathe diaphragmatically at will.
2. Put your hands on your diaphragm. Inhale slowly. Exhale and laugh, saying, *ha, ha, ha* through a complete exhalation. Notice the kick of the diaphragm.
3. Inhale and slowly exhale. Inhale. Say the letters of the alphabet until all the air has been exhaled. Repeat once or twice daily. You will gradually be able to increase the number of letters you can say during the length of one exhalation.
4. Try consciously to use diaphragmatic breathing whenever you speak.

The *vibrators*: The air coming from the lungs passes through the "voice box," or larynx. (See fig. 3.3.) The larynx is located at the top of the trachea. Inside the larynx are two vocal chords, or bands. The air must pass between these two bands. When we speak, the bands tense; as the air escapes between them, the bands vibrate—producing sound which we then form into words with other parts of our speech mechanism.

To have a pleasing voice, only enough air should be sent through the larynx to vibrate the vocal bands. Too much air produces a

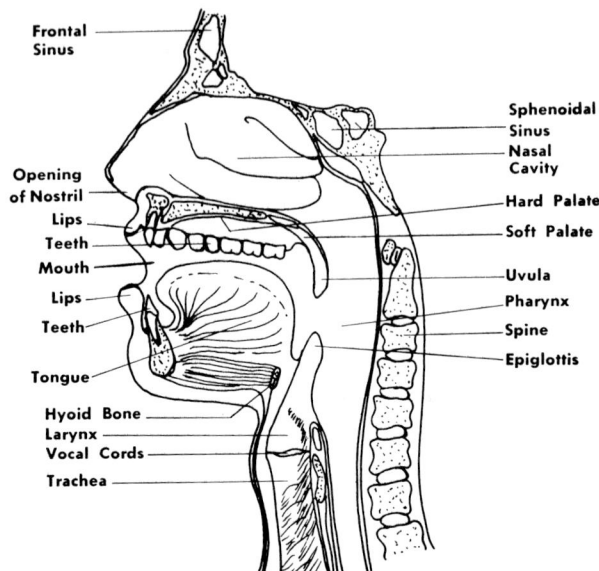

Fig. 3.3. Schematic drawing of head and neck

breathy quality due to air escaping and practically hissing as it leaves the throat. Practice the following exercises:

1. Practice the third exercise given for diaphragmatic breathing, making sure that no air hisses as you recite the alphabet.
2. Inhale and exhale, slowly saying *a—e—i—o —u.* Be sure you are breathing correctly and that the tone is clear—not breathy.

The *resonators*: Once the air becomes "voiced" by causing the vocal bands to vibrate, it must be increased in volume—or resonated. Whistle softly into a bottle. The sound is increased many times by the walls of the bottle. This is a simple illustration of a resonator.

In speech, resonance is produced primarily by the cavity at the back of the throat, known as the pharynx, and by the mouth, the nasal passages, and the sinuses. (See fig. 3.3.)

The *articulators*: The air that has been vibrated by the vocal bands and resonated by the resonators must be formed into words—or articulated. The articulators include the lips, teeth, tongue, hard palate, soft palate, uvula, pharyngeal walls, and jaws. (See fig. 3.3.)

Careful use of the articulators results in beautiful diction. Most frequently the sounds in our language are produced automatically—with no thought about the placement of the tongue, lips, etc. If you will listen to yourself and place the articulators carefully when you speak, you will be amazed at the change in diction. Listen to yourself speak—in front of a mirror. Do you say *doncha* or *don't you?* Can you hear the difference? Listen to your speech and eradicate as many of the slurs as you can. (Some examples are: *d'ya* for *do you*, *git* for *get*, *cuz* for *cause*, *jist* for *just*, *cancha* for *can't you*, and *wudja* for *would you*.) Also, try to eliminate the slang expressions you use. Check the dictionary for the correct pronunciation of words with which you are unfamiliar. Be sure that you know how to correctly pronounce simple words such as *Italian*.

To improve your diction, practice the following exercises daily, until you are conscious of how you use your articulators. Then a drill once a week should be sufficient to remind you of beautiful speech.

1. Open your jaws as wide as you can. Put the three middle fingers of your right hand between your teeth. The index finger should touch the upper teeth; the ring finger the lower teeth. If you cannot open your mouth this wide—and many people can't—exercise your jaws until you can. Open and close them several times, stretching them as far as possible. After several days of practice, some progress should be evident. Work until your mouth opens easily to a three-finger width.

   Clear speech depends, to a great extent, on a mouth that opens so that the articulated sounds can be released. The jaw must be relaxed and must move freely. Your lower jaw will feel as if you are exaggerating its use if you are speaking correctly and clearly.

2. Try to say as rapidly as possible all the tongue twisters you know. Here are a few examples:

   She sells sea shells by the seashore.

   Theophilus Thistle, the successful thistle sifter, thrust three thousand thistles through the thick of his thumb.

   Peter Piper picked a peck of pickled peppers.

   Rubber baby buggy bumpers.

These four sections of the body, then, *produce* the voice; but what kind of voice—pleasant or unpleasant, loud or soft, . . . or just right?

Four Characteristics of a Pleasing Voice

Let us think of the characteristics of a pleasing voice. It takes more than mechanics to make people enjoy hearing you speak. There are four characteristics of a pleasing voice: pitch, force, quality, and time.

The *pitch* of your voice is its relative highness or lowness. Your own pitch may be pleasing without effort. If so, you are fortunate. Medium pitch is usually considered most pleasing. If someone who will tell you the truth says that your voice sounds high, perhaps you need to lower your pitch. Use a piano for accompaniment. Sing up and down the scales, finding the highest and lowest notes you can sing. The note midpoint between the high and low extremes is the normal pitch of your voice. If you have been speaking above that pitch, practice using the new note as your "home base." Practice these exercises:

1. Inhale; repeat *a-e-i-o-u* on your key pitch as you exhale.

2. If your new pitch is lower than your former speaking voice, get a copy of Alfred Tennyson's "Crossing of the Bar" or "Break,

Break, Break" and read aloud, keeping your pitch low. It will help you express the meaning of the poems and allow practice in your new speaking range.

3. If you need to raise your pitch (a very unusual occurrence for a woman), use Lew Sarett's "Hollyhocks" and A. A. Milne's "The King's Breakfast."

With your new home-base pitch in mind, develop a wide range of pitch in speaking so that you do not speak in a monotone (on one note only). Practice reading selections you like—to be sure that you use a wide range of notes to make your voice interesting.

The *force* or *energy* with which you express yourself is another factor in attaining a pleasing voice. When you speak intensely, you are using much force. It may not be loud because a whisper can be intense. It depends on how hard and how suddenly you allow air to hit the vocal cords. For office work, force should not be applied, generally speaking. Keep the airstream well controlled without sudden bursts of vigor. You will sound relaxed and agreeable.

Most office speech occurs among two, three, or four persons and can be conducted quietly. Any intensity of tone tends to arouse emotion in listeners and may disturb some patients unpleasantly.

The normal *quality* of voice is largely determined by the resonators. It is important to use them correctly in pronouncing vowels in order to have full vocal quality. A round, open mouth when you say *ah* returns a beautiful sound. A partially closed mouth with a tense throat does not produce a quality enjoyed by your listener.

There are vocal qualities with technical names such as nasal quality, pectoral quality, oral quality, and orotund quality. While these are effective when portraying characters in a play, they have no place in a business office.

For improvement of vocal quality, exercise to relax, then exercise to add tone:

1. Drop the head to the chest, roll it to the right, and let it drop back; roll it to the left and let it drop forward. This makes a complete circle. Repeat several times.
2. Yawn to relax the throat and jaw. (Open your mouth wide enough, hold it, and you will yawn!)
3. Inhale, exhale, saying *mee-mee-ah*. Repeat until no air is left. Keep one tone for the exercise and listen to the quality. Make it as rich as you can. Repeat the exercise, using the vowels *o* as in *low, oo* as in *soon,* and *i* as in *high. Mee-mee-o, mee-mee-oo, mee-mee-i.*
4. Repeat the chorus of "John Brown's Body."

The final element is *time*. Our speech rate is determined by how long we hold sounds and by pauses between words or phrases. How cheerful you feel at the moment affects how rapidly or slowly you speak. Most of us tend to speak too rapidly. Speak reasonably slowly. Too fast a rate of speech causes poor diction and thus interferes with understanding. It also builds tensions in the listener. He tends to feel hurried.

Practice reading aloud selections of poetry which have a slow pace, as "O, Captain! My Captain!" by Walt Whitman, and selections needing pauses for emphasis, such as Lew Sarett's "Wind in the Pines" and John Masefield's "Sea Fever."

In summary, then, let us say that you need a well-groomed, animated, relaxed body and a controlled voice which has pleasing quality, and that you use good English, correctly and clearly spoken, at an unhurried rate, with adequate breath control.

Now you are ready to apply these skills to the office situation in which you find yourself. You ought to have something to say with your pleasing voice, housed in a well-groomed, animated body.

Selection of Pleasing Words

It is possible to phrase what is to be said to patients in ways which will please them and, therefore, make them remember. Language is made of symbols, and the symbols do not necessarily have the same meaning for all people. There are many meanings for words. Words have connotative and denotative meanings. Some words are more likely to have connotative meanings than others. Denotative words have meanings from the dictionary. The word *table* is denotative. For a test of whether a word has a denotative meaning, see if you can point to an object and have people understand what you mean.

Connotative meanings are a little different. They exist because you have an emotional feeling about the words, such as "The clouds reminded me of the gray dust rolls under my bed."

Difficulty in communicating is due to the fact that words which are normally thought of as having only denotative meanings really do have connotative meanings. For example, if someone says *chair,* what do you visualize first? The chair you sit on at work? a contemporary dining chair? an overstuffed armchair? a folding chair for a card table? a ruby red tapestry seat on an Early American cherry-wood rocker? Your personal vision of *chair* is present because you have had experiences which cause your mind to select a *specific* chair to remember. The person sitting next to you has another vision, colored by his experience. The symbol *chair* can have as many meanings as there are people present to hear the word.

We must remember that even words which we think of as factual, reportive words have different meanings for different people. If

words have an emotional meaning, this, too, colors the individual's reaction. For example, what does *watermelon* mean to you? Does it mean a delightful treat enjoyed especially on the Fourth of July? Does it bring back memories of wonderful family picnics? Most people think of watermelon as a happy memory. Let us consider the case of eleven-year-old Suzy. She had developed this wonderful feeling about watermelon. It was a treat reserved for such special occasions as Fourth of July. One Saturday, shortly before the Fourth, her father called Suzy and her brother and sister to the kitchen "for a treat." It was watermelon. Suzy could scarcely contain her joy and excitement. She popped a huge piece of the heart into her mouth and let the juice run all around until she could scarcely keep it from trickling down her throat and choking her. While Suzy was enjoying the sweetness and texture, her father said, "Children, your mother and I are going to get a divorce. You will have to decide which of us you wish to live with."

Suzy began to cry, and soon the salt tears, the thick saliva, and the watermelon sweetness mingled until she could hardly swallow. Years later when Suzy was grown, the mention of watermelon reminded her of her parents' divorce, not consciously, but unconsciously. Her reaction to watermelon was unpleasant. Its meaning for her was different from its meanings for others whose emotional memories were not so unpleasant. She didn't even know why!

This is a risk you take with every person you engage in conversation. He may have had some life experience which makes his emotional response to a word different from yours.

There is no "one word, one meaning." All words are surrounded by a cloud of experiences and emotions inside each individual, namely the connotative meanings the words have acquired *for that individual.* It is necessary for each individual to sort out from this cloud of meanings the one he thinks is the meaning intended by the speaker. How many times does he guess correctly? This is one of our most difficult communication problems.

Another problem with connotative meanings is that many of our words have several meanings. Let us take the word *fair* (including *fare* since the communication is oral and the spelling cannot be seen). If I use this word in sentences, the meaning is clearer to you.

He went to the *fair*.	That was a *fair* grade.
He didn't play *fair*.	A *fair*-haired boy.
The *fare* went up.	The sky was *fair*.
It's a *fair* day.	He left a *fair* estate.
She has a *fair* face.	She is *fair* game.

The dictionary gives at least nine definitions for this one word. Obviously the meaning changes with the use of the word in a sentence.

A third problem is that some words create emotional responses of hate or love reactions. Some communications experts refer to these words as "snarl" and "purr" words. Some words create negative prejudice, such as "Jack is a *rotter*" or Jack is *yellow*." Some words create affirmative prejudice, such as "Mr. Smith is a *noble, kindly* person." Some words are inclined to shock you—*nigger, wop, hick, Red,* and others.

How can you, a dental assistant, communicate effectively with patients since patients are likely to be affected by factors of which you are unaware? Meet each encounter by asking yourself why the patient *feels* as he does, rather than either agreeing or disagreeing with him. It is important to respond calmly to all emotion-charged words. You may or may not agree with the patient. You must try to understand *why* he makes the statement.

It doesn't matter whether the patient thinks the President of the United States is the best President we ever had, or the worst. What is important is that the negative emotions be allowed to exhaust themselves harmlessly and

that you understand *why* he makes such extreme statements about any subject mentioned.

Remember that it isn't what you say as much as *how* you say it. Much of our speech is not to give any factual information; it is simply to break silence, to socialize. "How are you?" "So nice to have met you," "Come see us!" are typical examples of speech which communicates little, yet to refrain from these phrases is to be rude. When someone says "How are you?" your correct answer is "Fine," not an account of how much you ache and dread the removal of the sutures from your recent surgery.

Talking is one form of human communication. Subject matter may be of secondary importance. The *warmth* of friendly talk is often more important. Greet your patients warmly. Listen to them attentively.

Listening—An Important Link in Communications

How do *you* listen? Attentively? Absent-mindedly? Do you half-listen? Perhaps you think you are listening attentively, but you fail to hear all of the message. Perhaps the nonverbal message is stronger than the verbal message, that is, what you *see* overpowers what you hear.

Communication is a two-way process. The person who is speaking wants to reach the listener and get a response from him. The listener hears what the speaker says, *interprets* it in his mind, and responds according to his interpretation of the speaker's comments. He may or may not remember what the speaker said. Thus, listening is a complicated process. Hearing and listening are not the same thing. First we have the *hearing* of the sound, then we have the *interpretation* of the sound, followed by a response of some kind. If the *interpretation* has been important enough to the listener, he remembers what the speaker said. Thus, listening really has three parts: the hearing of the sound, the interpretation of the sound, and the remembering of those interpretations which are important to the individual.

In addition, listening really starts even before the person begins to speak. The instant the listener *sees* the speaker he begins to assimilate (absorb) impressions about that person. The first *sight* begins the absorbing. He continues to formulate his impression during and following the speaker's presentation. This applies whether the situation is a formal speech or a conversation between two people. If the speaker is depressed, his depression will affect his entire appearance as well as his speech. If he happens to be resentful of his niche in life, his resentment will show in his bearing and in his tone of voice. The listener responds involuntarily to this emotional communication even before he responds to the verbal message of the speaker.

It is important in the dental office that you control your emotional reaction to people and give them *all* a warm, attentive reception, regardless of the "messages" they may be sending your way by their actions.

Research studies in listening have indicated strongly that the most important single attribute in a manager is *listening to the individual employee.* The principle behind this discovery is just as applicable in the office situation. The most important thing you can do to help relations with patients is to listen to them attentively. Concentrate on what the patient is saying. Try to evaluate (1) *why* he is saying what he is saying and (2) what his emotional state is at the moment. You will respond better with empathy for his particular problems if you try to see the situation from his point of view.

Observation, a Necessary Tool in Human Relations

It is necessary to observe carefully the people you meet. The keen observer can recognize little movements (a twitch of a muscle, the blink of an eye) and be more aware of what the person being observed is actually thinking. It is wise for a dental assistant to develop this ability. It is rather easy to do if you can discipline yourself to keep your mind on the subject you wish to consider. If you can concentrate on listening attentively to the patient who is speaking to you and at the same time be observant of his expression, his posture, his ease or lack of it, you are much more aware of what he is trying to tell you. You are also discovering much about that patient which you would otherwise miss entirely.

To train your powers of observation, examine some little object for a minute and then try to list everything you can remember about it. Then look at the object again and see how accurate you were. It can be a leaf from a tree, or any object with which you are familiar. When you have done this exercise to your satisfaction, try concentrating on a person—a classmate, a co-worker, or someone you see on the bus. Make a mental note of everything you can about that person in a specific length of time—like one minute.

Gradually you will sharpen your powers of observation. If you listen carefully to a patient and observe his physical movements and expressions, you will eventually be able to guess with fair accuracy what his next comment will be.

One of the greatest satisfactions in life is found in the interaction of human personalities with each other. Your day will be far more satisfying if you are able to be an observant, sympathetic, and attentive listener.

Office Conversation Technique

"Conversation occurs when two or more people *exchange* ideas of interest to themselves."[3] In normal conversation, the emphasis

3. C. Gilbert Wrenn, Reinhard Hein, and Shirley Schwarzrock, *Planned Group Guidance,* part 2, p. 1.

is on the word *exchange*. In the dental office, your job is to keep the conversation centered on the patient and his interests and to make dentistry one of his interests. Instead of expounding *your* ideas, therefore, you should continue to make remarks and ask questions which draw the patient out. You must be careful, however, to see that conversation does not interfere with dental work. Use it wisely—just enough to make the patient feel appreciated—and sparingly enough so that you do not interfere with the proper functioning of the dental office. Greet the patient with a personal comment and, after his answer, change the interest to dentistry—the purpose of his trip to your office.

To attain this mature status as an expert conversationalist under the specific conditions of the dental office, you must be a good listener, be alert to the interests of the patient, and be able to make the patient the center of interest. Your comments should be made in a sincere and straightforward manner.

Since your patients are apt to be interested in a wide range of topics of conversation, try to be informed about as many currently interesting subjects as possible: sports, national events, movies, plays, books, international affairs, business conditions, styles, interior decoration—to mention several. The object is to know enough to make a personal contact with the patient on his favorite subject. It is not intended that you expound on it. Actually, to be informed requires little effort on your part beyond reading the newspaper and glancing at a magazine or two. This will also make a delightful difference in your social life.

Elsewhere it is mentioned that a note clipped to the patient's record of an important family event gives the office staff something personal to mention at the next visit of the patient.

A note listing a patient's favorite subjects of conversation and clipped to the record is also a great aid to the dental assistant when the patient comes in for a recall. Example: Some women love to talk fashions, and a simple note clipped to the record of the one word, *fashions,* or *hats* if she specializes in this one area of fashions, allows the dental assistant to ask a question casually about some current fashion, to the delight of the patient.

After you have asked a patient a question, *appear interested* in the answer. Attention at this moment is the basis of being a good listener. It also gives you an opportunity to learn to read the behavior of the patient. Only by learning what to expect can you anticipate situations which could be problems unless they are properly met.

Most of us go through life without observing other people's reactions to what we do and say. The first step in learning to know what the patient is thinking is to listen to him and watch him closely.

When you talk with a patient and he reacts unfavorably, remember what you said that brought about this reaction from the patient. Later, analyze your remarks. Try to recall the particular phrase you used that caused the trouble. Find a substitute phrase. The next time you have a similar situation, try the new phrase which you have worked out. Keep experimenting until you know that what you say to patients is pleasing.

Co-workers and Communication

Understanding and communicating with office personnel are also areas of importance. For patients, one ordinarily plans and follows through with planned communications; but co-workers are another matter. One is inclined to feel that planning communication with them or working to express a message in the most diplomatic terms is unnecessary, but barriers to communication exist in all phases of life.

Communicating with co-workers may be even more difficult than with patients because a close working relationship exists in a dental office, and the exposure to co-workers is usually for eight hours a day. Any personal frictions can create attitudes which form barriers to understanding.

The person who attempts to do an effective job of communicating with people remains alert for these three barriers to communication:

1. *Misunderstanding.* Never assume meaning. Always ask for clarification. *Ask* "What do you mean?" and *listen* to the response. Ask for explanations of expressions which could be interpreted in several ways. When something is described as *satisfactory* or *unsatisfactory,* try to discover *how* it is satisfactory or unsatisfactory. Under what circumstances? In what way? Try saying, "Let's see if I understand you." Repeat in your own words the message you have just received. The speaker then has an opportunity to correct your interpretation of his message. The difference in meaning may surprise him—and you.

   It may help you understand the problem if you remember that of the 2,000 words most frequently used by Americans, 500 of them have 14,000 dictionary definitions! There is possibility for misunderstanding simply because a word has two different meanings to the persons trying to communicate.

2. *Disagreement* may also build barriers to communication. Occasionally some of the office personnel have purposes they wish to accomplish which they may never share with the rest of the staff. For example, if Mary wishes to keep the spatulas in drawer *A* and Susie wishes to keep them in drawer *C,* this *can* become a barrier to communication, although it doesn't have to—but the principle is there. Disagreement may be about something as simple and as small as spatulas. It may also be a fundamental disagreement about the philosophy of working in a dental office. Unless the disagreement can be aired and resolved, problems may arise in communicating.

3. *Misinformation* can cause barriers to communication, also. If Sally thinks Doctor said he was dissatisfied with her arrangement of the recall file, whereas what he really said was that it would have to do until something better was discovered, Sally may not be able to communicate effectively about the file until she learns that what she has done with the file is acceptable for now.

Listening—actually listening—can probably do more for staff accord than almost anything else that can happen. We simply do not listen well to others. Usually we are planning what we are going to say while the other person is talking. To be able to listen, think, and then answer takes self-discipline. But without having heard what the other person had to say, how can one understand and respond effectively?

Try to give the same attentiveness to your co-workers as has been suggested for your patients.

Summary

Two of the most common problems in the communication of ideas are understanding others and being understood.

Communication is more than words. It is emotions, behaviors, sounds, and gestures in addition to words. Often an individual is unaware of the message he is transmitting.

Dental assistants can plan some of the communications which are necessary in the office.

A message is transferred from one person to another by a process which includes the need for recognition of the message, formation of the message, giving the message, receiving the message, translating or interpreting the message, and giving the response (which becomes a form of feedback). Feedback is a way of judging whether the message has been received as intended.

Complexities of person-to-person communication include these problems: variations occur in interpretation of the message; meanings are in people, not words; treatment of persons during communication varies; and misunderstandings are to be expected.

Skillful use of the speaking mechanism should be developed.

Communication with co-workers is often neglected, but it is very important. Ask "What do you mean?" rather than permit a misunderstanding to occur. Try to repeat the message for clarification.

Listening is vitally important for staff accord.

Study Questions

1. What is a basis for understanding?
2. What steps are necessary for one person to effectively transfer a message to another person? Illustrate with the skills used to encourage Janie to leave her mother and go with the assistant to the operatory.
3. What problems can be avoided by giving thought to the complexities of communication?
4. What three factors build barriers between staff members?
5. How can barriers to effective communication be avoided?

Bibliography

BOSMAJIAN, HAIG A. *The Rhetoric of Nonverbal Communication: Readings.* Glenview, Ill.: Scott, Foresman & Co., 1971.

BROWN, RONALD, and NICHOLS, RALPH G. *Practical Speechmaking.* Dubuque, Ia.: Wm. C. Brown Co. Publishers, 1970. [The authors recommend the entire Speech Communication Series published by Wm. C. Brown Co.]

FABUN, DON. *Communications: The Transfer of Meaning.* Beverly Hills, Calif.: Glencoe Press, 1968.

FAST, JULIUS. *Body Language.* New York: M. Evans & Co., 1970.

GIFFIN, KIM, and PATTON, BOBBY R. *Fundamentals of Interpersonal Communication.* New York: Harper & Row, 1971.

HALL, EDWARD T. *The Hidden Dimension.* Garden City, N. Y.: Doubleday & Co., 1966.

————. *The Silent Language.* Greenwich, Conn.: Fawcett Publications, 1959.

WRENN, C. GILBERT; HEIN, REINHARD G.; and SCHWARZROCK, SHIRLEY PRATT. *Planned Group Guidance.* Circle Pines, Minn.: American Guidance Service, 1961.

ZIMBARDO, PHILIP, and EBBESEN, EBBE B. *Influencing Attitudes and Changing Behavior: A Basic Introduction to Relevant Methodology, Theory and Applications.* Reading, Mass.: Addison-Wesley Publishing Co., 1970.

4 | Reception Procedures for All Who Contact the Office

Introduction

The warmth and cordiality, the friendliness of the staff are necessary attributes in the reception procedures for *all* who contact the office. One never knows who the stranger entering the office is, what his business is, and *what he will say about his reception in that office once he is again outside.* Advertising in the usual sense of the word cannot be purchased by dentists. To do so is considered unethical. Therefore, word-of-mouth advertising by persons who contact the office either personally or by telephone becomes extremely important. Cordial treatment of all persons is one of the best ways to establish good empathy with the public.

The treatment of patients is one of the important aspects of dental assisting. The patient appreciates a cheerful, pleasant attitude from the assistant and feels he has a bonus in relations if the assistant also treats him as a *person.*

It is important, then, that you learn to work well with patients and to make them like you and your office. Some of the treatment which has been accorded waiting patients is shocking. We who serve the public in the health fields should view these instances of rudeness with concern.

Recently a garage mechanic was heard to say in a vicious tone, "Let him wait! It'll make up for some of the time my wife has spent sitting in doctors' waiting rooms." He was referring to a doctor who was waiting for his car.

There was real animosity in his tone. He didn't even know the doctor in question. Perhaps this doctor did not keep patients waiting, but as long as some do, the profession as a whole is condemned.

In a milder form this same resentment is expressed by housewives. Contrary to the opinion of most people who receive a paycheck for their working hours, a housewife's time is just as valuable *to her and to her family* as the office worker's is to him and his employer. It is important to take patients on time insofar as it is humanly possible. If delays are encountered, it is exceedingly important to be fair to all patients—housewives and children as well as office workers . . . or your best friend.

The garage mechanic was generalizing that since some doctors have no respect for patients, all doctors have no respect for patients and therefore should be treated with disrespect. This is not true, but it is necessary for all the personnel in dental and medical offices to help change this idea so prevalent among lay people (the general public) today.

Actually observed in a *waiting* room was this example of disrespect for people. It was standing room only. The receptionist looked at the group impassively. Names were called indifferently. The waiting period beyond an appointment was close to two hours. She glanced coldly over the group and said, "You, there in the green chair by the lamp, come here."

There was no trace of common courtesy in her tone. There was no consideration of the people there as individual human beings *with*

obligations and appointments beyond this office. This might have been a herd of cattle—and not even her own herd of cattle. She was totally distinterested in anything except that she had to call the next patient.

You may feel that this is an extreme example, and certainly in our better-administered offices this treatment does not occur, but it does exist in enough offices to create a negative impression for some of the public.

We have also heard assistants complain of the treatment they have received from patients who have been rude. We are not suggesting that only the office personnel are inconsiderate. We know that patients can be very inconsiderate and rude. Some of them will even try to run the office. However, there is one extenuating circumstance in connection with patients. Remember that most of them are apprehensive, which in itself denotes fear. They may also be dreading the treatment they are about to receive. Their ability to be pleasant is directly limited by their physical and mental conditions.

It is your job to make such a person as comfortable as possible and to refrain from responding to rudeness with rudeness. One can be firm and remain courteous regardless of the attitude of the patient. The most important attitude to develop with patients is to make them feel that each one is a VIP whose health and welfare receive top priority in your office.

It is the objective of this chapter to help the dental assistant become aware of and develop the skills which permit her to treat patients to this well-deserved care.

Let us avoid treating people as impersonally as if they were chairs. Let us remember that they have obligations beyond this office and will appreciate a well-planned schedule of appointments. Only rarely will a patient object to waiting due to some unforeseen emergency—provided every day is not an emergency. It is the business of treating every day as an overload which upsets patients.

Reception Room Procedures

A reception room for receiving guests—rather than a waiting room where nonpersons are allowed to sit until they are called—is the important differentiation to be made in your work with patients. Try to maintain the important concept that you are *receiving* VIPs. Think and speak of the *reception* room.

Everyone should be greeted warmly with a smile, as you would receive people who call on you at your home. They should be greeted promptly *upon arrival.* When the doorbell rings, indicating someone has entered your reception room, *respond* as quickly as you possibly can. Be a very gracious hostess to all who enter the office. Remember that the patient who returns does so because he likes the way he was treated on previous visits.

What you do after the initial greeting depends on the nature of the caller's business.

Receiving Previous Patients

Know the name of the patient you are expecting to arrive. Use it when you greet him. The schedule for the day will have it listed. Know the name; use the name.

One of the finer touches in hostessing which you can use, if time permits and your dentist agrees, is to greet the patient with a coat hanger in your hand and hang up his coat for him. This moment, if available, gives opportunity for that personal contact you wish to make with the patient and makes him feel very important while you are asking him about his particular interest—or commenting on her stylish hat. Elderly women especially appreciate such assistance, and it is not out of place for any patient—as it would not be out of place for you to do at your home. In cold climates, the really heavy work of dressing children for

travel to the dental office, removing their outer clothing for the appointment, then dressing them again for the trip home is extremely tiring for the mother. Assistance with children under these conditions is more than appreciated. It also gives you the opportunity to remove overshoes or boots which otherwise might be left on to track snow or mud into the operatory. Mothers would not leave them on the child at home, but frequently the work of removing and replacing them is such that the temptation to leave them on the child supersedes.

If for any reason the dentist will be late in beginning work for the patient who has already arrived at the office, inform the patient of the fact. Include the probable time of waiting involved—do not say "just a few minutes" when you are actually twenty minutes behind. You *say,* "I'm sorry, Mr. Jones, we have been delayed. We will be ready for you in twenty minutes."

See that the patient is seated, with reading matter available. If children are present, see that they are entertained. A few coloring books and a supply of soap crayons (which will wash off from almost anything) can do much to keep most children occupied for short periods.

If patients have the habit of dropping in, expecting the dental work to be done right then, always make an appointment for them in the future—even if your dentist *could* see them. Explain that scheduled appointments come first, and there are only so many hours in a day. It wouldn't be fair to take others ahead of scheduled patients. The reason for never permitting a drop-in patient to receive dental attention is that once he has succeeded in accomplishing his goal, he will continue to expect such treatment. Thus, he must never be given an opportunity to drop in for dental care—even if you have had a cancellation and your dentist is idle.

Receiving Strangers

"May I help you?"—said with a smile. The first thing to discover is the purpose of this stranger's visit to your office.

The New Patient

If the stranger indicates that he is a potential patient and is having pain of dental origin at the moment, ask him to be seated, hand him the Acquaintance Form[1] on its clipboard, and say: "Will you please fill this out? I will ask Doctor Smith how soon he can see you." Appraise the individual as best you can.

Immediately notify your dentist, by note if he is operating. He will suggest your next step. It is helpful if the assistant can inform him of the patient schedule at the moment. For example, the dentist may be finishing his present patient and the next appointment may not have arrived.

If the stranger indicates that he is a potential patient but is having no pain or discomfort, ask him to be seated, hand him the Acquaintance Form on its clipboard, and say, "Will you please fill this out for Doctor Smith?"

Have possible appointments in mind. When you have received the completed form, check it rapidly. Note which day of the week is preferred. Then say, "Doctor Smith would like to see you for examination on................(day) at................(hour), or................(hour). Which time will be more convenient for you?"

Proceed to give him an appointment card for that date and hour, filling in his name in the appointment book first, then on the appointment card, double-checking the date and hour as you make it out to be sure you have written the same date and hour as you marked off in the appointment book. Give him the card, and use his name when you say goodbye.

1. See figure 16.1, p. 181.

Receiving Salesmen or Detail Men

Salesmen should rarely see the dentist except by prearranged appointments. Almost all sales can be handled by the dental assistant. If it is desirable for a salesman and the dentist to talk, make an appointment. Make the salesman feel that his time is valuable, and it is much better for both the salesman and the dentist to have appointments with specified lengths of time. You must limit his time with the dentist and make certain he understands that such is the case. According to the day's schedule, you say, "Doctor can see you at 1:50 for ten minutes" or "Doctor Smith is free from 1:50 until 2:00." Make the appointment between patients—not at the beginning of the dentist's lunch hour nor at the close of the day. It is much wiser to be able to interrupt the conference at the end of the allotted time. When that time has arrived, you say "Doctor Smith, your patient is in the chair."

Of course, the salesmen seen by the dentist during office hours should be salesmen of dental products and equipment. Insurance salesmen should be seen at home, as well as any salesman selling products for the dentist's personal life rather than for dentistry.

Protect your dentist from detail men whom he does not wish to see. Detail men often show a new product to stimulate sales. Remember that if you continue to politely refuse to allow the detail man to see the dentist, he will stop coming. Several refusals should convince even the most obtuse individual.

Perhaps your dentist prefers to see dental salesmen as soon as it is convenient for him to do so. In this case, the suggested handling of the stranger who is a salesman will be altered. The salesman who has entered the office should be informed of the time-wait involved or of a more opportune time to call.

No matter what method of dealing with salesmen is used in your office, *all* salesmen should be treated courteously. They earn their living by selling and very often can be helpful.

The Professional Man

If the stranger who enters your reception room introduces himself as "Doctor Jones," immediately ask him to be seated and excuse yourself. In a clear, distinct voice tell your dentist immediately that Doctor Jones is in the reception room. Your dentist will tell you what he wishes you to do. Unless your dentist specifically indicates otherwise, always remember that the privacy of the patient in the chair should be respected. Ordinarily, any other professional man, or any person not a member of the office staff, is *not* brought to the chairside without the express permission of the patient beforehand.

The Unidentified Caller

There will be occasional individuals who merely indicate that they would like to speak to Doctor Smith, without giving you either name or business. Usually this would indicate in itself that if the dentist knew the reason for the visit, he would refuse to see the caller. Some judgment is required in these situations, but if you do feel doubtful due to the appearance of the individual and his reluctance to tell you his name and business, inform him firmly and courteously that you must have his name and the subject of his visit, indicating that you will then be able to ask Doctor Smith if he will see the visitor. Should he refuse again, say, "I'm sorry, but in that case you will have to reach Doctor Smith at his home after office hours." Then leave him.

This same technique is used with telephone callers who insist on speaking to the dentist and refuse to give their name or business after you have gone through the regular routine.

Once in awhile, an individual will ask a question (in response to your greeting) such

as, "Are you the only employee in this office?" or, "How long have you worked for Doctor Smith?" Such an approach, a rapidly given personal question, is often the device used to gain the initiative in the conversation and is widely used by door-to-door salespeople. Merely keep in mind that personal questions are not the privilege of a stranger; do not follow the impulse to answer.

Reply with a question of your own, such as "What is it you are selling?" Or simply say, "What is it you wish, please?" Do not waste your time or your employer's time unnecessarily.

Dismissing Patients

Helping a patient to leave the office feeling worthwhile and valued is also important. Frequently the dismissal *begins* at the dental chair. (Duties of the chairside assistant will be discussed in chap. 45.)

The receptionist's duties usually include escorting the patient from the operatory back to the reception room. All possible assistance should be given with coats, boots, and gathering of personal belongings. If the patient is elderly, helping him put on his coat is often appreciated. If a mother has small children, she can be very grateful for assistance at the time of departure.

These courtesies to patients can only be performed when time permits and the dentist approves. One of the advantages of this type of reception and dismissal of patients is that it permits the receptionist to "protect" her dentist from a problem situation which might develop. The dentist cannot afford to spend too much time of day with patients, salesmen, insurance men, or anyone else. He must confine his contact with the patient to the time allotted, making certain that during the time of the patient's appointment the patient is made to feel his value to the dentist and his importance as a person. When that allotted time has elapsed, the dentist must be ready to devote his undivided attention to the next patient. At this point the receptionist or other staff member can give the departing patient attention so that the patient leaves the office feeling appreciated.

Telephone Procedures

A patient enters a dental office by one of two methods: either he appears in person or he calls on the telephone. The usual procedure is to telephone prior to coming to the office; thus, the telephone becomes a most important means of entry. The dental assistant whose assignment includes answering the telephone must possess skillful techniques in telephone usage. She must be aware of the factors which encourage patients to take the next step—appearing in person at an appointed time.

The success of a telephone contact is dependent on how well the two persons involved understand each other. All the physical factors which are present to help that understanding in a person-to-person contact are missing in a telephone conversation. It is possible to have just as satisfying an interaction over the telephone, provided the message content is carefully selected and effectively presented. The individual who is gracious, sincere, and courteous while interacting on the telephone usually creates a favorable impression.

Telephone Technique in the Professional Office

The telephone is such a common part of our everyday life that some of us are apt to treat its use carelessly. In a professional office, care must be taken to use this instrument properly. The fact that the physical management of the telephone can be stated simply does not lessen the importance of following the instructions for its effective use.

The telephone should be held so that the transmitter is one-half to one inch from the lips. Since the telephone transmitter is as sensitive as a microphone, the voice must be directed into it. A person must be especially careful not to let it slip under the chin, or to cover the transmitter with the hand.

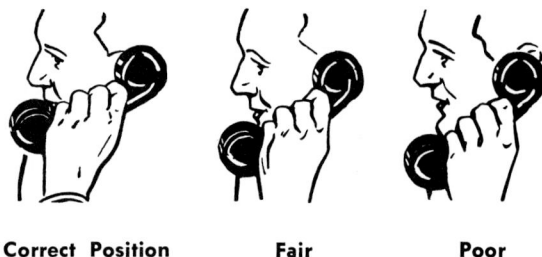

Correct Position   **Fair**   **Poor**

Fig. 4.1. Hold the telephone correctly

A well-modulated conversational tone of voice carries best over the telephone. Of course, it goes without saying that impediments—like a pencil or gum—should not be placed in the mouth when talking. This could lead to annoyance or misunderstanding and create unfavorable impressions.

Care should be taken to hang up gently, since banging the receiver is unpleasant to the ear and is like slamming the door in someone's face.[2]

Following the rules set forth in the foregoing quoted paragraphs will care for the mechanics of telephone usage. In addition, when speaking on the telephone, always speak as you would if the person were standing before you—the same courtesy, the same warmth of expression, and the same friendliness of manner. Try smiling while speaking. Only your voice contacts the person with whom you are speaking. You must make it so cordial that the person on the telephone feels the warmth of your personality just as though you were

2. *Teletraining (Effective Use of the Telephone)*, published by the Bell Telephone System for use within the system in training employees.

speaking to each other in the same room. Remember that *how* you say what you say affects the person on the telephone more than in a person-to-person conversation.

The Professional Telephone Call

A professional telephone call may be divided into four parts:

1. Identification of caller and person called.
2. Purpose of call, including any specific arrangements to be made.
3. Conclusion of business, including verification of information or specific arrangements.
4. Termination of call, including courteous closing remarks, such as "Thank you for calling."

Additional suggestions to render effective telephone service include the following:

1. Answer the telephone promptly, thus making the caller feel that he is important, that this is an efficient dental office, and that you value his time as well as your own.
2. When you make calls, allow time for the person to answer. A minute is a very short time for a housewife to reach the telephone if she is in the yard or upstairs and has but one telephone. In one minute the telephone will ring about *ten times.*
3. Try to avoid calling a wrong number by having the correct number at hand and then dialing carefully after you have heard the dial tone. If you do receive a wrong number, apologize and hang up gently.
4. Give information regarding an appointment slowly.
5. If it is necessary to leave the telephone to get information, remember these three items:
   a. Be sure to excuse yourself and indicate that you will return in a specific length of time, such as a few seconds, one minute, or two minutes.
   b. Return to the telephone to assure the caller that you haven't forgotten him if it takes longer than you said it would to find the information.
   c. Attract his attention on your return by saying his name or "Thank you for waiting, Mr. Jones." Then give him the desired information.
6. Always close *any* telephone conversation with a pleasant, "Thank you, Mrs. Jones," or "Thank you for calling, Mrs. Jones." The first phrase applies if you called Mrs. Jones; the latter phrase applies if Mrs. Jones called your office.
7. Upon completion of a call which a patient made to your office, the caller definitely should be the first to hang up his receiver. It is courteous to let the other party be the first to hang up.

Recording Telephone Calls

Often it is necessary to take messages from telephone callers. The telephone notebook is the ideal record of telephone calls. A bound notebook used for this purpose means that every call which is written in the book remains there to be seen later. It is impossible to lose a telephone message if it is bound into a telephone notebook which is much like a receipt book. A carbon copy of the written message remains bound in the book for future reference; the original copy is removable. This means the message can be kept for future reference and, at the same time, be given to the person who is to receive the message. A notebook listing the telephone calls received should be kept whether or not the dentist for whom you work wishes to use the telephone book with carbon copy. A sample page from a telephone notebook is shown in figure 4.2. Notice that specific information is given for each call.

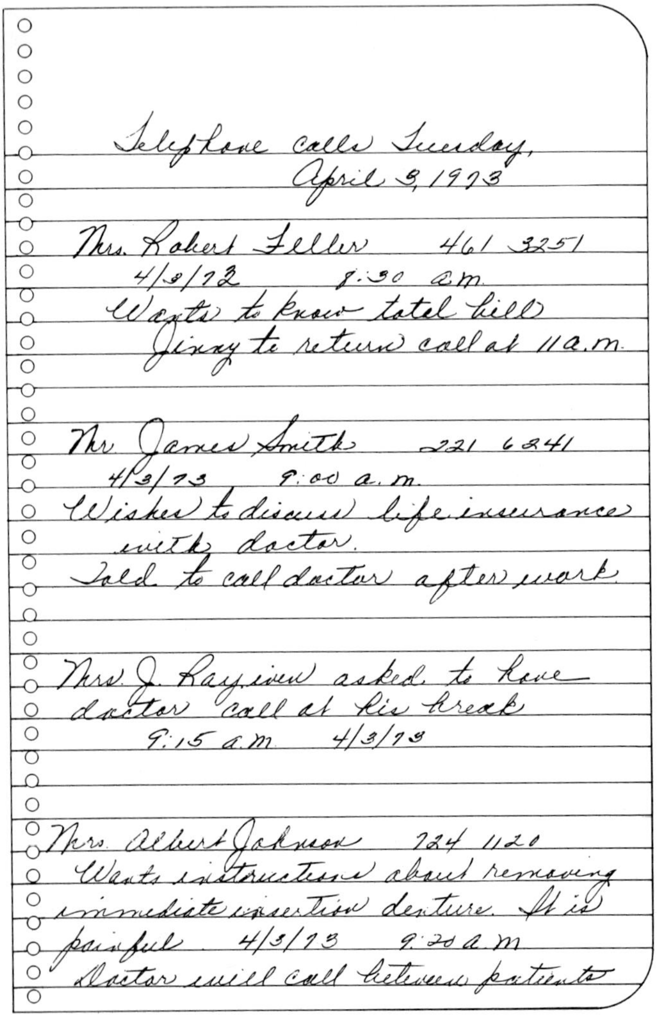

Telephone calls Sunday,
April 3, 1973

Mrs. Robert Feller   461-3251
4/3/73   8:30 a.m.
Wants to know total bill
Jinny to return call at 11 a.m.

Mr. James Smith   221-6241
4/3/73   9:00 a.m.
Wishes to discuss life insurance
with doctor.
Told to call doctor after work

Mrs. J. Ray, ... asked to have
doctor call at his break
9:15 a.m   4/3/73

Mrs. Albert Johnson   724-1120
Wants instructions about removing
immediate insertion denture. It is
painful   4/3/73   9:30 a.m
Doctor will call between patients

Fig. 4.2. Sample page from a telephone notebook

Taking the Message

Be helpful if you are taking a message. Be certain that you have the name, the telephone number of the caller, the date (with year), and the time of the call—written legibly. Agree on an approximate time for you to report back to the caller or have him called by the person he wished to contact. Be certain that this information is recorded on your note of the call:

1. name of caller,
2. telephone number (can you read it?),
3. date and time of call,
4. desired information,
5. time at which his call will be returned, and
6. who is to return the call.

Specific Suggestions for the Dental Office Telephone Problems

1. *Answering routine.* In answering the telephone, say "Doctor Smith's office." Your dentist may like you to add, "Miss Jones speaking." Use an agreed-upon wording and do not alter it.

2. *Expressing competence.* You must give the telephone caller the positive assurance of your ability and that you know what you are doing. You do not say so, but you give this assurance by using a tone with no rising inflections at the ends of sentences. A calm, low voice is good, provided it is cheerful.

3. *Visualizing the caller.* Try to put yourself in the caller's place. Think what he is thinking—and treat him as *you* would want to be treated. Be pleasant!

Individuals who telephone the office will occasionally abuse this form of entry and become discourteous. Never give anything but courtesy in return, even under the most trying circumstances.

4. *Two jobs at once.* If the telephone rings while you are caring for a patient—welcoming, dismissing, or accepting payment, for example—answer the telephone after excusing yourself, ascertain the name of the caller, then courteously ask the telephone caller to wait until you have finished with the patient in the office.

You say, "Mr. Jones, will you please wait while I complete an appointment?" If he indicates he is too busy, then you may say, "May I call you in a few moments?" and take his number and call him immediately after you finish the business with the patient who is standing in front of you.

However, most callers will be willing to wait, understanding that you are working with another patient. In this case, finish your business with the patient in the office as quickly and as courteously as possible; then return to the telephone, saying, "Thank you for waiting, Mr. Jones. Now may I help *you?*" It is extremely irritating to a patient to find his business with you interrupted by a telephone call and to have you give the telephone call precedence in your attention. It is discourteous to the patient who is present in person.

If a patient enters the reception room when you are telephoning, smile at him and bring your business conversation to a close as quickly as possible to care for the needs of the patient in the reception room. If your conversation is personal (a *rare* occasion), immediately terminate it and finish your personal business later.

5. *Insulating the dentist.* Should the caller ask to speak to the dentist, your reply is, "Doctor is with a patient. May I help you?" Ascertain the reason for the call. The dentist is always "with a patient" never "busy," even though he may be preparing a case in the laboratory or reading a journal in his private office at that moment. Always secure the name of the caller. If you cannot take care of the business of the caller (and that is rarely the case), ask for his telephone number, note it and his name, and ask if you may have the dentist call back when the dentist is free.

6. *Know to whom you are speaking.* It is important that you know to whom you are speaking before you give any information or answer any questions. It is customary to identify the office and state your name, then ask for identification of your caller unless the person has already given it. Refer to the proper professional call procedures.

7. *What NOT to say.* Do not inadvertently give out information to a caller if that information is not necessary. It is very easy to do. If the dentist, for example, is taking two days away from the office, it is not necessary to tell a patient that the doctor won't be in on the twenty-second or twenty-third, but he can see the patient on the twenty-fourth at three. Say, rather, "The first appointment we have available for you, Mrs. Jones, is Wednesday, the twenty-fourth, at three o'clock in the afternoon."

There is one exception to this procedure, however. If your dentist is attending a convention, a study course, a postgraduate course at a school, or a dental committee meeting, always be sure to state the cause of his absence: "Doctor Smith will be attending a postgraduate course at the University that week, Mrs. Jones. The first appointment available is the following Wednesday, the twenty-fourth, at nine o'clock in the morning." This information indicates to the patient that Doctor Smith is refreshing his education and therefore must be a good dentist.

8. *Fees.* A discussion of fees has no place in a telephone conversation. Should a patient telephone to discuss anything related to a fee or an account, invite him to stop at the office to see you. Make a definite appointment with the patient for this visit—an appointment with you, not the dentist. Inform the dentist of the call when convenient and get the details of the account or charges for use during the appointment.

9. *Confidentiality.* When you telephone a patient about an overdue account or payment or any other strictly personal matter, never give this information to anyone but the patient personally. Other members of the patient's family may be quite insistently curious about the subject of your call. For example, if the patient is a young adult who still lives with parents, brothers, or sisters, it may be difficult

for him to maintain privacy. Your only statement in these circumstances is, "This is Mary at Doctor Smith's office. Will you please ask John to call me as soon as possible?"

10. *Shoppers.* Individuals who call various dental offices to ask what it costs to have a "tooth filled," "a tooth pulled," or "plates made" are called shoppers. Should someone call and ask such a question, respond with the question, "May I ask who is calling please?" A shopper will usually not give his name. If he should, he will also repeat his question. Your answer is, "I'm sorry, Mr. Jones, but Doctor Smith would have to examine your mouth before he could give you an estimate. Would you like an appointment for an examination?"

11. *SOS for dentist.* At times there may be a telephone call which you cannot personally care for nor delay until your dentist is free. Note legibly the name of the caller and the subject of this emergency. Show it to the dentist, preferably so that the patient on whom he is operating is unaware of the process. Your dentist will tell you what he wishes done or will give you an answering note.

12. *Cancellations.* Should a patient call to cancel an appointment, ask if you may make another appointment. The purpose of this approach is to avoid having the patient say that he will call you. Memories can be short—and then you have lost contact with a patient. If the time involved is a matter of weeks or even months before the patient expects to be available for another appointment, ask if you may call at that time. The patient will usually agree to this arrangement. Immediately make a note of the call to be made—in the appointment book, in pencil, on the proper date, or on another calendar of the note type used for this purpose. See that these calls are made promptly.

13. *Expectations.* In order to preserve the value of any set routine in handling telephone calls as well as in-person calls at the office,

it is necessary that your dentist keep you informed of personal calls or visits which he expects. He will indicate his willingness to accept these contacts immediately. If this routine is followed, you will be aware of calls, which some individuals may imply are personal but are really commercial in nature, for which your dentist does not wish to be disturbed.

14. *Keeping the dentist away from the telephone.* The dentist should not come to the telephone except to speak with another professional man regarding professional work.

A patient rarely needs to talk on the telephone with the dentist. You can relay most messages, even in an emergency.

In an emergency you ask about the trouble, getting its location and other pertinent information. If you need advice regarding hot or cold packs, or other relief measures, write the message and hold it up for the dentist to see. Take the answer to the telephone, while the dentist continues working. If the emergency requires an appointment, you can give it, in most instances, without having the dentist come to the telephone.

15. *When to be uninformed.* Often, the patient who has had an examination and is called after X rays have been read may immediately say, "How many cavities do I have?"

To the patient, this means "How much work do I need?"—as a basis for estimating probable costs.

To the dentist, the number of cavities does not indicate the amount of work. A cavity may require a one-surface restoration or it may require a full crown.

One example of effectively meeting the problem is illustrated in this conversation:

Dental Assistant: Doctor has studied your films. You need to have some work done. Would you like to come in the morning or in the afternoon?
Patient: How many cavities do I have?

Dental Assistant: About an hour's time will be required, Mrs. Jones.

Patient: But how many *cavities* are there?

Dental Assistant: Mrs. Jones, I'm not qualified to read these films, but Doctor asked for an hour's time for your work.

There are times when it is wise to be uninformed, and this is one instance.

16. *Keeping your promise.* If you tell a patient that you will perform some service (call him back, etc.), *write yourself a note immediately!* Don't trust your memory. There are too many things to remember. Write notes!

17. *Mind your job.* None of the conversations which you hold with people can be "stiff" if you are to be successful in leading them or in keeping them as patients. All this has to be automatic. You must be on your toes and a jump or two ahead of everyone. Your mind must be on your work in the office.

18. *A habit to avoid.* Answer the telephone as promptly as possible. Remember that it forms one of the main entrances for new patients into your office and should be kept as free as possible for this purpose. Using it for personal calls, while occasionally necessary, is a habit to be avoided.

19. *Retain the initiative.* The ideal in patient control is to retain the initiative, whether on the telephone or in person, without hurting the patient's ego or being discourteous in any way. The easiest way to achieve this end when you are inexperienced is to have a set routine which is used without variation to resist the usual pressures some patients will exert for special consideration. As you gain poise in your office, you may vary the routine to suit the occasion.

Either *you* manage the patients or the patients will all too willingly manage your office.

If you lead, the patients will follow. It must be done lightly. Inject humor occasionally, yet let the patient know that you mean what you say.

For example, a dental assistant was confronted with a longtime patient who always insisted on personally talking with the dentist to make an appointment. In previous conversations, the dental assistant had mentioned that *she* was making all appointments now, so this particular day she avoided mentioning it again.

The dentist happened to be at *his* dentist's office having some necessary work done from noon to one o'clock.

Dental Assistant: No. Dr. Smith is not in. Who is calling, please?

Patient: Do you expect him back today? (*Refusal of patient to give his name*)

Dental Assistant: Yes, I expect him back. May I help you?

Patient: I'll call later. (*Still wants the dentist*)

Dental Assistant: It would be better if he were to call you—otherwise you may call when he is unable to come to the telephone. (*Said with a smile*)

Patient: This is Mr. Appleby. (*Capitulation*)

Dental Assistant: John's father! Oh, yes! May I help you? (*Recognition*)

Patient: Well, I want to see the doctor at five tonight.

Dental Assistant: What seems to be the difficulty? (*What do you want to see him about?*)

Patient: Well, . . . I have a sore spot. (*Reluctant capitulation*)

Dental Assistant: Doctor Smith could see you for your emergency at a quarter of two, Mr. Appleby. That will be so much better than your having to wait around all that time after work. Doctor has a five o'clock patient so he would not be able to see you today after that hour.

Patient: All right, I'll be in at a quarter of two. Thank you very much.

Dental Assistant: Goodbye, Mr. Appleby.

The purpose of the dental assistant's approach was to keep the patient from doing what she did not want done: to overcrowd an already overloaded late afternoon and to prevent the patient from speaking with the dentist. (The dentist might have felt it necessary to say, "Come when you want to.") She saw the opportunity to work in this emergency at a better moment and proceeded to set it up her way instead of allowing the patient to set it up his way.

She did it with lightness in her voice—tricky business to make an "old" patient satisfied with taking orders from the assistant rather than from the dentist.

Had the dentist been in the office, she would still have proceeded as she did—preventing the patient from contacting the dentist directly. What the patient desired—an appointment—is the business of the assistant, not the dentist.

In reviewing this conversation, we see the attempts of the patient to achieve his desire to talk with the dentist, and the assistant's deft sidestepping to avoid an open clash as she frustrates his intent—and satisfies him sufficiently to keep him as a patient.

Assisting New Patients Who Call by Telephone

The assistant should start an Acquaintance Form for the new patient who calls by telephone. Ask the caller's name, home address, home telephone, and the name of the person who referred this individual to your office. Then you ask, "Do you wish an appointment for an examination, Mr. Jones?"

If the caller is having pain, he will so inform you at that time. If such is the case, make whatever arrangements are customary in your office for emergency care, and at that appointment complete arrangements for an examination appointment. If you should ask the caller if he is having any pain, this very frequently serves as a suggestion to that individual to claim discomfort as a means of securing an earlier appointment with your office. If you suggest an appointment for examination and do not mention pain, you will experience less pressure of this sort.

Should your caller indicate that an appointment for examination is the purpose of his call,

ask what day of the week is usually most convenient. Check for a possible appointment time in the appointment book, then say, "Doctor Smith will see you for an examination on .... (day) at .... (hour), or .... (hour). Which time will be more convenient for you?"

There is always the problem of training new patients psychologically to the manner in which you run your dental office. Many individuals are quite accustomed to dictating the time of their appointments, the date, what needs to be done, and how it shall be done. For that reason, if the first date offered the caller is not satisfactory at either hour, offer another date and another choice of two different hours—but no more. It is generally preferable to tell the caller that you will place his name on your "call" list and telephone him as soon as you have a date available. When you do call, a few days or a week later, again offer a choice of two different hours occurring on the preferred day of some week ahead. In this manner you favor developing a relationship in which the patient does not attempt to run your office for you. This applies to new patients in the office or on the telephone.

Appointments for Children

Should you receive a telephone call from a parent desiring an appointment for a child, the responsible person's name should be asked (usually the father's), whose first name, middle initial, and last name should be placed on the Acquaintance Form. The name of the child, date of birth, the child's nickname, and whether or not the child has been to a dentist previously should be ascertained and noted. If the answer to the last question is yes, ask if the child objected to seeing the dentist. Note the reply.

At times, should you merely ask for the name of the child's father, you may receive some objection. Estrangements or divorces do occur. Should you note any resentment at the question, merely indicate that your office wishes to know the name of the person responsible for the child. This is a reasonable request.

Keep the age of the child in mind as you check your appointment book. In accordance with the suggestions given under "New Patients Who Call by Telephone," offer a choice of two appointments. One of the parents should accompany the young child for his examination visit.

Children can be very pleasant to have as patients. Some dentists enjoy working with them, some tolerate them, and some do not care to work with them at all. Discuss this question with your dentist.

Difficult Calls

Callers sometimes present difficulties for the assistant. A patient may request information which you are not at liberty to give, a patient may be upset about a bill, someone may call to inquire about a patient, or a "shopper" may call to quiz you about fees.

It is a good idea to think of as many of these difficult calls as possible and try to have some answer ready in your mind or in a file by the telephone. After you have worked awhile, these calls become much less difficult.

The patient who is easily upset by change in routine may call and be disturbed because you are not the assistant she talked with before. Listen for the name carefully, use it soothingly in speaking with her, and assure her you will see that she has careful attention. She should soon become accustomed to your presence.

A patient may call to shift his appointment. Be sure you make it clear that your dentist sees patients by appointment and give the caller a specific appointment at a time which is open. He should not be allowed to crowd into an already filled day simply because he

has an appointment which he cannot keep. Find another appointment for him.

A patient may call to complain about a bill. Courteously ask the patient to wait. Pull the patient's financial card and clinical record from the file. Return to the telephone and be courteous about the matter.

Sometimes you will receive a call asking about the dentistry performed for one of your patients. Never give information to anyone about a patient. Tell the caller that you will have your dentist return the call.

Outgoing Calls

It is frequently necessary for the assistant to call patients or other dentists. Before you make one of these calls, have at hand all the materials necessary for completing the business of the call. Be certain that you have the correct telephone number. Try to place the call at a time when you anticipate the least amount of interruption within the office. (If you know your dentist is within a minute of needing you, it is *not* a time to place a call.)

If you are calling a patient, a dentist, or a physician with whom your dentist wishes to speak, be sure that your dentist is available before you place the call. If you are calling a patient about an appointment, have the appointment book in front of you. If it is necessary for you to change the appointment, give the patient all the consideration possible. A mother may have already engaged a baby-sitter, or an employed person may have already asked for the time off. An explanation of the reason for the change is courteous.

It may be necessary for you to call a patient with instructions. Be certain that your information is accurate before you make the call.

When you use the telephone to make a series of outgoing calls, for example, when calling to remind patients of the next day's appointments, space them out well. Make one or two calls, then wait ten minutes or so before making the next one or two calls. This procedure allows time for incoming calls to be received. If your office has two or more in-coming telephone lines, this precaution is not necessary.

Be certain to review the discussion of the professional call in this chapter and try to have all your calls conform to this procedure.

Telephone Answering Service

Today dental offices may have some type of telephone answering service which cares for calls during the periods when no one is in the office. The answering service is notified when the receptionist leaves the office. The information to be given to callers is given at that time. It may be the telephone number where the dentist can be reached, or the answering service may be requested to take the name and telephone number of the callers for the receptionist until she can return her calls.

Summary

Friendliness, warmth, and cordiality are necessary attributes in the reception procedures for *all* who contact the office—whether it be by telephone or through the reception room door.

Be prepared for previous patients as they enter the reception room. Greet them as old friends. Strangers must be identified and given attention on the basis of the purpose of their visit. The new patient is given an Acquaintance Form and eventually an appointment. Salesmen receive an appointment. Professional men are either ushered into the dentist's business office or given immediate care in the reception room. Unknown callers are identified or are not permitted to see your dentist.

A reception room for receiving guests rather than a waiting room where nonpersons are allowed to sit until they are called is the important differentiation to be made in your work with patients. Try to maintain the important concept—that you are receiving VIPs. Think and speak of the *reception* room.

If a patient does not enter the dental office through the reception room door, he does so by means of the telephone. The success of the telephone conversation depends on how well the two persons understand each other. Since the only contact is by voice, there is room for misunderstanding which doesn't exist when two people can see each other as they speak.

General technique of telephoning demands the same courtesy and warmth as one would express in a personal contact. Speak directly into the telephone with a normal voice and good diction.

A business call can be divided into four parts: (1) identification of caller and person called, (2) purpose of call, (3) conclusion of business, and (4) termination of call.

Prompt answering, care in writing messages received, ascertaining name and number of the caller—all are important points to remember in using the telephone.

It is important that there be an agreed-upon method of answering the telephone in the dental office. Special care should be exercised when the telephone rings and you are working with a patient in the reception room. Other important ideas to be remembered in working with the telephone are the following:

1. When the dentist is with a patient, refrain from calling him to the telephone.
2. Give only the information necessary to the business of the moment.
3. Do not discuss fees over the telephone.
4. Answer the telephone as promptly as possible.
5. Close every call with a "thank you" in one form or another.

6. Confer with your dentist by note about telephone matters which cannot wait until he is free.
7. Allow time between outgoing calls.

Lead the patients rather than allow them to lead you in matters of appointments and office routines. Emergencies can be handled by relayed messages rather than by interrupting the contact your dentist has with the patient in the chair—a very important person who is paying for that undivided attention from your dentist.

Study Questions
1. Why are reception procedures so very important?
2. Discuss the fundamentals of reception room techniques for the dental assistant.
3. Discuss the variations in reception for (1) previous patients, (2) strangers, (3) unidentified callers, (4) salesmen or detail men, (5) professional men.
4. Discuss the best form for a professional telephone call.
5. Discuss telephone courtesies and routines.
6. What information must you secure in case of an emergency?
7. What routine do you follow when a new patient calls on the telephone?
8. What information do you need when a parent calls for an appointment for his child who is new to your practice?

Bibliography

BERSCHEID, ELLEN, and WALSTER, ELAINE HATFIELD. *Interpersonal Attraction.* Reading, Mass.: Addison-Wesley Co., 1969.

BLASS, J. LEWIS. *Dentistry as Personal Service.* Philadelphia: J. B. Lippincott, 1963.

BREGSTEIN, S. JOSEPH. *Handbook for Dental Assistants, Hygienists, and Secretaries.* Englewood Cliffs, N. J.: Prentice-Hall, 1961.

GERGEN, KENNETH J. *The Psychology of Behavior Exchange.* Reading, Mass.: Addison-Wesley Co., 1969.

LAING, R. D., et al. *Interpersonal Perception: A Theory and a Method of Research.* London: Tavistock Publications, 1966.

Pamphlets Which Can Be Ordered

How to Win Friends by Phone. Northwestern Bell Telephone Co. Call the telephone company and ask for it.

What Every Telephone User Should Know. General Telephone System, publisher. Call or write business office for a free copy.

PART TWO | ADMINISTRATION OF THE BUSINESS OF DENTISTRY

The administration of the dental office—with all its minute details—is the job of the dental assistant, the office receptionist, or the office administrator or manager, depending upon the size of the staff. The dentist should be kept busy producing dentistry. He has given some six or more years of his life in attending college before he ever practices dentistry. He continues to study his profession as long as he is an active dentist. Since no one else in the office possesses his skill, it is the staff's responsibility to see that he spends his time doing what no one else in the office can do—namely, practice dentistry. All jobs which can be done by someone else should be done by someone else. In addition, in an office in which there is an oral health care delivery team, each member is skilled in a specific area of service and should perform that service.

The responsibilities of the office administrator are:

(a) to keep the dentist producing dentistry, that is, to keep his time properly organized,

(b) to keep other members of the oral health care delivery team optimally performing their skills,

(c) to keep proper records so that the dentist is protected professionally and financially, and

(d) to organize all other details so that the office functions smoothly.

5 | *Administrative Planning*

A Dental Office Administrator

Whenever two or more people work together, some form of cooperation and communication is necessary. If these two or more people are working together to provide a service to others, the cooperation must be organized and administered to avoid confusion and to encourage efficiency.

As dental offices increase in size, and as dentistry becomes the oral health care delivery team operation, the coordination of the services provided must be accomplished without making it necessary for the dentist to devote his precious time to administrative duties instead of professional skills.

Result: A dentist may hire an office administrator or coordinator—or assign the administrative duties to some staff member. Depending on the delegation made by the dentist, this staff member will perform (or assign to other employees to perform) certain duties.

The delegation of these tasks should result in at least three advantages:

1. More efficient dental service to patients.
2. Less mental, emotional, and physical strain for all members of the oral health care delivery team.
3. Lowered operating costs.

Although a dental office administrator will have little opportunity to plan the office layout, his ability to recognize efficient work patterns and good office floor plans can be helpful. Thoughtful evaluation of traffic patterns and office arrangements can often indicate some slight shift which will produce a far more efficient use of space, equipment, or time. While it is not the business of the employee to institute such changes, he can tactfully present his ideas to the dentist who can decide whether or not the suggested changes appeal to him.

The purpose of having an office administrator (no matter by what title that position is designated) is to increase the efficiency of the entire staff, permitting more pleasant relationships to be maintained while promoting more efficient dentistry. The administrator will attempt to gain an overview perspective of this particular dental practice as outlined by the dentist-employer. It is her/his duty to continually appraise the office routines in an effort to maintain the highest quality service to patients.

Visualization of the office organization through the use of the diagram in figure 5.1 may be helpful. The relationships between staff members can be understood. This diagram does not necessarily apply to all dental offices. It is important that the dentist give careful thought to his needs and develop his own plan of organization.

Coordinating the Office Staff

Perhaps one of the most difficult problems in a large office—or even in an office with only two employees—is to coordinate the work of the staff members in order to avoid over-

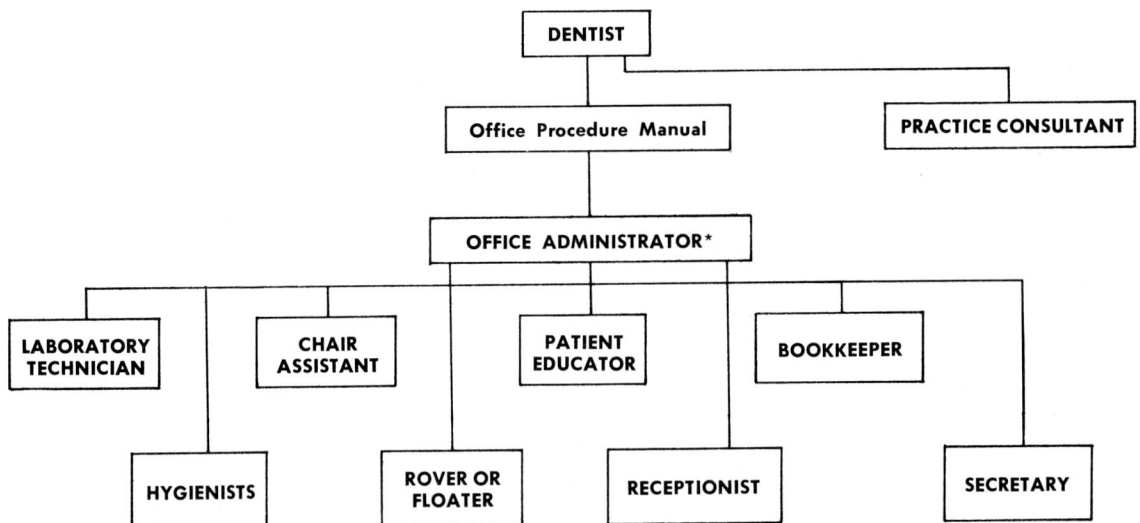

*However the dentist wishes to designate this function. The employee may perform only administrative tasks or may have another responsibility, such as reception or bookkeeping. The concept is that some form of administration must occur if the dentist is to spend his time practicing his profession.

Fig. 5.1. Functions in the dental office organization

lapping of duties. The dentist should be given the assistance he needs when he needs it by the one person appointed to give this specific assistance. Two employees should never be standing around, each waiting for the other to give the necessary assistance. It is important that each employee *know* what is expected of her/him and when.

The ideal is to have the coordination of the staff explicitly stated in a procedure manual. However, even when the duties are carefully written in a procedure manual, a certain amount of attention must be given to the staff to see that the directions as set forth in the manual are kept in operation in the office. *Writing something on paper doesn't necessarily make it happen in working relationships between people.*

The employee who is assigned to coordinate the efforts of the oral health care delivery team must have a sense of timing which allows her/him to manage intuitively to keep the traffic flowing. This type of intuition is developed with practice, alert observation, and notation of details such as the amount of time:

1. the dentist uses for specific preparations,
2. the chair assistant takes to prepare the operatory,
3. the hygienist spends with a four-year-old patient, and
4. the laboratory technician needs to complete certain operations.

A knowledge of traffic-flow studies is helpful. In such studies, the observer uses a floor plan of the area and draws the walking pattern of the individual(s) involved. A study of this pattern may lead to improved ways of performing specific tasks. Perhaps steps can be eliminated by rearranging materials or equipment.

The goal of the well-coordinated office is to keep the dentist occupied in providing care for patients which no one else can provide. The employees perform all other tasks.

Some of the employees may perform specific services which no one else on the staff can provide. The employee may be certified in a specific area of oral health care. No matter what the job differences are, the central idea is that each team member performs the tasks for which he is trained and any other tasks which are assigned him in the overall plan as visualized by the dentist. The duty of the coordinator or administrator is to utilize this previously-agreed-upon plan.

Procedure Manual

A manual of office procedures is important *regardless of the size of the office staff.* It is most helpful in acquainting a new employee with the office routines. It is also helpful in that each member of the staff knows what is expected of him because it is carefully written in the procedure manual. If the office in which you work does not have such a manual, you would be wise to convince your dentist that he should permit you to make one. Each duty of every assistant should be listed, and detailed instructions should be given about the dentist's preferences in the way certain routines are performed.

Part one of the manual should contain statements about the following:

1. Salary.
2. Working hours for each employee, including exact working hours, an indication if an employee is expected to remain in the office as long as the dentist is there. (If this qualification is listed, arrangements for some time off or added income can be stated, too. In some instances a dedicated employee accepts the fact that her hours are those of her dentist and expects nothing in return. In such a case

the dentist is usually wise enough to see that her annual pay is commensurate with her services.)

3. Coffee-break periods.
4. Lunch-hour regulations.
5. Vacation policy. If there is accrual vacation time for length of employment, this should be stated.
6. Sick leave and absenteeism, with or without pay.
7. Fringe benefits.
8. Grooming of the staff members.
9. Uniforms—whether uniforms are to be worn, who furnishes the uniforms, who cares for the laundry.
10. Use of the telephone for personal calls. Calls may be limited to before and after office hours, or there may be a specific statement that *no* personal calls are to be made or accepted except in case of an extreme emergency. It is possible to make your personal telephone calls on coffee break at a nearby public telephone so that the office telephone is available for the office business, including emergencies which, of necessity, form a part of every day in a dental practice.

Part two of the manual should list the duties of each employee in the office, including the following:

1. Dusting and tidying the office, assigned by *area*. The receptionist in a large office may have the responsibility for the care of the reception rooms; a chair assistant may have the responsibility for the operatories; the laboratory technicians may be responsible for the laboratory, and so on.
2. The assignment of the care of telephone calls with phrases listed for the more common telephone conversations.
3. The assignment of the appointment book which ideally should be controlled by only one person.

4. Laundry records, sorting and verification of laundry.
5. Autoclaving and related duties.
6. Inventory and ordering of supplies, both dental and business.

The Staff Conference

Plans of operation are just that—plans. The successful administration of a plan necessitates action. In the dental office, cooperative action is necessary. One of the most efficient methods of assuring the success of an action plan by a group is to set aside a time when the team members can confer about the problems which arise—about irritations as well as pleasant experiences. A regularly scheduled meeting of the staff can become one of discussing mutual problems and of making suggestions to improve the efficiency of the entire staff.

The decision to conduct staff conferences is the responsibility of the dentist. He should be given every opportunity to discover that his working conditions are more satisfying when his team can meet to successfully coordinate their efforts.

The meeting should be *scheduled at a regular time each week.* It is not to be treated casually nor held when some patient cancels an appointment. This meeting can become the key to successful team cooperation and should be treated as one of the most important occurrences during *each* week.

Each staff member should make notes during the week of the subjects he/she wishes to discuss. In a normal office relationship, frictions often occur. Each member of the team is better prepared to handle his irritations in a mature way if he knows there is a time when this closely interdependent team can sit down and discuss how they can work together more effectively.

The dentist should also be prepared to make his comments. Comments should not make one poor staff member uncomfortable and "at fault" for a problem. Comments might be, "The cooperation of the entire staff was excellent on Wednesday when we inserted Mr. Jones's immediate denture. Everyone was alert and did an excellent job"; or "The schedule was really fouled up Wednesday. What happened? Can we avoid it another time?"

This allows for an evaluation of the activities on Wednesday without making poor Suzy the brunt of the criticism even though it was caused by careless appointing on her part. She will perceive the problem.

In addition to a time to air one's feelings and improve working relations, the staff conference is a time for the dentist to teach his staff whatever he feels they need to know. It may be a talk for five to ten minutes on his philosophy of preventive dentistry. It may be that a new product has been introduced which he feels his staff should understand. He can talk about it, or have a detail man do so. Perhaps he has information from a dental consulting firm which he wishes all staff members to understand.

Perhaps he will want his staff to know more about the psychology of working with patients and will spend some time for a few weeks giving them thimblefuls of practical psychology. There is a great deal of merit in being prepared, through better understanding, to handle the emotional problems you must face when working with the public.

To use some staff conference time to further this kind of understanding is a wise investment for any dentist or oral health care delivery team.

Sources of Information

No one can know everything it may be necessary to know in any career you may care to mention. One of the marks of being an edu-

cated person is to know where to find information which you do not have.

In the dental office there are books which will prove invaluable in looking up some item. There are periodicals which will be delivered to the office. The *Journal of the American Dental Association* is one; *The Dental Assistant*, the journal of the American Dental Assistants Association, may be another. In addition, many of the pharmaceutical houses send out bulletins and pamphlets which are helpful. "Throw away" magazines about dentistry will be delivered free in the mail, and your dentist may subscribe to others.

A dictionary is one of the most valuable aids—to know a thing is the ability to describe and understand it. If one can define a term, he usually has insight into its full meaning.

There are specialized dictionaries and terminology books which are valuable and ought to be found in your office library. Use them frequently. One which is most pertinent to dentistry is Boucher's *Clinical Dental Terminology*. Blakiston's *New Gould Medical Dictionary* and Dorland's *Medical Dictionary* are also helpful.

If you are uncertain whether some piece of information is available, consult the local county dental society or their library.

Succeeding as an Administrator of the Dental Office

An office administrator maintains a perspective of the entire office operation, attempts to provide an equitable division of labor, and facilitates the team operation. How? The personnel functions diagram (fig. 5.1), the procedure manual, and the staff conference are three tools to which can be added certain organizational procedures for the business office which are discussed in the succeeding chapters of this section of the text. Careful organization and supervision of these details will permit the office administrator to concentrate her/his attention on people and problem situations.

The operation of a well-organized, pleasant office cannot be left to chance. It must have constant attention. An open-minded attitude, a willingness to challenge the present system, and an attempt to try out new ideas to develop better ways of doing the "dailies" are very important to successful administration.

Keep a list of your problems. Keep it current. Add to it. Keep it in your desk drawer, but take it out frequently and look at it. Then rank the problems in order of importance. Try to do first things first.

First, ask yourself which problem causes the greatest difficulty to you, to your dentist, or to the patients who come to your office. This is the problem to attack first.

Second, ask yourself, "How severe is this problem? Is it worthy of the time it will take to solve it?" To answer your question, you might try to count the number of times this irritating situation recurs in a day, a week, or a month. Walk through the routine if necessary. (Suppose it is the interference of two assistants when one is trying to remove materials from the file and the other must move past her to another part of the office.) List the number of times the problem occurs in a specified length of time.

Third, ask yourself how soon the problem must be solved. If it is a serious matter which requires immediate attention, it must receive priority in the thinking process which occurs in problem-solving.

Fourth, if some problems can be solved, which problem, if eliminated, will give the greatest benefits to the dentist, the patient, and you? This is the process we can call investigation of the problem; that is, selection, or recognition of which problem to attempt to solve. Now that you have decided on one problem to solve first, examine this problem.

Keep a record about this activity which is causing problems. A chart which lists the activity in question and has columns for listing the time, the distance involved, and any other notes needed will help clarify the situation. A diagram showing the floor area and the traffic pattern is also helpful. Make the diagram after watching the interference for a period of time.

Next, ask questions to try to discover an alternative method of accomplishing the task. Ask *what, why, where, when, who,* and *how.* If a file is the object of interference because the assistant who is filing is in the way of those who must pass back and forth to assist the dentist, or if patients must pass by her to get to the operatory, a listing of the number of interruptions of her work per hour—of the number of times she must push in the file drawer, straighten up, and lean against the file—should be made. The office should be reexamined critically and creatively. There may be another location for the file which would eliminate the crowding of the passageway. Lacking this, perhaps the filing could be done prior to the patients' arrivals and after their departures.

Through the creative process, the members of the office staff can take the problem as outlined on paper and find some better methods of meeting the situation. One of the most important things to remember in any administrative work is to keep asking questions about the present routines. Usually there is room for improvement no matter how effective the past thinking has been.

Suppose you have now arrived at a solution to the problem. The next step is to sell your idea to your dentist. He must be agreeable to the change.

Some methods of approach work better than others. *Timing* is exceedingly important. When your dentist is tired, hungry, or frustrated is no time to ask for a change. If he is having difficulty with the problem you are concerned about, perhaps this is the moment to suggest a change. If he must wait by the file until the file clerk has placed a handful of papers in the drawer in order to avoid spilling them on the floor, and then closed the drawer, this is a good time to suggest that perhaps a new place could be found for the file. Stress those ideas which will interest him . . . those solutions which will appeal to him. Be enthusiastic, but don't push. Let him sell himself. Use a question approach—ask him, don't tell him. When he accepts the idea, you can establish a timetable to get the approval of others for your idea.

Improvement cannot be left to chance. Constant attention must be given to the office problems. There must be open-minded attitudes to challenge the status quo if new ideas are to be developed. Remember that the greatest strides have come from creative thinking about a problem—sometimes brought on by necessity. New methods of teaching foreign languages were developed during World War II when it was discovered that there wasn't time to spend two or three years in developing mastery of a language. New ideas can be developed and used if people are open-minded and willing to experiment.

Orderly Office Routines

There are routines which, when regularly performed in a dental office, allow the office staff the pleasure of working without the frustration caused when certain duties are overlooked. The patients and the dentist are directly as well as indirectly benefited when these details are performed regularly as an orderly routine.

Posting the Day's Work Schedule

The day's work schedule is a list of the patients who are coming to the office, the time of their appointments, and the service for which you must be prepared for each patient.

After all appointments are verified and any cancelled appointment time is filled, type the day's schedule on four-by-six-inch paper, using carbon to make as many additional copies as you need. List the time of appointment, name of patient, and the work planned for each (fig. 5.2). One copy is for the private office, one for each operatory—in a place not visible to patients—and one for the laboratory. Commercially prepared forms are also available for this purpose (fig. 5.3).

8:30 John Doe	insert immed. dent.
9:30 Flo Smith	set crown
10:15 Jean Brown	inlay preps

Fig. 5.2. Method of listing the day's work schedule

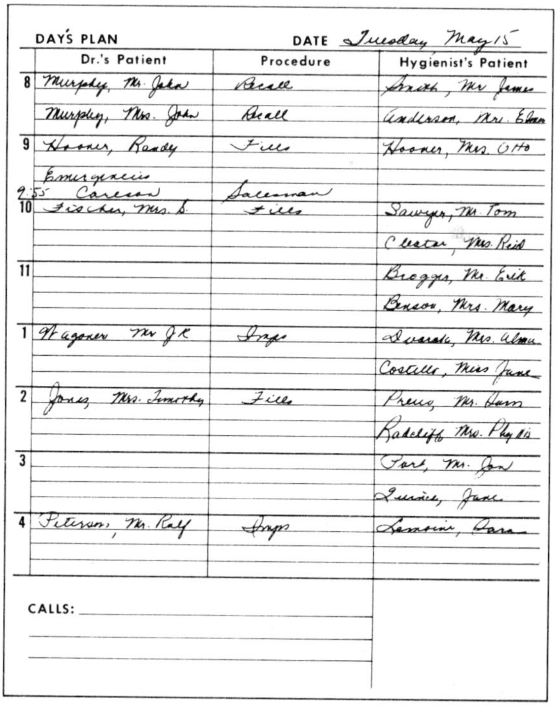

Courtesy Spillane's, Inc., Minneapolis

Fig. 5.3. A commercially available form for posting the day's work schedule.

Folders or records for the next day's patients are placed together in the proper operatories. Blank record cards and folders clipped to the Acquaintance Forms for new patients are also placed in the operatories. These forms were either filled out by the patients when they came to the office to arrange their first appointments or were begun by the assistant who received their calls on the telephone.

If we were to type up a day's work schedule for the Tuesday, March 18, appointment book sample we have worked out in chapter six, our four-by-six-inch paper would include the following information:

SCHEDULE, Tuesday, March 18

8:00	Murphy, Mr. John, Recall
8:30	Murphy, Mrs. John, Recall
9:00	Hoover, Randy, Fills
9:30	Emergency break
9:55	Carlson, S. J.—Salesman
10:00	Fischer, Mrs. S. T., Operative
12:00	Lunch
1:00	Wagoner, Mr. J. R., Impressions
2:00	Jones, Mrs. Timothy, Operative
4:00	Peterson, Mr. Rolf, Recall
4:30	Smith, Miss Mary, Impressions
5:30	

Remember that proper management of dental chair time is an art in itself. It means much in producing dental work efficiently. Try to become expert in managing this aspect of dental office routine.

Laboratory Schedule

The work performed in the laboratory can be roughly divided into *two general classifications*: (1) cases which are carried to completion entirely within the dental office and (2) those which are forwarded to a professional dental laboratory for all or part of the processing. Depending upon the individual dental office, varying degrees of preparation will be involved in cases which are forwarded to the professional dental laboratory. Some dental offices may perform very few of the laboratory procedures for any cases; others may perform all procedures for their requirements.

A laboratory schedule for all cases, whether accomplished in the dental office laboratory or the professional dental laboratory, should be maintained properly and should be posted in the laboratory. This schedule should include the name of the patient, the type of case to be completed for that patient, and the date the case must be finished. If more than one professional laboratory is used, the name of the one which has each particular case should be indicated. As cases are completed, they are removed from the laboratory schedule. As new cases are started, they are added to the schedule.

Verification of Information

Form the habit of casually verifying the home address, work address, and telephone numbers when the patient comes in for his regular recalls. If there have been changes, the corrections on the record card and envelope should be made immediately. A recommended procedure is to keep a record of the old address on note paper placed in the record envelope. When this procedure is followed, it is wise to date each note completely so that the chronology of addresses is not lost. Any note or information made on a separate piece of paper should be dated with the month, day, and *year*. Once the habit is acquired, you will find it most convenient to have dated notes.

It is very reassuring to be able to look at your own writing and know that Mrs. Brown moved on January 10, 1970, to 124 South Elm Street or that it was on Tuesday, February 9, 1971, that the laboratory called to ask about a particular bridge and told you it would be delivered on Friday, the 12th. You won't have to guess about the day of the call nor the date of delivery.

Thank-you Notes

A thank-you note sent to all individuals who have referred patients to your dentist is a gracious gesture. Preferably, these notes should be written by hand if the job is delegated to you; however, many dentists prefer to write these notes themselves. The assistant should not sign the dentist's name to such a note whether a printed form or a handwritten note is used.

Current Invoices

It is a convenience to have a file folder labeled "Current Invoices" in your subject file. All invoices received may be kept in this folder until the monthly statements arrive. This procedure will prevent the misplacement or loss of any invoices before the arrival of the monthly statements.

Come-up Card Files

A Come-up card file, or reminder file, is merely an easy method for controlling duties which would otherwise be overlooked or would require more cumbersome reminder methods. The basic idea has been used in business for many years for exactly this type of control of details and is admirably suited in several ways for application to the dental office. This method of control can be applied to equipment maintenance, general office tasks, recall control, and birthday card lists and can serve as a reminder method for any detail which is to receive future attention. For its successful operation there is but one requirement: *the file must be checked each day.* Variations in the manner of setting up the reminder cards are numerous, but the cards used for any one type of reminder—for example, the recall control—should be of the same color and same layout form.

The Come-up card file is best used in a file drawer at the desk or in a drawer converted to operate as a file drawer in the desk. For general use in the dental office, four-by-six-inch cards are perhaps the best size to use for all purposes, although three-by-five-inch cards are satisfactory. The size must be the same for the entire file. A different color is used for each classification of detail: one color indicates equipment maintenance and general office tasks; another color indicates recall control cards; a third, birthday card reminders; and other colors are used for other classifications.

Patient Recall Control

If the dental office in which you work does not enter recall appointments directly in the appointment book, this type of control is necessary and desirable. On or before a patient's last appointment for work he needed as a new patient, the dentist or the assistant will explain the desirability of regular examination and prophylaxis visits. At this time good intentions are highest in the patient's mind. He is determined that never again will he so neglect himself that he has any serious amount of dental work to be done. Therefore, *now* is the time to obtain a definite commitment, phrasing your question exactly: "Mr. Jones, if you wish, we will be happy to place you on our recall list and send you an appointment in six months. Would you like us to do that for you?" The patient who will answer negatively at that particular time is very unusual.

When a patient gives his consent to the recall arrangement, check with him immediately, if you do not already know, to discover the day of the week and time of day which are usually most convenient for him to come to your office. This is noted in pencil on his recall control card (4″ x 6″). Place a check beside the address to which his notice should be sent—the business address or the home address. The re-

Jones, Mr. John J.	*645 Elm St.*	*332-7070*
Name	Home Address	Home Phone
May 23, 1920	*204 Main St.*	*822-4114*
Birthdate	Business Address	Business Phone
Recall due:	*6 Mos.*	
Preferred time:	*Mondays, early afternoon*	
Due for recall:		
May 1972 ✓ 27		
Nov 1972		

Fig. 5.4. A recall control card. Entries are written in pencil to facilitate easy change.

call control card is made out as shown in figure 5.4.

Note in pencil the month and year in which he is due to be recalled. The recall control card is then filed in the Come-up card file behind the appropriate monthly index tab. Recall control cards should be filed in the Come-up card file behind the monthly card index *one month before* the month noted for the recall. This is done to allow for the lapse of time necessary to place an appointment in the appointment book and for mailing the recall notice to the patient two weeks before the appointment date. Therefore, in the sample shown, the recall control card would be filed behind the *April* index tab.

When the first of April arrives, all cards behind the April index tab are removed. Our sample recall control card will be in this group. This patient is then dated in the appointment book for his recall during the month of May, accommodating his preference for day of the week and time of the day as nearly as possible. Since you will be arranging *all* the May recalls at this time, it is possible to control their appointments throughout the month to balance the workload as you desire.

The patient's recall control card is then marked with the actual date of the appointment, in pencil, following the previous indication of month and year already written on the card. The recall notice, which is to be sent to the patient two weeks before the appointment, is made out at the same time and checked twice against the appointment book entry for accuracy. The recall notice is placed in its envelope, addressed as indicated on the recall control card, and the *date of mailing* is written in pencil in the upper-right-hand corner of the envelope, where it will be covered by the stamp when the card is mailed (two weeks before the actual appointment date).

The recall control card for this patient is then filed behind the *May* index tab, and when May 1 arrives, the card is placed behind the correct *date* tab. When the patient records are pulled for the day on which this recall comes, the recall control card is clipped to the patient's record and, after the examination and prophylaxis are completed, the dentist will indicate the month and year when the patient should again be recalled, if not according to the interval noted on the recall control card. The month and year are written in pencil below the former entry. Since our sample patient was recalled in May, 1972, and is to be in at six-month intervals, the next penciled date is November, 1972. The recall card is then filed behind the *October* index tab in the Come-up file.

The patient was asked about participating in the recall system by a carefully phrased question, "Mr. Jones, if you wish, we will be happy to place you on our recall list and send you an appointment in six months. Would you like us do that for you?"

The psychology behind the wording is obvious in the phrasing of the recall notice which is mailed to him. (See fig. 5.5.)

The patient will remember, as he reads the recall notice, that he *did* ask for it voluntarily.

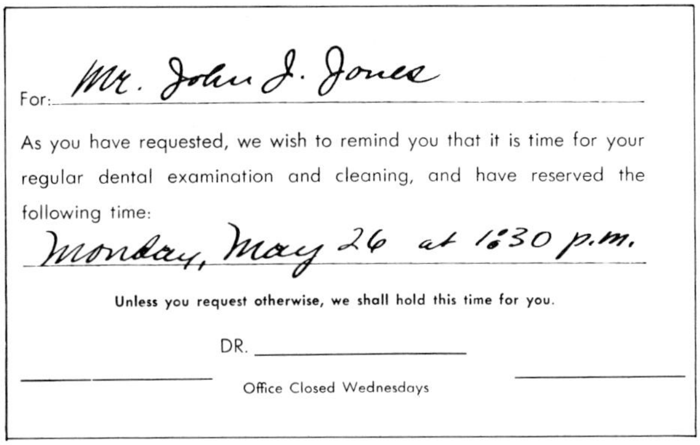

For: *Mr. John J. Jones*

As you have requested, we wish to remind you that it is time for your regular dental examination and cleaning, and have reserved the following time:

Monday, May 26 at 1:30 p.m.

Unless you request otherwise, we shall hold this time for you.

DR. _____

_____   Office Closed Wednesdays   _____

Fig. 5.5. The recall card as sent to the patient. This particular phrasing is used only if the patient has been asked at the time of his last previous visit whether or not he would like to be placed on the special recall list and has indicated that he would like to be notified. The details, such as giving a definite appointment time, are explained to him at the time he first indicates his desire to be notified.

The sense of pressure from the dental office is eliminated, while the tendency to keep the appointment, since it is by his request, is increased. The patient may call to change the time or date of the appointment, but very few will not be in your office for a recall. The average patient will require little or no dental work at this time. A comparison should be made between the amount of work necessary on his first contact with the office and the amount necessary now. The case of maintaining oral health by regular recall will please the patient, and his acceptance of regular dental care will be established.

The dental office which employs a dental hygienist can maintain a separate recall control file under the care of the hygienist.

The profession of dentistry performs a service to the patient in restoring the mouth to good health and in teaching good oral habits and care. Dentists should assume a moral responsibility for the regular care of their patients by making it possible for them to have recall appointments promptly and as frequently as necessary.

Office Task Control Cards

This classification of cards to be used in the Come-up file should be a different color from those used for the patient recall control cards. The average dental office will require but one color for one copy of this classification. In the large office or clinic type of practice which has an employee in charge of general office duties, it is more convenient to have each card of this classification in duplicate, preferably in two colors (neither color the same as used in any other classification, however). These cards list the regular recurring duties of maintenance of equipment and periodic work such as changing X-ray solutions, cleaning sterilizers, cleaning and waxing equipment, and cleaning surgical cabinet and instruments, laboratory cabinets, and storage shelves. The cards as used in the multiple office should be numbered to facilitate handling and matching the original with the duplicate card. The supervisor can give the original card to the assistant delegated to take care of the particular task and can leave the duplicate out of the file, on her desk, as a reminder that this task has been assigned for accomplishment. When the task has been completed, the assistant gives the original card to the supervisor, who returns original and duplicate cards to the Come-up file under the proper index card for the next date on which that task will be performed again. (See fig. 5.6.)

The office task control cards may be typed or printed in the following form: at the extreme top left, the frequency of the task, such as daily, weekly, semimonthly, monthly, six weeks, bimonthly, quarterly, semiannually, or annually; at the extreme top right, the name of the item to be serviced, such as dental unit, X-ray tank, or laboratory; and at the top center, the day for which the job is scheduled.

```
QUARTERLY          First Friday of March,      DENTAL UNIT
                   June, September and
                   December.




Remove and clean water supply screen.
```

Fig. 5.6. An office task control card

Working out the proper arrangement to balance the workload throughout the year is a very important feature—and not too difficult to accomplish.

In any dental office there are so many duties to be performed that it is imperative to arrange recurring office tasks so they may be accomplished as required without overloading any one period of time. Because of incompetent work schedules, some dental offices neglect the majority of these tasks which would increase the efficiency and smoothness of operation. For example, examine the card in figure 5.6. Failure to perform this simple task on a quarterly basis results in an accumulation of gravel particles and other foreign material from the main water-supply pipe, which gradually chokes off the water supply to the unit. The lower the volume of water supplied through this screen, the poorer is the operation of the saliva ejector, the water syringe, and the amount of water available for the cuspidor. When you have learned to do the job, however, it takes but a minute or two to accomplish. The screen may be difficult to remove the first time because it may not have been removed for many months, or even years.

All daily tasks should be typed on four-by-six-inch cards and kept behind the *Daily* tab in the Come-up file. This procedure relieves the assistant of memorizing daily routine jobs and leaves her mind free for other tasks.

When all cards for the Office Task classification are made out, sort them according to the upper-left-hand notation, the frequency of the operation.

DAILY TASKS   Cards for these duties are filed under the *Daily* guide card for daily checking. An alternate method of handling daily tasks, which may be preferred in the smaller dental office, is discussed on pages 87-88.

WEEKLY AND BIWEEKLY TASKS   These cards are filed according to the *date* the work is to be performed. Assume that a job is scheduled for Tuesday of each week. The calendar is referred to for the date of the next Tuesday. This card is then filed behind the guide card of that particular date, in the 1 to 31 section of the Come-up file. When the work has been completed, the card is filed under the date of the next Tuesday. If the first Tuesday was the seventh, the job is completed on that date and the card is refiled under 14, the date of the next Tuesday.

MONTHLY, BIMONTHLY, QUARTERLY, SEMI-ANNUAL, AND ANNUAL TASKS   These cards are filed behind the monthly guide cards of the particular month in which the work is to be done. On the twenty-seventh day of each month, the cards filed under the following month are removed from the monthly section and refiled behind the 1 to 31 guide cards, under the particular date shown by the calendar for the day given in the upper center of the card. When the job specified on the card has been completed, the card is filed behind the next appropriate monthly guide card. Thus, the sample card shown in figure 5.6 would be filed under March. On February 27, it is removed, along with the other March cards, and this particular card is placed in the 1 to 31 file behind the date of the first Friday in March. If that should be March 3, you file it behind 3. On March 3, the card will be removed and the job accomplished. The card will then be filed in the monthly file behind June, the next month this task is to be performed.

ALTERNATE METHODS FOR DAILY TASKS

Tasks to be performed on a daily basis may be listed on a stiff-backed paper and either posted in the laboratory or kept in the desk for ready reference. If the list is posted in the laboratory, it may be protected with a transparent plastic or Celluloid cover.

The following are lists of daily tasks described in this textbook. The dental assistant may use these lists as guides to make up a copy which will apply to the office in which she is employed. Add items necessary in your office.

DAILY TASKS UPON OPENING THE OFFICE

1. Thoroughly air the office.
2. Turn on all necessary switches to place equipment in readiness.
3. Run sterilizer if necessary.
4. Have instruments replaced correctly or have trays ready for use.
5. Dust office thoroughly.
6. Check waiting room and its magazines.
7. Check entire office for proper lighting.
8. Patient records should be placed in the proper operating rooms.
9. Lists of day's patients should be in operating rooms, private office, and laboratory.
10. See that dental chairs are clean.
11. Wipe with a damp cheesecloth pad all enameled surfaces of equipment. Do not forget X-ray arm.
12. Wipe off all dental unit glassware (cuspidor, tumblers, spray bottles). Use a nonabrasive cleanser if necessary. Refill necessary containers with fresh water.
13. Very carefully wipe engine arm of dental unit, if present on unit, to remove accumulated dust. Check all the way up from engine pulley to handpiece pulley.
14. Use cotton saturated with chloroform to clean dental unit gas burner cup of wax drippings.
15. Check medicine bottles in cabinets for a workable daily supply in each bottle.
16. Check the Come-up file for today. Lay out office task cards.

DAILY TASKS TO BE PERFORMED DURING THE DAY

1. Polish outside of sterilizers with soft cloth or chamois. Wash with soap and water or use a nonabrasive cleanser, when necessary.
2. Check operation of sterilizers. Solution levels should be checked several times daily.
3. Weigh and load silver-filing capsules whenever necessary, if used.
4. Take care of the jobs for the day as indicated by the Come-up file. This includes recall notices, birthday cards to be sent, and office tasks to be accomplished.
5. Call patients scheduled for the next workday to remind them of their appointments. Space out calls so that the office telephone line is not monopolized.
6. Keep as current as possible on the required bookkeeping entries.

DAILY TASKS UPON COMPLETION OF APPOINTMENTS FOR THE DAY

1. Call any patients not already reached to verify the next workday's appointments.
2. After all appointments for the next workday have been verified, type the required number of copies on four-by-six-inch

paper, listing time of appointment, patient's name, and the work scheduled for that patient. (See fig. 5.2.)

3. If necessary, sterilize any instruments needed for the first patient in the morning. Set up required trays of instruments.

4. Flush a glass of slightly soapy water through the cuspidor hose and/or through hose of the low-pressure evacuator.

5. Relieve tightness of belt on dental engine arm, if present.

6. Clean up after last patient.

7. Run chairs all the way up, if motor-driven. Pump up once a week for proper lubrication if foot-pump style.

8. Turn off all switches.

9. Close windows.

10. Leave radiators turned on in cold weather, if required.

11. Put all records out of sight, filing in the proper section of the files those not needed for the next workday—after all bookkeeping is completed for which they may be required.

12. Refile the Come-up cards under their proper dates if you have not already done so.

13. Double-check to see that all sterilizers, units, lights, and water valves are off and that no X rays are left in the washing tank.

14. Take all outgoing mail.

15. Be certain that the files are locked, if supplied with locks.

16. Be certain that the office door is locked when you have closed it.

Recall and Birthday Card Control

In any office which cares for children, the benefits derived from sending birthday cards to children through the age of ten are often surprising. Children have such little personal mail that the birthday card from someone outside the immediate family carries a tremendous psychological impact. Children have

been known to take their dentist's birthday card on a tour of their neighborhood to be displayed in proud fashion. Young families have been most grateful for the personal touch of a card for a youngster who happened to be ill on his birthday. When cards are purchased by the box, sending them is not an expensive item for the promotion of goodwill. The type of birthday card which displays the age is preferred because it adds another personal recognition of this individual child, and he can identify himself with the card even more completely.

This classification, again, should have a different color from any other used in the Come-up file. Whenever a new child under the age of nine years is registered with the office— that is, through the age of eight so that he will receive at least two cards from the office—a birthday control card is made up for him. The letter *B* is placed in the lower-left-hand corner of his personal record envelope to indicate that a birthday control card has been made out. The form followed for this classification is shown in figure 5.7.

When the birthday card is prepared for mailing, the year and age are indicated on the con-

Jones, Kay	June 5, 1966
Name	Birthdate
146 Any Street Anytown, Anystate	
Address	*55506*

Cards sent:

Year	Age	Year	Age
1969 ✓	3	1972 ✓	6
1970 ✓	4	1973	
1971 ✓	5	1974	

Fig. 5.7. A birthday control card

trol card as an indication that the card has been prepared for mailing.

As with the recall control cards, it is preferable to file these control cards under the month previous to the birthday to insure mailing the cards in sufficient time to arrive before or on the birthday—*never late*. The birthday control card can be ignored each month until about the twentieth if the dental assistant will keep a reminder card under the date "20" in the 1 to 31 guides. This card should state that the birthday cards for the next month should be prepared at that time for mailing. The dentist can then sign the entire month's birthday cards in one group. The assistant places them in their envelopes and marks the mailing date for each card in pencil in the upper-right-hand corner of the envelope where the postage stamp will cover it.

The recall control cards may be handled in one group in a manner similar to that suggested for the birthday control cards. It is necessary, however, that the reminder card for the recall classification be kept under 15 in the 1 to 31 guide in order to complete and have ready for mailing those recalls which may be dated for the first of the following month, since the notice must be mailed two weeks prior to the appointment.

Recall notices and birthday cards prepared in advance for mailing later may either be placed behind the proper date in the 1 to 31 guides or, if too bulky, may be arranged in mailing sequence and kept in a separate desk drawer. In this event the assistant must be certain that the cards are mailed as intended on the proper dates.

Summary

The coordination of the efforts of the oral health care delivery team is extremely important and can be accomplished best by the appointment of an office administrator.

The first goal of the well-coordinated office is to keep the dentist occupied in using his unique professional skills which only he can perform. The second goal is to so delegate duties that the other members of the oral health care delivery team provide services for which they have been uniquely trained. Each team member ought to be enabled to accomplish his responsibilities in dental care, and all team members should relate to each other in the total office production schedule.

The delegation of tasks should result in three advantages:

1. More efficient dental service to patients.
2. Less mental, emotional, and physical strain for members of the oral health care delivery team.
3. Lowered operating costs.

The office administrator is charged with the responsibility of administering a plan which will accomplish these goals. An office procedure manual which acquaints new staff members with office routines is one useful tool. The manual should list each duty of every staff member and certain statements about working conditions, fringe benefits, and salary.

A regularly scheduled staff conference allows the office team to become an efficient, harmonious unit and permits instruction of the staff about new materials or team operations.

Every dental assistant should be aware of sources of information such as clinical dental terminologies, periodicals, reference manuals, medical dictionaries, and texts.

A dental office administrator can succeed by being constantly alert for problems. Such problems can be listed and considered for solution. There are four questions which the administrator can ask in determining which problem to attempt to solve. Timing is important in presenting the suggested solution to the dentist.

Maintenance of certain written schedules and Come-up files assists in the performance of office routines.

Study Questions

1. Describe a procedure manual and tell why it is valuable.
2. Explain the office administrator's role on the oral health care delivery team.
3. Describe a good staff conference.
4. What are sources of information and why are they valuable?
5. Describe a Come-up file system.
6. What are a number of orderly office routines which assist in administering a dental office?
7. What information is included on a day's work schedule?
8. What are the two general classifications of work performed in the laboratory?
9. What information is included on the laboratory schedule?

Bibliography

KILPATRICK, HAROLD C. *Work Simplification in Dental Practice*. Philadelphia: W. B. Saunders Co., 1964.

STINAFF, ROBERT K. *Dental Practice Administration*. St. Louis: C. V. Mosby Co., 1960.

Pamphlet Which Can Be Ordered

How to be a Super-Secretary. Published by Remington Rand Office Machines, Division of Sperry Rand Corporation, 1962). (No author credit)

6 | *Time Control...*
the Appointment Book

The Importance of Time Management

Your first responsibility in office administration—to keep your dentist busy—revolves around a thorough understanding and use of the appointment book and its related records. The success or failure of the individual dental practice depends, at least in part, on the proper management of the appointment book. Its correct use, control, and effect upon efficiency are worth much study.

The Appointment Book

The appointment book may be a bound book, a loose-leaf folder, or a spiral-bound book. It lists the months of the year, the working days of the month (Monday through Saturday), and the time available each working day, usually in fifteen-minute intervals. Some appointment books list each week on a double page. An entire week can be seen at a glance. Appointment books may be purchased from any dental supply house, numerous stationery supply companies, or the American Dental Association, Chicago, Illinois, as well as from practice management companies such as Professional Budget Plan.

New appointment books dated for the proper year are usually available during the autumn of the preceding year. Obtain one as early as possible. The first procedure is to go through this new book, drawing a red-penciled x through those days which are regular days off in your office. Next, place a similar x through those holidays on which your office is closed. Remember the half-days on which most dental offices are closed, such as the afternoons prior to Christmas Eve and New Year's Eve. Check with the school board clerk or the local school for the regular school holidays and write "School Holiday" over the appropriate days in the new appointment book. These days are used to accommodate school children as often as possible.

Your dentist may be a member of one or of several groups which meet regularly. The schedule of these meetings for the full year should be indicated in the new appointment book. This suggestion applies to luncheon groups, study clubs, and dental society meetings.

Some appointment books are loose-leaf bound. On the last day of each month, remove the used sheets from the past month and insert the same number of new ones. Be sure to mark off the days on which the office is closed and properly indicate others as mentioned.

The Long Appointment

Research studies have indicated that there is economy in long appointments. The following explanation may help you see the value of the long appointment.[1]

It is very easy to lose ten minutes each time you change patients. It is possible to keep this lost change-over chair time to a minimum of three minutes, but that is unusually low.

If you multiply the lost chair time by the number of patients seen during the day, you

may be startled at the bulk of unproductive time which your office has experienced during one day. If the number of patients is 16 (16 half-hour appointments), you have lost 10 times 16, or 160 minutes or 2 hours and 40 minutes.

Many offices feel that seven patients per day is a good working day. This cuts the lost time to a seventy-minute maximum. It is obvious that by working with one patient for an hour, more dentistry can be accomplished than if you were to use three patients to fill that hour.

For the purpose of this explanation, let us say that it takes twenty minutes to do a two-surface amalgam restoration but that six surfaces can be done in forty minutes and twelve surfaces in eighty minutes. Greater economy in the actual work performed is accomplished during a longer appointment, in addition to the fact that time is saved by not changing patients every half-hour. The most efficient way to organize the dentist's time is to use longer appointments—including one lasting the entire day.

For example, Mr. Wilson needs thirty-two surfaces of amalgam restorations. If you book him in two-surface units (for 20-minute appointments), he must make sixteen trips to the office for a total of 320 minutes' chair time. If Mr. Wilson is booked for appointments at which six surfaces can be done (40-minute appointments), it will take slightly over five appointments with a total of 240 minutes' chair time. If you arrange two appointments of 80 minutes and one of 60 minutes (twelve surfaces in each of the 80 minutes, and the balance on the last appointment), he has spent 220 minutes in the chair and made only three trips. This is a saving of 100 minutes of the dentist's time over two-surface appointments.

Not everyone will agree with this breakdown of time in the performance of dental operations. The unit of time necessary to pre-

---

1. Dr. A. T. Thorson, formerly director of the Dental Assistants Training Program at the University of Minnesota, has worked out this explanation for lost time in the dental office after consultation with numerous dentists and contacts with hundreds of assistants.

pare a two-surface amalgam restoration is un-important—that will vary with each dental office—but the principle of time economy in the long appointment should be recognized.

If you, the dental assistant, can so organize your dentist's time that he works with little free time between patients, you will be helping to eliminate the lost chair time. You must learn to be accurate in judging how long his operations take and have patients booked for specific amounts of work to be done. Always try to make the appointment long enough to complete *all* the work of the patient. This sometimes presents problems. You may find a space in the appointment book for forty-five minutes' work. A particular patient requires sixty minutes. Find another appointment during which the dentist can actually complete the patient's work. If you book him for that forty-five-minute appointment and the patient has to return for another appointment, you have lost time for your dentist and your patient.

It is important to consider the patient. In the foregoing example, the travel time which Mr. Wilson saves by coming to the office three times instead of sixteen times is considerable. Depending upon the community in which he lives, he may save as much as thirteen hours. This consideration for the patient's time is one he appreciates.

There are, in general, two ways of managing an appointment book. One method restricts the length of time filled in with future appointments to a definite period, such as three weeks or one month ahead. All patients needing appointments who cannot be entered without exceeding this limit are listed on a *call* list. This list gives the name, address, and telephone number of the patient, the work required by that patient, and the time needed to complete this work. As appointments within the three-week or one-month limit become available, patients are contacted from the call list.

The other alternative is to date each patient for the amount of time necessary to complete the required dental work, regardless of how far ahead the appointment book is filled. When this method is used, it is wise to leave occasional time open for unforeseen requirements. In addition, the dentist must arrange his time for meetings or vacations well in advance.

Some dentists have objected to this method because they feel their time is so organized that it is impossible to break away on short notice for some special occurrence. This very real objection can be overcome if the patient is given only the next appointment in his series. The entire series of appointments is written in the appointment book, but you inform the patient of his *next* appointment at the time of each visit. Then should it be necessary for the dentist to be away from the office on short notice, it is possible for you to change the appointments without having to notify the patient since he is unaware of the complete series of appointments.

Regardless of which method of operating the appointment book is used in the office in which you are employed, you and your dentist must know the amount of time it takes to perform specific operations. One recommended way of organizing time is the unit system. You and your dentist decide on a specific amount of chair time to be called a *unit*. This may be fifteen minutes since most appointment books are divided into fifteen-minute intervals. There is nothing, however, to prevent your office from using ten or twenty minutes as the *unit* figure. Your dentist looks over the work to be done for a specific patient and writes for you or tells you the number of units he will need to complete the work. With practice it is possible for the dental assistant to learn the amount of time required for the various dental operations and thus be able to figure the units of time required without conference with the dentist.

The use of the unit system has an advantage because you can mention the number of units in front of the patient without calling attention to the specific time about which you are speaking or indicating to the patient how much time it will take for his dentistry, allowing him to figure an hourly rate for his work without regard for other factors involved in the cost of dentistry. It is wise to disassociate the necessary amount of chair time from the charges for services rendered. The preferred emphasis should be on services performed for the patient in relation to charges. Once the patient knows what is to be done and what the cost will be, together with the plan for payment, usually his desire is to get the work done as rapidly as possible.

Until you become familiar with the time factors in dental procedure, your dentist should indicate to you the amount of time or number of units required for each appointment of a patient. For your permanent reference, a list of time required for all dental operations performed in your office, placed either inside the cover of the appointment book or at a convenient location at the desk where appointments are made, is helpful. Practice using this list to verify the dentist's instructions until you no longer need to be told the length of appointment to make and the intervals between appointments for various types of work. If time for laboratory work is required between appointments, your dentist should inform you of the necessary time-lapse before the patient is again appointed.

The responsibility for management of the appointment book is best left entirely to one individual in the office. The greater the number of individuals allowed to make appointments, the greater will be the inefficiency in management of the appointment book.

Scheduling Appointments

If you are going to do the finest kind of time organization for your dentist, you will find that, insofar as possible, appointments should be scheduled when you are alone, with a number of them to make, and without being pressed for time. It is only under such circumstances that you can really see how to organize the time to the best advantage. It takes careful planning to arrange appointments so that there are no unused units of time in your book.

Some appointments must be made when a patient is present, but you can keep them to a minimum if you will follow these suggestions about making appointments.

The New Patient

The new patient is first given an appointment for an examination. In this example, the appointment is for one hour, or four units. Indicate by a red pencil that this is a "new" patient appointment. (The word "new" circled in red is easily seen.) At the close of this appointment, the patient is given an appointment for a "conference" (case presentation) at which time the dentist will explain the necessary work, allowing the patient to choose the service which he desires. The length of this conference will be determined by the dentist. A fifteen-minute period spent in the dentist's private office is usual. At the close of the dentist-patient conference, the dentist is able to inform his assistant of the number of units required for the patient's work. With the unit figure in the dental assistant's possession, it is possible for her to make the necessary number of appointments to complete the patient's work. If at all possible, schedule all the work during one appointment.

If it is necessary for this patient to have a series of appointments, give him just one while he is waiting for you. Be sure that you know the most convenient day and time of day for that patient. Plan the rest of the appointments when you are alone and not under pressure.

Not all offices use a patient conference. Necessary dentistry is scheduled as soon as the X rays are read. The assistant is informed of the number of units of time needed for the patient. She appoints the patient while he is present or calls him if he has left the office.

The Recall Patient

At the time of a recall, the patient is told that he will be called when the X rays have been read. (Most recalls today include at least bitewing X rays.)

The dentist studies the findings of the oral examination and X rays. He indicates the necessary amount of time to complete the patient's work. The assistant appoints the patient and calls to inform him of the appointment.

Some offices call a patient whether or not he needs additional work. It affords a person a wonderful sense of satisfaction to be told, "I thought you would like to know that there is no further dental work necessary at this time. You will hear from us in six months." Patients so treated usually respond with a "Thank you for calling!"

Your relationship with patients determines whether this type of call should be made. Time-pressed patients can be told, "Unless you hear from me next week, we won't be seeing you for six months."

The Emergency Patient

When a patient calls and is in pain, he is to be seen as soon as possible. If your office has an emergency period reserved each day, the patient is asked to come at that time only. If your office operates without such a break, look over the schedule and select the most likely looking break in time. If it is a true emergency, the patient will come at that time. If it is not, there is no need to crowd your schedule.

In any emergency, the patient should be told that the dentist will see him to *take care of the emergency* or *to take care of the pain.* No patient should be permitted to crowd into the day for work other than a real emergency. If further work is required following the relief from pain (and there usually is), the patient should be appointed for an examination, and the procedure for regular patient care should be followed.

Courtesy Service
(for a Patient of Another Dentist)

Occasionally a vacationing dentist asks your office to care for his patients during his absence. These appointments are almost always emergencies. When the patient calls, you explain that you work by appointment, that you can see him at ....(time) to care for the emergency. Give the patient an appointment as you would for an emergency among your own patients. After the appointment which gives relief from pain or irritation, no further appointment is given. It is your dentist's responsibility, ethically, to see that the patient returns to his regular dentist as soon as that dentist's vacation is over. Usually this emergency service is given without charging a fee.

Patients Not on Recall

Some offices do not run a recall system. They allow some of their patients to take care of making their own appointments for checkups instead of placing all patients on recall. When these patients call in, appoint them for an examination as you would a recall patient.

Salesmen

Appoint salesmen according to the instructions already given in Reception Procedures or see them on available emergency time.

School Children

Many school systems have some arrangement for the release of children to keep dental appointments when necessary. When such an arrangement has been worked out, it is usually between the local dental society or group and the school board or superintendent. The requirements of these arrangements should be scrupulously kept by your dental office.

At the beginning of each school year, the assistant can usually secure, through the local dental society office or from the school office, a list of the holidays for the coming school year. These days should receive all the preference possible for appointments with school-age children.

If your office is open on Saturdays, either all or part of the day, there will be considerable pressure to make appointments available on this day for practically all the patients in your practice. A good policy to use is that of approximately proportioning Saturday appointments equally among the different groups in your practice.

The time of day selected for the dental appointment is extremely important. Preschool children should generally be given only early morning appointments, the time of day during which they are most able to adapt themselves to cooperation in the dental office. The average child under ten is preferably seen before noon. The early school years demand a great deal of energy from the child in relation to his stamina. Appointments after school for this child will usually be difficult, from the standpoint of cooperation, because he has expended so much energy during the course of the school day that he has little ability left to cope with the tensions he will undergo in the dental office. Recall appointments for this group, after they are thoroughly adjusted and acquainted with the dental office, are frequently satisfactory during after-school hours. Any appointments for operative procedures, however, are best held to the morning hours.

Discuss dental appointments for children with your dentist and learn his wishes. Try to use this information, then, as a set routine in arranging such appointments.

The Appointment Book Entries

Let us assume that you have arrived at the time when you can sit down with the appointment book and make appointments for several patients. It is March 1 and you have just pulled from the recall control file the recalls to be appointed between March 15 and 31. You also have the records on several patients who have had conferences or case studies with your dentist. *What must you remember as you schedule these appointments?*

1. Schedule appointments for as long a sitting as possible. There is an exception to this rule, however. Some patients are exceedingly sensitive and dread dentistry so much that they are emotionally unable to endure long sittings. It is then necessary to schedule their work in shorter units of time until you have overcome their fears. Your dentist will recognize any such serious emotional disturbance. (Premedication is frequently used for such tension.)

2. Be sure that you know the length of time needed for the dentistry to be completed and give your dentist that much time, but no more!

3. Include, insofar as possible, a variety of types of dentistry in the day. Work is more interesting then.

As a general rule in arranging appointments, each day should follow, as closely as possible, a regular sequence: that work which requires most concentration and effort should be scheduled for morning hours, with a gradual trend toward work requiring less tension and concentration. Thus, appointments for operative work, bridgework, denture impressions, and preschool children should be scheduled for the morning hours. The first two types of work mentioned are usually given long appointments.

The early afternoon hours can best be devoted to the shorter operative appointments; the recall appointments for prophylaxis and examination; new patient appointments (except for children); denture work necessary between impression and final insertion appointments; and appointments with new patients for discussion of necessary work (appointments for case presentation).

It is not always possible to adhere strictly to such an arrangement of dental appointments, but the general thought in giving appointments should be to take the greatest advantage of those hours during which the dentist is best able to concentrate on difficult work.

4. Write only in pencil in the appointment book. (It is easier to correct or change, should this be necessary.)

5. If a patient has a complete mouth reconstruction or some operative work, bridgework, and perhaps a partial denture to be done, he will require appointments over a considerable period of time. No one likes to continue going to the dentist for three months. Try to organize these appointments into a four- to six-week period. Use the longest sittings possible considering the nature of the work to be accomplished.

6. If a series of appointments is to be given, it is preferable to give the patient an appointment on the same day of the week at the same time of day until the series is complete. It helps him remember his appointment more easily.

7. Your dentist may want a "break" period left open both in the morning and afternoon, or just in the morning. A period so maintained is very useful either for emergency work when required or for a relaxation period. There are times when an unforeseen difficulty prolongs an appointment beyond the original plan, and the "break" period will be of help in maintaining the balance of the schedule. However, some dentists prefer to work without such a break, risking their lunch hour if necessary. Be sure that you set up the appointment book on the basis which pleases your dentist.

8. In arranging appointments try to organize the time so that the unused time is easy to fill. For example, if your patient requires a one-hour appointment on a morning which is open from 8:30-11:30, give that patient either 8:30-9:30 or 10:30-11:30, rather than giving him an appointment in the middle of the open time. If he is given 9:30-10:30, the remaining time is cut up into periods which are difficult to fill. It is more efficient to leave the remaining time in a larger single period.

9. Remember to schedule children according to their age and physical ability.

10. Certain information is necessarily entered in the appointment book to run an efficient office. Check this list as you fill in the appointment book. Until you are more familiar with the list, perhaps you could copy it and put it on the appointment book cover as a reminder to be sure you have all the necessary information.

1. The patient's full name (in order not to confuse him with some other patient whose name may be very similar).
2. Telephone number (so that you may reach him in case of emergency or necessity to change the appointment).
3. Time of appointment.
4. Length of appointment.
5. The nature of the work to be done.

A Practical Example

Now you are ready to write the names and times in the appointment book. Although you will work with a much larger group of patients and many more days in such a planning session under ordinary office conditions, we will limit our list for this example to nine pa-

NAME	AGE	WORK	BEST TIME
Andrews, Mr. K. B.	30	Bridge impression 10 units	Tuesday, mid-mornings
Hoover, Randy	5	Fills, 2 units	Tuesday mornings
Jones, Mrs. Timothy	45	Operative—8 units	Tuesday, p.m., Friday a.m.

(Conference revealed she needs 48 units of work, five separate appointments, allowing one week between each of the last three for laboratory work to be completed. First appointment for operative work prior to impressions should be for 8 units.)

NAME	AGE	WORK	BEST TIME
McIntosh, Mr. Kenneth	25	Recall—2 units	*Early* Tuesday mornings
Murphy, Mr. John	38	Recall—2 units	*Early* Tuesday mornings
Murphy, Mrs. John	36	Recall—2 units	Tuesday mornings
Peterson, Mr. Rolf	60	Recall—2 units	Tuesday at or after 4 p.m.
Smith, Miss Mary	55	Denture impressions 4 units	Tuesday, late afternoon
Zambolini, Mr. I. F.	21	Operative—4 units	Tuesday, late afternoon

Fig. 6.1. Entries for completing sample appointment book page (fig. 6.3)

tients, all desiring Tuesday appointments. For the purpose of this example, a unit will be fifteen minutes. A recall takes two units. Our cast of characters with the information you would normally know about each patient appears in figure 6.1.

You also have a note stating that S. J. Carlson, the S. S. White salesman, makes his regular call on Tuesday (5 minutes). Your dentist likes to see this particular salesman.

Before arranging appointments for this cast of characters, the page of your appointment book will look something like the one in figure 6.2. There probably will be three single columns (each from 8:00 to 5:45) on a page, a double page making up the total week in order that you can see the week's schedule at a glance.

Select the patients who are to come on Tuesday. Fit them into the schedule on the basis of the most efficient work plan which you can visualize. If it is impossible to schedule all the Tuesday patients on this one day, some may have to be postponed to the next week. With the entire appointment book before you, that is possible.

Tuesday, March 18

8:00	1:00 Wagoner, Mr. R: Imps
8:15	1:15 331 6600
8:30	1:30
8:45	1:45
9:00	2:00
9:15	2:15
9:30 Emergencies	2:30
9:45	2:45
10:00 Fischer, Mrs. J. : Fills	3:00
10:15 588 3620	3:15
10:30	3:30
10:45	3:45
11:00	4:00
11:15	4:15
11:30	4:30
11:45	4:45
12:00	5:00
12:15	5:15
12:30	5:30
12:45	5:45

Fig. 6.2. Appointment book page prior to organizing appointments.

Already filled in from previous appointment-making sessions are 10:00-12:00 and 1:00-2:00. Notice that lines are drawn from the patient's name downward through the hours consumed by his appointment, with an arrow indicating the last unit.

Look at the list of people to be scheduled for Tuesday. Mr. K. B. Andrews needs a ten-unit period in midmorning. Since that time is already filled, leave his work for the following Tuesday. Randy Hoover, age five, needs a morning appointment. Schedule him for 9:00. This leaves one hour between 8:00 and 9:00 —a good time to recall the Murphys, who like to come on the same day. Schedule Mr. John Murphy at 8:00 and Mrs. Murphy at 8:30, leaving Mr. Kenneth McIntosh until the following Tuesday in order to give him the 8:00 appointment which he desires. As you look at the morning, you see that there is a fifteen-minute break after the emergency period this office happens to maintain. Schedule your salesman for the *last five minutes* of that fifteen-minute period. Mark the corrected time in your appointment book. This completes the morning.

In the afternoon, Mrs. Jones is scheduled at 2:00 for two hours of operative work, with additional appointments made at this time on successive Tuesdays and Fridays to complete her work. She will not be informed of the additional sittings, however. (The notice of these appointments will be in her folder so that you can find them easily on her successive trips.) Mr. Peterson can be scheduled at 4:00, which he will appreciate since it means that he doesn't have to wait for his appointment but can come right after work. It is important to start a denture patient who must have additional appointments; therefore Miss Smith is chosen over Mr. Zambolini for the later afternoon appointment. Mr. Zambolini will be appointed the following Tuesday. Miss Smith can come at 4:30 to finish the working day

by 5:30—a half-hour longer than it ought to be, but some days this happens.

As you work with a large group of patients and several days in which to appoint them, you will learn to adjust the time to the patients' needs. Sometimes you may turn up with an unused unit. Try to avoid this if possible. Schedule on a different day to avoid wasting a single unit. Be sure that you allow time for laboratory work to be completed between appointments.

In pencil on the patient's record write the time of his next appointment or appointments. You can then find this information quickly when the patient is again in the office and you are to make out an appointment card for him.

Your appointment book page will look like figure 6.3 when you have finished writing in

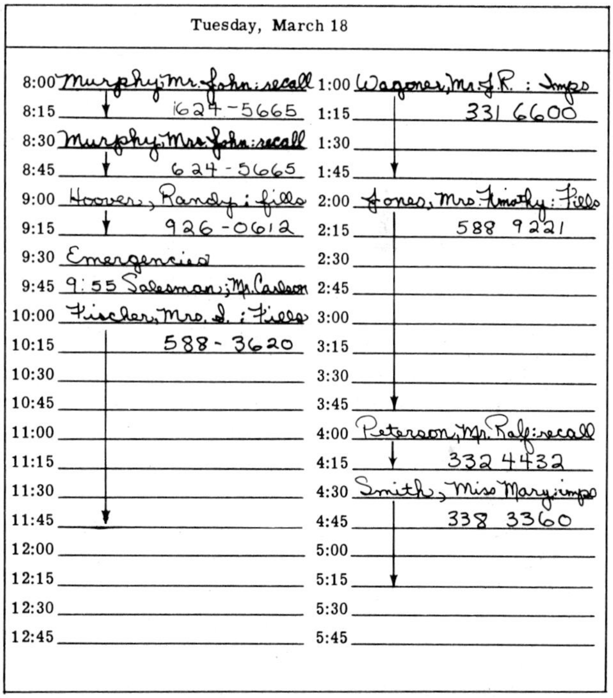

Fig. 6.3. Appointment book page after organizing appointments.

the names. Note that the *complete* name and telephone number are given for each patient appointed. This saves time when the reminder telephone call is made the day before the appointment.

Evening Meetings

Occasionally your dentist has evening plans —a professional dinner meeting or a social engagement—which may mean that he must leave the office at a certain time. At the hour at which he must stop work in order to keep his engagement, write: "No more. District Dental Dinner, 6 P.M." or "Dinner party at 6 P.M." This should be called to the dentist's attention earlier in the afternoon as an oral reminder. It should also be written on the bottom of the Day's Work Schedule which is posted in each operatory and in the business office.

Patient Awareness of the Importance of Appointment Time

Writing the appointments in the appointment book is important. Still more important is to see that the patients keep these appointments—on time. What can you do?

You can help patients become aware of the importance of the appointment time.

When the patient is orally informed of an appointment, it is possible to stress the importance of keeping the appointment. Perhaps a patient whom you do not know or one who is habitually late can be told to be a few minutes early. Stress the facts that the time is reserved for this patient only, and if doctor cannot begin his work on time, he may not be able to complete it because another patient is due immediately following this patient's appointment. It is also well to tactfully remind patients that an early cancellation permits another patient to receive treatment.

The Appointment Card

An appointment card reminds the patient of his appointment in writing. It may be as small as a calling card or it may be somewhat larger. Some offices use appointment slips made out in duplicate, with a carbon copy kept at the office for verification in case of confusion about an appointment. Some offices may have the patient write in his name and time of appointment so that the carbon copy shows the patient's handwriting.

The appointment card has spaces for the patient's name, the date, and the time of appointment. It gives in printing the name of the dentist, his address, and his telephone number. Some cards have a statement that twenty-four-hour notice must be given if the appointment cannot be kept. Sample cards are shown in figure 6.4.

When the patient is present in the office, the dental assistant copies the appointment date and time from the appointment book onto the appointment card. The card is then given to the patient. Some offices mail the cards to patients whose appointments have been made by telephone.

Reducing Appointment Failures

After making the appointments, it is also necessary to see that appointments are kept, or your dentist will be resting when he should be operating. As you have time during the day, call the patients who have appointments for the following day. (Their telephone numbers should be in the appointment book by their names.) A postcard should be mailed as a reminder to patients living beyond the local telephone exchange—mailed early enough to reach them a day or two before the appointment.

If a patient scheduled for a recall appointment has previously telephoned to verify his appointment (when he received his recall no-

_____

has a reservation with

DR. _____

_____

For_____

at_____o'clock

This time is reserved for you. If, for any reason, the appointment cannot
be kept, notification should be made 24 hours in advance, please.

PHONE: _____

_____

M _____

HAS AN APPOINTMENT

MONDAY	AT	O'CLOCK
TUESDAY	AT	"
WEDNESDAY	AT	"
THURSDAY	AT	"
FRIDAY	AT	"
SATURDAY	AT	"

THE ABOVE MENTIONED TIME HAS BEEN RESERVED ESPECIALLY FOR
YOU. IF UNABLE TO USE THIS RESERVATION PLEASE GIVE TWENTY-FOUR
HOURS NOTICE IN ORDER THAT ANOTHER PATIENT MAY USE THIS TIME.

TELEPHONES: OFFICE _____ RES. _____

Fig. 6.4. Appointment cards. The appointment
should first be written in the appointment book,
then copied from the appointment book to the appointment card, and, finally, double-checked for
accuracy.

tice specifying a definite day and time), his
recall appointment in the appointment book
is marked with a red x. This patient is not
reminded by telephone the day prior to his
appointment, since he has indicated his awareness of it.

It is preferable not to call a new patient
scheduled for his first appointment with the
office. A good test of his interest and appreciation of dental service is whether he keeps
his appointment promptly. If the new patient
should fail to keep this appointment without

notification, he is probably not sufficiently interested to be a good patient. The sooner this
is made evident, the better. Your dentist may
not want this type of patient in his practice.

The telephone call requires only a simple
statement: "This is Dr. Smith's office calling
to remind you of your appointment at 10:00
tomorrow morning, Mr. Jones."

Mr. Jones will usually respond with an indication that he will be there as scheduled.

"Thank you, Mr. Jones," is a correct response. Wait for Mr. Jones to hang up his
phone first.

In the event that Mr. Jones is ill or for some
reason cannot keep his appointment, the office
will have sufficient time to arrange to use Mr.
Jones's appointment time either for a patient
from the call list or to extend the work, when
possible, scheduled for the patient preceding
Mr. Jones's appointment.

If you will remember to give a patient who
needs several appointments to complete his
dental treatment an appointment on the same
day of the week, the same time of day, he is
less likely to forget it.

Summary

Proper management of the appointment
book is one of the factors which contribute
to the success or failure of the dental practice.
It keeps your dentist busy or allows him to
be idle. It should be managed by one person
rather than by several people.

Good management includes using a unit
system of measuring time for dental operations, knowing the amount of time needed for
each operation, appointing a sizable group of
patients at one time in the quiet and privacy
of an inner office where it is possible to pay
attention to time organization, and seeing that
general rules for the use of time are followed.
Appointments should be as long as possible for
the benefit of both the patient and the dentist.

If possible, include a variety of work in each day. Include a break period each day in order to allow for emergencies, unless your dentist specifically dislikes this procedure.

The following information is to be included in the appointment book: the patient's full name, his telephone number, the time of appointment, the length of appointment, and the nature of the work to be done, Adults' names are preceded by Mr., Mrs., Ms., or Miss. "New" patients are so indicated for statistical use, also.

As soon as a new appointment book is received, the holidays, vacation days, professional meeting days, and any other days on which the office will be closed should be marked off with a red-penciled x. School holidays should be so indicated at the top of the page.

An appointment card offers the patient a reminder of his appointment.

Reducing appointment failures is an important part of dental assisting. Patients should be called one day in advance of their appointment to be reminded of the appointment. Recall patients need not be called if they have telephoned their acceptance of the date.

Proper management of the appointment book is an art and a skill. A well-managed appointment book allows a dentist to produce more dentistry and serve more people.

Study Questions

1. Discuss the importance of time management in the dental office.
2. What is important to remember in making appointments for (a) the new patient? (b) the recall patient? (c) the emergency patient?
3. What are your responsibilities in rendering courtesy service to a patient of another dentist?
4. Discuss appointments for school children.
5. Explain the ten steps to be remembered in making appointment book entries.
6. What is an appointment card?
7. How can you help patients become aware of the importance of being present on time for their appointment?
8. How can you help reduce appointment failures?

Bibliography

Bregstein, S. Joseph. *Handbook for Dental Assistants, Hygienists and Secretaries.* Englewood Cliffs, N. J.: Prentice-Hall, 1961.

Kilpatrick, Harold C. *Work Simplification in Dental Practice.* Philadelphia: W. B. Saunders Co., 1964.

Stinaff, Robert K. *Dental Practice Administration.* St. Louis: C. V. Mosby Co., 1960.

7 | *Mail Services and Care*

Just keeping up with the mail in a dental office can be a time-consuming job. Today the quantity of advertising by mail is enormous. Some of this material is valuable to the dentist and/or the office staff. Some of it is best deposited in "file 13," commonly known as the wastebasket.

Classes of Mail

It is important for you to understand the classes of mail because an experienced person examining the mail can quickly discover advertising which is designed to look like first-class mail of a "personal-for-your-doctor-only" nature.

First-class mail is usually sealed. It is handwritten or typed material. Letters, of course, are first-class. In addition, if you send any reports which are *typewritten,* they are considered first-class mail and must bear the correct first-class postage. If the material is mimeographed or printed, it is not considered first-class mail. If you are sending eleven or more packets in the same mailing, you may be entitled to a special rate. Consult your post office under such circumstances.

First-class mail is classified as letters and postcards, all matter wholly or partly in writing, except authorized additions to second-, third-, and fourth-class mail, and matter sealed or closed against inspection unless carrying the proper label for inspection.

Second-class mail includes newspapers and magazines which are registered with the post office as such. There are special rates for these items. If you, as an individual, mail a copy, it costs somewhat more than if the publisher mails it.

Third-class mail includes books and catalogs of twenty-four or more bound pages, circulars and other printed matter, proof sheets and corrected proof sheets with related manuscript copy, keys, identification cards, all other matter of eight ounces or less not included in first- or second-class mail.

Fourth-class mail includes merchandise, printed matter, mailable live animals, and all other matter not included in the first-, second-, or third-class mail.

There is a special rate for books of twenty-four or more pages and for films. These items must be specially marked on the outside to be eligible for the reduced rate. There are weight and size limitations which vary somewhat with the postal regulations. If your package weighs more than forty pounds, you had better consult your local post office for directions. Some packages of heavier weight may be sent under special circumstances. The same is true of size. Packages exceeding seventy-two inches in length and girth may be too large under some circumstances. Since these restrictions vary from time to time, it is wise to consult your post office.

Airmail is a very special class of service. It is the fastest service available. Mail is carried by air and by the fastest connecting surface carriers and is given the most expeditious handling in dispatch and delivery. It is not given special delivery to the addressee unless a special delivery fee is paid in addition to the airmail postage.

Registered mail is mail which is protected because it is personally registered as having been delivered. The mailman must have the recipient sign a card which states that the mail was received at the address given. For an additional fee it is possible to ask that the card be signed by the person to whom the mail is addressed. This card is then returned to the sender.

It is also possible to *insure* mail which you send, except first-class mail. The fee for insurance depends on the value of the package.

Cash on delivery (*COD*) is a way you can send an item for which you have not been paid, and the receiver will pay for it upon its delivery. The money for its purchase is then returned to you by postal money order.

Certificates of mailing furnish evidence of mailing only. A receipt is not obtained upon delivery of the mail.

Special delivery is a service which means that the mail is delivered immediately upon receipt at the post office. A special car takes it to its destination.

Special handling is a service available for fourth-class mail. It speeds the service somewhat but does not mean the package is delivered by special delivery.

Certified mail provides for a receipt to the sender and a record of delivery at the office of address. It is handled in the ordinary mails and no insurance coverage is provided.

Money orders, by which it is possible to send money to someone else, may be purchased at the post office.

First-class mail will be forwarded, provided the person has left a forwarding address.

There are special regulations for international mail. Postal rates are higher than domestic mail rates, and it is wise to call your post office and verify the correct postage for individual foreign countries.

Mail that is undeliverable is returned to the sender if there is a return address on the envelope. If there is no return address, it is sent to the dead-letter office.

A zip code directory for your local area should be obtained from the post office and *used*.

Mail which fails to reach its destination within a reasonable time can usually be traced. Receipts from the post office for money orders and insured or registered mail should be kept until you have received notification from the person to whom the mail was sent that he has received it in good condition. Should mail be undelivered, consult your post office for the proper forms to complete. The post office will then make every effort to find the lost mail.

Since postal regulations do change with the passage of time and with current conditions, it is wise for your office to obtain the special bulletins which the post office prints. The *Postal Manual* may be purchased from the Superintendent of Documents, Government Printing Office, Washington, D. C. In addition, the post office supplies a number of bulletins about mailing services. You can find the following publications at your local post office.

POD Publication 2: *Packaging and Wrapping Parcels for Mailing*
POD Publication 3: "Excerpts from Chapter Number One," *Postal Manual.*
POD Publication 13: *Mailing Permits*
POD Publication 14: *Combination Mailing.*

Incoming Mail

Processing incoming mail is an important part of your job. This task should be performed with speed, handled with accuracy, and completed in a minimum amount of time. Upon starting employment in the dental office, ask the dentist what he wants you to do with various types of mail ordinarily received in a dental office. The large majority of pieces received will present no problem. It is important, however, to develop the discretion and judgment to protect the dentist's time and inter-

ests. To conserve time, incoming mail may be classified into three groups.

1. Mail which should be placed on the dentist's desk:
    a. Personal mail.
    b. Letters from other professional men.
    c. Announcement of meetings.
2. Mail which the assistant should care for as completely as possible:
    a. Letters from patients (other than questions of accounts).
    b. Letters dealing with statements or accounts, other than payments.
    c. Payments on account.
    d. Letters soliciting contributions.
    e. Invoices for dental supplies or business suppplies.
    f. Monthly statements for the office bills for supplies, etc.
    g. Magazines.
    h. Laboratory cases (if mailed).
    i. Insurance forms.
3. Advertising matter, to be handled with discretion by the assistant.

As you sort the mail, place the personal letters in a pile and do not open them. Open the rest of the mail at one time. Minutes can be saved each day if you will use a letter opener to slit all the envelopes first, without removing the contents until all envelopes are cut. Tap the envelopes against the desk to be certain that the enclosures are away from the edge before you use the letter opener. When all the envelopes are opened, lay down the letter opener and carefully remove the contents of each envelope in group one. Be certain that nothing is lost. Clip the contents and the envelope together. If any of the letters require records or previous correspondence to be available for the dentist, attach these materials to the letter. Add these letters to the unopened personal letters and place the entire group on the dentist's desk immediately.

As soon as time permits, carefully remove the contents from the envelopes in group two. Again, be certain that nothing is lost. Always clip the envelope to the enclosed material until you have had time to check the address on the envelope with that on the enclosed material and with your records, where indicated. Some letters request information. If it is information which you personally are able to furnish and it is ethical for you to do so, answer the letter the day it is received. Sign your own name to the answer—not your dentist's name, initialed by you.

Letters from a patient, especially concerning any complaint, should be placed in the patient's record envelope after noting the date upon which an answer was mailed to the patient. Should you have any doubt about the handling of such a letter from a patient, it should be brought to the attention of the dentist for his recommendation.

If any mail refers to previous correspondence, this correspondence should be removed from the files and placed with the current letter. Be certain to read the letter thoroughly enough to know whether you have removed all the necessary records. (Your dentist may have to examine an X ray or reread an examination record to intelligently answer the mail. He will need the previous correspondence file if the letter refers to one he has written first.)

Be alert for remittances and give them special attention. Examine checks and money orders carefully to see that they are properly filled out, that all necessary information is given so that you can credit the proper accounts with the payments. There are basic requirements for a check which must be met before a bank will accept it for deposit. It must be dated no later than the date of deposit; that is, a check for deposit October 1 must be dated on October 1 or earlier, not October 10. The amounts of money, written

and numerical, must agree, and the check must be properly signed. If any of these items is missing or incorrect, the bank returns the check to you and will not deposit it to your account until corrected. Thus it is important that you verify these items carefully before attempting to deposit each check.

A check cannot be cashed by anyone if it is endorsed on the back, "For deposit to the account of Doctor ...." Thus, for protection, endorse a check as soon as it is received. Most dentists have a bank stamp which states this type of endorsement, and it is only necessary to stamp the endorsement space on the back of the check. No other writing is required. Should the check be lost or stolen, it cannot be cashed with this note on its reverse side.

Most invoices for dental office supplies will accompany the merchandise at the time it is received in the dental office. Occasionally, however, they will be forwarded in a separate envelope through the mail. The assistant should be sure that all the merchandise for which her office is billed has been received. The invoice is then placed in the file folder labeled "Current Invoices" until the first-of-the-month statement is received, when the invoice will again be needed.

Statements for dental office bills are received near the first of each month. The invoices relating to the statement are removed from the Current Invoices file folder, checked against the items on the statement, and the total verified for correctness. The assistant should then make out a check for the proper amount, according to the practice of the office. Some dentists prefer to review the complete statement with its invoices. In this case, the assistant may make out the check without signature, clip it to the statement and invoices, together with an envelope ready for mailing, and place it on the dentist's desk along with all other statements when they are received by the office. If possible, invoices should be paid no later than the tenth of the month.

Laboratory cases received in the mail should be opened and the invoice located. Many dentists like to have the laboratory charge indicated on the patient's record card. If this procedure is desired in the office in which you work, it should be done as soon as the invoice is received for each case, before it is placed in the Current Invoices file. Laboratory cases which consist either partially or wholly of processed acrylic, such as jacket crowns, full crowns with acrylic veneer, facings on bridges, or denture bases, should be removed from their protective wrappers and placed in water in the laboratory as soon as unpacked. A slip of paper identifying the patient for whom the case is constructed should be placed in such a manner that it cannot be separated from the proper laboratory case. Items which do not require immersion in water are placed in small plastic, metal, or cardboard boxes in the laboratory, with the identifying slip of paper containing the patient's name clipped to the box with a paper clip. Large plastic boxes may have the name written directly on the box with a "china" pencil which will wipe off when the box is to be reused.

Any supplies received through the mail should be cared for as directed in chapter eight.

In today's practice, insurance forms will consume a large block of time. If you know the regulations concerning these forms and keep a separate file of them, you can expedite your time when such a form comes in the mail.

The third group of mail, advertising matter, is examined only after group two has been completed. Some advertising material is definitely desirable in the dental office because it may acquaint the dentist with a new product which he should know is on the market. On the other hand, some advertising material

is not related to the practice of dentistry, is of no interest to the dentist, and is devised to look like personal or first-class mail. If one of the end flaps of the envelope is merely tucked in for closure and carries a statement in fine print that it may be opened for postal inspection if necessary, it is advertising. In addition, such mail will usually have a "permit" postage mark rather than an attached postage stamp or a "metered" postage mark, due to the large number of pieces the originating office will place in the mail at one time. Open this mail and place it on the bottom of the pile for your dentist.

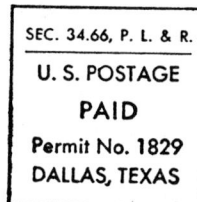

Fig. 7.1. A "Permit" postage mark often used on circulars and other advertising mail.

SEC. 34.66, P. L. & R.

U. S. POSTAGE

PAID

Permit No. 1829

DALLAS, TEXAS

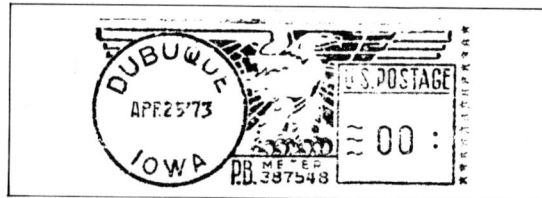

DUBUQUE
APR 25 '73
IOWA
U. S. POSTAGE
00
P. B. METER
387548

Fig. 7.2. Pitney-Bowes metered postage used on first-class mail quite frequently, as well as on some advertising. The amount of postage indicated in the square at the right corresponds with the rate for the particular classification of the piece of mail on which it appears (first-class, second-class, etc.).

Your dentist should brief you on the types of samples he wishes to see, the advertising literature he wishes to read, and what you should do with the rest of such mail. Samples not used in your office can be given to a charitable organization.

In a large dental clinic, after the mail is sorted into groups, each group may be delivered to the person responsible for that part of the mail. For example, the bookkeeper will receive all payments and accounting complaints.

Outgoing Mail

Mail to be sent from the office must also receive care. When letters have been dictated, typed, proofread, and signed, they should be properly folded and prepared for mailing. It is wise to see that enough postage is used on any mailing. The last person to leave the office should be certain that there is no mail waiting to be mailed. Sometimes a report is finished late or the dentist signs a letter just before he leaves.

Care of Mail During Dentist's Absence

When the dentist is on vacation or attending a meeting, it is important that he have a complete understanding with his assistant about mail. It may be that the personal mail should be opened and contents noted so that the assistant may decide what needs to be communicated to her dentist.

If he is to be away for a long enough period, some mail may need to be forwarded to him. In any event, if a delay may occur in an answer, it is wise for the secretary to write a brief note of explanation that the dentist is away from the office and will answer the letter personally as soon as he returns. If it is a matter which the assistant can handle, she should write a letter stating that she is caring for the matter in the absence of her employer, including a statement that should any question arise, the correspondent should write again for further clarification.

Some mail can wait for the return of the dentist, without seeming to delay too long.

If some mail—and occasionally there is some—demands an immediate decision by the dentist, perhaps he will arrange with you before he leaves to call him at the meeting he is attending. In the absence of such an arrangement, use your best judgment about any action you think necessary.

If you are to send any mail to your employer while he is away, *make a copy of it to send him.* If it is lost in transit, you will still have the original.

If your dentist does not want you to open letters marked personal in his absence, send a note to the return address on the envelope, explaining the dentist is away and will receive his mail on his return. Also, indicate that if there is anything which you can do to help, the writer should contact you personally. Sign your name.

A Closed Office and Mail

Notify the post office or mail carrier if your office is to be closed for any length of time. The mail can be held at the post office until your return. It will eliminate lost mail and and possible loss of income through theft of the letters which contain payments. In addition, any large pile-up of mail at the door of the office is indication to a would-be thief that now is the time to break into the office.

Summary

There are several classes of mail which the dental assistant should recognize and understand both for classifying the importance of mail received and for understanding which type of service to use for mail to be sent. These classes include first-, second-, third-, and fourth-class mail, airmail, registered mail, COD, special delivery, special handling, certified mail, and money orders. Zip code is necessary on all mail sent.

A postal manual which will contain the correct regulations may be purchased.

Incoming mail must be sorted and processed according to its urgency. Mail which must be seen by the dentist should be opened and placed on his desk, with the most important pieces on top.

Outgoing mail is to be proofread by the secretary before it is mailed. It should be mailed just as soon as possible after the dentist has signed the letters.

Special care must be taken of personal mail for the dentist during his absence from the office while on a trip. Mail which can be answered by the secretary should be answered. Mail which the dentist wishes to remain unopened should be placed on his desk or in a special file for his return. The secretary should send a note to the return address on each envelope, explaining the absence of the dentist and indicating that if the matter is urgent, the addressee can write the secretary direct.

If the office is to be closed for any period of time, such as a week, the mail carrier should be notified so that the mail can be held at the post office for the reopening of the dental office

Study Questions

1. Why is it desirable for the assistant to recognize the classes of mail?
2. Describe the proper sorting of mail.
3. Why should outgoing mail be proofread by the secretary?
4. Describe the special care of mail during the dentist's absence while he is attending a convention.
5. Why should you notify the mail carrier if the office is to be closed for a two-week period?

8 | *Supplies and Their Control*

Introduction

Few businesses can be run effectively without control of the supplies which are used. In the dental office, one of the dental assistants usually is responsible for supplies of all types. She should manage them efficiently.

Supplies used in a dental office are varied. Some indication must be given of exactly what supplies are needed in order to facilitate the work of the assistant who is responsible for ordering them. Dental supplies depend on the type of practice. Business supplies depend on the type of bookkeeping and dental record system preferred by your dentist.

Materials in the dental office are either expendable or nonexpendable. For all practical purposes and bookkeeping for federal income tax reporting, it is wise to consider as expendable all items which cost less than fifty dollars and have a life of less than three years. All materials costing more than fifty dollars which will last longer than three years are then automatically nonexpendable. Thus, your chair, unit, and X ray are all nonexpendable, while burs, cotton pliers, mouthwash, and X-ray films are all expendable.

Probably no dentist will demand that you classify the items in his office as equipment, instruments, and supplies, but you should know that some things are used once or for a short period of time; other things last for longer periods of time, perhaps up to ten or twenty years in the case of some large pieces of equipment.

No matter what the life expectancy of the supplies, at some time it is necessary to order replacements. While the dentist probably will not ask you to order a new chair, he may expect you to call to his attention anything in the office which needs replacing. Careful records are the best way to keep him and yourself informed of the need for any item.

There are two types of supplies used in the office: professional and business. The professional supplies are all materials which are used in the practice of dentistry as such—operative or laboratory. Business equipment or supplies are items which are not used in the actual practice of dentistry. Thus, silver amalgam alloy is a professional supply, while stationery is a business supply. Business supplies include cleaning supplies, materials with which to conduct the business side of dental practice, coffee supplies if coffee is served by your office, and magazines and flowers for making the office attractive.

Selecting the Supplier

Dental materials are usually ordered from a dental supply house. If your office is in a city where a supply house is located, the desired item can be in your office in a matter of minutes. If your practice is not so favorably located in relation to dental supply houses, it is necessary to keep a more careful check on supplies and to write well in advance of need. Some supply houses have salesmen who call on dental offices, and orders can be placed orally rather than by letter.

Drugs are usually ordered from a pharmacy. Your dentist will probably have a preference.

Business supplies are more generally available near the office. A stationery store will provide the necessary office supplies, with the exception of those items used specifically in a dental practice such as patient records, business record sheets, and appointment books, which are ordered through your dentist's bookkeeping service, dental supply house, or directly from a firm which specializes in this type of material. Your dentist will know where he prefers to purchase these items.

Cleaning supplies, coffee, etc., can be purchased in nearby grocery or department stores.

Control of Supplies

Bulk purchasing of supplies can mean a considerable savings over a period of time. The degree of bulk purchasing used by the dental office depends upon whether or not the dentist desires to make the savings which such purchasing can gain and upon the amount of room available in the dental office for storage. Many dental items require little space, however, and purchasing in dozen, gross, or other quantity lots which provide savings of ten to twenty percent over the single unit price should always be considered whenever possible.

For good control of supplies, make up a number of four-by-six-inch cards, each headed with the name of a material or an item of expendable supplies used in your office. When any item is purchased, make note on the proper card of the date, the quantity, where purchased, and the price. Once this information has been collected for any item of supply, re-order merely involves a check of the card. The rate at which a material is used up will indicate the desirability of purchasing in the same quantities or in lesser or greater quantities. An item which has proved unsatisfactory is also easily identified, and its reorder can be prevented. Supply control cards may be kept as a separate file at the desk or in the labora-

BIBS				
DATE	QUANTITY	FIRM	BRAND	TOTAL PRICE
6/8/59	1 case	John Marans	K.P. (260)	$8.00
9/15/59	3 cases	"	K.P. (each)	22.80
10/1/60	12 cases	"	K.P.	87.50
11/10/64	20 cases	"	K.P.	120.00
2/2/71	20 cases	"	K.P.	144.00
4/10/73	20 cases	"	K.P.	154.00

Fig. 8.1. A supply control card. Useful information is easily collected by keeping the supply control cards: rate of consumption of various items, your dentist's preference for certain brands, help in re-ordering in order to replace with an identical item, and some assistance in cost-of-operation detail.

tory, if preferred. They should be arranged alphabetically by item name.

A "running inventory" of supplies on hand is kept by making a list of each supply item. Try to post this paper on the laboratory wall, or convenient to the storage area. Listing by storage section is of help in locating items more rapidly. Each time an item is removed from the storage space, the amount indicated on the list as "on hand" should be corrected. Sufficient warning is thus available to reorder materials as required. Keep in mind the desirability of spreading supply purchases as evenly as possible throughout the year.

Your dentist should indicate at what level of supply he wishes you to reorder. When the "running inventory" indicates that any particular supply is at his reorder level, you add it to your list of supplies to be ordered.

Check the supply control card to determine how much you should order. Proper use of control cards will tell you the best bulk purchase rate. It is wise to check the bulk rates

occasionally. You may discover that a somewhat larger purchase will give you a much greater discount. Your dentist may decide to increase his storage of that particular item. Special prices on many items are often available at convention time each year.

Care of Supplies Upon Delivery

The package of supplies arrives and you open it. Inside there should be an invoice (see fig. 8.2). Check the supplies received against the invoice to see that you have received everything for which you have been charged. This invoice should then be filed in the Current Invoice file (see page 83). The supplies are stored in their proper places in the office. Be sure you have not received damaged merchandise *before* you store it.

If some item is damaged or incorrect, it should be returned. If your dental supply house is in your city, they will send someone for it if you call them and explain. If your office is located beyond such direct service, it will be necessary to mail the merchandise back with a letter of explanation. This letter may be placed inside the package if you write "First-Class Mail Enclosed" on the outside of the package and attach a first-class postage stamp to the package in addition to the required postage for the merchandise.

You should receive a credit slip for the item returned. Be sure to see that you do. File it with the current invoices for the firm from whom you received the credit slip.

If you receive a note saying an item is out of stock and will be shipped later, the word "Back-ordered" may be used. This is a business term meaning that the firm will send the item as soon as they have received it from their supplier. If you need this item immediately, you may try to acquire it from some other firm. If you succeed, you should let the first firm know that the back order is cancelled.

John Marcus Dental Supply Company

3037 LYNDALE AVE. SO. • MINNEAPOLIS, MINNESOTA 55408 • PHONE 827-6125

TO

Doctor James A. Raywin
104 Any Street
Anytown, Anystate 12345

Salesman   Dick

Customer

Date   April 8, 1973

MANUFACTURER	BACK ORDERED	QUAN. ORDERED	QUAN. SHIPPED	DESCRIPTION	UNIT PRICE	AMOUNT
K.P.		3	3	Bibs (Rate for 3 or more cartons)	$8.00	$24.00
Eastman	3	6	3	Kodak D.F. 58	$8.70	$23.49
				(Less 10%)		
					SUB TOTAL	$47.49
					TAX	1.74
					SHIPPING	---------
					TOTAL	49.23

ITEMS APPEARING IN BACK ORDER COLUMN WILL FOLLOW SHORTLY

Courtesy John Marcus Dental Supply Co., Minneapolis

Fig. 8.2. A dental supply invoice

Proper Storage

The majority of dentists have preferences for storage of supplies; but whether your dentist decides the placement or leaves it to you, you are expected to see that everything is orderly and that the oldest materials on hand are used first.

When new supplies arrive, items on hand must be removed from storage. The new stock is placed in the back or on the bottom of the space assigned to each item. Then the older stock is placed in front where it will be used first. One method is to write a number or date on the packages as a double check so that the older materials are surely used first. Certain materials age and are less effective after a certain time limit.

There are supplies which must receive special storage care: for example, X-ray film must be stored in a lead-lined box unless it is stored in a cool, dry place, well away from the area in which the X-ray machine is used; X-ray developer and fixer must be stored in a dark, cool area; and gypsum materials (artificial stones and plaster) must be kept dry. Check with your dentist to see what arrangements he has in his office for special storage.

Care of Laundry

Your office may send its towels to the commercial laundry. Some offices send all uniforms as well. Some laundries furnish linens as well as launder them; sometimes the dentist owns the towels and uniforms.

If your office uses a commercial laundry, it is important to know how to manage this service. The driver usually stops at regular intervals, such as every other day. Before his scheduled arrival,

1. count all the soiled linens,
2. record the number of each kind for your future reference,
3. count the number and type of uniforms if you are sending them with the linens, and
4. record the number of each kind.

When the driver returns the clean laundry,

1. count the linens (the figures should agree with your note of the number of pieces sent),
2. check the charge to see that it is correct, and
3. file the invoice.

If your office uses linens furnished by the laundry, these three steps are all you need to follow. If your dentist owns his own linens, they should be marked for identification. Make certain that the linens returned from the laundry belong to your dentist. The quality and age of towels sent to a commercial laundry vary considerably. Sometimes an entire bundle of laundry will be sent to the wrong office. The only way the laundry can discover their error is if one of the recipients informs them of the error. Quite possibly the towels received in such an error will not be of the same quality nor in the same condition as those of your office. The package may even contain uniforms which are not the correct size for your office personnel. It is of help to the laundry if you report such an error immediately.

After you have determined that the correct amount of laundry belonging to your office has been returned to you and that the charges are accurate, store the laundry in its proper place.

Summary

Supplies must be managed efficiently. Dental supplies must be carefully stored and plainly labeled.

Supplies are expendable if they cost less than fifty dollars and have a life expectancy of less than three years. They are nonexpendable if they cost fifty dollars or more and have a useful life of more than three years.

Supplies are also classified as business and professional. The professional supplies are materials used in the practice of dentistry. The business supplies are those used to keep the dental office operating as a business.

A control system for all supplies, both business and professional, is desirable to keep the office supplied with all materials needed to operate the office.

A 4" x 6" card is made for each material ordered, and the date of purchase, quantity, supplier, and price are listed for each purchase.

A "running inventory" of supplies is made by listing the supply and quantity on hand. Whenever any material is taken from the supply cupboard, the quantity removed is written in the appropriate column. Simple subtraction indicates the quantity on hand.

When supplies are delivered, the package is checked for (1) the invoice and (2) damaged or incorrect contents. Any damaged or incorrect merchandise is returned. Whatever merchandise is correct is stored. It is necessary to rotate stock so that the oldest supplies are used first.

Proper storage for all items is necessary (refrigerator for some; dark, cool areas for others; and so on).

Laundry should be counted prior to sending, counted on return, and inspected to see that it is your laundry if the supplies belong to your office instead of to the commercial laundry. After verification of the laundry and charges, the laundry is stored in its proper place.

Study Questions

1. Why do you carefully store and plainly label dental supplies?
2. What supplies are expendable?
3. Differentiate between business and professional supplies.
4. Why is a control system for supplies desirable?
5. Describe a control system.
6. How do you make a "running inventory" and what is its use?
7. Describe the assistant's duties when a package of supplies is received.
8. Describe your care of the laundry from the time you gather the soiled items until you place the clean ones in their proper storage places.

9 | *Preservation of Written Records... Filing*

"Business is floundering in a sea of filed materials—materials which simply take up storage space."[1] While it is true that many written records are filed and forgotten, there are important records to be preserved. Judgment must be used in deciding which materials are to be retained and, later, in selecting materials to be destroyed when they are no longer deemed useful.

Dental Record Preservation

In a dental practice, all patient records must be saved until the statute of limitations has expired for the particular patient. (See chap. 13.) Complete records about a patient, dating from the first visit to the latest, can be of invaluable assistance to the dentist in planning a course of treatment and in observing gradually changing physical conditions. Thus, patient records must be preserved until the dentist is positive that they are of no further use to him or to his patient.

In conducting a business, files are *indispensable*. They are the memory of a business. Files are containers in which papers are

1. Ernest G. Bormann et al. *Interpersonal Communication in the Modern Organization*, p. 8.

stored. Many years ago *vertical files* were invented when it was discovered that papers placed on end in a folder were easier to locate, remove, and return to the file than were papers stacked in a pile on a spindle. Today there are many versions of vertical files, but the principle of vertical filing is still considered the most efficient method of storing papers.

The basic function of filing is the storing of records in a safe place in a way which permits finding them quickly when needed. It means to file only papers which ought to be kept and file them so they can be found. The filing equipment should conserve time and space and should provide adequate protection of records. Cabinets are available for storing every standard-size record including X rays. Filing cabinets can be obtained with or without locks; shelf filing cabinets are also obtainable with slide-out covers with or without locks.

Filed materials consist of records or papers which come into the office and must be kept, copies of materials which leave the office, and records made in the office for use within the office. The employee to whom the task of filing is delegated must understand how to organize the filing system, must use good judgment in what is filed, and must decide when to dispose of filed material. Usually the employer sets policies for preservation and disposition of the records.

It is important for the employee responsible for filing to have a written list of classifications used in the subject matter file. This list will include such subjects as taxes, dental supplies, office supplies, bank records, A.D.A. correspondence, and any organization with whom the office personnel correspond. Many other subjects will be used. A typed list of file subjects, with notations concerning the material to be filed under each subject, is necessary to prevent misfiling of materials.

All records or papers which require filing in the dental office should be filed accurately and immediately on completion of any service which required their use. In other words, all records should be filed promptly when your work with them is completed. There should be no stack of records on your desk for days awaiting action—posting of charges, for example. The records may be needed in the operatory, and someone else of the office personnel may search for many minutes for a record which has not been returned to its proper place in the files. File accurately and immediately on completion of work with all records.

Types of Filing in the Dental Office

Three types of filing may be used in a dental office. The *alphabetic* file is exactly what its name implies—a set of records filed in the same sequence as the letters of the alphabet —and is most commonly used for patient records. A *numeric* file is one in which records are given a number and placed in numerical order. With this method a numerical guidebook or file of names is used—the names listed in alphabetical order with the number assigned each name listed therein. The assistant checks this alphabetical file for the correct number and then removes the folder from the numeric file. The third type of file which may be used in the office is the *subject* file. Records concerned with taxes, dental supplies, bank records, etc., will be filed under guides labeled by these subjects. The subjects will be in alphabetical order, and the correspondence and materials within each subject will also be in alphabetical order. The size of this file and its use will depend entirely upon your dentist's approach to his practice of dentistry.

There are advantages to each type of filing. The alphabetic file means the clerk looks immediately for the name of the person whose file she wants. The disadvantages are (1) that the spelling of a name may cause problems in finding the record and (2) that some of the letters of the alphabet are more common beginning letters of surnames, resulting in uneven distribution behind the various guide cards.

The numeric file requires the file clerk to look on a visible file for the name of the patient in order to find his number, and she then must be certain she has the correct number before she looks up the record number. The advantage is that the records may be distributed more evenly on the shelves. The users of this system feel that less time is spent in finding a record. They believe it is faster to locate a name on the *visible* file, where names are quickly seen (several at a glance), and to pull a folder from the numeric file than it is to find a record filed in an alphabetic file. It also allows for more accuracy in filing because numbers seem to be easier to read than letters in a name.

A *visible* file is one in which the name of the patient is entered on a "name" line provided on a 3″ x 5″ card. The card is inserted in a protective plastic folder and arranged in a rack or flat drawer so that the "name" line of each card shows. The cards either hang or lie flat, depending on whether the file is a rack or a flat drawer. (See figs. 9.2, 9.3, 9.4.)

Indexing

Materials to be filed are usually put into folders which have a raised tab on them so that the name or filing classification can be written on the tab for easier reading. Indexing is then accomplished by sorting the materials according to the information written on the tabs. The name, subject, or number on this tab is called the *caption*.

Cross-referencing

A record is filed under the caption most likely to be used. However, sometimes the record could be requested under a caption of secondary importance (fig. 9.1).

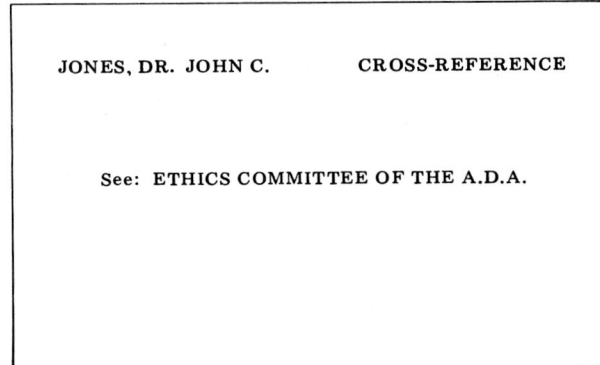

JONES, DR. JOHN C.   CROSS-REFERENCE

See: ETHICS COMMITTEE OF THE A.D.A.

Fig. 9.1. A cross-reference index card

For example, your dentist may be chairman of a committee on ethics for the American Dental Association. He corresponds with a number of dentists who are on this committee, and this correspondence is filed under *Ethics Committee of the A.D.A.* One day your dentist wishes to see a letter from Dr. John C. Jones about the Ethics Committee, but he may not be specific enough to add the last phrase. You look under *Jones, Dr. John C.,* but you do not find the letter since it is filed under *Ethics Committee.* However, you do find a cross-reference index card in the file. The caption is headed *Jones, Dr. John C.* On the card is written "See: Ethics Committee of the A.D.A." This card has been placed in the file with the caption *Jones, Dr. John C.* at its top. When you look for *Jones, Dr. John C.,* you are directed to the *Ethics Committee* by *cross-referencing.*

Steps in Filing

When the material is ready to be filed, the assistant should complete these duties:

1. She should *inspect* it to be certain that it is worthy of filing and that it is ready to be filed. To determine whether or not the material ought to be saved, she should ask herself these questions: (*a*) Will the information in this letter be needed later? (*b*) Is this record required by some government service? and (*c*) Is there a legal necessity for keeping the record? If the answer to any one of these questions is *yes*, the letter should then be readied for filing. As soon as the requests in the letter have been accomplished, it is ready for storage.
2. She should *index* it under the caption most likely to be used when a request to see it again is received.
3. She should *code* it; that is, underline the words on the letter which are used for the caption.
4. She should *sort* it, alphabetically or numerically, depending on the filing system.
5. She should *store* it in the proper folder in the proper file.

Removing Filed Material

As important as proper storage of filed materials is the appropriate way to remove the filed materials for work. Proper safeguards prevent the loss of materials or the misfiling of some item, which is the same as loss in many instances.

The bookmark method of removing a file from its normal position is a time-saver. The folder is raised until the left end can rest on the edge of the file drawer. The right bottom edge is now at the bottom of the drawer, or slightly higher. The folder is somewhat diagonally exposed. It is easy to extract or insert a paper and replace the folder without having to relocate the proper place for that folder.

In another filing system in which folders must be removed for use, colored cardboards are placed in the file at the place the folder is removed. When the folder is to be replaced, it is easier to find its exact location. At this time the cardboard is removed from the file.

Charge-Out Methods

When a patient record folder is removed from the file, or an entire folder from the correspondence file, an out-guide or out-folder should be placed in the file to replace the missing folder. When a single paper is removed from the folder which is left in the file, a substitution card should be placed in the folder.

The date and name of the person removing the file should be written on the charge-out form attached to the guide.

The charge-out system has three reasons for use:

1. It shows the records are being used, and are not lost.
2. It tells the file clerk whom to contact for return of records.
3. It makes refiling easy by marking the place from which the material was removed.

Rules for Alphabetic Filing

A few carefully observed rules for the alphabetic file will establish a smoothly operating memory system in the dental office.

The importance of obtaining the correct spelling of a new patient's name can hardly be overemphasized. Once it has been obtained, it should be carefully printed or typed to avoid errors in transcription. Although original mistakes may be discovered later, it is difficult to rectify errors which have been recorded in a number of different places—recall files, birthday files, radiograph files, patient service and account records, and even visible index files which are used in some offices. Meticulous care at the *first* visit will save much needless work later.

Equal care with respect to the spelling of the name on return visits will save much lost time in searching for previous records.

In addition, it is essential to adopt a standardized method of *filing* names, many of which could conceivably be filed in more than one way. The choice may be somewhat arbitrary, but once adopted the method must be followed consistently. Some of the examples presented here come in this category. Following are a few basic rules to observe when filing:[2]

1. As alphabetical files of names are traditionally arranged according to the surname, it is important to determine which *is* the surname, and which are the first and middle names, and to record and file them in that order. A great many names, of course, offer no problem.

   Example: John J. Brown
   Filed as: BROWN, John J.

2. It is also customary to file a married woman's record by her own name and add her husband's name as a cross-reference.

   Example: Mary Williams Brown
   Filed as: BROWN, Mary Williams (Mrs. John J.)

   As an optional method in the smaller dental office, a name such as this is often filed:

   BROWN, Mrs. John J. (Mary Williams)

3. In some names—including many of foreign derivation—the surname is not always so obvious.

2. Adapted from *Medical Radiography and Photography*. Courtesy of Roscoe E. Miller, M.D.

When it can be determined, it is filed according to rule 1.

Example: C. D. Abd El Naur
Filed as: ABD EL NAUR, C. D.

Otherwise, it is recorded as written.

Example: Ah Hap Akee
Filed as: AH Hap Akee

4. Hyphenated names are filed as one name, disregarding hyphen and second capital.

   Example: Richard Baron-Opits
   Filed as: BARON-OPITS, Richard

5. Prefixes of one or more syllables, with or without capitals and apostrophes, are considered part of the surname.

   Example: Charles M. DeLacy
   Filed as: DeLACY, Charles M.

   Example: Joseph P. D'Agostino
   Filed as: D'AGOSTINO, Joseph P.

   Example: Alfred de la Durantye
   Filed as: de la DURANTYE, Alfred

   Example: James R. McKenzie
   Filed as: McKENZIE, James R.

6. The alphabetical filing of names means that alphabetical order is used throughout the entire group of names, such as Abbott through Zenith. It also means that the same order is used from the first to the last letter of the name when filing names beginning with the same letter.

   Example: John M. Anderson and George L. Abbott
   Filed in this order: ABBOTT, George L.
   ANDERSON, John M.

   b in A*b*bott precedes *n* in A*n*derson.

   Example: Jane Anderson and Mary Andersen
   Filed in this order: ANDERSEN, Mary
   ANDERSON, Jane

   e in Anders*e*n comes before *o* in Anders*o*n.

If there are several identical last names; the given name is used, and if necessary, the middle initial.

Example: Paul K. Anderson and Paul J. Anderson

Filed in this order: ANDERSON, Paul J.
ANDERSON, Paul K.

If the middle initials are the same, the middle name is used.

Example: Paul John Anderson and Paul James Anderson.

Filed in this order:
ANDERSON, Paul James
ANDERSON, Paul John

If there is no middle initial, the rule that nothing comes before something is followed.

Example: Mary Brown and Mary A. Brown

Filed in this order: BROWN, Mary
BROWN, Mary A.

Initials precede a full name.

Example: J. Phillip Sorenson and James Bruce Sorenson

Filed in this order:
SORENSON, J. Phillip
SORENSON, James Bruce

Titles are disregarded in filing but are included in parentheses at the end of the name.

Example: Dr. J. Phillip Sorenson

Filed as: SORENSON, J. Phillip (Dr.)

Finding Filed Records in the Alphabetic File

In order to find names, it is necessary for the searcher to know the rules by which they have been filed. There are inevitably a certain number of occasions when records filed alphabetically cannot be found, either because the name was originally misspelled and hence misfiled

or because the name given at return visits was in error. In searching for these records, time can be saved if you understand and keep in mind the likely sources of error and search in a logical manner. The majority of errors in names are caused (1) by failure to ascertain the correct spelling of names pronounced, (2) by errors in transcribing from handwriting, and (3) by transposition of first name and surname. A few typical situations follow:

1. Incorrect spelling.
   a. Names pronounced alike, or almost alike, but spelled differently.

      Examples: Jeffrey / Geoffrey
      Catherine / Katherine
      Kohn / Cohn
      Acheson / Atchison
      Kennedy / Canady
      Miller / Mueller
      Caine / Kane
      Bach / Bock
      Atkins / Adkins
      Carroll / Carrol
      Schwarzrock / Schwartzrock
      Reed / Reid

2. Errors in transcribing from handwriting.
   a. Initial letters that may look alike.
      Examples: *C/G; K/R; A/O; U/V; G/Y*
   b. Internal letters or combinations of letters which may look alike.
      Examples: *u/ei/ie/n; a/o; i/e; m/ni*
   c. Transposition of letters in typing
      Examples: A*d*ler / A*l*der
      Deigert / Diegert

3. Wrong designation of surname.
   Examples:
   Henry James, / HENRY, James
   Craig Douglas / CRAIG, Douglas

Occasionally problems arise that are not due to errors in recording or filing the name. One source of trouble is a change of name since the previous visit. A patient of foreign birth may have Anglicized his name. A woman may have married or resumed her maiden name. A child's name may have been changed by adoption. A man may have begun to use a middle name rather than his first name. When a record cannot be found for a patient who claims previous examination, tactful questioning may be necessary.

Shelf Filing with Numeric System

Some dental offices are accepting a new approach to filing called the shelf file. The filing cabinet consists of a vertical series of open shelves. (See fig. 9.2.) The records are filed edgewise on these shelves, with a patient's number or name on a visible outer end of the patient folder. A sliding door which locks in

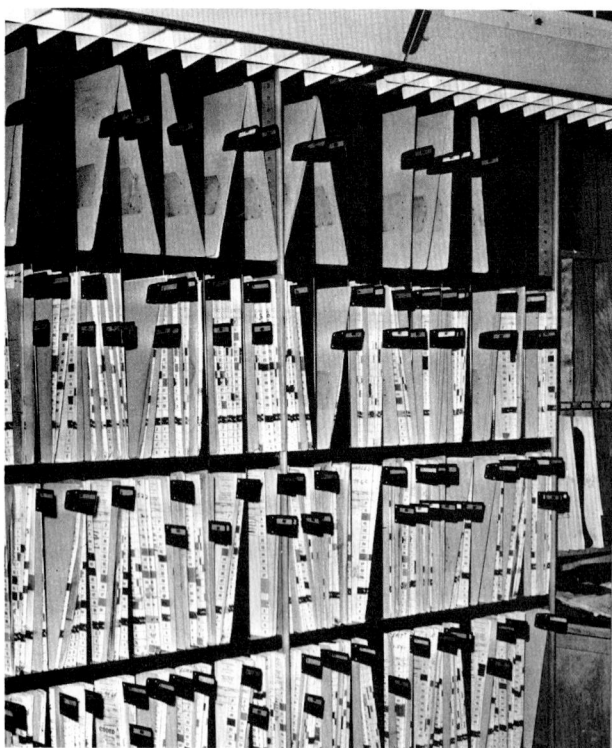

Fig. 9.2. Open-shelf files

place over the records when desired can be part of the file purchased from some manufacturers.

This method lends itself very well to numeric filing.

Numeric Filing

Straight numeric systems do not lend themselves to dental office use, but one variation of numeric systems is extremely useful in the large clinic practices which have thousands of patients. This variation is known as "terminal digit" filing in which a number, usually consisting of three pairs of digits (such as 72-56-34), is given to each patient in a master control listing. The advantage of the terminal digit method is the elimination of the difficulty of filing many nearly identical names and the consequent frequency of error, as well as the tedious relocating of a particular patient's file. This method is also very convenient to use with shelf files, which are more compact and less expensive than cabinet files when a large installation is required. The method also results in a uniform distribution of patient records throughout the filing area rather than a very heavy load, for example, behind the letter *B* and a very light load behind the letter *Y* in an alphabetic file.

A brief description of the working of the terminal digit method may make it sound complex, but it is actually a simple method of indexing and filing. The number is read from right to left. The first two numbers on the right are known as the primary or terminal digit numbers. The second two numbers from the right are known as secondary digits. In a terminal digit system, the number given previously, 72-56-34, would be filed behind a guide showing "34" as the terminal digit number. In "guiding" terminal digit, terminal numbers (primary guides) are arranged from 00 to 99. Further breakdowns are made by secondary

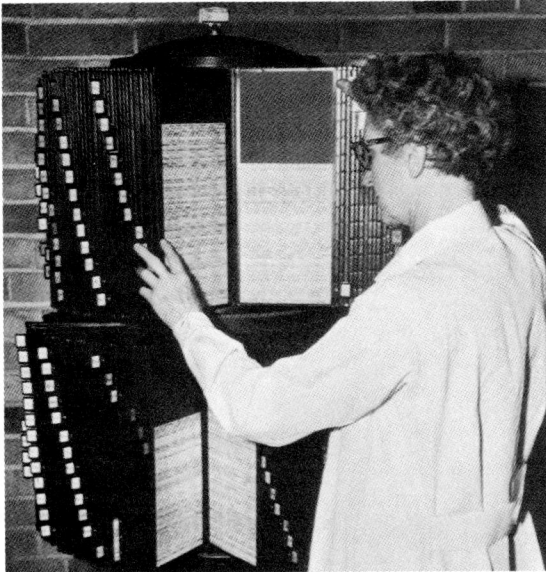

Fig. 9.3. Master (cross-index) file of patients and their terminal digit numbers.

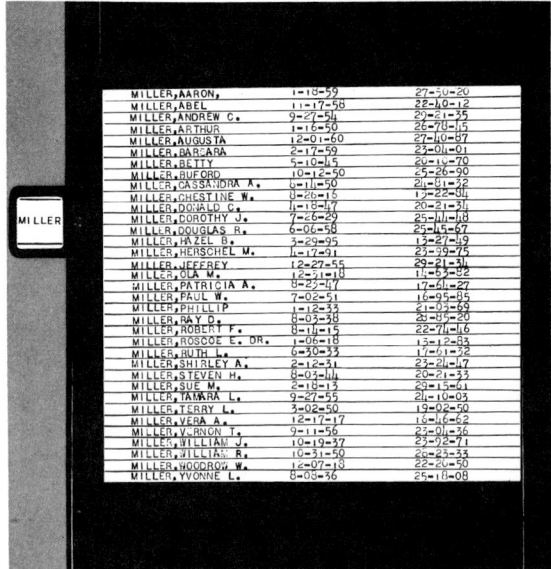

Fig. 9.4. One portion of the master file shown in figure 9.3.

digits, from 00 to 99 behind each primary guide, a maximum of 100. In many cases the secondary digit guides can be less than a complete set because of the tremendous capacity of this arrangement. In large filing applications, this method is simple, fast, and accurate.

Filing Color Slides

The enthusiasm for photography with dentistry indicates a need for well-filed slides. The number of slides collected usually grows rapidly. To have them properly filed makes them useful when your dentist wants them.

Slides are used to show a patient "before" and "after" shots of his mouth and to help him see the need for improvement in dental health or appearance. Slides are also used to help educate patients about dental conditions. Sometimes your dentist talks to a high school science class or other meeting, and these slides are very helpful for his speech.

It is important to file them properly. An excellent system for such filing has been explained by Edward T. Wentworth, D.D.S.[3]

Filing Patient Records

The manner of classifying patient records for filing will depend, to a large degree, on the method of bookkeeping and billing employed in your office. Patient records are usually filed in two or three groupings. The separation of the patient records into these groupings is to place in a file for ease of access the records of patients who are currently being treated. Records of patients who have not been in the office for a long period of time are filed separately. The files of patients are usually referred to as *active, accounts receivable,* and *inactive* or *dead.*

3. Edward T. Wentworth, "Filing Color Slides," *Dental Radiography and Photography,* pp. 36-37.

The *active* file contains the service folders of all patients who are considered by the dentist to be included in his practice.

The *accounts receivable* file contains the records of all patients whose work is complete but who have not completed payment for services rendered. When a patient has finished paying for his dentistry, his file is transferred to the active file.

The *inactive* file contains the envelopes of patients who are not expected to return to the office as patients in the future and whose accounts are paid in full.

When a patient's record is placed in the inactive file, the reason for this placement should be entered. The X rays are removed from the mounts and placed in a coin envelope labeled with the date the X rays were taken and the patient's name. All paper clips are removed to eliminate bulk. The small envelopes of X rays and all the cards from other files, such as recall control and/or birthday control cards, are placed in the patient's envelope.

If the office uses a separate patient service record and patient account record, there will also be a patient account record (usually a 4″ x 6″ card) in the patient account file. If a patient's service record is transferred to the inactive file, the account record is placed inside his service record envelope for storage.

Thus, the entire data on the patient is filed in one envelope in the inactive file, including the reason the record is in this file.

In some offices, the dentist makes a distinction between *inactive* and *dead*, keeping in the inactive file records of patients who are not currently patients but who were seen in the office during a specified period of time. He transfers to the dead file the records of those patients who have not been seen during that length of time. For example, the dentist may decide that records of patients who have not been in the office in two years are to be placed in the inactive file. When five years have passed and the patient has not been in the office, the records are then transferred to the dead file.

Retention of Records

Why keep patients' records when they have presumably left the practice? One reason is that patients sometimes return to a practice which they left as long as ten years before. It is helpful to have a record of the last contact with these patients. Sometimes patients move out of town but eventually return to resume living in the community, and they return to the same dentist.

The legal reason for keeping a patient's records in an inactive or dead file is that a patient can sue the dentist for malpractice any time before the statute of limitations expires. This limitation is regulated by the state governments, and it is wise to know the length of time specified in your state.

The records of a deceased person should be retained, as well as the records of patients who no longer come for dental care, until the statute of limitations has expired. Minors are privileged to sue for a period of time (after they reach their majority) equal to the statute of limitations. Records of minors must therefore be kept until they are no longer considered minors and then for the number of years specified in your state statute of limitations law. Consult an attorney who is familiar with this law.

If space is not a problem, it is wise to keep all the records of all patients, except perhaps those of a deceased person, for as long as it is possible to store them.

Since patient records must be kept as long as the statute of limitations indicates in your state, problems in filing can become a burden. To keep the folders of inactive patients with the active ones means handling hundreds of records to find the comparatively few to be used. Thus, a vault or storage room for the safekeeping of inactive records is most desirable.

Transfer of Records

Transfer of records to the dead storage area should occur on a planned schedule, such as quarterly.

Decisions as to when a record is transferred must be made by the staff member assigned this responsibility. A card index file of the names of patients whose records are in dead storage should be kept.

Transfer cabinets of inexpensive materials are available for storing old records which must be kept. Some of these cabinets are corrugated fiberboard. The records so filed are kept in these transfer boxes in the same alphabetical or numerical order they had in the office.

A card should be prepared to indicate the transfer of the records to dead storage. This card should include the name and the address of the patient, the date of transfer, reason for transfer, and the date the statute of limitations expires so that the dead file can be cleared periodically of records which are no longer useful. Such a transfer file is kept in a special drawer in the files.

Patients' Account Records

Some patient account records are filed on cards for posting. They are vertical files or visible files (cards standing upright or cards laid in a drawer with the front edge of each card showing—see fig. 9.4).

Both visible and vertical files are used to refer to existing information and to record new information. These files are frequently used for patient account records because new entries can be added easily, payment habits of the patient can be readily ascertained, and the amount owed by any patient is easily seen.

In some very large clinics a motorized rotary file may be used in which the drawers are brought into position by motor. (They rotate inside a huge metal compartment.)

Summary

Filing is the arranging of papers or records in methodical order for preservation and convenient reference. Papers or records should be filed promptly when work with them is completed in order that they can be quickly located again.

Three types of filing may be used in the dental office: *alphabetic, numeric,* and *subject.*

Care must be taken to accurately spell names to be put in the file. Rules for filing sequence in your office should be established and followed.

Dental offices usually have active, inactive, and accounts receivable files where the folders of patients are kept. They also have a subject file where headings such as Current Invoices, Taxes, and Bank Records will be found.

Indexing is accomplished by sorting the materials according to the information written on the tabs. The name, subject, or number on this tab is called the *caption.*

Cross-referencing is used when a material could be filed under two or more headings.

There are five steps in filing: inspection, indexing, coding, sorting, and storing.

Removal of filed material must be accomplished according to rules which allow personnel to know where the materials are.

Shelf filing is a more recent addition to the area of storing materials. The vertical series of open shelves allow easier access to the materials.

A *numeric system of filing* known as terminal digit filing is commonly used in large medical offices. A *rotating visible file* is used with this system.

Patient records must be kept as long as the statute of limitations indicates in the state in which the dentist is practicing. *Dead storage filing* is used to hold records of patients not currently in the practice until such time as the statute of limitations expires at which time the materials can be destroyed.

There are three questions which you can ask yourself to determine whether or not to retain a record.

Transfer of the records to dead storage should occur on a planned schedule, such as quarterly. A card indicating the transfer should be made out and kept in a file in the office.

Vertical or *visible files* frequently are used for patient account records.

There are three reasons for using a *charge-out system* for removing records from the file: to show the records are being used, to tell who has the records, and to make refiling easy by marking the place in the file from which the material was removed.

Study Questions

1. List the three types of filing which may be used in the dental office.
2. Explain indexing.
3. Define cross-referencing and explain when it is used.
4. List the five steps in filing.
5. State three reasons for using a charge-out system.
6. Describe a terminal digit file.
7. Describe a visible file.
8. How long must patient records be kept?
9. How do you determine which material is to be placed in dead storage?

Bibliography

BORMANN, ERNEST; HOWELL, WILLIAM S.; NICHOLS, RALPH G.; SHAPIRO, GEORGE. *Interpersonal Communication in the Modern Organization.* Englewood Cliffs, N. J.: Prentice-Hall, 1969.

KAHN, GILBERT; YERIAN, THEODORE; and STEWART, J. R. *Progressive Filing and Records Management.* New York: McGraw-Hill, 1962.

MILLER, ROSCOE E. "Radiography Filing Facilities and Loan Service," *Medical Radiography and Photography* 38, no. 2 (1962).

WENTWORTH, EDWARD. "Filing Color Slides," *Dental Radiography and Photography* 37, no. 2 (1964). Rochester, N. Y.: Eastman Kodak Company.

10 | *Written Communications*

The Right Impression

Earlier in the text we discussed the importance of greeting new arrivals in your reception room with warmth and cordiality. We spoke of creating the right impression on the public and of considering everyone as a very important person in whom you are interested.

The same philosophy in working with people is necessary in written communications. The letters, reports, and statements which leave your office tell a tale about you, your dentist, and the way your office operates. What sort of impression is being created?

If the paper used to write the letter is the dollar-per-ream cheapest typing paper available, if there are no printed letterheads, if the typist has struck over her errors, erased some and left smudges, used no planning in creating the format of the letter or report, misspelled words, and used incorrect punctuation and incorrect grammar, what is the receiver going to think about the office?

Obviously he will be suspicious. He may feel sorry for the dentist who is unable to hire any better help, but he may also wonder whether the dental assisting in the office is of the same poor quality—whether instruments are sterile when they need to be. He may also wonder whether this dentist is capable of providing his patients with adequate care.

A dental office ought to use a bond paper of fine quality for its reports. It should use the same grade of bond paper for letterhead stationery on which the dentist's name, address (plus zip code), and telephone number, including area code, have been printed or engraved. The stationery should be businesslike in appearance. This does not necessarily eliminate an artistic, beautiful design, nor even the use of sophisticated color. Some men use an off-white or slightly grayed, blued, or other-colored paper and do so without seeming unbusinesslike or effeminate. Some men have an effective design developed which distinguishes their stationery. The minimum requirement is a printed letterhead giving the name of the dentist with his degrees after his name, his street address under his name, and his city, state, and zip code under the street address. This is usually centered on the paper. The typist can then align the date of the letter under the city and state, or type it in the conventional place on the right-hand side of the page, or use the newer left-hand block form.

Envelopes to match the stationery should be available, with a printed return on them, also. Envelopes for other purposes should be available, too. Window envelopes are often used for billing purposes. The dentist's name and address should be printed in the upper left corner.

A satisfactory grade of paper should be kept for carbon copies. Plenty of high-quality carbon should also be available. Correction sheets and fluids are excellent aids in making neat, almost unnoticeable corrections. Erasers are also helpful.

It is possible to purchase copy paper for which no carbon is necessary. Simply place the sheet behind the original letterhead you are to type on, and the copy appears on the second sheet. This paper is somewhat more expensive but is perhaps worth it when you consider the cost and bother of carbon paper.

The typing area within the office should be equipped with a very well built desk of proper height for typing, drawer or cabinet space for all the supplies which are needed at the typewriter, a rack on which to rest copy (whether the copy be a report or a secretary's notebook), adequate light, a good typewriter, and a chair which encourages the best posture for typing.

Should any of these items be missing, consult your dentist and try to acquire the necessary equipment to make it possible for you to do an excellent job of public relations via the written communications from your office.

The administrative dental assistant who is assigned to secretarial duties should keep the same kind of inventory of stationery supplies as the chair assistant keeps of the dental supplies. Prior to running out of stationery, an order should be placed in ample time to receive the new supply before it is needed.

It is possible to obtain such aids as *25 Typing Shortcuts* and *155 Office Shortcuts and Time Savers for the Secretary.*[1] These booklets have excellent suggestions for more efficient use of your typewriter and other office equipment.

In today's dental office not only is the typewriter a necessity, its effective operation is essential. Certainly courses in the use of this type of equipment are desirable, if not essential. If you have had a basic course in typing, there are many shortcuts you can learn from the booklets already mentioned.

If you are skilled in using shorthand, you know the supplies which you need to keep available. If you work in an office in which a dictaphone or tape recorder is used instead of shorthand, the typing center must also contain the necessary equipment for playing tapes or records and listening to them without the patients in the reception room or any of the

1. Cf. Bibliography.

rest of the staff being able to hear. Head-phones are usually provided, or an earpiece similar to a hearing aid.

There are some aids for working with a dictating machine which can be helpful. For example, if the dictator has not keyed his letters or commented at the end of each letter about the enclosures for that letter, it is a good idea to keep a notebook handy and list the enclosures as he comments on them during the dictation of the letter. It is also desirable to listen once to the tape before beginning to type the letter. In this way, you will pick up the corrections and have a good idea of the length of the letter before you make that excellent copy which is to leave the office.

Methods of Assisting Your Dentist When Taking Dictation

Although letter writing may be infrequent in the dental office, it does occur in some offices.

A planned time for dictation is a part of good office organization.

You can help your dentist most if you will adopt the attitude that you are not expected to assume *anything*. Ask him about anything you do not understand. Ask immediately, or if he objects to being interrupted, ask at the close of the document he is dictating.

Be certain that you understand names: full names, spelling, titles, and addresses. After you become acquainted with your dentist and his activities, most of these names will be familiar to you and will not present the problem they do the first time you hear them.

When your dentist gives you instructions about the correspondence, put a number by the part of the letter to which the instructions apply and write your instructions as an additional note to your work with the same number by it. In this way each instruction will be numbered, and there can be no mistake about which instruction fits which piece of dictation.

Be sure your dentist dictates slowly enough for you to be accurate in your work. It is inconceivable that anyone would attempt to take dictation from a dentist without first having mastered the most frequent dental terms used by this particular dentist.

When you are certain you know just what is expected of you and that your dentist has finished his dictation for this period, take with you the material to be answered and your notebook and pencils, being certain to leave the chair in which you sat in its proper position. Be a good housekeeper. Keep looking for straightening-up jobs as you work around the office.

Prompt transcription of shorthand notes, dictaphone records, or tapes is most desirable. If the dentist has not indicated which material is most important, it is necessary for the secretary to use her best judgment in deciding the order in which she types up her notes.

At least one copy is made of every paper which leaves the office. Sometimes a dentist prefers to have two copies. This is usually true in an office which uses a follow-up file.

Occasionally it is necessary for a secretary to correct a statement which she has in her dictation. If the statement is unclear, if the grammar is incorrect, or if for some reason it is necessary to reevaluate the statement, it is important that her dentist be consulted before any change is made in his dictated notes. It is absolutely necessary to correct any errors before the transcript leaves the office, even if this means an extra consultation with the dentist.

Shortcuts to Note-taking

Sometimes it is necessary for an employee who has not had shorthand to take dictation or notes about an employer's dictation. The trick is to work out a system of abbreviation which may be unique to you, but which you can understand.

You can learn a system like Gregg Notehand or you can make your own from longhand abbreviations. The longhand abbreviations are not as fast, it is true, but if you haven't already learned a system, longhand abbreviations will help you until you can learn one. The only caution is to be sure to write legibly.

For example, drop all unused letters.

learn = lrn	can = cn
abbreviations = abrvns	communications = cmcns
	may = ma
true = tru	become = bcum
be = b	our = r
you = u	are = r
for = 4	

This system can be used for dental terminology which is long and hard to write. Be sure you have a medical dictionary for unscrambling the abbreviations at the time of deciphering.

Business Letter Form

Design the letter which is to leave the office so that it is an excellent representative of you and your dentist. From one point of view a letter is an ambassador—it *represents* the office. Sometimes it is the only criteria by which the receiver can judge the quality of dentistry and professionalism of the office.

Following are some helpful suggestions:

1. A letter should be a beautiful work of art —even margins at both right and left sides and preferably the same margin on the top, with a slightly larger one at the bottom whenever possible. Consider the letterhead as part of the letter when planning composition of the page to look like a picture (fig. 10.1).
2. All business letters have the writer's address and the date at the top. If your den-

tist's stationery has his name and address printed at the top in the center, type the date below the address. If your letters are written on plain typing paper, the address and the date are typed on the right-hand side of the paper, at the top. (See fig. 10.2.)

3. The name of the person to whom the letter is written and his address are placed on the left-hand side. This information is often referred to as the "inside address." (See figs. 10.1 and 10.3.)
4. In formal business letters the salutation is still "Dear Mr. Blank," or "My dear Mr. Milquetoast"; *but*—a new trend in letter writing is to drop this meaningless phrase and substitute one which is both appropriate and cordial. For example:

   "It is a pleasure, Doctor Smith ....
   . . . . . to respond to your letter addressed to Mr. Cawley."

   or

   "Thank you, Mr. Jones ....
   . . . . . for your frank statement regarding your account."

5. The body of the letter is then typed.
6. A complimentary closing follows, but instead of the formal "Yours truly," more and more businessmen are substituting "Sincerely" or "Cordially yours."
7. A space should be left for the dentist's signature. Type his name below the space. Correspondence should be signed by the dentist, unless the assistant writes the letter personally. Never sign the dentist's name and initial it. Sign only those letters which are written by you.
8. Be certain to consult your dictionary if you are in doubt about the spelling of any words. See that the letter is correctly punctuated, also.
9. Avoid typographical errors. If they are unavoidable, make a neat erasure of the

incorrect letter and then lightly strike the correct typewriter key. The erasure will be less obvious than if you strike heavily or try to restrike all the letters in that word. Your eraser must be of good quality and do a clean job. You may prefer to use Typerase which allows you to correct without erasing.

10. Single-space letters of normal length. Double-space between the paragraphs. If a letter is very short, double-space it.

11. Decide on the form of the letter. If you prefer to use block form, there will be no indentation. The division between paragraphs is recognized by the double-spacing. If you wish to use an indentation at the beginning of a paragraph, this is acceptable form. The first sentence of the paragraph is usually indented five spaces from the left margin. Double-spacing between the paragraphs then becomes a matter of choice rather than necessity.

12. The length of a letter determines the margins and placement of the letter on the page. If there is any speculation that a letter is too long for one page, widen the margins and make it a two-page letter rather than crowd it all on one page. Normally, the second page of a letter is written on plain paper of the same quality as the stationery, with the dentist's name imprinted on it. It is numbered —2— at the top and frequently bears a line of type giving the names of the addressee and sender and the date.

13. It is sometimes necessary to type up a rough draft for the dentist to read prior to final typing.

Signatures

After you type a letter, *proofread* it. If it is perfect, clip the enclosures and the envelope to it. Place all letters on your dentist's desk

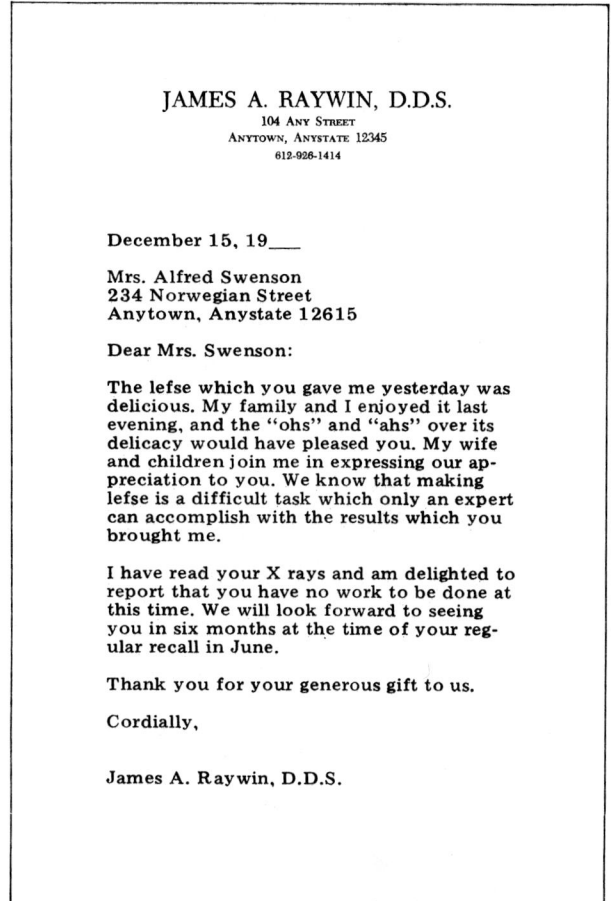

JAMES A. RAYWIN, D.D.S.
104 ANY STREET
ANYTOWN, ANYSTATE 12345
612-926-1414

December 15, 19___

Mrs. Alfred Swenson
234 Norwegian Street
Anytown, Anystate 12615

Dear Mrs. Swenson:

The lefse which you gave me yesterday was delicious. My family and I enjoyed it last evening, and the "ohs" and "ahs" over its delicacy would have pleased you. My wife and children join me in expressing our appreciation to you. We know that making lefse is a difficult task which only an expert can accomplish with the results which you brought me.

I have read your X rays and am delighted to report that you have no work to be done at this time. We will look forward to seeing you in six months at the time of your regular recall in June.

Thank you for your generous gift to us.

Cordially,

James A. Raywin, D.D.S.

Fig. 10.1. A well-planned letter with even margins

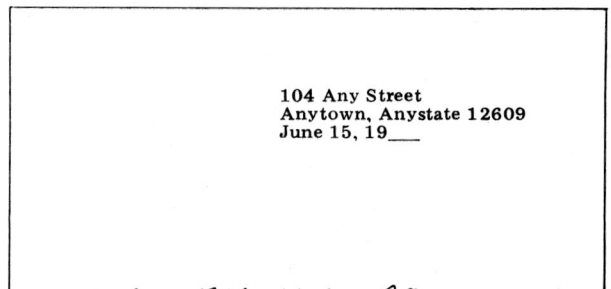

104 Any Street
Anytown, Anystate 12609
June 15, 19___

Fig. 10.2. A letterhead typed on plain typing paper

JAMES A. RAYWIN, D.D.S.
104 ANY STREET
ANYTOWN, ANYSTATE 12345
612-926-1414

June 15, 19___

Mr. James R. Jones
251 South Magnolia Avenue
Anytown, Anystate 12610

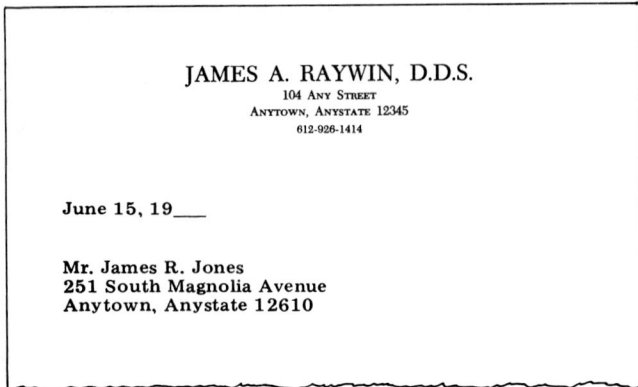

Fig. 10.3. Letterhead stationery properly dated and addressed.

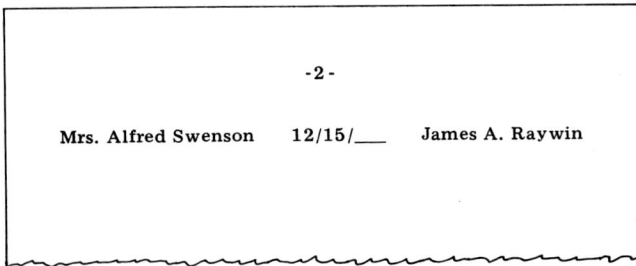

-2-

Mrs. Alfred Swenson   12/15/___   James A. Raywin

Fig. 10.4. Sample top for second page of letter

for his signature. The dentist should always sign his own letters. Never sign his name and your initials.

After he has signed the letters, fold them and put them in the envelopes with the proper enclosures. File the carbon copies and the letters which prompted the dentist to write.

Be sure to weigh any letters which are more than two sheets of paper to be certain you have the correct postage on them.

Written Communications Created by the Dental Assistant

During your career as a dental assistant, you may be required to write some original memo-

randa and perhaps some original letters of your own. The composition of such letters is important.

Most letters are written with the purpose of getting someone to do something willingly. The advantage and desirability of the action suggested must be "sold." The letter should be planned to bring about willing cooperation—persuasion rather than force—inducement rather than threats. The grammar and punctuation must be correct, and the sentences must be complete.

The wordiness and complexity of many business letters are carry-overs from the old days when letters were serious documents. They were often semilegal evidences of contractual offer and acceptance. A pattern of stereotyped expressions was developed, and the pattern has persisted to this day.

The formality and stiffness we encounter in many letters are similarly due to the influence of the past. Letters were often addressed to one's social superiors. For example, a tradesman wrote to a nobleman and thus used almost apologetic language. Letters were written infrequently, but when written, they became matters of the greatest importance: "I take pen in hand, . . . etc.," "Yours of the 24th inst. has been received." Endings frequently began with a participle—*Hoping, Trusting,* or *Thanking*—all in the vein of humility.

Business correspondence today aims for simplicity and conciseness. Letters are supposed to tell a story in the fewest number of words. Expression is direct and to the point. At the same time, business letters play an important part in developing good public relations; therefore, the qualities of friendliness, courtesy, and thoughtfulness are necessary.

The business letter can be divided into three parts: the opening—to prepare the reader for a favorable reception; the middle—to give the reasons why the reader should do as you wish;

and the closing—to stimulate the desired action.

Business letters must sell before they can tell. The reader must be prepared for a favorable reception of the message. As every person is interested primarily in himself or herself, the beginning of the letter should be about the reader.

A good opening gains the attention of the reader. It is the golden and fleeting opportunity to make a good impression. Don't waste the opening on trivialities. Capture its full value.

How? *By thinking—and writing—of the reader's interest.* By putting the reader in the center of the stage. By searching for the point in the particular letter you are writing that will please, attract, and even flatter the reader.

Just as the salesman relies on a friendly smile and a cordial handshake to win his prospect before making his sales presentation, so also should letter writers use the letter opening to "set the stage" for what they have to say.

Imagine the jolt to the reader receiving a letter which begins:

We have made many requests for payment of your delinquent account, and your failure to respond is very disappointing. You have not kept your word. We must take strong action to force payment.

Admittedly, this paragraph might be contained in a letter sent to a person whose account is in poor condition. However, if he were to come into the office personally to discuss the account, do you suppose the conversation would begin so abruptly? Surely some pleasantries would precede "getting down to brass tacks."

Yet the majority of collection letters swing into offensive action with the first sentence. The thunderbolts are shot without any preliminaries. The usual result is that the reader

is upset and angered, and chances of securing favorable action are much lessened.

Here, for example, are two openings selected from letters dealing with the partial-payment problem:

1. We regret that we have been unable to secure your cooperation in maintaining your account according to our established terms.
2. Your partial payments on your account show a splendid spirit of cooperation. For that we thank you.

Which one do you suppose would make the patient more inclined to mend his ways? Actually, there is not too much difference in words, but there is a great difference in the approach and attitude of the writer.

The Beginning

Letters written from the *We, Me, Us, Our, I, My* viewpoint are less likely to bring results than those which begin with the readers' interests. Examples of such letter openings include: "I feel sure that you overlooked this statement," "I am afraid that you have overlooked us in the matter of payment," and "We need money in order to pay our own bills."

The Middle

The message—why the reader should do as you wish—should be stated clearly; however, few business letters should be more than four paragraphs in length. Just looking at a full sheet of solid type discourages attention. Cluttering a letter with unnecessary explanations or arguments lessens its effectiveness. Ask yourself, What does this mean? Can I say the same thing more simply? Remove all unnecessary wording, but do write what you feel must be communicated. Use a separate paragraph for each main subject or argument.

Preserve the patient's dignity and self-respect. It is easy to make strong statements in your letters, but nothing is gained by such actions. Keep your own temper; the reader will more likely keep his. Some writers tend to hide under the cloak of imagined safety in writing letters—writing what they would not dare say in person. Even so-called "tough" letters should be written with restraint.

The Ending

The ending of the letter is the climax. The ending idea should be fairly short and a paragraph by itself.

It is at the ending that you leave the reader with the definite idea of what you want him to do. Be positive. Avoid weak, negative, and apologetic endings. Courteously, but firmly and unmistakably, point out the action you wish taken.

End the letter with one choice, if possible. Alternative proposals confuse the reader. He isn't quite sure what you want done.

Select the best possible action you wish the reader to take. End your letter with that. Together with the positive ending, the appeal to immediate and definite action, try for some statement that builds goodwill. Those two direct words *Thank you* can be used much more often than they are.

The effective letter, then, begins on the *you* note. It attracts the favorable attention of the reader. Something is said to create a favorable atmosphere for the message. In the middle, the reasons why the reader should follow a course of action are stated. The last paragraph is the ending and the *we* angle. It is here that the reader is told what the writer wants done. *You—Why—We.*

Writing a letter using this formula is more likely to produce the desired results in action and in relationships.

The sample letters which follow are not meant to be copied. They are examples of the form which might receive good results. You may use them as a guide, but make your letter to *your* patient a personal letter in your own style of writing.

Figure 10.5 is a sample of a mild letter to be used after a sticker or stamp "impersonal" series has brought no results and it is felt a letter would be more effective and quite sure to obtain payment.

The same principles of writing business letters can be applied in a letter which is not about collections. Consider the example in figure 10.6. Here the dentist has opened with a pleasant reference to the firm of the man to whom the letter is addressed. This is the *you* approach. He has put his reader in the center of the stage. The middle paragraphs are the message. However, he presents the message to coincide with the interests of the reader, encouraging him to want to do as the writer wishes. The last paragraph, the closing, asks for *action* and attempts to make it as easy as possible for the reader to comply. This letter illustrates the three steps in a business letter: interest, explanation, and action.

Typing Reports

Some dentists use a tape recorder to record their initial examination of a patient. A dentist will often have this recording typed as a case study and included in the patient's record envelope. Whether it is typed on a special report form or on plain typing paper, be sure to proofread the record for accuracy before you file it.

Reports to other dentists, to physicians, or to hospitals require careful typing on appropriate paper. The finished report should be typed with neat margins, no errors, and no smudges. Each page of the report should bear the title and page number. (The title may be a patient's name if the report is a case study.)

You may also type reports on special forms. Use the skills which you have learned in adjusting the typewriter platen so that you can type on the lines provided on the form.

JAMES A. RAYWIN, D.D.S.
104 Any Street
Anytown, Anystate 12345
612-926-1414

Mr. John C. Patient
000 Any Street
Anytown, Anystate 12345

Dear Mr. Patient:

Just a note to tell you that if we can be help-ful in the matter of your account, we would welcome the opportunity.

The usual reminders have been sent to you, but we have had no word from you. Perhaps you have been waiting until you could pay the whole bill at one time.

Sometimes, in every family, unexpected cir-cumstances arise that upset well-laid plans. We certainly would be willing to make spe-cial arrangements with you should that be the case.

In any event, it is important that you come in or write us as soon as possible. You will find us most cooperative.

Cordially yours,

James A. Raywin, D.D.S.

Fig. 10.5. A collection letter

February 22, _____

Mr. Fred J. Schwaemmle
Delta Air Lines
Atlanta Airport
Atlanta, Georgia

Dear Mr. Schwaemmle:

It's a beautiful day in Chicago this morning and a per-fect day for Delta to be flying.

Our American Academy of Dental Practice Administra-tion is looking forward to your Delta-ing to Chicago to speak before us at 9:00 A.M., Friday, February 2, 1968, at the Conrad Hilton Hotel.

I have personally admired the advances of Delta through the years and felt they had a story to tell about the philosophy of Communication and Motiva-tion in developing the wonderful personnel presenta-tion they offer to the public.

You are probably aware that dentistry is one of the greatest needs of modern man. All we in dentistry have to do is to make people want that need. In other words, it is our challenge to make them aware of their problem and create a want of their needs. This re-quires the type of mental attitude that I have wit-nessed in Delta personnel nationally.

It is hoped that the foregoing two paragraphs give you an understanding of the objectives I have in mind. Would you please correspond with me and give me the title of your presentation. Also, would you require one or one and a half hours to present your story? Please do not hesitate to telephone me if you have any per-sonal concern that we could better handle by direct communication.

With kindest regards,

Herbert Gustavson, D.D.S.

Fig. 10.6. An excellent example of letter writing

Courtesy Dr. Herbert Gustavson, Skokie, Ill., and Delta Air Lines

Lengthy reports of committee meetings should be carefully prepared, single-spaced, and properly indented. The object of indenta-tions is to provide ease in reading.

Form letters, prepared individually as a per-sonal letter, are often sent from the dental of-fice. The dentist may have composed several special letters to use when responding to spe-cific requests. When he asks you to use one of these form letters, type it as carefully as you type a letter he dictates. An example of such a form letter might be a thank-you note for re-ferral of a patient.

Insurance reports must often be completed. It is important to keep a carbon copy of each report for future reference.

Other Writing

There are other types of original writing to be accomplished in the dentist's office. He may be conducting some research and thus needs help in gathering data and bibliographical material. He may ask you to help in this work. It will require good note-taking on the books and sources you read in the dental library. Be sure you prepare the bibliography correctly, copying the author, title, publisher, date of publication, place of publication, and any page numbers to which you refer in your notes. Copy the page numbers of the material you read so that your dentist has a reference if he should need to refer to some passage.

SUBJECT: DIET

Nizel, Abraham E. *Nutrition in Preventive Dentistry: Science and Practice.* Philadelphia: W.B. Saunders Company, 1972. pp. 63-64.

"There is indirect evidence that dietary fats may have an anticariogenic effect in humans. For example, Eskimos, whose conventional diets are almost solely of animal origin and furnish about 70-80 percent of their total calories as fat, experience little, if any, decay."

Fig. 10.7. Example of notes for research

When it is necessary to type the final manuscript, follow the rules in whatever procedure manual your dentist uses. There are several, and different universities require different manuals.

When you have completed the typing, proofread *with care* to be absolutely certain your copy is correct.

Sometimes your dentist may be asked to read a paper before a society or study club.

He will need special typing preparation for this. If you have a Selectric typewriter, you can purchase an Orator ball of type which is enlarged print. Or you can rent a special typewriter with "convention" type which prints the large letters used to make name tags at conventions. The use of this size type, triple-spaced, makes a very readable manuscript. However, the capital letters of your own typewriter and proper spacing of the sentences will also facilitate the reading of a paper. Adequate space around the sentences allows the reader to see them in units and lessens the possibility that he will lose his place in the manuscript. See figures 10.8 and 10.9.

Summary

A proper impression should be created by the written materials which leave the dental office. Adequate and proper supplies are necessary. Shortcuts should be visualized and used for accomplishing the tasks necessary to project this impression.

When taking dictation you can assist your dentist by asking questions about anything you do not completely understand.

Prompt transcription is essential.

A business letter must conform to specifications. Thirteen suggestions are given.

Typing reports will be a necessary part of the work of the dental assistant and should conform to the preference of the dentist. All typed materials must be proofread for accuracy.

After the dentist's signature has been placed on mail, promptly fold, insert, seal, and mail the material.

Shortcuts in note-taking are desirable. Omit all unnecessary words such as *the, a,* and *an.* Work out a system of abbreviation which you understand.

I WANT TO TALK TODAY ABOUT INTEGRITY,

I HOPE THAT AFTER I AM THROUGH

WITH MY REMARKS SOMETHING OF

THE SHINING AND WONDERFUL QUALITY

OF THIS VIRTUE WILL REMAIN WITH US.

Fig. 10.8. A readable sample manuscript with enlarged type

I WANT TO TALK TODAY ABOUT INTEGRITY.

I HOPE THAT AFTER I AM THROUGH WITH MY REMARKS

SOMETHING OF THE SHINING AND WONDERFUL QUALITY

OF THIS VIRTUE WILL REMAIN WITH US.

INTEGRITY IS A LATIN WORD

WHICH MEANS UNFLAWED,

UNCORRUPTED, UNTAMPERED WITH.

Fig. 10.9. A readable sample manuscript using capital letters on a standard typewriter

The dental assistant who writes letters signed by herself should use care in the composition of these letters.

A dentist who is doing research may have his assistant gather data and bibliographical material. Careful note-taking and references are important. The use of a manuscript manual in typing these reports is desirable.

Study Questions

1. Why should you ask your dentist about anything which you do not understand during dictation?
2. Why is prompt transcription essential?
3. Describe a well-written business letter.
4. Describe a system of shortcut note-taking.
5. Describe a well-written letter composed by an assistant.
6. What must you include in your notes when you are gathering data and bibliographical material for your dentist?

Bibliography

How To Be a Super-Secretary. Remington Rand Office Machines, Division of Sperry Rand Corporation, 1962.

155 Office Shortcuts and Time Savers for the Secretary. West Nyack, N. J.: Editorial Staff of Parker Publishing Company.

Punctuation in a Nutshell. Prudential Insurance Company of America.

Speak When You Write. Pamphlet on letter-writing, Human Relations Program. Hartford, Conn.: The Connecticut Mutual Life Insurance Co. No charge.

25 Typing Shortcuts. Remington Rand Office Machines, Division of Sperry Rand Corporation.

11 | *Arrangements for the Meeting-Minded Dentist*

When your dentist attends a meeting of a dental society, he may need special preparation for this meeting. A notice of the meeting is usually received through the mail, together with a request for notification of attendance; and sometimes a reservation for luncheon or dinner is to be made.

If your dentist is to attend the meeting, the necessary time must be blocked off in the appointment book and the proper notifications returned to the secretary of the society. If your dentist is an officer of the organization, there may be additional activities for you—secretarial notes to be typed (and even mimeographed), treasurer's reports to be prepared, dues to collect, and programs to prepare. Should your dentist be responsible for a program, it is sometimes necessary for you to contact the speakers and arrange for their accommodations. If he is president, he is responsible for the agenda (plan of what is to be discussed at the meeting), and this agenda should be typed in advance.

Convention and Travel Reservations

Your dentist may attend conventions, study courses, and association meetings held in some other city. Such trips require considerable planning to make all the necessary reservations for travel, hotel, and attendance at the meetings. This is detail work which you can do. You may be asked to take care of such details for other travel as well.

Let us assume that one day your dentist lays a folder on your desk and says, "I plan to go to this convention. Please make the necessary reservations." It will be necessary for you to learn how he wishes to travel and what class accommodations he desires (first-class or tourist).

You must then learn whether he prefers to stay in hotels or motels and whether he desires the *minimum* accommodations or something more costly. If the trip is to a distant large city, he may want to rent a car at the airport. This can be arranged in advance.

Information can be obtained from travel agencies about methods of travel and accommodations in the city to which he is going. It is also possible for you to acquire the information from timetables and schedules found at the airlines. If he is a member of the American Automobile Association, you will find them most willing to make the reservations for you.

Look over the convention material. Write the following information on a sheet of paper:

1. The date the convention begins and the hour on that day.
2. The date and hour the convention closes.
3. The location of convention headquarters (both building and city).
4. Any special events that require reservations and/or extra fees.
5. Where the convention fees are to be sent if it is wise to register in advance—and what those fees are.

With your list in hand, ask your dentist the following questions and write down the answers:

1. Do you wish to arrive by the opening hour?
2. Do you plan to stay until the conclusion of the last meeting?
3. Do you have any preference for hotels?
4. Are you an associate member of the organization holding the meeting? (Associate members have some special privileges and often pay lower fees. Some dentists belong to out-of-state organizations as associate members.)
5. Do you wish to attend any of the special events? (Ask this question only if there are any courses or luncheons requiring advance registrations.)
6. How do you wish to travel?

   a. If air travel is to be used, ask whether he wishes to use limousine service to the airport.
   b. If he is using the limousine, ask where the limousine should pick him up.
   c. Ask whether he wishes to travel first-class or air-tourist.
   d. If he wishes to travel by car, ask whether you should have some service plan a routing.

7. Do you plan to travel alone, or for how many shall I make reservations?
8. Have you any instructions about the cost of transportation and hotel rooms?

With the written answers before you, you can send your dentist to the convention and return him to his office without disturbing him again except for check-signing.

If he is a member of AAA, call their office and give them all the information necessary regarding travel and hotel reservations. They will make all the arrangements for you except registration at the convention.

If you are called upon to do the reservation work yourself, call the airport for information regarding departure and arrival times. Make any necessary reservations. Pick up the tickets as instructed by the ticket office, or use a travel service.

Hotel Reservations

Write directly to the hotel which is your dentist's first choice. You will need to include this information:

Name of your dentist.

Number of persons in his party.

Type of room and beds desired (accommodations).

Date of arrival.

Time of arrival.

Number of nights room is needed.

Indicate whether the confirmation of the reservation should be made by mail, telegram, or a long distance telephone call, depending upon the time at your disposal in finding your dentist a room. Some hotels require a deposit to hold a reserved room. It is therefore wise to include a sentence which states that a deposit will be sent if it is desired.

You will receive a reply. If there are no rooms available, try his second-choice hotel, and so on until you locate a room.

If the convention is the national convention, blanks for hotel reservations will be found in the *Journal of the American Dental Association*, the issue published approximately six months prior to the convention.

Convention Reservations

Advance registration at a convention may not always be possible. In the event that it is possible to register early, it may be very desirable to do so. In such a case, write to the convention headquarters, as listed in the pamphlet your dentist gives you, and register, sending any necessary fees.

Itinerary

Now you are ready to write an itinerary for your dentist. It tells him in outline form just what to do from the time his transportation leaves. An example is shown in figure 11.1.

Dr. Raywin:

Your plane leaves from the International Airport at 3:30 p.m., VA Flight 762, Sunday, November 19.

You arrive in Convention City at 4:30 p.m. (3-hour trip, cross 2 time zones).

You have a room at Convention Hotel. A $5.00 deposit has been made on it. Your registration for the special course is attached.

You leave Convention City on Thursday, November 23, at 4 p.m., on VA Flight 681 and arrive at International Airport at 9 p.m. (lost 2 hours).

Fig. 11.1. A short itinerary

Attach all tickets, necessary papers, and convention pamphlet.

If it is your job to write checks, it may be desirable to see that your dentist has the necessary convention expense money in checks, cash, or traveler's checks which may be obtained from any bank for a small fee. Traveler's checks are a safe method of carrying large sums of money. They must be purchased by the traveler himself and signed in the presence of a cashier. On cashing the checks, the traveler must again sign them, and the two signatures must be identical.

Your dentist should have traveler's checks, credit cards, or money orders available for his use.

Ordinarily the convention hotel will cash checks for small amounts for a registered guest, but should some emergency arise, added funds may be needed. Credit cards offer considerable help in providing the extra funds.

Sunday 2/11/73	Lv. Minneapolis Ar. Portland (overnight in Portland)	3:15 p.m. 5:47 p.m.	flight #77 (dinner flight)	Northwest Orient
Monday 2/12/73	Lv. Portland Ar. Klamath Falls (overnight in Klamath Falls)	9:00 a.m. 11:35 a.m.	flight #727	West Coast
Tuesday 2/13/73	Lv. Klamath Falls Ar. Medford (overnight in Medford)	10:15 a.m. 10:45 a.m.	flight #726	West Coast
Wednesday 2/14/73	Lv. Medford Ar. Eugene (overnight in Eugene)	10:58 a.m. 11:45 a.m.	flight #860	United Air Lines
Thursday 2/15/73	Lv. Eugene Ar. Portland	sometime in a.m. sometime in a.m.		Private car
Friday 2/16/73	Lv. Portland Ar. Spokane	7:00 a.m. 7:50 a.m.	flight #236 (light breakfast)	Northwest Orient
	Lv. Spokane Ar. Minneapolis	8:25 a.m. 12:45 p.m.	flight #714 (full breakfast)	Northwest Orient

Fig. 11.2. A sample itinerary for a long trip

It is important for you to keep a copy of your dentist's itinerary and know how he can be reached in an emergency. Perhaps he will even set up specified times when you can talk with him during his absence. The sample itinerary (fig. 11.1) is a very simple one.

It is possible that your dentist may travel to several places on the same trip. Then an itinerary might look something like figure 11.2.

Preparation for Return

While your dentist is away is an excellent time to do some of the thorough housecleaning tasks which are difficult to accomplish when patients are constantly present. In the one-dentist office, many accumulated tasks can be accomplished.

If you have more than one dentist in your office, there probably isn't a slack time, and your only concern becomes proper appointing of patients for the return of the dentist who is away.

Be sure you have cared for the mail in his absence and have it ready—grouped according to importance—for him to see upon his return. It would help if when he reads his mail you stand by to take notes about replies.

Homecoming

When a dentist returns from a trip, he is usually somewhat fatigued from travel. The patients who have been unable to see him in his absence are anxious and sometimes pushy about seeing him *now*. You will do your dentist and the entire office staff a favor if you will see that the schedule is *light* the first two or three days after the dentist has returned to the office. There will be more emergencies those days (because he has been away) which will help absorb any slack time you may feel is present if you schedule lightly. Your dentist will appreciate the opportunity to ease back into his tough schedule, rather than feeling he has been scheduled for two days' work each day.

The same is true of the last two days before he leaves. Give him a little time to prepare for the meeting or vacation so he doesn't start on the trip exhausted.

Give him a leisurely send-off and a cordial but easy welcome back. Hold the unpleasant things out of the way, if you can, until he has control of his routine again.

"Doctor, the autoclave broke while you were away and the water pipe upstairs leaked all over the lab ceiling and we're simply going to have to turn Mrs. Jones's account over to the collectors and Mr. Gray says he's going to sue" is *not* the greeting your dentist should receive on his return. Give him a chance to feel pleasant about the office before you discuss the problems which arose during his absence. (Most of them will keep a few hours.) Then take them, one at a time, please.

Meetings and Conference Arrangements

If your dentist happens to be deeply involved in organizational work, it may be necessary for you to make arrangements for meetings for large groups of people. The secret of having successful meetings is to preplan for them. The reservation of the meeting place on the proper date and at the proper time is the first step. Your dentist should tell you when the group is to meet and how many members are anticipated. He may specify the place where the meeting is to be held. He may ask you to find a large enough space for the meeting. Usually the place of meeting will be determined by the members of the group before your dentist requests that you make the space reservations for the next meeting.

Call the hotel manager, or the resident manager if it is a meeting hall rather than a hotel, and give him the name of the organization, the anticipated size of the group, and the date and time of the meeting. Ask for a written verification of the space, the cost, and any other information your dentist may need to have. Ordinarily, if the group is having dinner or luncheon at the hotel, a meeting room is furnished with the meal; that is, there is no additional cost for the meeting place.

A small group will often meet in the library or study rooms of the local dental society. If this is the plan for the meeting for which you must obtain space, call the executive secretary of the local dental society and ask for the reservation for the time and date for which your dentist has made a request. Be sure you have written confirmation of the time and date for any meeting.

If you should be asked to make reservations for a very large meeting, the procedure is the same. The difference comes in the person with whom you make such arrangements. However, very large meetings, such as state dental society meetings, are usually arranged by a special employee of the dental society—frequently one who does nothing but arrange for meetings, handles displays and advertising for these meetings, and so on. Do not allow the size of the group to disturb you. It is the same principle regardless of whether the group be half a dozen or 60,000 people.

The second step is to see that the notices of meetings are properly prepared.

To accomplish this task, be sure you have the correct time and place of the meeting. If someone is to speak, be certain that you have the correct spelling of the person's name and the topic. When you have the copy accurately prepared for reproduction, it is wise to check with your dentist to see whether he has any corrections to offer before the meeting notice is printed.

If the notices are to be sent to a small number of people—say ten—perhaps you will simply type them in the office. However, it is possible that a letter service or a printer will be engaged to print or mimeograph enough copies of the notice. Be sure to have this order prepared in ample time.

The third step is to have an accurate mailing list of the correct names and addresses, including zip codes, of all the persons to whom the notice is to be sent. With the mailing labels now available, it is probably easier to type the addresses on labels and attach them to the envelopes or postcards. Many of the labels are self-adhering so that it is very simple to attach them to the envelope. The labels are addressed and attached to the notice of the meeting.

If your dentist is president of the meeting, it is usually necessary to have an agenda—a typed listing of what is to occur at the meeting. It begins with calling the meeting to order and proceeds through the order of business to be considered. Since this order is determined by the rules of order in conducting a meeting,

it would be a good idea to have a reference copy of a rules-of-order book in your library. A sample agenda appears in figure 11.3.

If your dentist happens to be secretary of the organization, there will be minutes of the meeting to be prepared and usually distributed. He will bring you the notes or the tape of the meeting. You will transcribe it and have him read it for approval. Then it will be duplicated by whatever method is correct, depending on the number of copies to be made. If the number is large, perhaps the preparation will not be made in the office; that is, a printer will do this part of the work.

The distribution of the minutes may be your job. If so, address another set of labels and mail out the minutes as soon as you are told to do so. Some organizations do not mail them out. Instead, the members are expected to pick up the minutes of the last meeting at the current meeting. If this is the case, you must see that the minutes of the last meeting are ready for your dentist to take to the meeting.

AGENDA

CALL TO ORDER

MINUTES OF THE LAST MEETING

TREASURER'S REPORT

OLD BUSINESS

    Report on school Examination program

NEW BUSINESS

    Consideration of new members' applications

    The Memorial Scholarship Fund

    Report of the Committee on Flouridation of the Water Supply

COMMITTEE REPORTS

    Finance

    Publications

ADJOURNMENT

Fig. 11.3. A sample agenda

Summary

Special preparation for a meeting of a dental society includes proper reservation of time in the appointment book, preparation of any materials for which your dentist is responsible, preparation of his itinerary, and collection of reservations, ticket, and the like, should the meeting be in another city.

The preparation for his return should include special cleanup of the office, should this be possible, and light appointing of patients the first two or three days in order to give him a chance to readjust to the workload.

Conference arrangements are made by the dental assistant should her dentist be in charge of some area of preparation for such a meeting. He should be prepared with any papers for which he is responsible.

Study Questions

1. Describe an agenda. Under what circumstances might you be asked to prepare an agenda?
2. List the things you must do if your dentist attends a convention in another city.
3. What is an itinerary? Why should you have a copy?
4. What can you do while your dentist is away to make your work easier on his return?
5. Why should the schedule be light the first two or three days after his return? Prior to his leaving?
6. Your dentist is responsible for calling a meeting of ten members of a committee who will meet in the dental society rooms. What are your responsibilities?
7. Your dentist is secretary of the dental society. What are your responsibilities?

PART THREE | *DENTAL LAW*

It has been said that law is the system by which society gives order to our lives.

An assistant who is well informed in the area of dental and medical law is an asset to any practice. It is important for her to know how the laws affect the practice of dentistry, the legal relationships which exist between a dentist and his patients, the dentist's liabilities in the practice of dentistry, and his public duties.

Just in knowing the dangers which exist, the alert dental assistant can prevent an unjustified legal entanglement by her care of certain office responsibilities. It is to this purpose that part three is devoted—education in the area of the legal relationships and responsibilities of the dentist and his staff.

12 *The Dental Practice Acts*

The Need for Regulation

That some people are eager to diagnose the problems of others and prescribe treatment for the "cure" of these problems is a reality which has existed almost as long as civilization. However, sometimes those who are eager to diagnose and prescribe are not educationally qualified to do so. There have been instances recently of the exposé of unlicensed and uneducated persons who have perpetrated a hoax on innocent lay persons.

The history of dentistry is so intertwined with the history of medicine that it is necessary to examine the two legal histories simultaneously. Many problems in licensure and those of legal concerns are similar.

A dentist (as well as a physician) is sometimes responsible for the life or death of a patient. The judgment of the professional doctor may determine what happens to that patient. And so it is that society has come to be rightfully concerned with the preparation of the health care professionals.

In early history there were some laws aimed at improving medical care, but these were largely repealed until no laws existed by 1850. Because so much quackery developed, all the states passed dental and medical practice acts by 1900. There was much discussion and contention about these laws—some people protesting that persons were denied their constitutional rights if they were not allowed to practice medicine. The Supreme Court ruled in 1889 that the states had a right to pass licensing legislation because:

The power of the State to provide for the general welfare of its people authorizes it to prescribe all such regulations, as in its judgment, will secure or tend to secure them against the consequences of ignorance and incapacity as well as of deception and fraud.[1]

This statement simply means that the state is given power to protect its citizens from harm by persons who are not qualified to perform certain functions such as *diagnose* (determine what is wrong) and *prescribe* (specify the use of a remedy or treatment).

Following this decision, licensing requirements for the health professions have been upheld by the courts in the interests of protecting the general public. Any state may use any requirements which are not "arbitrary, unreasonable or discriminatory"[2] in issuing licenses for the practice of the health professions. Requirements are not considered "arbitrary, unreasonable, or discriminatory" if they are attainable by reasonable study or application, are appropriate to the profession, and are available to all persons of like age and condition.

Inasmuch as this decision by the Supreme Court set these criteria, any state may reasonably increase educational requirements, raise the licensing fees, and radically revise qualifications by action of the state legislature as time goes on.

The power of the national Congress to license dentists and physicians federally has never come to the attention of the Supreme Court, but the right of Congress to require a federal permit for narcotics has been conceded.

You will hear of "dental jurisprudence" which may be defined as the science which concerns the principles of positive law and legal relations concerning dentistry. Sometimes this law is clear and sometimes it is doubtful.[3]

American Law

We have commented that it is difficult to separate medical and dental law. It is also difficult to separate dental law from general law. Thus, the awareness of how American law came to be is important.

There are three general sources of American law: federal law, which includes the United States Constitution; state law, which includes the state constitutions; and judicial decisions. Federal laws (also called statutes) are laws which apply to the entire country and regulate everyone who is within the domain of the United-States. These are written laws and can be found in the *United States Code*. Unless these laws contradict the United States Constitution, they represent "black letter law," the hard and fast rules of the United States.

State laws differ only in that they must also be in accord with the constitution of the state of which they are a law. They apply only within the boundaries of that state.

In addition to these two well-known areas of law, there is judge-made law (often called common law). This law is applicable within the jurisdiction of the judge who issues the decree. The only requirement is that it does not conflict with the constitution of the state in which the judge presides and the Constitution of the United States. There are differ-

---

1. *Dent* v. *West Virginia*, 129 U. S., 114, 9S. Ct. 231 (1889).
2. The quotation marks denote legal language.

3. Sarner, *Dental Jurisprudence*, p. 3.

ences in judge-made laws within a state. For example, a local judge in the northwest corner of a state may create a common law which states that all dogs must be kept on a leash, while a judge in the southeast corner of the same state may decree that dogs may run loose so long as they do not attack anyone. Since neither of these common laws is in conflict with the constitution of that state or the United States Constitution, they both can be part of the body of common law of that state.

The *areas* for which the federal government can make laws are definitely established by the Constitution of the United States. The Constitution also states that all other areas are to be controlled by the states. Police power (in its broad sense—*regulation*) is one of the areas which the states control. This means that the states control the practice of dentistry.

Common law simply means that the courts must fill in the gaps between the laws which the legislature makes. It is not possible for the legislators to anticipate all the possible problems, and therefore laws are generalized. The judges (courts) then have to interpret and also decree certain regulations. These decisions become "common law"—that "body of those principles and rules of action, relating to the government and security of persons and property, which derive their authority solely from usages and customs of immemorial antiquity, or from the judgments and decrees of the courts recognizing, affirming and enforcing such usages and customs." (Black's *Law Dictionary*)

The dentist is controlled by:

1. *federal law* if he prescribes medicines containing narcotics. He must have a federal license to authorize the pharmacist to dispense any narcotics;
2. *state law* in the state in which he practices. This state law is the dental practice act. It governs licensing; and

3. judge-made, or common law, in his professional relationships with his patients.

The legal relationships of dentistry and medicine are intertwined and dependent on each other because judges usually follow *judicial precedents* (earlier decisions by other judges) set in similar cases within their own state.

Common law is difficult to amend. Appeal to a higher court is one way. Another way is to have the legislature of the state enact new legislation which voids the common law.

Since common law is the law which usually affects the dentist and his relationships with his patients, it is very important that all members of the oral health care delivery team become aware of the precautions necessary to avoid malpractice claims.

Laws Regulating Dentistry

Dental practice acts are regulatory statutes (laws) which prohibit the practice of dentistry by any person without a license. This means that anyone who indicates he is able to perform dentistry—diagnose, treat, prescribe, or operate for any disease, pain, injury, deficiency, deformity, or physical condition of the teeth, jaws, or adjacent structures—must acquire a license. The individual state dental practice acts may word the definitions differently, but each defines the area of dentistry. Most acts indicate that the use of the title *dentist* (or any of its other forms such as oral surgeon) or of the letters *D.D.S.* or *D.M.D.* is reserved for those individuals who have been licensed by the state.

Most of the states agree that the applicant for a dental license must meet certain conditions. He must:

1. have graduated from a dental school which has been approved by the State Board of Dental Examiners and/or the Council on

Dental Education of the American Dental Association,

2. be twenty-one years of age or older,
3. be a citizen of the United States,
4. be a resident of the state,
5. be of good moral character,
6. not have committed a crime involving moral turpitude,
7. not be addicted to drugs or alcohol, and
8. pass an examination both written and oral, both theory and practical, given by the State Board of Dental Examiners.

As long ago as 1928, the Council of the National Board of Dental Examiners of the American Dental Association began promoting the idea that a certificate issued by this Council should be acceptable to the State Boards of Dental Examiners in place of the written theory examinations. About seventy percent of the states now accept this certificate. It means that a student trained in one state can move to another state, using the certificate issued by the Council of the National Board of Dental Examiners to replace the theoretical examination the new state might require him to pass.

In addition to this courtesy, *reciprocity* (or *licensure by endorsement*) has been established in about three-fifths of the states. Reciprocity means that the two states involved will acknowledge that a student who has passed the State Boards in one state will be eligible to practice dentistry in the other state.

Requirements for Licensed Dentists

Once a dentist has been licensed to practice in a state, and continues to practice, he must renew his license annually by payment of the licensing fee as determined by the state. This fee must be paid promptly at the proper time each year. A yearly certificate is issued. The *original license* and the *annual certificate* should be displayed in the office.

A dentist must also have a *narcotics license* if he is to dispense drugs which contain narcotics. This license is obtained from the federal government. It is the only medical function which the federal government licenses. The narcotics license is obtained by application to the Bureau of Narcotics, United States Treasury. It is sent to the district branch of the United States Treasury in the district in which the dentist practices. A stamp with the narcotics license number of this particular dentist is then issued. The number must appear on each narcotic prescription blank. The license is renewed annually on June 30, which is the end of the federal fiscal year.

Revocation of License

Since licensing occurs, there are situations where revocation of license becomes necessary. The rules vary from state to state. However, suspension or revocation of a dental license can occur:

1. if the dentist is convicted on a felony (narcotic violations, murder, and rape are specifically included);
2. for unprofessional conduct (such as permitting an unlicensed person to perform dentistry or permitting employees to perform duties not specifically permitted by law, advertising which is unethical or misleading to public morals or safety, giving or receiving rebates, and habitual intemperance in the use of narcotics or alcohol);
3. for personal or professional incapacity. (If a dentist has been judged insane or incompetent, his license may be revoked. If a dentist insists on continuing to practice when he is senile, his license might be revoked because he is personally or professionally incapable of performing dental service of value to his patients. In all probability, every effort would be made to

persuade him to retire voluntarily before denying him his license.)

The power of revocation or suspension is given the Board of Dental Examiners by the state legislatures.

Summary

The eagerness of people to diagnose and prescribe for others has made it necessary to establish controls over who is entitled to practice in the health sciences.

There are three general sources of American law: federal, state, and judicial decisions. Federal statutes are found in the *United States Code*. Federal statutes must not contradict the United States Constitution; state statutes must not contradict the constitution of that particular state. Judicial or judge-made law is often called common law. It applies within the jurisdiction of the judge who issues the decree.

Police power (in its broad sense of regulation) is the privilege of the states; therefore, states control the practice of dentistry by licensure.

The dentist is controlled by (1) federal law if he prescribes narcotics, (2) state laws in the state in which he practices, (3) judge-made or common law in relationships with patients.

The dental practice acts are regulatory statutes which prohibit anyone from practicing dentistry without a license.

Licensing is by state, National Board of Dental Examiners, and by reciprocity.

The annual certificate and original license must be displayed in the dental office.

Narcotics may not be prescribed without a narcotics license.

Licenses can be revoked for specified actions. The power of revocation belongs to the State Board of Dental Examiners of each state.

Study Questions

1. Why should a dental assistant understand the basic laws relating to dentistry?
2. Why are there laws regulating the practice of dentistry?
3. What are the sources of American law?
4. Who licenses dentists?
5. What body of law regulates the relationships with patients?
6. What are causes of revocation of license?

Bibliography

The bibliography for part three, "Dental Law," is given at the end of chapter fifteen.

13 | *Legal Relationship of the Dentist and His Patient*

A definite legal relationship exists between a patient and a dentist. This relationship can be, and often is, upheld in a court of law. Eleven commonly accepted duties of dentists to their patients are implied by law, while only two such duties of patients to their dentists are implied. Failure to fulfill any of these duties can become the basis for a lawsuit. Thus, it is imperative that all members of the oral health care delivery team become aware of their obligation in order to minimize the opportunity for a lawsuit.

As a dental assistant you should be aware that emergency care is being refused by some dentists and physicians. An atmosphere of caution about treating strangers has developed within the health care professions because claims for damages have been filed by some unscrupulous persons following such "good Samaritan" treatment.

Creation of a Contract

The first step in any dentist-patient relationship is the creation of a contract. A dentist is not required to accept everyone who asks him to serve as his dentist. The legal decisions from our courts have indicated that a dentist may arbitrarily refuse to accept anyone as a patient, even though there is no other dentist available.

The dentist-patient relationship begins when the dentist performs services after a patient has requested him to do so, either by implication or by direct statement. Administering emergency care does not create the relationship. The dentist must use his skill and care when treating an emergency, but this act does not create the dentist-patient relationship. The dentist is also free to limit his care to a specific time or place or to one specific treatment. However, after the patient-dentist relationship has been established, there are certain obligations on the part of both patient and dentist.

What Is a Contract with a Patient?

A contract is an agreement with an individual patient which indicates the patient is placing himself under the care of this dentist for a specific treatment of a specific condition or placing himself in the dentist's care for whatever services the dentist may deem necessary (as a patient does who engages a family dentist). This agreement may be *verbal*; it may be implied rather than specifically stated.

When a patient is unable to make this arrangement himself, an *agent* makes it for him. The agent may be the parent of a child; or in the case of an aged parent, an adult son or daughter; a near relative in the case of a mentally incompetent individual—someone this individual has engaged to act for him or a court-appointed guardian.

A dentist and his staff should know the laws governing financial responsibility. A husband is responsible for his wife's debts, but a wife is not always responsible for her husband's debts. A father is responsible for his children's debts if they are minors, but children are not responsible for the debts of their parents.

Know the laws governing financial responsibility which apply to the practice of den-

tistry in your locality. Be certain you are dealing with the correct person when you attempt to collect a fee.

The Assistant as Agent for the Dentist

Whenever an employee is able to act for his employer, he is considered an *agent*. The dentist must, of necessity, empower (direct) his employees to act for him in some circumstances, usually under his specific direction. For example, the dentist directs his hygienist to perform prophylaxis for his patients. The hygienist, in this case, is acting as the dentist's agent. (She is performing a treatment for the dentist according to the regulations he has instructed her to follow.)

Since someone must be responsible for any treatment given a patient, it also follows that the dentist is responsible for the actions of his agent. If the hygienist accidentally injures the patient, the patient can sue the dentist for the damage rather than sue the hygienist; or the patient may sue them jointly.

Generally, a dentist is responsible for injury if his assistant, apprentice, agent, or employee does not have the proper skill or does not exercise the proper care. However, one employee is not responsible for the negligence of another employee. Thus, if the dentist employs another dentist who in turn gives orders to the hygienist to perform some treatment and the patient is injured, the employed dentist is not held responsible for the negligence of the hygienist because he is an employee, as is the hygienist.

This area of responsibility for an agent's actions is difficult to define completely because so many factors enter the conditions under which the service is performed.

The dental assistant will be the agent of the dentist in her work in the office. She is acting under his direction, and therefore he is responsible for the conduct and treatment of patients. It is essential that anyone engaged as an oral health care delivery team member be constantly alert to see that the directions of the dentist are accurately followed and recorded for future reference.

Duties to Patients

What are the duties a dentist has to a patient with whom he has made a contract (either written or oral)? The implied duties are the following:

1. The dentist must be licensed. Anyone who attempts to practice dentistry without being properly licensed to do so is liable to court action.
2. The dentist must use reasonable care and skill in diagnosis and treatment according to the standards of care provided by other dentists in the same type of community.
3. The dentist must use standard drugs, materials, and techniques in treatment and postoperative care.
4. The treatment is to be completed within a reasonable length of time.
5. The patient is to be given instructions for any postoperative care, including instructions to return for postoperative observation when necessary.
6. The dentist may not abandon a patient. Once the contract has been established between a dentist and a patient, it is necessary for the dentist to care for that patient. If the relationship becomes impossible for the dentist, it is his duty to give the patient sufficient notice for the patient to be able to find another dentist.
7. The patient is to expect a reasonable charge for services rendered. This fee may be different for different patients, but the dentist is obligated to charge a reasonable fee for services rendered.
8. The dentist is obligated to see that patients have care during his absence from

his office. If some patient is likely to need care during his absence, it is advisable for the dentist to tell the patient before he leaves and to make arrangements with a colleague for this care. (Most dentists make arrangements for the care of emergencies with a nearby colleague prior to being absent from the office.)
9. The patient has a right to a reasonably satisfactory result from his dental care.
10. The dentist is to refer a patient to a specialist for proper treatment if such care is necessary.
11. The patient-dentist relationship is a confidential relationship, and any information disclosed to the dentist must be treated confidentially. This rule applies to financial matters as well as health and/or any personal information which is disclosed.

Duties of the Patient

In contrast to this lengthy list of dentist duties, the patient is only required to do the following:

1. Pay a reasonable fee for the dentistry which has been performed.
2. Follow instructions and cooperate with the dentist in whatever treatment is required.

This contrast of duties only emphasizes the responsibility of *all* the members of the oral health care delivery team to be aware of the dentist's legal obligations and to be certain that these obligations are met insofar as it is possible for each individual member of the team.

Remuneration for the Dentist

The dentist may charge the patient directly for his services and receive payment from the patient. Frequently, however, *remuneration* (payment) may occur through insurance, prepayment plans, union contracts, employee benefit contracts, and government agencies.

The various plans differ in coverage and method of remuneration. It therefore becomes necessary for the dentist's office staff to understand these differences clearly. Inasmuch as the benefits vary from full coverage to deductibles and percentages, accurate understanding of the particular plan is essential, and in some instances the plan must be explained to the patient. In all cases, for complete detailed assistance the patient may be referred to the specific insurance carrier or government agency.

Considering the premium, the patient is remunerated according to some established fees, payable by the insurance company but not necessarily accepted as full payment by the dentist. He may charge more for his services than the allowance made by the carrier. In the final analysis, the contract is between the dentist and his patient rather than a third party, the insurance company. Therefore, the responsibility of the dentist and the patient to each other is of paramount importance.

Payment through a government agency may be handled somewhat differently. If a patient states that the government is responsible for his dental bills, the dentist must determine that his patient is eligible for such governmental care and must then file the proper forms and reports. Failure to report the case according to government regulations may mean loss of fee. The various governmental agencies have often refused to pay a claim because it was improperly reported. Workmen's compensation laws in your state should be examined very closely, because some states do not permit the patient to choose his dentist if his care is to be paid for by his employer under workmen's compensation laws.

The amount a dentist may charge for his services is a subject of controversy. Some courts in the United States have refused to permit a dentist to charge fees based on the patient's ability to pay when a case is brought to court. Other areas do permit just this approach to setting fees. It is important for a dentist to know the decisions in his state in regard to the setting of fees. A dentist is the sole arbiter of his fees. They are based on usual and customary charges made by him for specific services and are more or less in keeping with similar services rendered by others in his community.

Termination of a Contract

Once a dentist enters into an agreement with a patient to care for him, he is under an obligation to continue to care for the patient. The contract continues until it is *terminated* (ended) by either the dentist or the patient. Either one may terminate the contract by indicating that the relationship no longer exists.

For his legal protection the dentist needs to complete certain papers when a relationship with a patient is terminated. It is well to have these forms available in the office.

A contract with a patient may be created *verbally,* but the dentist had best terminate it in written form. The patients have a responsibility in the dentist-patient relationship of following the instruction of the dentist and appearing for the requested examinations. Failure of a patient to uphold his part of the contract is reason for a dentist to dismiss the patient and terminate the contract, but it should be done with a written statement.

There are certain letters with which a dental assistant should be familiar concerning the dentist who is faced with termination of the patient-dentist relationship. The dentist is under an obligation to care for the patient unless he gives notice of his intention to withdraw from the case. Thus, one form which a dental assistant must understand is the letter of withdrawal issued by the dentist. The dentist must give the patient reasonable notice if he intends to withdraw from the case. This varies with the conditions of the community in which the patient lives (fig. 13.1).

Another way in which services are terminated is at the instigation of the patient. In this case, the dentist's office should issue a letter of confirmation of this discharge (fig. 13.2).

Other notifications to the patient or authorizations by the patient are illustrated in figures 13.3-13.5.

These letters should be sent by *registered* mail. A copy should be kept in the dentist's files, along with the return signature card which the post office will send to you after the patient has signed it as having received the letter, until the statute of limitations has ex-

---

JAMES A. RAYWIN, D.D.S.
104 ANY STREET
ANYTOWN, ANYSTATE 12345
612-926-1414

July 17, 197—

Mr. John H. Smith
734 Poplar Lane
Anytown, Anystate 12610

Dear Mr. Jones:

I wish to inform you that I will no longer perform dentistry for you because you have failed to follow my dental advice and treatment program concerning your home care.

If you so desire, I shall be available to attend you for thirty days after you have received this letter. This should give you ample time to select a dentist from the many competent practitioners in this city. With your written approval, I will make available to the dentist of your choice your case history and information regarding the diagnosis and treatment which you have received from me.

Very truly yours,

James A. Raywin, D. D. S.

Fig. 13.1. Sample letter of withdrawal from case

JAMES A. RAYWIN, D.D.S.
104 ANY STREET
ANYTOWN, ANYSTATE 12345
612-926-1414

July 17, 197—

Mr. John H. Smith
734 Poplar Lane
Anytown, Anystate 12610

Dear Mr. Jones:

This will confirm our telephone conversation of today in which you discharged me as your dentist.

In my opinion, your condition requires continued treatment by a dentist. If you have not already done so, I suggest that you employ another dentist without delay. You may be assured that, at your written request, I will furnish him with information regarding the diagnosis and treatment which you have received from me.

Very truly yours,

James A. Raywin, D. D. S.

Fig. 13.2. Sample letter of confirmation of discharge of patient.

pired. (The sample letters should be used as guides but are not to be copied verbatim.)

The dentist who uses these letters and statements of his relationships with patients who leave his care or fail to cooperate places himself in the position of having established the written facts that (*a*) he did not abandon the case or (*b*) he was discharged by the patient or (*c*) the patient refused to follow his advice.

I have refused to permit Doctor_____
to take X rays (roentgenograms) of my teeth for
his diagnosis. He has told me that it is advisable
to use X rays for this diagnosis. I waive any claim
for damages because roentgenograms (X rays)
were not taken.

Date:_____

_____SIGNED:_____
WITNESS   Patient

Fig. 13.4. Form for refusal to permit X rays

JAMES A. RAYWIN, D.D.S.
104 ANY STREET
ANYTOWN, ANYSTATE 12345
612-926-1414

July 17, 197—

Mr. Albert M. Sorenson
652 Maple Avenue
Anytown, Anystate 12622

Dear Mr. Sorenson:

At the time that you brought your son, William, to me for examination this afternoon, I informed you that I was unable to determine without X-ray pictures whether a fracture existed in his jaw. I strongly urge you to permit me or some other oral surgeon of your choice to make this X-ray examination without further delay.

Your neglect in not permitting a proper X-ray examination to be made of William's jaw may result in serious consequences if in fact a fracture does exist.

Very truly yours,

James A. Raywin, D. D. S.

I hereby authorize Doctor_____
to disclose complete information to_____
regarding his dental diagnosis and treatment of the
undersigned from_____ 19___until the
date of the conclusion of the treatment.

Further, I authorize him to testify, without limitation, about all his dental findings and treatment of the undersigned, in any legal action, suit, or proceedings to which I am, or may become, a party; and I waive on behalf of myself and any persons who may have an interest in the matter all provisions of law relating to the disclosure of confidential dental information.

_____   _____
WITNESS   Patient

_____   _____
Date .   Address

Fig. 13.3. Sample letter to a patient who fails to follow advice.

Fig. 13.5. Authorization for disclosure of advice

The Dentist's Public Duties

A dentist has some public duties which he must perform simply because he is a dentist. He must have a narcotics license to dispense or prescribe narcotics, and the quantity he prescribes is registered by the licensing bureau. It is necessary to keep an inventory of the narcotics in the possession of the dentist. Daily records must be kept of certain drugs dispensed. These drugs are listed by the federal government. Only a qualified person may administer narcotics. The type of records to be kept will be discussed in the section on administration of the office. Reports on addicts must be made.

A dentist may be called by the courts to serve as an expert witness. An expert gives an opinion on a subject as an *expert* for the benefit of the jury and the court. This testimony has nothing to do with an individual patient of the dentist. He may not know the defendant or plaintiff in the case. His judgment is being used for court education.

It is also possible that he may be called to testify in behalf of his patient who is involved in a damage suit. He is expected, in this instance, to explain his diagnosis, findings, progress of treatment, description of the patient's residual problems, amount of suffering the patient has experienced, and probable permanent impairment.

The statute regarding patient-dentist privilege affects what the dentist may say in court. If the patient does not waive his privilege, the dentist may not testify.

If the dentist must appear in court, it is important for his assistant to discover the exact date and time, the courtroom number, and the judge's name. Most attorneys are very cooperative in judging the exact time at which the dentist must appear.

It is important that he take his records of the case along so that he can refresh his memory when asked questions about the case. Occasionally it is necessary for the assistant to testify as to what was said and done in her presence.

Sometimes a subpoena is required when a dentist is called to testify. A *subpoena* is an order from the court which requires that the person named in the paper appear in court to testify. A penalty is dealt if the person named does not appear. This subpoena helps waive the confidential patient-dentist relationship.

Summary

A definite relationship exists between a dentist and a patient and is upheld in a court of law. A contract is created when a dentist agrees to perform services for a patient who requests such care. The dentist may limit his care specifically or agree to provide continual care. This agreement may be verbal, but a wise dentist terminates such an agreement with a written document. An agent may complete the agreement if a patient is unable to do so for himself.

Financial responsibility laws should be understood by the dentist and his staff. The dental assistant is an agent for the dentist. The dentist is responsible for the conduct and treatment performed by his employee.

It is important that the dentist and his staff make proper arrangement for payment for services if an agent requests dental care for anyone.

Insurance programs, prepayment benefits, and government agencies present specific problems in collections. The staff should be acquainted with the regulations pertaining to such plans in their locale.

A contract must be properly terminated if a dentist is not to be held liable for neglect. Forms for such terminations are available through medical protective insurance companies. These termination letters should be sent registered mail.

Termination can occur if the dentist gives notice of intent to withdraw or if the patient indicates he no longer desires the services.

Public duties which a dentist must perform include reporting narcotic addicts and recording the use of narcotics in the office.

Study Questions

1. Why must dental assistants understand the rights, privileges, and laws concerning the care of patients?
2. What is a contract with a patient?
3. Discuss laws governing financial responsibility.
4. What is meant when it is stated that the dental assistant is the agent of the dentist?
5. What knowledge must a dental assistant have about insurance programs?
6. Why should a dentist terminate a patient contract in writing?
7. What public duties must a dentist perform?
8. For what two reasons might a dentist be called to appear in court?
9. Why is the use of narcotics recorded so accurately in the dentist's office?

Bibliography

The bibliography for part three appears at the end of chapter fifteen.

14 | *Liabilities... Professional and Criminal*

There are many ways a dentist may be sued in a court of law. It is important that the assistants to the dentist understand the problems and use care to see that insofar as possible there are no incidents which might give a patient an opportunity to sue.

The matter of patients suing dentists has become a serious problem. Until 1930 the number of cases was insignificant, but from 1930 on, suits for injuries began to increase in many fields. A contractor was sued for injury to children playing in his partially constructed home, even though they were trespassing. A washing machine manufacturer was sued for injury to the user who had failed to read the directions. The claims against physicians and dentists began to increase, also. It is estimated that they rose twentyfold between 1930 and 1950.[1] Since then the claims have continued to rise, and frequently the judgments awarded have been in six figures. The indications from the larger medical professional liability insurance firms are that the number of suits is still increasing. This means that the dentist and his staff must exercise extreme care to prevent this type of legal involvement.

1. Committee on Mediocolegal Problems, *Malpractice and the Physician* (Chicago: American Medical Association, 1951).

Personal Injury Claims

Everyone who has a place of business or a home is responsible for any injury which occurs on its premises. The large department store is responsible for any conditions within its premises which cause accidents. If an injury occurs within a building but not within the office space rented by an individual, the owner of the building may be responsible.

Everyone needs protection against this personal injury liability, including the dentist who maintains an office—perhaps most of all the dentist.

Since the dentist can be held responsible for everything which happens in his office, it is essential that the staff be alert to common problems and do all they can to eliminate accident-inviting conditions. For example, if there is a screwhead on the doorknob which cuts anyone in opening the door, the dentist is responsible for the injury. If a nylon stocking is caused to snag and run by a rough spot on a chair, the dentist is liable for the cost of the nylons. If a rug causes someone to trip or a waxed floor causes someone to fall, the dentist is responsible. This is *personal liability,* and a dentist must be protected from such claims by insurance and by extreme care exercised by his staff to eliminate all possible hazards.

Medical Professional Liability (Malpractice Claims)

However, personal injury claims are usually not as serious nor frequent as medical professional liability, commonly known as medical *malpractice* (bad practice) claims, for which a dentist may be sued if the patient feels he was detrimentally affected by a treatment, was injured by treatment, or that the diagnosis was incorrect.

The term *medical professional liability* is preferred because it best describes the area in which the claims actually arise. Furthermore, malpractice has a special meaning (connotative meaning) which causes people to think in terms of criminal acts or disreputable conduct and can cause prejudgment of the issues in a court case.

Medical professional liability describes all the civil liability "which a dentist can incur by any of his professional acts"[2] or by his failure to properly perform his duty to a patient if this failure results in some injury to the patient.

Black's Law Dictionary defines medical professional liability as follows: "bad, wrong, or injudicious treatment resulting in injury, unnecessary suffering, or death to the patient, and proceeding from ignorance, carelessness, want of proper professional skill, disregard of established rules or principles, neglect, or a malicious or criminal intent."[3]

Malpractice claims can be listed under three legal classifications which will help your understanding. There are *malfeasance* claims in which it is said that the dentist has wrongfully treated the patient—for example a dentist extracted the wrong tooth. This is *malfeasance*—wrong treatment.

The *misfeasance* claims involve lawful action done in the wrong way. If the dentist extracted the correct tooth but did not use necessary care to prevent infection or failed to properly treat the area, a claim could arise out of *misfeasance*—what he did was lawful, but he didn't perform it correctly.

The third group of claims are *nonfeasance* claims—failure to do anything. If a dentist does nothing about a patient's complaints—a wait-and-see policy—or leaves town and does not provide someone to care for his patient's tooth, he can be sued for *nonfeasance*. If, for

2. C. J. Stetler and A. R. Moritz, *Doctor, Patient, and the Law,* p. 305.
3. *Black's Law Dictionary,* 3rd ed., 1933.

example, the dentist looked at the tooth and said, "Let's wait and see if the infection spreads," and the patient went home and soon became seriously ill, the dentist could be liable for nonfeasance.

All medical professional liability claims can be classified under one of these three actions or nonactions by dentists. This complicated area of medical law can be clarified if you are aware of this classification. The dentist may be attacked for not helping, for trying to help in the wrong way, or for trying to help in the right way but performing the procedure incorrectly.

The dentist is expected to use reasonable care, and the tendency is to bring suit for failure to use such care because such actions can result in larger awards.

The basic standard of reasonable care is one which exists for every citizen in relation to his fellow citizens. In the case of a dentist, this means that he is required to possess and use the same knowledge and skill used by other dentists in good standing who have the same general training in the same or similar neighborhoods under similar circumstances. Thus the generalist would be compared with generalists of similar background, but not with specialists, such as oral surgeons. The specialists generally are expected to have a higher degree of skill in the area of their specialty.

Breach of duty is a broad term which covers a number of actions or a lack of action by a dentist for which a patient may sue:

DIAGNOSIS requires that a dentist use ordinary skill in acquiring all the data necessary to a complete diagnosis. Should he fail to make the necessary tests, take essential X rays, or observe all unusual conditions as his colleagues do under similar circumstances, he can be sued for negligent diagnosis.

STANDARD PROCEDURE refers to treatment as commonly performed by most dentists of similar training.

PRIOR DENTISTS need protection. When a patient terminates a contract with one dentist and becomes a patient of a different dentist, the new dentist must not, by inadvertent gestures, looks, or comments, give the patient any idea that he might sue the prior dentist. The present dentist cannot know what the circumstances were at the time of treatment, and any indication that the prior dentist was not skillful must be carefully avoided.

INSTRUCTION OF PATIENTS. Patients must be properly instructed about home care of themselves and what symptoms to report to the dentist.

REFERRAL OF THE PATIENT. If a dentist feels a specialist is necessary to adequately treat or diagnose the patient's problem, he is expected to make a proper referral.

EXPOSURE OF PATIENT. The exposure of the patient to the public can also bring a lawsuit. The dentist must be very careful that the patient is seen by no one but him and his necessary office staff without the patient's express permission. This *includes* being seen by another dentist or being photographed for scientific purposes.

ATTENTION TO PATIENT. The patient must receive the attention his symptoms require. Failure of a dentist to give the patient the proper amount of attention has resulted in court actions.

Proof of Negligence

It has been historically true in the courts of the United States that the plaintiff has to *prove* negligence. Recent court decisions have on occasion cast the burden of proof on the defendant dentist, causing him to prove that he was not negligent. Interpretations of laws are changing, and it is wise to protect oneself with all the written documents possible.

However, there are some comforting facts to be remembered. An error in diagnosis is not enough evidence by itself that a dentist was negligent. A dentist cannot be held accountable for poor results for dental treatment. Other circumstances, such as nonsterile instruments, must be part of the evidence to obtain a verdict of negligence. X ray is one cause of numerous claims.

The *burden of proof* requires that the patient offer more proof that the dentist was negligent. If the jury decides the two groups of evidence are equal, they must decide in favor of the defendant (dentist). The dentist is not considered negligent until proved so by overwhelming evidence. The patient must prove the standard of care dentists in good standing exercise and then prove that this dentist does not exercise that care.

Expert testimony formerly was necessary to prove negligence. However, in recent years there have been two areas of suits in which expert testimony has been judged unnecessary in many courts. They are cases which are tried under *res ipsa loquitur* and the doctrine of common knowledge.

It is said that the jury, from its fund of common knowledge, is able to decide without expert testimony whether or not the defendant is guilty. It is generally felt that some of the court applications abandoning expert testimony are creating unfair situations for the settlement of court claims.

Admissions

It is conceded that no dentist should ever admit error unless his attorney and insurance company tell him to do so. Frequently the dentist does not know the facts in the situation. Perhaps there were some concealed symptoms at the time of examination. Regardless of what the dentist and his office staff think about the case, absolutely no information should be given to anyone but the dentist's attorney and insurance company, unless the attorney so instructs the dentist.

Proof by Res Ipsa Loquitur

This term literally means "the thing speaks for itself." The character of the accident and surrounding circumstances determines whether *res ipsa loquitur* applies. If an accident is inexplicable in terms of ordinary and known experience except by negligence, then negligence is either presumed or inferred. Circumstances surrounding the accident must amount to evidence from which the jury can *infer negligence*. It differs from circumstantial evidence in that the evidence points to no specific fault.

Three conditions necessary for *res ipsa loquitur* are as follows:

1. "The accident must be one which ordinarily doesn't occur unless someone is negligent.
2. "It must be caused by something within the control of the defendant.
3. "It must not have been due to any voluntary action or contribution on the part of the plaintiff."

Proximate Cause

The negligence of the dentist must be the "proximate cause" of the injury or death. This negligence must be shown to be such that the injury would not have occurred if the dentist had not acted as he did. For example, if the dentist fails to sterilize his instruments and the patient develops an infection or dies, the dentist is liable because the proximate cause is obviously the nonsterile instruments.

Additional Tort Liability

Tort is a term used in legal discussions and means "conduct which constitutes a civil wrong," making it possible for the injured individual to collect damages from the person who caused the injury. In dentistry the most common liability is the tort of negligence.

Other liabilities are the following:

1. Assault, battery and false imprisonment, personal restraint.
2. Fraud or deceit.
3. Defamation, libel, and slander.
4. Invasion of privacy and breach of confidential communication.
5. Liability for the acts of others.

The last item means that the dentist is responsible for the acts of anyone who is employed by him. If an employee injures a patient, it is the dentist who is responsible and can be sued. The employee may also be sued, but usually secondarily.

Negligence ordinarily means that the dentist had permission to treat the patient but the treatment did not measure up to the standards imposed by law or that this particular dentist did not perform his work as effectively as members of similar standing in the dental profession in his community.

Breach of Contract

Another area to consider is breach of contract in which a dentist promises to correct or promises to perform a service for a patient.

If a dentist agrees to achieve a particular result or effect for a patient and fails to do so, he is liable for breach of contract even if he has used the highest degree of professional skill in his work.

It is also in this area that one dentist promises another not to compete in the practice of dentistry and then violates this promise. The court case concerns two dentists, one of whom had for some reason agreed not to practice dentistry within a certain restricted area (such as within a certain town or within fifty miles of that town) and then reconsiders his promise. Usually one of these dentists has been employed by the other or has purchased the records and space of an older dentist who leaves the community. Eventually the older dentist

decides to reopen an office somewhere nearby, and his former patients return to him; or the younger dentist decides he likes the area too well to leave and opens his own office too close to the dentist for whom he worked. Patients who like the younger man soon leave the practice of the older dentist and make their way to the younger man's new office.

Professional Liability Insurance

It is important that a dentist carry liability insurance, the amount being determined by his particular vulnerability. In view of the six-figure settlements which are being awarded, it is wise to carry maximum insurance. Inasmuch as the added cost for complete coverage beyond medical professional liability insurance is slight and the possible need for such coverage is real, it is very wise to have all-inclusive insurance coverage. The actions of assistants should most assuredly be included in the coverage.

Criminal Liabilities

Another form of liability which a dentist can experience is *criminal* liability. In criminal liability cases, the dentist must be guilty of a crime punishable by the court which has jurisdiction over this form of crime.

A crime is an act which wrongs the public as a whole instead of injuring one specific individual. Crimes are classified as misdemeanors or felonies. The classification is important to a dentist who is unfortunate enough to be accused of a crime, because state medical practice acts usually revoke the license of a dentist convicted of a felony. Crimes of moral turpitude (such as willfully evading income taxes) can mean suspension of a dentist's license to practice.[4]

4. C. J. Stetler and A. R. Moritz, *Doctor, Patient, and the Law*, p. 331.

Criminal liability is more difficult to prove than civil liability. In civil action the injured party simply has to show more evidence of injury than the dentist shows lack of proof of injury. If the plaintiff can show more evidence, he is usually able to collect damages.

In a criminal action the government must prove that the defendant is guilty beyond a reasonable doubt and must convince every juror of it. The defendant is guaranteed the right to a trial by jury and is presumed innocent until proved guilty. He need not even try to defend himself. He can remain silent, and the government must prove him guilty beyond reasonable doubt. He can then appeal to a higher court.

Criminal abortions, narcotic violations, and birth control statute violations are some of the subjects of criminal actions. More serious is that of unlawful homicide. Negligence which causes death is sometimes labeled manslaughter. It can occur due to misfeasance, malfeasance, or nonfeasance (a lawful act without due caution, an unlawful act, or failure to perform a legal duty). To be charged as a criminal the dentist must have been "willful," "wanton," "gross," or "culpable" in his negligence.

Another area of possible serious concern to some dentists is tax evasion. Criminal prosecution and conviction for evasion of tax payment can result in loss of license. It is very important that accurate records be kept to prevent the slightest doubt of the accuracy of income statements.

Summary

It would be unwise for an assistant to look with suspicion on all persons who enter the office—they are not all intending to sue your office for personal liability or medical professional liability. It is wise, however, for the assistant to be alert to conditions which encourage such suits, because in the course of seeing hundreds of people, it is only logical that some of them may become claimants.

We cannot urge you too strongly to be alert to the dangers which exist in your office. Be constantly vigilant. Watch for safety features: furniture, fixtures, rugs, waxed floors, sharp edges, frayed electric cords, furniture which tips easily, step stools which are weak or do not have a wide base. Never leave a patient alone in a room in which there is equipment which could be inadvertently activated, such as X ray if the controls are in the room.

To avoid malpractice claims, see that your records are accurately and clearly kept and that all assistants observe the regulations which are so necessary in preventing these claims.

Criminal liability means an act has been committed which wrongs the public as a whole rather than one individual. Such crimes usually result in loss of license to practice dentistry. Among the crimes in this classification is evasion of taxes. Careful records must be kept to prevent the slightest doubt of accuracy of income statements.

Study Questions

1. Why is it so necessary today to be alert to dangers in the office which may bring lawsuits?
2. What kinds of claims are filed?
3. Discuss malpractice claims.
4. What are breach of duty claims?
5. Discuss *burden of proof.*
6. What is *res ipsa loquitur?*
7. What is proximate cause?
8. What are the tort liabilities for a dentist?
9. Discuss breach of contract.
10. What protection does professional liability insurance provide?
11. Why is a criminal liability accusation more serious for a dentist?
12. What records must be carefully kept to avoid a charge of one kind of criminal liability?

Bibliography

The bibliography for part three appears at the end of chapter fifteen.

15 | *Avoiding Dental Professional Liability Claims*

(Minimizing the Danger of Unjustified Malpractice Claims)

In chapter fourteen, minimum explanations of the types of medical professional liability claims which have been filed against dentists were discussed. It is possible, by being careful of actions and records, to avoid to a large degree the danger of such suits. This chapter is devoted to the presentation of defenses of medical professional liability actions.

Three Defenses for Dental Professional Liability Actions

Contributory Negligence

If a patient does not cooperate with his dentist by following all reasonable instructions, and this failure on the part of the patient contributes to his problem—injury, worsened condition, or death—he cannot collect damages because it is classified as contributory negligence.

Assumption of Risk

Legally it is assumed that to knowingly pursue a course of action which involves certain risks means that the person cannot recover damages should injury occur. For example, a skier assumes the normal risks of injury while skiing. In dentistry the assumption of risk means that a patient assumes the risks of specific treatment, having been properly informed about them, but he does not assume risk from negligent treatment.

If experimental treatment is to be attempted (that as yet is not adequately proved safe), the patient must be fully warned and should sign a consent statement to relieve the dentist of liability for the possible detrimental effects.

Statute of Limitation

Time limits are established for the filing of court claims. These time limits vary from state to state. It is important to know the statute of limitations for your state. If a claim is not filed within that period of time, it can never be filed.

Minimizing the Danger of Unjustified Medical Professional Liability Claims

Some of the medical professional liability claims which are filed against dentists have legitimate bases. However, many of the cases are unjustified claims. In order to protect your dentist from such claims, there are certain basics which must be observed.

A grievance committee of the county dental society provides effective assistance to both dissatisfied patients and the dentist who might be sued by these patients. The committee hears the patient's complaints, investigates the problem, and is then in a position to establish better communication between the patient and dentist. *How* effective this committee is will depend on its local organization and methods of operation.

The *general standard of care* dispensed by a dentist should be the equivalent of like dentists practicing under similar conditions.

Experimental treatment should be performed only with the full knowledge and consent of the patient. A law exists that a dentist shall use only such methods as are generally approved by other dentists in the community. Thus, for any experimental treatment it is wise to have the written permission from the patient because the dentist is violating a law if he experiments on a patient without this permission. If the patient requests this care, he has released the dentist from the violation.

Diagnostic tests which are usually used for specific symptoms must be performed if the dentist is to escape the accusation of inadequate diagnosis.

Specialists and consultations should be used whenever the dentist deems it necessary and proper. Failure to request the care of a specialist for a condition which is not normally treated by the dentist could lead to a charge of negligence.

The maintenance of equipment used in the office is very important. Regular care of electrical and X-ray equipment will prevent injury and therefore medical professional liability claims.

Consent of the patient is necessary to perform treatment or surgery. A dentist who proceeds without the written consent of the patient is inviting claims of assault and battery. It is necessary for the dentist to inform the patient of the course of treatment and its probable outcome and to permit the patient to decide whether he wishes to undergo the particular treatment. The same is true for oral surgery. Any surgical procedure must be preceded by a specific consent for the particular surgery to be performed.

The employment of assistants creates an area which can be filled with hazards. A dentist must be exceedingly careful in the delegation of tasks to his staff. No one other than the dentist is licensed to practice dentistry, and any delegation of duties which legally can be performed only by the dentist can result in medical professional liability suits.

The dental assistant must be careful to refrain from statements which may invite a lawsuit. Suppose, for example, there has been an accident in which the dentist has inadvertently injured a patient in the presence of an assistant. Anything which the assistant says at that time is a part of the action, and the patient can quote the assistant in court.

A dental assistant should be very careful to avoid making any statement which might imply that she thinks the dentist made a mistake or was at fault. No comment should be made about the dentist's work at this time—even the comment "This never happened before" is an invitation to some patients to sue. *The dental assistant can best say nothing.*

It is also essential that assistants are careful not to prescribe for the patients in conversation with them, not to discuss the relative merits of methods of treatment, and not to pass *any* opinion about any dentist.

If you discuss medication or its effect, without specific instructions from the dentist, you are liable to be charged with practicing dentistry without a license to do so.

The dental assistant is permitted to take dictation from the patient or a member of his family concerning the effects of the treatment he has received. *However, she may not discuss the probable effects or predict what she thinks the dentist may do when he receives the report.*

Never permit the refill of a prescription without first consulting your dentist and receiving his permission for the pharmacist.

If you follow these suggestions, you may avoid doing or saying anything which would place you in the position of practicing dentistry.

The *instructions given a patient* must be specific, detailed, and clear. Some of them should be in writing to avoid misunderstandings. Frequently a medical professional liability claim is begun by a patient because of poor results of treatment. Be sure that the poor results are not due to the fact that the patient was not carefully instructed as to his obligations in home care.

Optimism, like courtesy, is infectious. Optimism is the inclination to anticipate the best possible outcome and leads to confidence on the part of the patient in the ability of his dentist and the anticipated results. It should be instilled into the minds of the staff and, in turn, be infectious to the recipient of services.

Dental records are of extreme importance. A complete, legible, carefully written clinical record is essential. It may make the difference between a verdict in favor of the dentist instead of one against him.

It is also wise not to correct nor write over these records. It is better practice to note the correction as such. Draw a single line through the incorrect statement so that the statement is still readable. Then note the correction and the date on which the correction was made. It is also helpful to initial the correction.

An example of incorrect care of records occurred in a situation where a dentist was sued. His prescription for the patient was well within the normal limits of the general prescription policies for that drug. However, this patient suffered a severe allergic reaction to it. When the patient's attorney approached the dentist, he became disturbed because the dosage was somewhat more than he usually prescribed. He erased the record of the amount of the drug administered and wrote over it. When the insurance company made a photocopy of the record, the erasure showed clearly. A quick out-of-court settlement was made because the record had been altered, not because there was anything wrong with the original dosage. Be certain that your records are neatly and accurately kept, and be certain all corrections are visible and noted as having been made on the date that you prepared the record, or close to that time.

Frequently a professional liability claim is begun by a patient due to poor results of treatment. Actually the poor results are due, at least in part, to the fact that the patient did not follow his dentist's orders, or the specific drug or dosage was inadequate. However, in a jury trial, the aggrieved individual is a far more appealing object to the jury than the dentist is. The complete, carefully written record, substantiated by letters to the patient indicating the need to follow the treatment schedule carefully, is one of the best defenders of the dentist in the courtroom. Be certain that your office protects your dentist as completely as possible by keeping such records and by writing the necessary letters which should be sent by registered mail.

Any record to be given to a new dentist requires a *written* request from the patient. A brief résumé of the history and treatment is then sent to the new dentist.

The patient can also request that the new dentist send to the former dentist for such records, but the dentist giving the information ought to insist on a written request signed by the patient.

Insurance Forms and Reports

It is possible to have an insurance report used against a dentist by both the patient and the insurance company. Examine insurance reports carefully. Call the attention of your dentist to any items which might cause trouble for him. Be certain that you have a copy in your file of every insurance report which leaves the office.

Some of the items you should think about as you look over an insurance form to be mailed are these:

1. A medical professional liability suit can start from an indication by the dentist that the problem encountered in the office was not entirely the fault of the patient. In this instance the patient collects from the insurance company and then sues the dentist.

2. Any statement which might be interpreted as placing the responsibility on your office for any accident or unfortunate occurrence should be rephrased so that it does not admit or assume blame.

3. A statement made by the dentist which uses the wrong words to describe the patient—words which can be termed libelous —should be rewritten. For example, the dentist should say he was "unable to discover any physical conditions which would account for the patient's complaints" instead of saying the patient is a "malingerer."

4. Be certain the insurance form is completed properly. An insurance firm can sue a dentist for incomplete reports.

   If you have *any* misgivings about these reports, it is far wiser to consult your dentist and gain his permission to present the papers to his attorney than to mail in a report which might create a legal problem. It is to be hoped that your dentist does maintain a relationship with an attorney.

Criticism of other dentists is considered unwise because only the dentist in attendance knew the conditions existing at the start of the treatment. Careless derogatory remarks about the treatment prescribed by another dentist or physician have started unjustified lawsuits. The reputation of the health profession suffers every time there is a lawsuit. The public certainly deserves to keep its faith in the health professions. You can help by not destroying that faith by careless remarks.

Attitude of the staff toward patients is extremely important in maintaining the desired atmosphere of thoughtful consideration of each patient. The tactful care of the patients by the entire staff can be a preventive measure when considering medical protective liability suits. If a patient seems to change his outlook (grumble, be somewhat antagonistic or withdrawn), it is time to *communicate*. A review of the case history in consultation with the patient may tell the dentist why the patient appears dissatisfied. In turn, this may prevent a medical protective liability suit.

Consideration of each patient as an individual human being with a life to lead and interests beyond your office will be one of the best deterrents to medical protective liability suits any dentist can have. A patient who feels kindly toward the entire staff is not going to start a suit. He thinks of his dentist as his friend.

A *substitute dentist* is sometimes necessary. Patients are to be informed should the dentist plan to be away. They should also be told whom to see in the dentist's absence. To some patients the discovery that their dentist is not present to care for them is very upsetting. Soothing, tactful reassurance is a strong deterrent to possible court actions.

Prescriptions have been the cause of some court problems. A written prescription by the dentist is the best insurance against being charged for an error in prescription for which the dentist is not responsible. Sometimes there is misunderstanding when a prescription is given verbally over the telephone and an error is made in filling a prescription. The problem can be avoided by insisting that the written prescription be presented to the pharmacist.

A *reliable witness, especially for examination of female patients,* is essential. The chairside assistant, for example, can be present in the operatory during the examination. She is rightfully there to write down the dentist's findings. A male dentist who examines female patients in the absence of a third person shows extremely poor judgment. Serious charges have resulted from such examinations. Without a witness, the dentist is suspect.

Discussion of Cases

A patient must confide in his dentist information which he may not wish known to *anyone* else. The law protects each human being by stating that he has a right to privacy. The dentist cannot reveal any information to anyone without the express permission of the patient. This also means that the dentist's staff is unable to divulge any information regarding any patient. Special circumstances such as insurance examinations require the listing of information. The patient must be made aware of this procedure before the information is released.

Never reveal information about a patient to an unauthorized person. It may surprise you to know that to be legally correct in giving information to an authorized person, it is necessary to have the request for information in writing. *Never* give information about a patient over the telephone. Ask the caller to write his request and mail it to you. Be sure to ask him to furnish the authorization by the patient or a responsible member of the family. Be certain that the written authorization is actually a document executed by the patient or responsible member of his family. It pays to double-check the authenticity of this request.

If a dentist is requested to give information to an attorney, he must have a release signed by the patient. The release includes the name and address of the person to whom the report is to be sent. It should be signed by the patient and dated. His signature should be witnessed by someone other than the dentist or his staff members.

It is interesting to know that in addition to the right to privacy, the patient-dentist relationship is one of *privileged communication*; that is, it is the privilege of the patient to request his dentist to keep the information private or reveal it in a court of law as the patient desires. The statute regarding privileged communication does not apply to the dentist's staff. No staff member can reveal *any* information at any time. They are all required to keep the records confidential.

One exception to the right to privacy and privileged communication is that of the dentist who is employed by an insurance company. He examines a patient with no thought of treatment, and reports his findings to his insurance company. The information from this examination is not privileged. The dentist may testify in a court of law about his findings without the permission of the patient.

Carelessness or negligence is one area to guard against by scrupulous care in the office. The alert assistant will maintain a constant vigilance against dirt, lack of order, and outworn materials. Records will be accurately maintained. She will frequently look at the office through the eyes of a patient to see wherein some detail needs attention so that the office looks immaculately clean and neat. The appearance of a tidy office is a deterrent to accusations of carelessness and negligence. Attention to patients' needs, considering each patient as a VIP (very important person), is important in establishing this office as one in which negligence does not occur because the staff is too interested in the welfare of the patient.

Fees should be discussed with candor and understood *before* treatment is begun. It prevents serious misunderstandings and is fair to the patient. The patient will appreciate this kind of consideration. Contrary to the opinion of many that a dentist is too important to discuss fees, the dentist who has satisfied patients will discuss fees because he has been communicating with his patients.

Lawsuits for Fees

Sometimes malpractice suits are really countersuits to a large dental bill or collection work by the dentist and his staff. The patient has decided the bill is too high or for some reason he doesn't want to pay when payment is due. The charge, of course, should be correctly just and owing before initial billing. In the event of a patient's dissatisfaction with the fee charged, the patient is urged to discuss this with his dentist. Should this discussion fail to produce any satisfactory arrangement for the patient to complete his financial obligation, it is wise to know the time limits on malpractice suits in your state. There is a law which outlaws a malpractice suit; and perhaps by careful consideration of just when you should apply pressure to collect an account, a suit may be avoided.

Withdrawal from a case is sometimes necessary or wise. As discussed in chapter thirteen, there are certain precautions which are necessary when a dentist wishes to withdraw from a case. It is necessary to send the patient a registered letter stating that the dentist is withdrawing and suggesting how the patient can find other dental help if he so desires.

Medical protective liability insurance is a must in today's practice of dentistry. There are several large firms who do nothing but look after the legal problems which dentists and physicians face. It is important to understand the regulations of malpractice insurance and to follow the suggestions of the insurance company. For example, no statement should be made nor letter be written about a medical protective liability claim by a dentist or his staff unless it is done at the instigation of and with the approval of his attorney. If a dentist is advised that he is to be involved in a suit, he should notify his insurance company at once.

Insurance companies urge dentists not to admit fault because frequently the dentist does not know all the facts regarding a patient's reaction to treatment. Many policies state that a dentist cannot admit fault without the express permission of the insurance company. It is wise for the assistant and the dentist to read the policy carefully and be certain that they both understand what the insurance company does for them and what they are expected to do to keep the insurance in force.

Legal advice concerning lawsuits should be accepted from the attorney whom the dentist employs. A simple list of rules about such matters ought to be posted where the staff can be reminded of their duties, such as refraining from discussing any cases and avoiding the temptation to inadvertently prescribe for the patient.

Settlement of lawsuits is a matter to be handled by the insurance company with whom medical protective insurance is carried and/or the dentist's attorney. Be very certain that no comment about any matter pertaining to a lawsuit is ever made by any staff member except as required by the attorney of the dentist or the court of law.

Summary

Defenses to medical professional liability actions are as follows:

1. Contributory negligence. (Proving the patient contributed by not taking proper home care of himself.)
2. Assumption of risk. (Proving the patient was informed of the risks involved.)
3. Statute of limitations. (Allowing the collection of the case to wait until the statute of limitations becomes effective and makes it impossible for the patient to start a suit.)

Minimizing the dangers of unjustified medical professional liability claims includes the following:

1. Using the local dental society grievance committee.
2. Practicing dentistry equivalent to the general standards of care provided by like dentists in the community.
3. Asking the patient to sign a written permission for experimental care.
4. Using known diagnostic tests for all diagnoses.
5. Calling in specialists for consultation when warranted.
6. Maintaining equipment in excellent condition.
7. Having written permission to perform surgery or institute treatment.
8. Being careful in delegating duties to assistants and being certain assistants do not practice dentistry inadvertently.
9. Giving patients detailed specific instructions for home care.
10. Being cheerful and optimistic about the outcome of treatment.
11. Keeping complete, carefully written clinical records.
12. Being accurate and complete in preparing insurance records.
13. Consulting your attorney when necessary.
14. Avoiding criticism of other dentists.
15. Treating patients tactfully and being certain communication is established.
16. Notifying patients of a substitute dentist when such substitute is necessary.
17. Writing all prescriptions, permitting telephoning of a prescription on an emergency basis only. Request a copy when this procedure is followed.
18. Using a reliable witness at all examinations of patients, especially female patients.

19. Avoiding discussions of cases . . . abiding by the law regarding patient's right to privacy.
20. Getting all requests for information in writing with signed consent by patients to release such information.
21. Remembering the statute regarding privileged communication.
22. Keeping the office scrupulously clean and neat to avoid charges of carelessness and negligence.
23. Discussing fees with patients *before* performing services.
24. Using written registered letters when withdrawing from cases.
25. Carrying medical protective liability insurance in a large enough amount to be worthwhile.
26. Using legal advice concerning lawsuits . . . as a prevention to lawsuits by consulting the lawyer *first*.

Study Questions

1. List the defenses to malpractice actions.
2. Write an explanation of the dental assistant's role in maintaining equipment in excellent condition as an aid to preventing lawsuits.
3. Discuss complete clinical records and their importance to the dentist.

Bibliography

HAROLDS, LOUIS R., and BLOCK, MELVIN, eds. *Medical Malpractice: The ATL Seminar.* Rochester, N.Y.: The Lawyers Cooperative Publishing Co., 1966.

HOWARD, W. W., and PARKS, ALEX L. *Carnahan's The Dentist and the Law.* St. Louis: C. V. Mosby Co., 1965.

MILLER, SIDNEY L. *Legal Aspects of Dentistry.* New York: G. P. Putnam's Sons, 1970.

SARNER, HARVEY. *Dental Jurisprudence.* Philadelphia: W. B. Saunders Co., 1963.

STETLER, C. JOSEPH, and MORITZ, ALAN R. *Doctor and Patient and the Law.* St. Louis: C. V. Mosby Co., 1962.

WORMSER, RENE A. *The Story of the Law.* New York: Simon and Schuster, 1962.

PART FOUR | PROFESSIONAL AND FINANCIAL RECORDS

Patients and dentists need accurate records of the dental services rendered and the financial transactions these services involve.

The dental assistant must understand how to keep such records, including all records concerning:

> services rendered patients,
> accounting of services rendered patients,
> financial arrangements for patients,
> credit and collections,
> office operating expenses,
> taxes,
> insurance, and
> office income.

The records which concern the rendering of dental services for patients are *professional* records. Sometimes this part of the record is spoken of as the patient's *clinical* record to distinguish it from a record of payment for the services received. The patient payment record is often called the *patient's account record*. The financial and professional records are usually kept separately.

Part four is devoted to a comprehension of basic record keeping.

16 | *Clinical Records*

The Purpose of Clinical Records

Clinical records are exceedingly important to your dentist for his professional protection. They are preserved in order that all the information your dentist may need at some future date is available. These records include written notes, radiographs (X rays), study models, and photographs.

A wise dentist makes a thorough case study before he begins treatment in order that he may have a complete written record of his diagnosis of the case. The subsequent "treatment" or "service" record, the diagnostic records of the case study, the study models, radiographs, and the color slides which he may make—all comprise the permanent record. This record is essential to the dentist for reference as he completes the prescribed dentistry for the patient. During the progress of the work, a patient may forget the original agreement and need to be shown records which will eliminate any misunderstanding which has developed.

Clinical records are considered legal records. Should a patient ever bring a court action against a dentist, the clinical records become vitally important in the dentist's defense. *Never* alter entries on clinical records. If an error has been made in an entry, draw one line through the incorrect entry and write the correct entry below. Be sure the incorrect entry can still be read.

Accurate, complete, neat records, properly filed, will be invaluable to your dentist and thoroughly appreciated by him.

We will now discuss in detail the types of records which will be found in dental offices. Not all offices will keep all records, but some of these records, or similar forms, will be used in most dental offices.

Patient Registration

The procedures used in various dental offices for the registration of patients range from an extremely detailed personal history, with a signed permission for the dentist to treat a case as he sees fit, to no requests for information whatsoever. In the office of an oral surgeon, or other specialist, there may be need for a detailed registration form. Every office will benefit from using some form of patient registration, however.

The information usually requested on a registration form commonly serves to definitely identify the patient, since the patient records the information himself. His name will be spelled correctly. If there is any question, the correct pronunciation of the name should be asked when the registration form is received by the assistant. The address will be the correct current one. Whatever information the particular office asks the patient to supply on such a form is more likely to be accurate because it is handwritten by the patient.

The information requested in a registration form should not be confused with that which the dentist may ask in the way of a dento-medical history before proceeding with examination and diagnosis. The registration form deals primarily with the information needed for effective conduct of the business requirements between the dental office and the patient.

For minimum requirements, it is desirable to know the patient's first name, middle initial, and last name; home address; home phone number; business address and phone number; the name of the person responsible for the account (who shall be billed?); the name of the person who referred the patient to your office; and the date.

Properly presented to the patient, a form with blanks provided for this information will be completed without question. Proper presentation means the manner used by the assistant to indicate that this form is routinely used by the office and is routinely filled out by all new patients.

One suggestion which has been made for the use of such a form is that it be headed "Acquaintance Form" rather than "Registration Form" or "Patient's Registration."

Patient's Individual Record Card

The patient records maintained by various dental offices vary from extremely simple records to properly detailed and maintained records of dental services.

There are several reasons for keeping a thoroughly detailed record of services performed for any individual patient. An accurate record of previous treatment is certainly an aid in providing the best dental service for the patient. Complete records are the best protection against malpractice claims or in defense of them.

For the purposes of training, one type of record keeping will be discussed here. It remains for any new dental assistant to adapt herself to the particular method of recording patient services, and all record keeping in general, used in the office in which she is employed.

The patient's individual record card, 8 1/2 by 11 inches in size, has headings across the top which should be carefully completed by the assistant. Information which is apt to be permanent is typed or written in ink. Tem-

Fig. 16.1. Acquaintance Form

```
ACQUAINTANCE FORM          Date_____

Patient's                                    Date of
Name_____  Birth_____

Person responsible for account_____

Residence Address_____

Business Address_____

Residence Telephone_____ Business Telephone_____
                                                    How
Employer_____  Long?_____

Occupation or type of work_____

Physician_____ Referred by_____

Relative or close friend_____

Former Dentist_____

Convenient Time for Appointments_____

_____

F204  REV. 4-63                    SPILLANE'S, MINNEAPOLIS 4, MINN.
```

Courtesy Dr. James Kershaw; with authors' modifications

porary information is written in pencil. Thus, in the proper spaces type or write in ink these items:

1. Patient's name, last name first, then first name, middle name or initial, and any title in parentheses.
2. Birth date.
3. Name of person who referred patient, preceded by the words "Referred by."

In pencil enter these items:

1. Home address and telephone.
2. Business address and telephone.

The body of the patient's record card contains ruled columns and lines, providing space for the following information relating to (*a*) the dental services performed for that patient, (*b*) year, month, and day, (*c*) service rendered (should be detailed well), (*d*) chair time and/or laboratory time required for the service, and (*e*) fee charged. Very frequently there is also room for amounts paid and the balance owing on the account. In some offices the dentist will complete the entries on this record; in others, the assistant is expected to copy the required information. In either case, it should be done as soon as possible after the service is given to the patient, while the information is remembered and can be entered in good detail.

Notes should be made on patient's records of emergency treatment, surgical procedures, and treatment of infections. They should include any warnings of possible complications or any instructions to report to the office on a specific date for observation which were given by the dentist or his staff. Should any legal action be started by a patient, these records are invaluable. Details of treatment should be complete, even though abbreviated wording is used.

Case History

Case history is a term applied to a collection of pertinent facts related to the examination, diagnosis, prognosis, and treatment of the patient. The examination portion may include such information as age, sex, marital status, nationality, occupation, spouse's occupation, educational level, history of systemic and oral diseases, medications, allergies, weight, height, complexion, physical infirmities, temperament, diet, dental history, and habits. Generally, it is common practice to do a thorough case history in university dental school clinics, dental public health clinics, and hospitals. In private dental practice, however, this questioning of the patient regarding his physical history is frequently reduced to a minimum. Six or seven questions can usually satisfy the important points of physical condition required by the dentist. The circumstances in private dental practice usually do not necessitate the detailed physical history, since most patients seen in a dental office are ambulatory and their physical condition is usually good. When the reverse is true, it is quite easily discovered by a condensed version, and further information can be elicited from the patient. A consultation with his physician will be requested if the dentist deems it necessary or desirable for the patient's welfare.

Color-Coding the Record of Special Patients

Regardless of what other information is sought, of utmost importance on any case history in a dental office is information relating to conditions which may require special medical attention. *Routinely* the dentist must know these facts:

1. Does the patient have an allergic reaction? If so, what causes that reaction and what drug or drugs must be avoided for the patient's safety and comfort? (If the patient is vague about allergies, consult his physician.)
2. Does the patient take a "maintenance dosage" of any drug? This drug may affect the individual's ability to tolerate certain dental treatment, may require the administration of some medication to make dental treatment possible, or may create a problem for even the most routine dental procedures. For example, cardiovascular patients commonly take anticoagulant drugs which prevent blood from clotting. Special treatments must be instituted with these patients *before* any dental surgery is performed.
3. Does the patient have any chronic condition which may develop into an emergency in the dental office? For example, the patient may be subject to epileptic seizures or may be a diabetic and, therefore, subject to insulin shock. Prompt medical attention is absolutely essential under certain circumstances.

Some dentists use an arresting color to mark the records of patients who may require special medical attention. The physician's telephone number is written boldly in a color which can be seen easily. Should an emergency arise, the physician can be contacted quickly if the number is so written. The color-coding of the record envelope and patient's service card reminds the staff that this patient may develop into an emergency requiring immediate attention.

Radiographs (X rays)

Patient records are the property of the dentist. X rays are a part of those records, although many patients misunderstand this relationship because many dentists state a charge "for X rays," rather than stating that the charge is for the "examination" in its entirety. If any treatment beyond examination and diagnosis is performed for a patient, the X rays should be retained as a part of the legal record of the office. In circumstances involving a request for the X rays by the patient, many dentists will send the X rays to another dentist for the patient if no actual treatment was involved beyond examination and diagnosis; or if a regular patient finds that he is to be transferred to another city, it is not unusual to supply him with his most recent X rays as a gesture of courtesy. It is preferable, however, to forward radiographs by mail directly to the dentist named by the patient as his new practitioner.

Radiographs must be placed in an X-ray mount to be properly examined. The name of the patient and the date of X rays are written in pencil on the mount. This provides for neat reuse of the mount when radiographs are made later. Mounts containing radiographs which are sent out of the office—for the use of a specialist, for example—should have the name of your dentist and all other data written in ink.

When X rays are no longer current, they are usually removed from the mount and placed in a coin envelope with the date and the patient's name on it. They can then be filed in the patient's record envelope or a separate X-ray file. How long they should be kept as a clinical record is a matter of your dentist's choice.

Mounted X rays are usually filed separately. One of three plans is used for filing: (1) They can be numbered and filed by number. A 3" x 5" file of the patients' names in alphabetical order lists the numbers of their X rays on the card; (2) The information may be kept in an X-ray guidebook which lists the patients' names and the numbers of the X rays; and (3)

Radiographs may be kept in the patient's record envelope.

Study Models

A dentist may use study models of a patient's mouth in order to study and diagnose the problems of the individual patient more accurately. These study models are casts made from impressions taken of a patient's mouth. They are carefully labeled with the patient's name and the date and are stored safely for future reference after the dentist has made his diagnosis.

Slides

Many dentists are aware of the importance of intraoral and extraoral photography and use both "before" and "after" color slides of patients who have a prosthetic case or a mouth reconstruction which affects their appearance.

The slides, both extaoral and intraoral, are filed by number. A number is placed on the slide mounting itself or on a gummed label. The gummed label is glued to the slide mount. The number of the slide is written on the patient's record. The slides are then filed in numerical order. A slide number book may also be used. In this book the patients' names are listed alphabetically with the slide number after the name.

Patient's Record Envelope

The envelope which is used to contain and protect the patient's record card and X-ray mounts is slightly larger than the record card. Whether or not it has ruled lines on it for entry of the various details required, it is important that this information be entered in exactly the same manner and in the same position on each patient's record envelope. The form used is the same as that used on the heading of the record card: patient's last name, first name, and middle name or initial, in ink or typed, in the upper-left-hand area of the envelope. This is followed on the same line by the home address, telephone number, city, and zip code in pencil. The second line has no entry under the name of the patient but has the business address below the residence address and business phone below the home telephone number, all in pencil. A 3-H or 4-H pencil is good for such entries. When changes are necessary, the use of an art-gum eraser will permit the envelopes and cards to last through many changes of address.

A minor's birth date is entered in ink on the third line, center, of the patient's record envelope. The name of the father or responsible adult is entered in ink in a routine place in the heading section of the patient's record card, just below the minor's name on the rec-

ord envelope, again in ink. Since the statement must go to the responsible individual, not to the minor, the information is necessary for billing.

If the patient is a married woman, her name is entered as Jones, Mrs. John J. (Mary). If she is divorced, widowed, or separated from her husband, she is correctly referred to as Jones, Mrs. Mary L. Mr., Mrs., Miss, or Ms. provides a simple method of indicating an adult or a self-supporting minor.

Many dental offices like to keep some additional information on the patient's record envelope. One item is the "yearly number" of each patient. Beginning with the first workday in January of each year, the first patient receives the number "1"—entered in ink on the left side of the patient's record envelope, below the top three-line area, thus: 19XX-1. The sequence of numbers is kept in order by noting

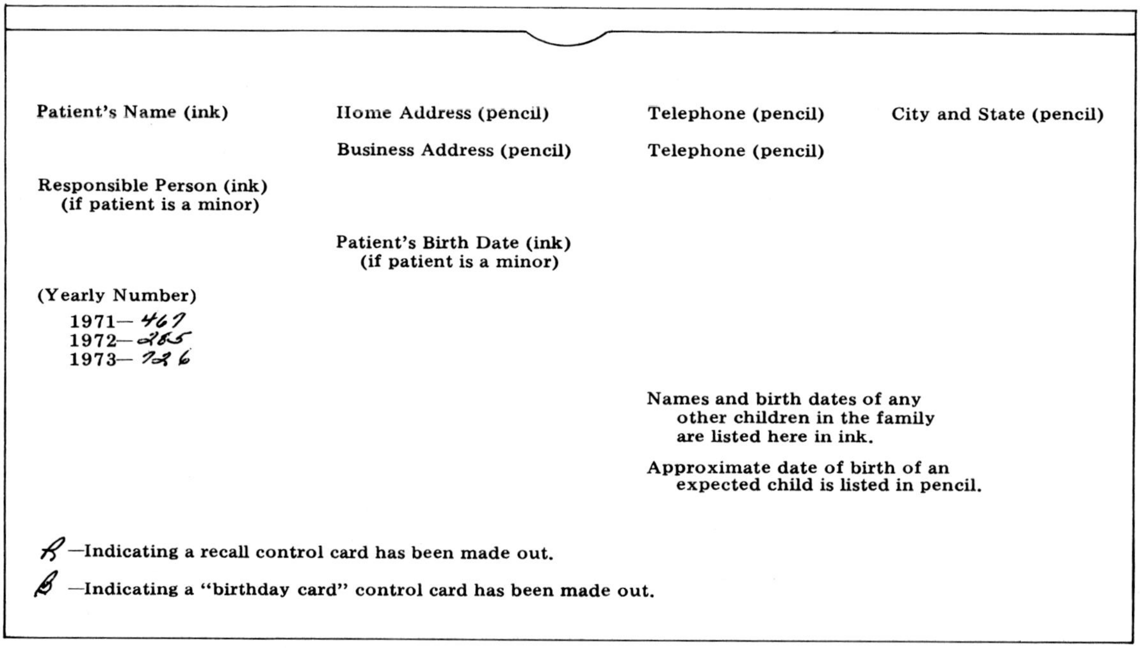

| Patient's Name (ink) | Home Address (pencil) | Telephone (pencil) | City and State (pencil) |
| | Business Address (pencil) | Telephone (pencil) | |

Responsible Person (ink)
(if patient is a minor)

Patient's Birth Date (ink)
(if patient is a minor)

(Yearly Number)
1971— 467
1972— 265
1973— 236

Names and birth dates of any
other children in the family
are listed here in ink.

Approximate date of birth of an
expected child is listed in pencil.

ℛ —Indicating a recall control card has been made out.

ℬ —Indicating a "birthday card" control card has been made out.

Fig. 16.2. Patient's record envelope

the *next* number to be used on the day sheet. For example, after placing "19XX-1" on the first patient's record envelope, the number "1" in the bottom margin of the day sheet is crossed off and the number "2" written after it. When number "2" has been assigned to the second patient's record envelope, it in turn is crossed off at the bottom of the day sheet, and the number "3" is written. At the end of each day the next number to be used is transferred to the day sheet for the next day. Thus the final workday in December will carry the figure indicating the total number of patients seen in the course of the year. The increase each month can be entered as a separate figure in that month's reports for comparison with previous months or previous years. A patient of some years' standing would have a vertical column of figures representing the first year he became a patient in the practice and each year he has been in as a patient thereafter. It indicates, in general, how regular he has been. The total figures are of use statistically to the dentist and, if kept at all, should be kept accurately.

Some dentists like to have the children's names and birth dates entered on the record envelope of a parent as a means of keeping up with the family and encouraging their entry into the practice at the proper time. Those entries are made in ink in the lower right quarter of the patient's record envelope.

If a separate recall card system is used in the office under a Come-up card file, the fact that a recall card has been made out from the patient's record envelope information can be so indicated by writing the letter *R* in the lower-left-hand corner of the envelope. If the dentist sends birthday cards to his young patients up to a certain age, a similar card for the birthday Come-up file is necessary and a letter *B* in the lower left corner of the envelope indicates that this card has been made out and is in the birthday card file.

New Patient Examination and Diagnosis Card

Another card which is often used in conjunction with the patient's record card is the new patient's examination and diagnosis card, also 8 1/2 by 11 inches in size. (See fig. 16.3.) This card usually includes a diagram of the teeth for entry of the necessary treatment pictorially, several entries for a history of the patient, space for entry of results of vitality tests of the teeth, and usually space for a written summary of the required dental work with the fees to be charged for the services. The manner of using this card, in those offices in which it applies, is much the same as the patient's record card insofar as information provided in the heading is concerned. The diagnostic part of the record might be completed either by the dentist entering the information as he conducts the examination or by the assistant as the dentist gives her the information verbally at the time. The estimate portion may likewise be made up by the dentist; or if the assistant has developed a familiarity with the procedures in the office in which she works, the dentist may delegate to her the work of making up the listings and estimates according to his directions.

Case Presentations

Now that all the patient records are gathered—including radiographs, models, case histories, photographs—the dentist may have an appointment with the patient for "case presentation" to help the patient understand his dental needs.

The case-presentation appointment is an appointment for the express purpose of discussing the dental needs and the treatment to be instituted with the patient or other responsible person. Some offices vary this routine by doing only the full-mouth and bitewing X rays and study models, if desired, on the first

DATE 19___	LOCATION R	L	SERVICE PLANNED	ESTIMATE #1		ESTIMATE #2		COMPLAINT
								PRESENT ILLNESS
								PREVIOUS HISTORY
								ORAL FINDINGS
								HYGIENE 1 2 3 4
								DEPOSITS 1 2 3 4
								PERIODONT. 1 2 3 4
								OCCLUSION
								RESTORATIONS
								ABNORMALITIES
								PROPHYLAXIS
								X-RAYS
								STUDY MODELS
								REMARKS:

NAME IN FULL ___ DATE
RESIDENCE ADDRESS ___ PHONE ___ AGE
BUSINESS ADDRESS ___ PHONE
EMPLOYED
REFERRED BY
RENDER BILL TO
FORMER DENTIST ___ PHYSICIAN
REMARKS

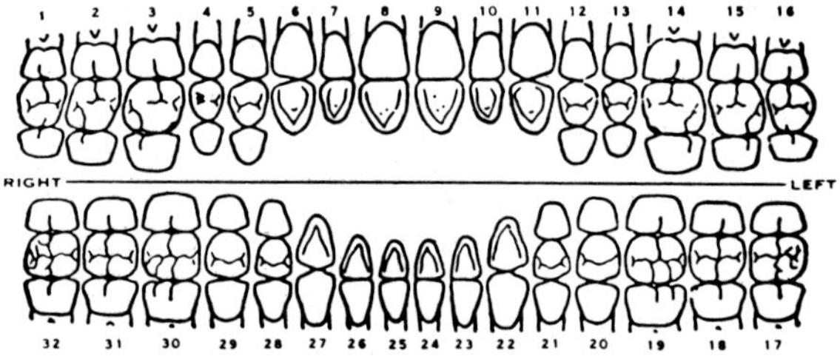

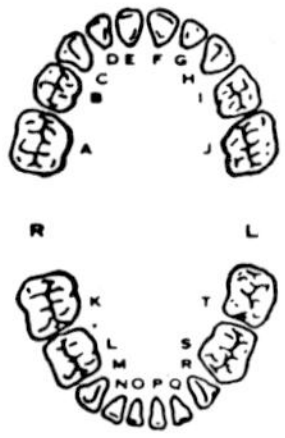

SPILLANE'S, INC. 2826 CEDAR AVE. MPLS. NO. 42

Courtesy Spillane's, Inc., Minneapolis

Fig. 16.3. Combination examination and estimate form

visit. The second appointment is a prophylaxis and oral examination, followed by a discussion with the patient, or other responsible person, of the dental needs and treatment.

Such procedures are not used by all dental offices, of course. The assistant should familiarize herself with the wishes of the dentist for whom she works and should perform all phases of office routine as her employer prefers.

The discussion with the patient or responsible person is referred to as a case presentation—the presenting of the case to the patient for his consideration and necessary decisions. The required dental work is discussed, the various ways of accomplishing the desired results, the recommendations of the dentist, and the costs involved in the various methods of treatment.

It is necessary that a case presentation be protected from any outside interference, such as other members of the office staff moving around, telephone calls for the dentist, or any distracting degree of noise. If a private office is available, it is usually the place selected for these discussions. Some dentists prefer using an operatory, however.

Everything pertaining to the patient's examination and diagnosis is made available beforehand, including X rays and a method for viewing them. Any models your dentist has which might be applicable to the case are placed for his convenience. Very frequently seating space is required for another person in addition to the patient.

There are many methods of presenting cases to patients and many variations in the part which the dental assistant is to play in this procedure. Your dentist may teach you to take over all arrangements once the patient has made a decision about the dental work to be performed. In that event, you will be instructed in arranging payment and scheduling appointments for the work.

If a minor is involved as the patient, the dental office must be sure that the parent gives written consent to the planned course of treatment in all cases.

In summary, then, be sure that no one disturbs the dentist and patient during a case presentation. When the dentist has finished his part of the conference, be ready with your appointment book and other materials which you may need to complete the presentation as your dentist desires. It is well to memorize thoroughly any instructions which he wishes to give the patient. Use notes, if necessary, to be certain nothing is omitted during case presentation.

Summary

Clinical records are exceedingly important to your dentist for patient treatment and professional protection. They include complete studies of the patient's dental health, his diagnosis, and treatment.

The *patient registration form* includes the patient's name, address, telephone number, person responsible for the account, and the individual who referred the patient to the dentist.

The *patient's individual record card* is a detailed record of the services performed. It also has the necessary information about the patient's name, address, telephone, birth, etc., entered at the top of the card. The detailed service record is to be filled in as soon after service as possible, including the date of service.

A *case history* is a detailed physical examination record and is usually used only in clinics or university dental schools. A condensed version is more applicable to the dental office because patients who enter the dental office ordinarily are ambulatory.

Radiographs are identified on the mount with the patient's name in pencil. If the radiographs are kept in a coin envelope, the patient's name and the date of X rays are listed on the envelope.

Study models are used to help diagnose dental ills. They are made from impressions taken of the patient's mouth.

Slides of "before" and "after" appearance of the patient are sometimes used when prosthetics or mouth reconstruction is performed.

The *patient's record envelope* is used to protect his records. It carries identifying information on the exterior: name, address telephone, minor's birth date, and other pertinent data.

The *new patient examination and diagnosis card* is used in some offices for each new patient. It is somewhat similar to the patient's individual record card and contains room for dental history and diagnosis.

Case presentations are conducted by many dentists to enlighten the patient about the condition of his mouth and what services are really needed. During this important interview, the dentist and patient should be undisturbed.

Study Questions
1. What are clinical records and what is their purpose?
2. Discuss the minimum requirements for patient registration.
3. Why are complete records of a patient desirable?
4. Who usually makes entries on a patient record card?
5. What is a case history?
6. To whom do X rays belong?
7. How are X rays stored?
8. What are study models and what does the assistant do with them before use and after use?
9. If your dentist uses slides, how do you care for them?
10. What information is usually found on a patient's record envelope?
11. What is a new patient examination and diagnosis card?
12. What is a case-presentation appointment? What is the usual responsibility of the staff during such an appointment?

17 | *Financial Records*

The financial records which will allow a dentist to know his income and outgo are just as important as the clinical records detailing the care he has given his patients. Remember, the patient will expect the same accuracy in billing as he does in dental treatment. In his mind they reflect one and the same capacity —that is, either accuracy or inaccuracy. It may be illogical, but accuracy in bookkeeping equals accuracy in dental treatment in the minds of many patients!

Business Services for Dentists

In addition to being professionally competent to practice dentistry, a dentist must also operate a business in order to be properly remunerated for his professional services and to provide the necessary organization to treat his patients. In the lengthy education of a dentist, little time can be devoted to business education. At the same time, our society is becoming more complex, and comprehension of business procedures is a necessity. The result is that dentists are increasingly hiring accountants to design and manage a method of keeping their business records. An accountant (hopefully a certified public accountant)[1] is a person who

1. A certified public accountant has served a period of apprenticeship and has passed difficult examinations. He is *certified* much as a dental assistant is certified after passing her examinations. The initials CPA are then used after his name as an indication of his skill in accounting.

has studied management and record keeping.

A dentist may employ the services of a *dental CPA firm*. These firms, whose owners are usually CPAs, perform all types of financial recording for dental offices. Usually a dentist has a choice of several services. The CPAs may prepare only the tax returns if the dentist so desires, or the firm may contract to furnish complete accounting for the office. The dental assistant will make receipts for money received and post the charges on the patients' account records. The CPA firm will assume responsibility at that point, and no further accounting is performed by any employee of the dentist. There are many "packages" of service offered by CPAs between these two extremes of minimal service to complete responsibility. The amount of outside assistance is determined by the dentist. He decides how much accounting service he wishes to purchase. If he plans to have an accountant prepare his income tax statements, he would be wise to permit the accountant to supervise his accounting during the year.

Another person a dentist might employ is a *management consultant* who may or may not be a CPA. The management consultant advises the dentist about his business, and sometimes about his investments. Initially he studies the dentist's way of practicing and his business records. He then sets up a system of accurate bookkeeping for the maintenance of the proper records. He follows through and works with the dentist on a monthly basis. Anytime it becomes necessary to do so, he trains a new assistant in the type of record keeping he wants in the office. He trains the dentist's office employee to keep the office records exactly as he wants them kept for his use in evaluating the business operation of the office, in preparing tax forms, and in periodically examining, analyzing, and reporting to the dentist about his business.

In addition to the accountant services, there are systems such as the Write-It-Once bookkeeping systems promoted by such firms as Burroughs, and the pegboard systems made by a number of firms including Little Press, Inc., of Minneapolis, and National Cash Register. These services ease the complicated problems of accurately keeping records and writing the same information several times.

With computers and rapid office machines, mechanization is overtaking the bookkeeping of the professional office. It appears that data processing (the name given the mechanized form of office accounting) will soon be responsible for the major part of accounting procedures in dental offices because these offices are being computerized.

The "Why" of Record Keeping

No matter how mechanized data processing becomes, each office must still have some method of maintaining day-by-day records which, in turn, can be stored in the computer. The initial data must be prepared by hand by some employee who is exacting and accurate in the preparation of these records. This employee's responsibilities include orderliness and accuracy. An accountant or management consultant will usually supervise the overall plan of keeping records. The record keeper will be told exactly what to do and how to do it.

Everything which exists in a business can be divided into

things that are *owned*,
things that are *owed*, and
that which is left over after these two
    are equaled.

That which is left over belongs to the owner of the business.

Things which are *owned* are called *assets*. They could be converted to cash. Things which are *owed* are called *liabilities.* They represent money owed and are claims against the business. The *cash value* of the difference between assets and liabilities is called *proprietorship* because the owner of a business is a proprietor, and this extra cash value belongs to the owner.

No matter what system of bookkeeping is used, every set of books (record keeping) has to reflect the fact that whenever you *get* something you *give* something, and whenever you *give* something you *get* something. Two things happen in every transaction. You *get* a box of X-ray film and you *give* cash; or you *give* a patient a treatment and you *get* cash.

Assets in a dental office include:

1. Any property owned by the dentist.
2. Accounts receivable.
3. Money in bank accounts.
4. Money already received but not yet deposited.
5. Cash on hand (petty cash and office change fund are examples.)

Liabilities in a dental office include:

1. Obligations to pay for goods already received (supplies to be used during the month ordered from a supply house).
2. Accounts payable (rent on a monthly basis).
3. Interest on debts.
4. Notes (such as a promise to pay for equipment over a period of time).
5. Bad debts (bills which will not be paid by persons owing the dentist money).

Proprietorship (net worth) refers to what the dentist owns after his assets and liabilities are balanced. If he has a thousand dollars in liabilities and two thousand dollars cash on hand and in accounts receivable, he has a proprietorship of one thousand dollars.

Assets equal liabilities plus proprietorship. This information is carefully recorded and studied by the accountant. He sets up the bookkeeping system so that he can watch the factors in this formula. Ordinarily the bookkeeping cycle which is used is called *double entry bookkeeping.* It starts with the keeping of a journal and proceeds through posting, adjusting, closing, and issuing financial statements. Some form of this system will be used in the office in which you work. If there is an accountant or management consultant, your work will be simplified. If you are expected to manage the entire matter yourself, you will need special training in bookkeeping and accounting prior to assuming such responsibilities.

Regardless of what system of bookkeeping is used, every assistant who works with the office records should be sure she keeps careful, formal, written records of

that which the office owes to others,
that which others owe to the office,
all money which is received, and
all money which is spent.

As a dental assistant, you should be aware that you must acquire and *keep all source documents.* (Source documents are the records of proof of billing or proof of payment.) If you order some impression material from the supply house, you must find and keep the invoice which either comes in the package or is mailed to you separately. This is a *source document.* (Fig. 8.2, p. 113, is a source document.)

When a patient visits the office, charges for the services rendered are recorded for the first time on the patient's service record and/or on a "charge slip" if a Write-It-Once bookkeeping system is used. This first record is a source document and must be kept permanently. Invoices for supplies received are also source documents. The record keeper must know where these source documents are. They are the "backup" documents—the proof that a service actually was performed or that a supply actually was received. An accountant or management consultant will expect the record keeper to have these documents available for proof.

Whatever system of bookkeeping is used in the office in which you work, be sure to ask questions and be certain that you follow directions. It is better to ask questions than to guess and do your work incorrectly.

It is also wise to ask your supervisor how you can check periodically to see how well you are doing. Write down any questions which occur to you during the first week you are working with a bookkeeping system and have them available for your supervisor when he comes to verify your work at the end of the week; or seek him out if he does not come to inspect your work.

You are not expected to be able to set up books for the running of a dental practice. You *are* expected to be able to follow directions and keep the records exactly as your dentist wishes to have them kept.

Basic Requirements in Financial Records

Bookkeeping systems in dental offices vary. As with patient records, some offices maintain a minimum of such procedures, some maintain an easily workable but completely adequate system, and some maintain quite complex systems. The successful management of a dental practice requires a bookkeeping system which is fundamentally sound in all its phases and designed to provide the information the dentist desires and the information necessary to make out income tax returns. This section will present *one* way of meeting these complete basic requirements.[2] Following the explanation of the basics is a section on pegboard or Write-It-Once bookkeeping.

2. Recommended by Andrew Froehlich, C.P.A., of the firm of Kuusisto, Froehlich, Borgfelt, and Segal, C.P.A. (medical and dental accountants), Minneapolis, Minnesota.

On page 191 we stated that every record keeper must maintain careful records of the following:

1. Money received and spent.
2. All things for which the office owes others.
3. All things others owe the office.

Records of importance for these classifications include:

1. Records of receipts.
2. An office change fund.
3. Patient service and account records (transactions with individual patients).
4. A day sheet (records of all service rendered and all financial transactions.
5. Discount records.
6. Statements to patients for services rendered.
7. Accounts receivable control to verify the record keeping.
8. Records of petty cash expenditures.
9. Invoices and statements for dental office purchases.
10. Disbursement records (where the money went).
11. A yearly summary of the entire business operation of the office.

In addition to these records, the process of banking and using the checkbook correctly must be thoroughly comprehended. We will divide financial records into three groups:

1. Records about money received and service rendered.
2. Records about expenditures.
3. Banking records.

The Write-It-Once bookkeeping system will then be described. Tax records, which must also be considered, will comprise another chapter.

Records About Money Received and Service Rendered

Receipt Book

A "receipt" (*ree-seat*) is a written acknowledgment of anything, such as money or goods, obtained from another person. In the dental office a receipt should be made out for each and every payment which comes into that office.

Receipts should be made in duplicate. The original copy is given to the patient; the carbon copy remains bound in the book as part of the permanent record for the year. The receipt book of carbons must show *every payment* which has been made in the dental office during the year; therefore it is necessary to make a receipt for each payment (regardless of whether the payment is by check or cash). The total amount of money shown on the carbon receipts for a year should equal the gross income of the dental office for that year.

The patient needs the receipt as proof of payment if he pays for his services by cash. The receipt is not so essential to him if he pays by check, although it is desirable for him to have proof for income tax purposes that he actually paid the dentist the amount which he has stated he paid.

When the patient makes a payment in person, give him a receipt at that time. Daily, when time is available, the payments received through the mail are entered in the receipt book. It generally is not necessary to send the original receipts to the patients whose payments were by check or money order, but some of them may request it. In any event, every payment must be entered in the receipt book so that you have an accurate record of your dentist's gross income.

The receipt should be made out to the individual to whom the account was billed. If the charge was made for six-year-old John and the account was billed to his father, Mr. James

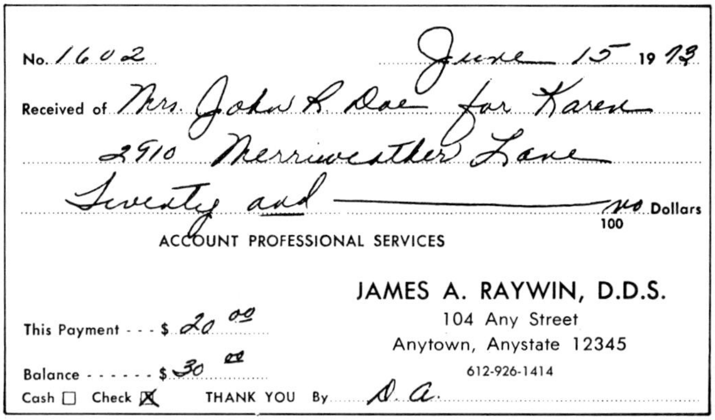
No. 1602 June 15 19 73

Received of Mrs. John R. Doe for Karen

2910 Merriweather Lane

Twenty and no/100 Dollars

ACCOUNT PROFESSIONAL SERVICES

JAMES A. RAYWIN, D.D.S.
104 Any Street
Anytown, Anystate 12345
612-926-1414

This Payment $ 20.00

Balance $ 30.00

Cash ☐ Check ☒ THANK YOU By D. A.

Courtesy Spillane's, Inc., Minneapolis

Fig. 17.1. A sample receipt

Jones, the receipt should be made out to "Mr. James Jones, for John." To insure against errors in crediting an account, the name on the receipt should be followed by the address on the next line. Indicate whether the payment was by check or by cash. When balancing the books at the close of the day, you will find it helpful to know which payments were cash and how much cash was actually received.

Be sure that the carbon copy is always legible. It is your permanent record. A few suggestions can help insure legible carbon copies. Use a good ball-point pen for writing receipts and write firmly. If your office uses receipts for which carbon paper is furnished, buy extra pencil carbon paper and change the carbon frequently. (Some offices now have receipts with carbon paper furnished for each receipt, or paper which duplicates without carbon.)

Office Change Fund

Patients who pay their bills by cash sometimes need change. It is desirable to keep ten to fifteen dollars in small bills in an office cash box—*separate* from the petty cash fund.

The dentist writes a check for the office change fund *once*. The money is permanently available; therefore, the record keeper must always remember to set this amount aside when totaling the cash received during the day. If it is included with the cash received during the day, the total will be greater by exactly the amount which should be in the office change fund.

Another difficulty commonly experienced is illustrated by this example: Suppose Mr. Johnson offers the record keeper, Miss Patrick, a twenty dollar bill and states that he wishes to pay fifteen dollars on account. Miss Patrick makes a receipt for fifteen dollars cash for Mr. Johnson. She now has a twenty dollar bill in her cash receipts, but five of it belongs in the office change fund. It will be necessary for her to make change during the day and replace the five dollars in the office change fund, or at the close of the day Miss Patrick will have five dollars more in the day's receipts than she has actually collected.

Patient's Service and Account Records

Each day several patients receive dental care for which they are to pay either immediately or within the near future, and some records of the dental service, the charges, and the payments received are necessary. These records are called the *patient's service record* and the *patient's account record.* Each is a record for an individual patient.

Some offices combine the patient's service record and the patient's account record and call it the *patient's service and account record.* With such a system the dentist enters in detail the services performed and the charges for them. The assistant enters the payments received and figures the balance. A special filing arrangement is used to keep all records of patients who still owe money in an active file. (See "Filing.")

For purposes of understanding these records more easily, the two types will be discussed separately. They may be maintained as separate records in your office—or combined on one record.

Patient's Service Record

The patient's service record shows the patient's name, address, and telephone number at the top. It may show both home and business telephones and addresses. If the patient

Business Address: Housewife
Business Telephone:
NAME: Doe, Mrs. T. K. (Mary)
Residence Telephone: 826-9172
Address: 6152 Alphonso Street, Anytown, Anystate 12345
Send Bill To: Doe, Mr. Thomas K.

DATE 19[illegible]	Tooth Number	Cavity Location	OPERATION Chair	DEBIT	CREDIT	BALANCE	DATE 19__	Tooth Number	Cavity Location	OPERATION	DEBIT	CREDIT	BALANCE
6/2	L5	MOD	Amal. Nav. 45	25 -		25 -							
6/10	R5	Full Crn	Prep. Nav. 55	40		65 -							

Courtesy Spillane's, Inc., Minneapolis

Fig. 17.2. Patient's service record

is a minor, there is space for his parent's name or other guarantor of the account.

The card provides space for the date and for detailed entry of services rendered. Each time a patient receives a service, the specific service is entered in detail, usually by the dentist. This card is kept in the patient's envelope.

Study the entries on the patient's service record in figure 17.2.

Patient's Account Record (also called Patient's Ledger Card)

A card is used with the patient's name, address, and telephone number at the top. It has spaces for date, item, charges, receipts, and balance.

When the patient receives services, the charge for these services is entered with the date. When the patient pays on account, the amount paid is entered in the receipts column, the balance in the balance column, and the date in its column.

When you transfer the services and charges from the patient's service record, you put a check mark on the patient's service record to indicate that the charge has been posted to the account record. Each day you transfer from your receipt book to the patients' account records all payments for which you have written receipts. As soon as you copy the figure on a patient's account record, you put a check mark on the carbon receipt to indicate that you have posted the payment. The balance is figured each time you post an entry (charge or payment) in order to have all patient account record balances current.

The Day Sheet or Daily Record Sheet

The dentist must have a detailed record of the services he renders, the charges for those services, and the money he receives from patients. This complete, detailed record, professional as well as financial, of the day's activities relating to patients is called a *day sheet.* Some dentists use a book called a "Daily Log," others a printed sheet or card called a "Daily Record"; but they are all classified as a day sheet.

The name of each patient, the service he received, and the charge for this service are written in the proper columns. Some dentists ask that the chair time be entered also. (Chair

NAME IN FULL DATE

RESIDENCE ADDRESS PHONE AGE

BUSINESS ADDRESS PHONE

EMPLOYED

REFERRED BY

RENDER BILL TO

FORMER DENTIST PHYSICIAN

DATE	LOCATION		SERVICES RENDERED	MINS.		DEBIT FEES	CREDIT CASH & DISCOUNT	BALANCE	NOTES
19	R	L		CHAIR	LAB.				

Courtesy Spillane's, Inc., Minneapolis

Fig.17.3. Patient's account record

time is the actual working time which the dentist spends with the patient at the dental chair.)

At the close of the day, total the receipts written and enter this figure on the day sheet. This method provides the least opportunity for mechanical error in bookkeeping because individual payment figures are not transferred. The receipts show the names of the persons who have paid money. All that is really necessary on the day sheet is the total amount of money received.

Also total the charges listed on the day sheet. At the bottom of the sheet, the total charges for the day and the total receipts for that day appear.

Study figure 17.4 for a typical day sheet.

Some dentists want the name of each patient who makes a payment written on the day sheet. If this is true of your dentist, the alternative method to the one just discussed is to enter on the day sheet all payments which you receive with the names of the persons who paid and whether the payments were cash or check. This includes all payments received by mail as well as from patients entering the office. (At the time you enter the payments in the receipt book, enter them on the day sheet.)

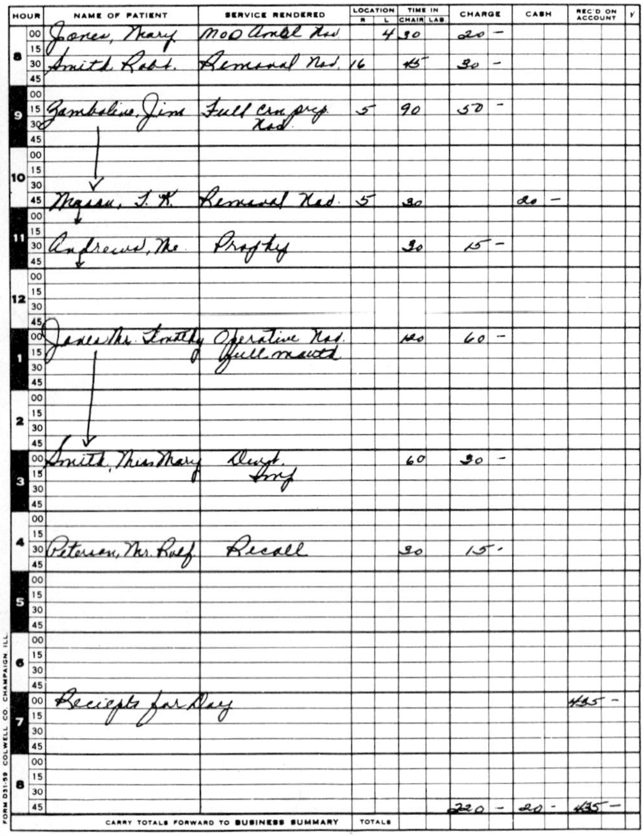
Wednesday
December 29

HOUR	NAME OF PATIENT	SERVICE RENDERED	LOCATION R	LOCATION L	TIME IN CHAIR	TIME IN LAB	CHARGE	CASH	REC'D ON ACCOUNT	✓
8:00	Jones, Mary	MOD Amal		4	30		20 –			
8:30	Smith Robt.	Removal	16		45		30 –			
9:15	Gambaline, Jim	Full Crn prep.	5		90		50 –			
10:45	Mason, T. K.	Removal	5		30			20 –		
11:15	Andrews, Mr.	Prophy			30		15 –			
1:00	Jones, Mr. Timothy	Operative, Full mouth			120		60 –			
3:00	Smith, Miss Mary	Dent. Imp			60		30 –			
4:30	Peterson, Mr. Rolf	Recall			30		15 –			
7:00	Receipts for Day								435 –	
CARRY TOTALS FORWARD TO BUSINESS SUMMARY		TOTALS					220 –	20 –	435 –	

Courtesy Colwell Pub. Co., Champaign, Ill.

Fig.17.4. Day sheet from "The Daily Log for Dentists"

The day sheet has columns for "Charges," "Cash," and "Received on Account." The charge for services performed for a patient who pays by the month or on open account is entered under "Charges." The charge for services performed for a patient who pays for the service in its entirety at the time it is performed is entered under "Cash" because he not only has work done, but he pays for it at that time. Any payments received on a monthly basis or on open account are entered under "Received on Account."

The total of the "Charges" and "Cash" columns equals the total work done during the day. The total of the "Cash" and "Received on Account" columns equals the total cash received during the day (income).

At the close of the day, total all three columns. The total of "Cash" and "Received on Account" must agree with the total of money actually received that day.

Discounts

Discounts are often given to patients, because some patients are financially unable to pay the entire cost of their care. Discounts are also given to college students, service personnel, clergy, teachers, and others. A discount must be properly entered in the bookkeeping system to show as a discount. The books should not read that Mrs. Gray paid $25 for complete X rays and Mrs. Jones paid $15 for the same service. Mrs. Jones's account must show the charge as $25. An entry must be made for a discount of $10, and the balance will appear as $15.

Frequently, dental services are provided for dental personnel for a specified discount such as twenty percent. The bookkeeping records must show this as a discount from the regular charges.

One of the pegboard systems has a special column for the express purpose of listing such discounts.

Statements for Patients

A statement is a bill, sent to the patient at the end of the month, which states the amount he owes the dentist for services.

It is important that these statements be mailed on time every month—the same time. It is wise to pick a date for closing accounts (such as the twenty-fifth of the month) and state that all charges and credits after that date will appear on the next month's statement. If the twenty-fifth is chosen, the dental assistant is allowed time to prepare the statements and have them mailed several days before the end of the month in order that all statements are received by patients on or before the first of the following month. In modern-day billing procedures of large stores, accounts for names beginning with different letters of the alphabet are closed on various dates throughout the month. People are quite accustomed to receiving bills during the month. The main purpose in closing the books early is to be certain that statements go out on the same date each month. Patients are less likely to treat payment of your statements in a haphazard manner if you are exacting in your habit of mailing the statement at the same time each month.

Statements, of course, achieve a more businesslike impression if they are typed rather than handwritten. The entire statement and envelope should present a neat and attractive appearance. (See figs. 17.5 and 17.6.)

JAMES A. RAYWIN, D.D.S.
104 Any Street
Anytown, Anystate 12345
612-926-1414

MR. JOHN JONES
246 YOUR STREET
ANYTOWN, ANYSTATE 12345

PLEASE RETURN THIS PORTION OF STATEMENT WITH PAYMENT

DATE	DESCRIPTION	CHARGES	CREDITS	BALANCE
FEB 4	PROPH & EXAM MARY	15.00	15.00	———
MAR 5	BRIDGE MARY	150.00		150.00
MAR 15	PAYMENT RECEIVED		75.00	75.00

Our books close on the 25th of the month and any charges or payments received after that date will be entered on next month's statement.

Courtesy Spillane's, Inc., Minneapolis

Fig. 17.5. Itemized statement form

STATEMENT

JAMES A. RAYWIN, D.D.S.
104 Any Street
Anytown, Anystate 12345
612-926-1414

ACCOUNT PROFESSIONAL SERVICES   Remaining balance $ 75.00

Mr. John Jones
246 Your Street
Anytown, Anystate 12345

Accounts Due and Payable Monthly as Services are Rendered.

Fig. 17.6. Simplified statement form

Payments by Check from Patients

Checks received from patients should be immediately endorsed. The assistant may endorse the check by simply writing "For deposit only" on the back and signing the dentist's name. Many dentists have a rubber stamp which is used for endorsing a check. Once a check has been stamped with this marking, it can be deposited only to the dentist's account.

Occasionally you deposit a check from a patient, and in a few days you receive the check back from the bank, with a note saying it is not acceptable because the patient does not have sufficient funds in his account to pay the amount of the check. Some people refer to this as "insufficient funds" or a "rubber check" (because it bounces). Whatever its label, it means that you have not received that money which the patient says he paid you. There are several methods of collecting when this happens. One is to call the patient and explain that the check was returned for insufficient funds. The patient will then tell you that funds are now available or give you a date when the check can be re-presented. At such time you redeposit the check and hopefully you receive credit for it. Or perhaps the patient will prefer to send you another check or a cashier's check.

Suppose you find the patient uncooperative, and it is impossible for you to collect the amount in this manner. The next step is to enter the check for collection with your bank. There is a charge for this service, depending on the size of the check. The bank will attempt to collect it for you. Should this method fail, it is time to turn the matter over to your attorney or your collection agency.

If a receipt has been given the patient for a payment by check, you will be wise to write the patient a letter immediately, stating that the check has been returned for insufficient funds and that the receipt which had been issued is not valid. This letter should be sent by registered mail with a return receipt requested.

Patient Records and Government Agencies

A dentist may perform dental services for patients whose bills are paid by one of several governmental agencies: Aid for Dependent Children, Family Welfare, County Relief Boards, and the Veterans' Administration. Most of these organizations have a set fee scale by which they pay for dentistry. It is necessary to contact them for the proper forms *prior* to performing the dentistry and to return to them an estimate of the work to be done and the cost. When the dentist has written permission to perform the dentistry as designated on the form, he is able to appoint the patient and perform the dentistry explicitly stated on the estimate form—and no more, unless approval is requested of the agency.

Should your dentist work for one of these agencies, become familiar with the forms to be completed for that agency and any instructions regarding their use and the patient's care.

Accounts Receivable Control

Statements must be sent to patients each month indicating the amount of money they owe and, in some offices, the services rendered. How can you know that you are sending statements to all the patients who owe money? The *accounts receivable control* permits a verification of these records.

Each patient account record shows the balance the patient owes. Total all the patient account record balances. Now total the amounts on all the statements to be sent. These two totals should agree. If they do not agree, it is necessary to recheck all records and arithmetic.

An accounts receivable control is figured thus:

To
Total accounts receivable from previous month: $43,300.00

Add
Charges for dentistry performed during current month: $11,100.00
$54,400.00

Subtract:
Current month's receipts: $11,300.00
and
Discounts given during month: $ 325.00
$11,625.00 $11,625.00

Total accounts receivable at end of current month: $42,775.00

The total amount of money billed on the statements should equal the final figure, $42,775.00. If there is a discrepancy between your statements and this control, there has been an error in (1) posting, (2) subtracting, or (3) adding. The error must be located and corrected. This control is necessary to ascertain that patients are being charged for the dentistry performed. Without accuracy in billing it is conceivable that a dentist would soon be unable to pay the salaries of his staff.

Records About Money Spent (Expenditures)

Records thus far have been records about money *received*. It is also necessary to spend money, and records of these expenditures are very important. There are petty cash expenditures and charge account expenditures paid by check.

Petty Cash Fund

Every dental office has some expenditures of a minor nature which do not warrant the writing of a check. Cash kept in the office for these expenditures is called a *petty cash fund*. To begin such a fund, a check is written to the dentist and endorsed by him. "Disbursement to the petty cash fund" is recorded on the stub, and the check is cashed. The cash should be kept separately from all other cash which comes into the office so that there will be no confusion of money. A small "Journal" may be purchased for the year's record; or a ruled sheet may be used for each month's record of the petty cash fund. A page is headed "Petty Cash Fund" with the name of the month. This page or sheet should have room on the left for the date, a broad column for detail entry, and three columns headed "Disbursements," "Receipts," and "Balance." The amount used in this fund will vary in different dental offices, but it should be sufficient to cover the largest month's minor expenses so that only one check need be issued each month.

The first entry on this sheet would be dated the first of the month. The detail entry would be "Check No. xxxx." The amount of the check would be written in the "Receipts" column.

Example: Suppose that on the tenth of the month a ball-point pen was purchased at the stationery store. This entry would be made, dated the tenth, "ball-point pen," and under "Disbursements" the cost would be entered. A receipt for the pen should be clipped to the petty cash sheet. This receipt is your *source document*. The balance remaining in the petty cash fund should be entered in the "Balance" column. (See fig. 17.7.)

At the end of the month, the actual cash in the petty cash fund is counted and checked against the petty cash sheet indication of "Balance." The amount of money in your fund and the figure in the balance column should agree.

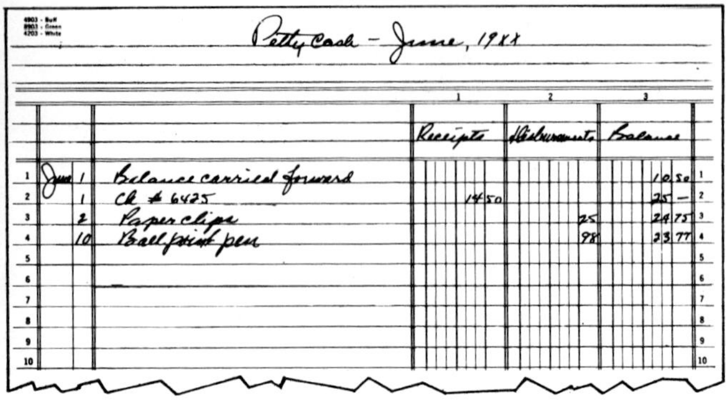

Fig. 17.7. Petty cash ledger sheet

An office check is made out for the amount necessary to return the petty cash fund to its original balance. The petty cash expenditures for each month are written on a separate page of the ledger. On the new sheet made out for the next month, the first entry carries forward the balance remaining in the petty cash fund at the end of the previous month, the second entry is for the check (and its number), the amount entered under "Receipts" and the new balance written in, which should be the original balance established for the petty cash fund.

There should be no cash expenditures from the office except through a petty cash fund. For every petty cash disbursement there must be a receipt!

Dental Office Charge Accounts

When a dental supply is charged, the payment is usually made at the end of the month. For charge accounts there will be both *invoices* and *statements* for office purchases. The invoices will be sent with the supply at the time it is ordered; the statement will follow at the close of the month.

Invoices for Dental Office Purchases

An invoice is a form included with an order of supplies. It usually has a number on it, the date, the name and address of the firm sending the supplies, the name and address of the dentist receiving them, how many and what supplies they are, and the price. This invoice is a source document.

During the month you receive invoices from various firms from which you have ordered supplies. Verify them when received to be certain that the charge is correct for the material which you have received and that you have received all material listed. File them in a folder marked "Current Invoices." Clip all invoices of each firm together in the file as they are received.

Statements for Dental Office Purchases

At the end of the month, each firm sends a statement listing all the items (sometimes by invoice number) which you have ordered and giving the total amount you owe the firm.

Upon receipt of a firm's statement, proceed as follows:

1. Remove the invoices for that firm from the current invoices file.
2. Compare the invoices with the statement to be certain that you have received the materials as charged and that the charges are correct.
3. Clip to this statement the invoices you have received since the previous billing.
4. Write a check for the correct amount.
5. Write the check number and the date on which you write the check on the lower half of the statement from the firm.
6. Tear off the upper half (which lists the firm name and your dentist's name).
7. Clip the upper half of the statement to the check.
8. Address an envelope if one is not furnished.
9. Put the statement, check, and envelope on your dentist's desk for his signature.
10. When the check has been signed, mail it.

11. File the lower half of the statement with the invoices in the permanent record section of the file. A file folder for the firm or for the month is commonly used.
12. At the end of the year, these statements are bundled, either by firm name or by month, and packaged in dead storage for future reference. The packages are clearly labeled.

Disbursement Record

The expenditures in the dental office must be recorded in permanent form much like the day sheet record of services for patients and moneys received. The record of the expenditures is called a *disbursement record*.

A disbursement record is composed of columns for recording certain information. Usually the column headings read: Date, Name of Firm (or Person) Paid, Object Purchased, Check Number, Amount of Check, Deposits, and Bank Balance.

In addition, most disbursement records have columns for classifying the purchases. The disbursement record will then continue on, after the Bank Balance, with columns headed: Taxes, Insurance, Rent, Laboratory Expense, Dental Supplies, Dental Equipment, Household Drawing, Contributions, etc.

A common form for a disbursement record is a thirteen-column ruled tablet on which the individual can write the headings he desires to use.

The Internal Revenue Service recommends a separate checking account for a professional man's personal expenses. It recommends that once or twice a month a check be deposited to the personal checking account and that all personal expenditures be paid from this account. The business expenses, which are legally deductible before the dentist's income is figured for tax purposes, are then clearly separated from those expenses which he must pay from his own income, such as clothing,

house payments or home rent, and medical bills. A column in the business disbursement record titled "Personal Account" or "Household Drawing Account," in which checks to the personal drawing account may be entered, keeps the business and personal expenses separated satisfactorily.

Usually there is a column on the disbursement record headed "Personal Deductions" or "Donations" separate from "Personal Account" or "Household Drawing Account," because this information is needed for tax purposes and is readily found if it is in a separate column. Generally speaking, personal donations are not deductible as a business expense but may be deducted from personal income taxes. However, some donations are properly considered business expenses—for example, contributions to a dental charity (assuming it is on the Internal Revenue Service approved list of deductible items) or a memorial to a recognized charity for a patient, etc. Sometimes it is necessary to make donations from the office which are not deductible as a business expense. It is customary to put all donations made from the office in the "Personal Deductions" column in the disbursement record.

Preparing the Disbursement Record

After the checks for office expenditures have been written, the disbursement record can be completed, using the check register. (See pp. 204-209 for a discussion of checking procedures.) Fill in the columns on the disbursement record as required by the particular check being recorded.

1. Start with the first check written in January.
2. Enter the date, check number, description (to whom and for what), and amount in the columns provided.
3. Now look across the headings and see what column describes this check. If it

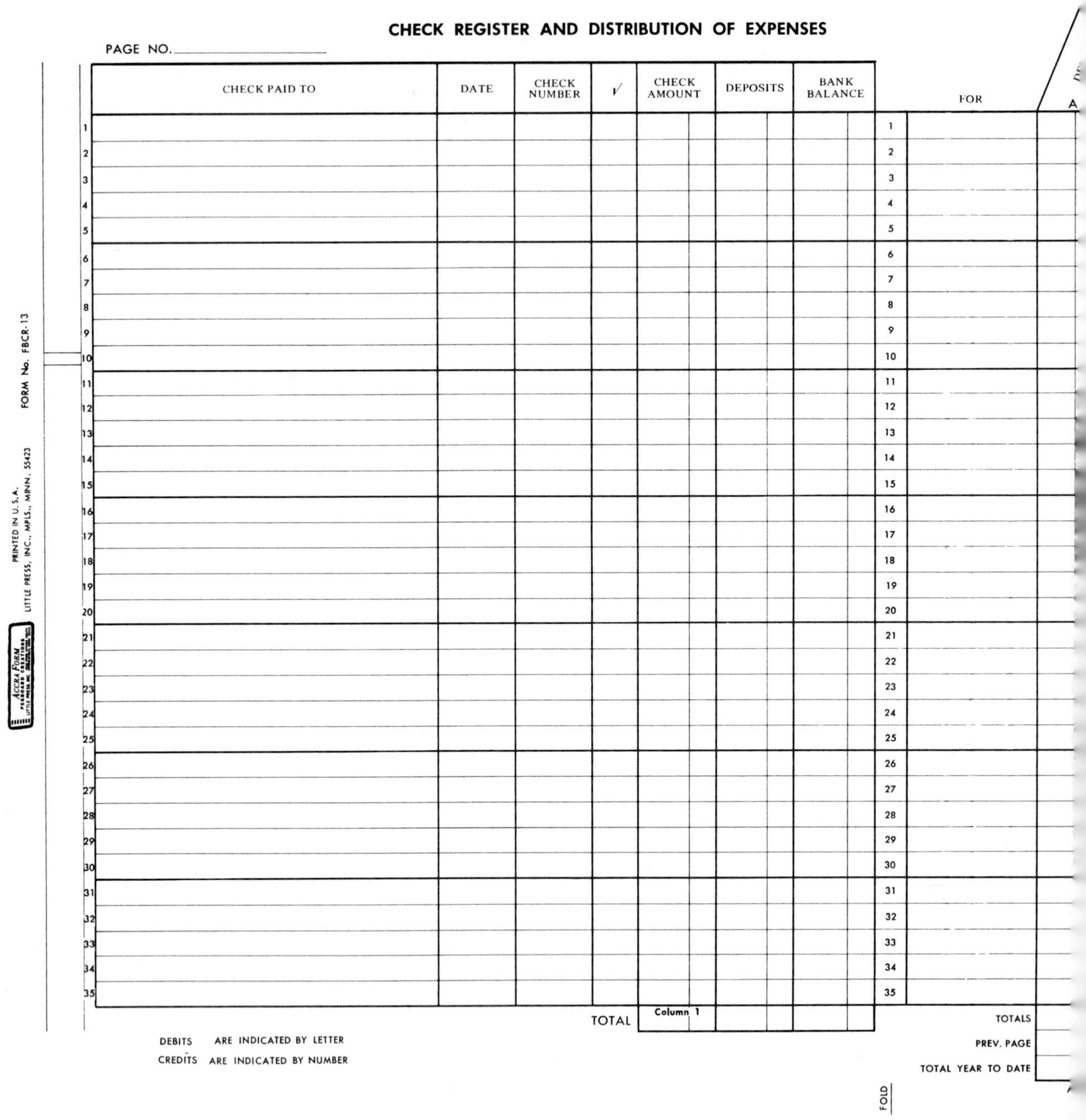

CHECK REGISTER AND DISTRIBUTION OF EXPENSES

PAGE NO. _____

	CHECK PAID TO	DATE	CHECK NUMBER	√	CHECK AMOUNT	DEPOSITS	BANK BALANCE		FOR		A
1								1			
2								2			
3								3			
4								4			
5								5			
6								6			
7								7			
8								8			
9								9			
10								10			
11								11			
12								12			
13								13			
14								14			
15								15			
16								16			
17								17			
18								18			
19								19			
20								20			
21								21			
22								22			
23								23			
24								24			
25								25			
26								26			
27								27			
28								28			
29								29			
30								30			
31								31			
32								32			
33								33			
34								34			
35								35			
			TOTAL	Column 1						TOTALS	
										PREV. PAGE	
										TOTAL YEAR TO DATE	

DEBITS   ARE INDICATED BY LETTER
CREDITS   ARE INDICATED BY NUMBER

FORM No. FBCR-13

PRINTED IN U.S.A.
LITTLE PRESS, INC., MPLS., MINN., 55423

FOLD

Fig. 17.8.   Disbursement record

YEAR ____________

MONTH ____________

SALARIES GROSS 1	SALARIES SOC. SEC. 2	SALARIES WITH. FED. 3	SALARIES STATE WITH. 4	HOUSEHOLD DRAWING C	OFFICE RENT D	LAUNDRY E	UTILITIES F	OFFICE SUPPLIES G	INTEREST PAID H	BUSINESS TAXES I	DENTAL EQUIPMENT J	CONTRIBUTIONS K	FED. INC. TAX L	STATE INC. TAX M	GENERAL LEDGER ACC'T NO.	GENERAL LEDGER DEBIT	
																	1
																	2
																	3
																	4
																	5
																	6
																	7
																	8
																	9
																	10
																	11
																	12
																	13
																	14
																	15
																	16
																	17
																	18
																	19
																	20
																	21
																	22
																	23
																	24
																	25
																	26
																	27
																	28
																	29
																	30
																	31
																	32
																	33
																	34
																	35
																	36
																	37
																	38
1	2	3	4	C	D	E	F	G	H	I	J	K	L	M			

Courtesy Little Press, Inc., with modifications

is a rent check and there is a column for rent, write the amount in that column. (See fig. 17.8.)

4. Continue this process until all the checks written have been recorded. It is possible to use a code system to be certain that each check has been recorded on the disbursement record.

5. Sometimes a check is written for an amount which must be divided on the disbursement record. For example, your dentist may purchase supplies and equipment from the same dental firm and make a payment by one check. It will be necessary to divide the payment on the disbursement record. For example, equipment costing $100 is purchased along with supplies totaling $52. The entire $152 is entered as the amount of the check the first time it is recorded on the disbursement sheet. Enter the $100 under "Equipment" and the $52 under "Supplies" in the disbursement record.

6. Divide the petty cash expenditures into their proper categories. When the petty cash fund is reimbursed, write the total amount of the check in the "Check Amount" column and write the amount of each type of expenditure in the proper column in the disbursement record.

7. At the end of the month, total each disbursement column.

8. Total the *totals* of the disbursement columns.

9. Total the check column. The total of the check column and the total of all the disbursement totals should agree.

10. The totals can be carried forward each month, and the dentist can know at the end of any month exactly what his expenses have been in relation to his income for the year or for any particular month.

Yearly Summary

At the close of the year, all income and expenditures must be summarized. A summary sheet, maintained monthly, brings the record up-to-date. Usually these forms have spaces for listing fees or charges, unpaid balance on accounts, and money collected in order to figure the gross income of the dental practice. There are also spaces for totals from the disbursement records, showing expenses such as materials, laboratory bills, general expenses, personal account, personal deductions, and permanent equipment. The total disbursements of a business nature (excepting personal accounts) are deducted from the total receipts to find the net income on which personal income tax is figured. Most yearly summaries have a section where general expenses may be broken down for further study. Depreciation on permanent equipment is usually figured when the tax returns are prepared.

Banking Procedures

The money has been received, and the receipts have been given to the patients. The money now must be deposited to the dentist's *office checking account*—and nowhere else.

Only by depositing every penny of income in the office checking account is it possible for an accountant to verify the income in the office. Internal Revenue Service agents are particular about accounting for income whenever money is collected in a business. A person who receives a salary check is a less likely object of concern than a person whose income is irregular. A dentist has an irregular income, with opportunity for failure to report some of it. Therefore, he must be especially careful to so conduct his accounting that there can be no question about the fact that all income has been reported. The easiest way to do this is to deposit all income in an office checking account. Checks can then be written for personal drawing accounts on whatever basis the dentist wishes.

Each day's receipts should be deposited as a unit. Verification of the accuracy of the day's receipts is thus provided.

Deposit Slips

At the end of each day, the total receipts on the day sheet should equal exactly the total of the cash and checks on hand. A deposit slip is then made out for the day's receipts, and the cash and checks are clipped to it. The deposit is made as soon as convenient. It is preferable to make a deposit for each day, but if this is not convenient or necessary, deposits should be made frequently enough to prevent the accumulation of checks or cash in the office. More frequent deposits are helpful in showing errors as soon as possible after they occur.

Deposit slip books are available from most banks in numbered, *duplicate* pages. This is the type which should be used for the office. Each deposit slip is used consecutively. It is recommended that the bank teller stamp the duplicate deposit slip at the time the deposit is made.

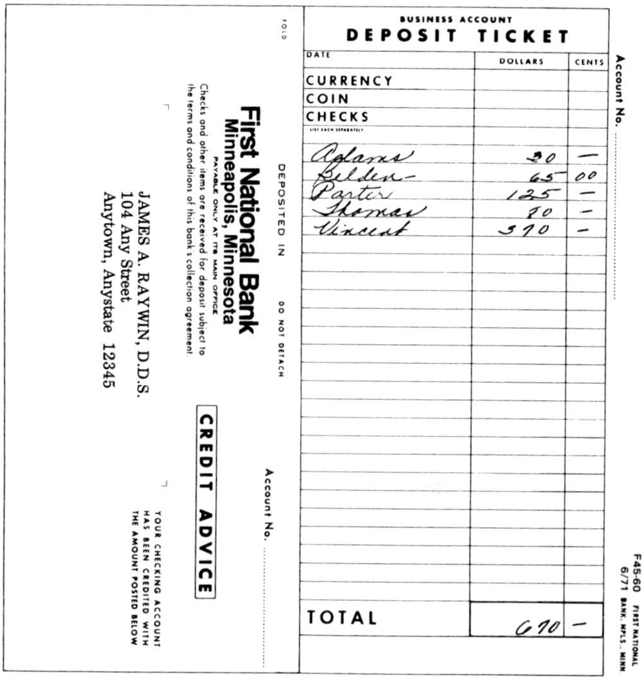

FOLD

DEPOSITED IN DO NOT DETACH

First National Bank
Minneapolis, Minnesota
PAYABLE ONLY AT ITS MAIN OFFICE
Checks and other items are received for deposit subject to the terms and conditions of this bank's collection agreement.

JAMES A. RAYWIN, D.D.S.
104 Any Street
Anytown, Anystate 12345

Account No. ....

CREDIT ADVICE

YOUR CHECKING ACCOUNT HAS BEEN CREDITED WITH THE AMOUNT POSTED BELOW

BUSINESS ACCOUNT
DEPOSIT TICKET

DATE	DOLLARS	CENTS
CURRENCY		
COIN		
CHECKS (LIST EACH SEPARATELY)		
Adams	20	—
Belden	65	00
Porter	125	—
Thomas	10	—
Vincent	390	—
TOTAL	610	—

Account No. ....

F45-60 FIRST NATIONAL 6/71 BANK, MPLS., MINN

Fig. 17.9. Deposit slip

Final deposits are made to cover any payments made through the last day of each month. While this deposit will usually be made on the first day of the new month, it is nevertheless made out as an individual deposit to close the preceding month. Any additional moneys for deposit at that time are listed on a separate deposit slip—the next consecutively numbered slip.

A new deposit slip book should be started with the first of each year in order that all records for the year just completed may be stored together.

Checkbook

The business checking account should be used *only* for the business, and the dentist should receive a check drawn on this account for payment to his personal checking account each month, or as he wishes.

A *check* is an authorization to the bank to pay a specified amount of money to the person named on the check from the account of the person who signs the check. Sometimes the person signs for a firm, and then the authorization is for the firm rather than the individual. (See fig. 17.10.)

The dental assistant is generally given the duty of making out checks for the payment of the various bills against the dental office and may or may not have her signature authorized for the checking account. If the assistant's signature is authorized by the dentist and entered at the bank in their records, the assistant may complete the entire procedure of paying bills for the office. If the assistant's signature is not

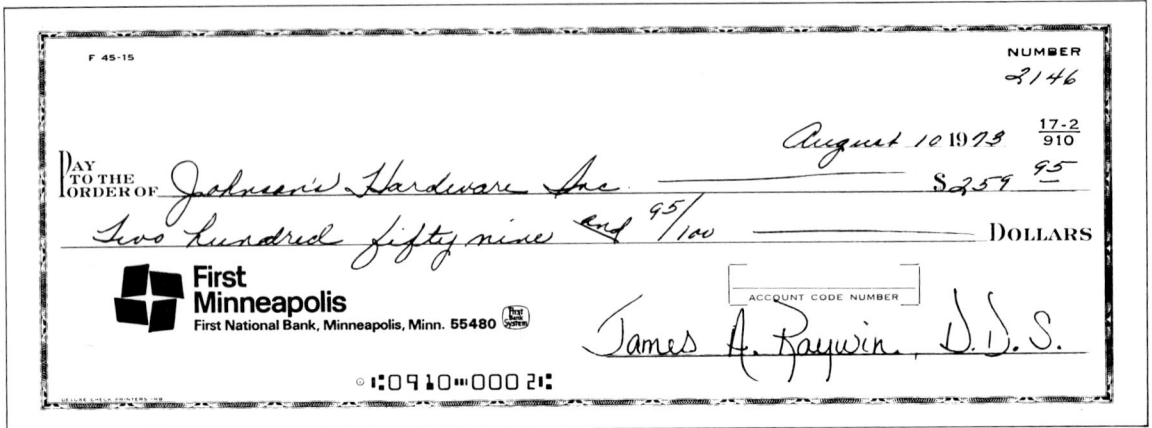

Fig. 17.10. A check correctly written

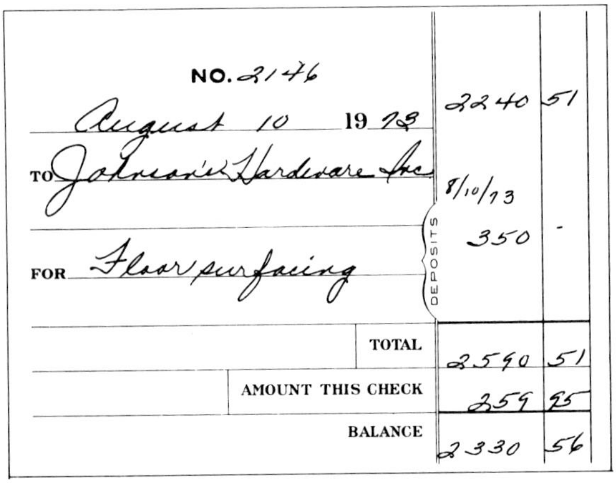

Fig. 17.11. A check stub correctly prepared for check in figure 17.10.

authorized for the checking account, the dentist must sign the checks.

Dental office records, including the checkbook, should be written with a permanent ink. The only exception to this rule is that receipts and deposit slips which require carbon copies are made with a ball-point pen.

The *check stub* or *check register* is a record retained in the office. It includes this informa-

tion, either on each individual check stub or on each page of the check register: (1) the number of the check, (2) the date, (3) to whom the check is written, (4) for what the check is written, (5) the checkbook balance, (6) recording of any deposits, (7) date of deposits, (8) total of the checkbook balance and deposit combined, (9) amount of the check just written, and (10) new checkbook balance (subtract the amount of the check from the previous balance). Thus, after writing a check it is possible to know how much money is still available in the checking account.

It is highly recommended that the check stub or register be completed first, then the check, and that *both* these forms be verified with the statement of the bill being paid. Accuracy is essential.

If a dentist uses a Write-It-Once system of bookkeeping, he may also use the checks of such a system. The register (or stub) is a page, and the checks with carbon lines are placed over the page in the same way as the charge/receipt slip. One writing completes the check and register entries. (A discussion of the details of Write-It-Once bookkeeping begins on p. 210.)

CHECK NO.	DATE	CHECK ISSUED TO	IN PAYMENT OF	AMOUNT OF CHECK	✓	DATE OF DEPOSIT	AMOUNT OF DEPOSIT	BALANCE
						5/31/73	BALANCE BROUGHT FORWARD →	5240	—
2085	6/1/73	Baker Investment Co.	Rent	300	00			4940	—
2086	6/1/73	Jafy Narew Dent'l Supply	Supplies	35	50			4904	50
2087	6/1/73	Dahl Pharmacy	Drugs	48	50			4856	—
2088	6/1/73	Dr. James Rayview	W W Draw	500	—			4356	—
						6/1/73	350 —	4706	—
2089	6/5/73	Minn. Natural Gas Co.	Service	6	48			4699	52
2090	6/5/73	Northern State Power Co.	Elect. Service	42	58			4656	94
2091	6/5/73	N.W. Bell Telephone Co.	Telephone Ser.	48	50			4608	44

Fig. 17.12. A check register correctly maintained

Checkbook Reconciliation

At or near the close of each month, a statement of the account, together with the canceled checks listed on the statement, is received from the bank. The balance in the checking account as shown on the bank statement will not agree with the balance shown on the last stub in the checkbook.

These figures must be checked to determine the correctness of the figures. This is known as "reconciliation" of the bank statement balance with the checkbook balance. This reconciliation process is not confusing if you follow a set procedure in accomplishing it.

Canceled checks are those which were originally made out to pay a dental office account. The check was received by the company to which it was sent. The company endorsed the check for deposit to their account at their bank. Their bank put the check through a "clearing house" procedure, which ultimately meant that the money from your office's bank, on which the check was drawn, was transferred to the bank of the company to which the check was sent. In exchange for transferring this money, your bank received the check itself, and since the purpose for which it was

written has been accomplished, the check is "canceled" by means of a stamp placed on it (usually punching tiny holes) stating that the check has been paid. These "paid" or canceled checks are then listed on your bank statement and are deducted from the balance you have on record at the bank. In addition to deducting the paid checks, the bank will deduct bank charges and, in some cases, charges for "exchange"—a service charge for handling checks drawn on certain types of banks.

You will have deducted the amount of each check from your balance as you issued checks from your checkbook, but you will not have deducted the bank service charges or any "exchange" charges.

You will have added, on your checkbook stubs or register, the deposits which you made. The bank statement covers through only a certain day of the month, and deposits made on or after that closing date will not have been included in the balance which the bank statement will show.

You may have had an office account, which you paid by check, with a firm located in some other city, or some firm to which you sent a check may not have deposited that check im-

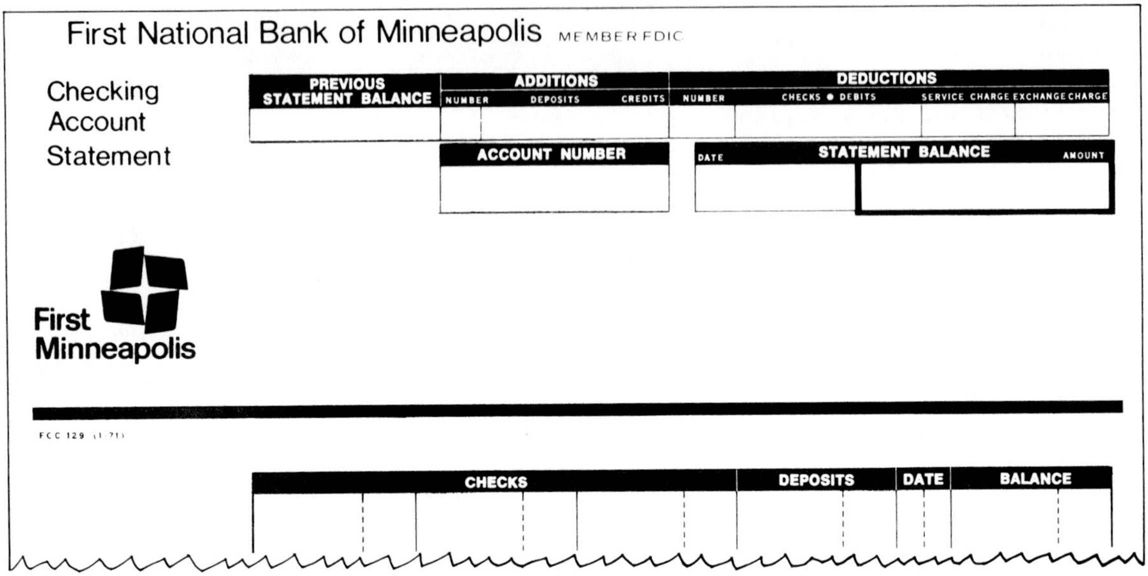

Fig. 17.13. Bank statement for checking account

mediately. Thus, it may not be canceled in time to appear on your statement. This check, of course, will not be deducted from the balance according to the bank's figures. You deducted it, however, when you wrote it out.

For this reason, the bank's monthly statement of your checking account is not always the exact figure which you have listed as the balance according to your last check stub. There are many figures to be carefully and accurately checked. *Do not permit the bank statement to go unreconciled.* Keep checking until it does correspond with your check stubs or register. Banks can make errors, and an error must be called to their attention within a specified time or the bank statement is assumed to be correct.

Checkbook Reconciliation Procedure

1. Arrange the canceled checks in numerical sequence.
2. Verify each canceled check with your check stub or register. Place a check mark

by the number on the register for each canceled check. If you do not have a check, do not place a check mark by that number on the stub.
3. Draw a line across the register after the last canceled check.
4. If your bank is computerized, the amount the bank actually deducted from your account will be typed on the bottom-right-hand part of the check. Verify that the typed figure is identical with the figure on your check register. (If they are not the same, on a sheet of paper note the difference and the rest of the information from the check. It will be necessary to call the bank and have them correct their records.)
5. Note each check number in your register which has no check mark beside it. These checks will be the outstanding checks— those which have not yet cleared the bank. Do not go beyond the line you drew. That line indicates the place at which the

checkbook should "reconcile" with the bank.

On the back of the bank statement (fig. 17.14), write the number of each outstanding check and the amount of the check in the appropriate columns in item 3. Total these checks as instructed on the statement.

6. Now verify that each deposit has been recorded by the bank. If the bank has not sent you the receipt for some of the deposits which you have already made, list each deposit. Write the total of these deposits in the appropriate column on the bank form.

7. Write the current balance, shown by the bank on the face of the statement, in the proper place on the back of the statement.

8. Total the bank's balance of your account and any outstanding *deposits.*

9. Subtract the outstanding checks from this amount.

10. Note any charges for bank services. Subtract this amount from the balance in your checkbook at the point at which you drew the line.

11. This amount and the bank statement of current balance should agree. For example:

Bank balance:	$1692.05	Your checkbook balance:	$1953.10
Plus outstanding deposits:	432.00	Less service charges:	1.05
	$2124.05		$1952.05
Les outstanding checks:	$ 172.00		
	$1952.05		

(A detailed practice example of checkbook reconciliation will be found in the workbook to accompany *Effective Dental Assisting.*)

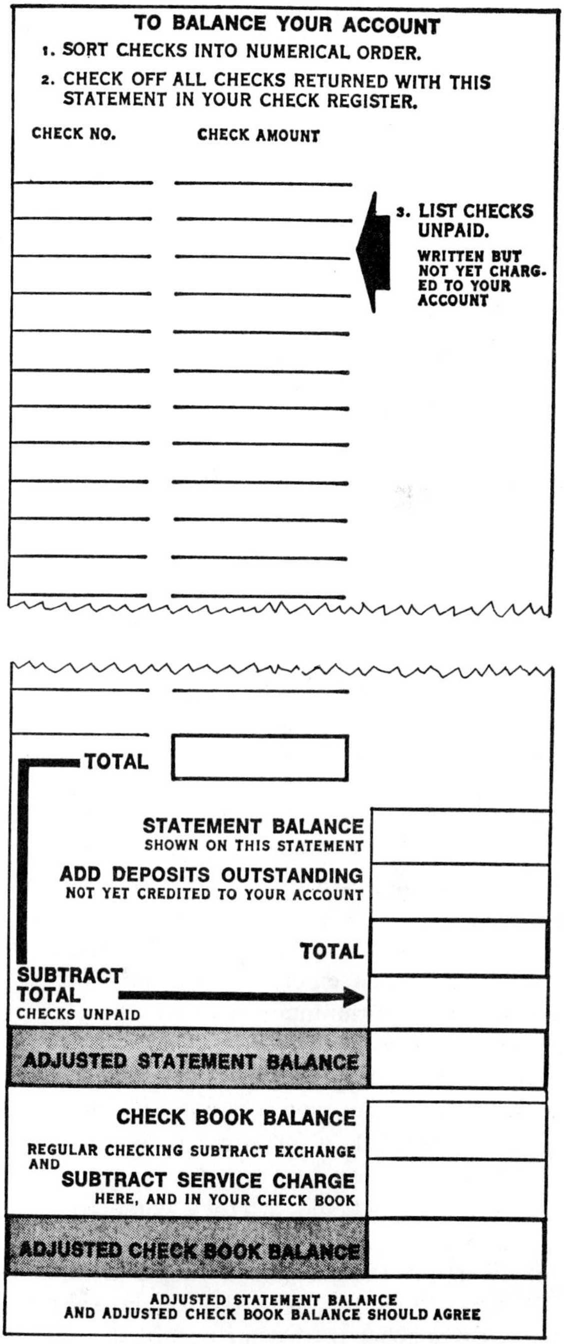

Fig. 17.14. Reverse side of statement shown in figure 17.13.

TO BALANCE YOUR ACCOUNT
1. SORT CHECKS INTO NUMERICAL ORDER.
2. CHECK OFF ALL CHECKS RETURNED WITH THIS STATEMENT IN YOUR CHECK REGISTER.

CHECK NO.   CHECK AMOUNT

3. LIST CHECKS UNPAID.

WRITTEN BUT NOT YET CHARGED TO YOUR ACCOUNT

TOTAL

STATEMENT BALANCE
SHOWN ON THIS STATEMENT
ADD DEPOSITS OUTSTANDING
NOT YET CREDITED TO YOUR ACCOUNT

TOTAL

SUBTRACT TOTAL CHECKS UNPAID

ADJUSTED STATEMENT BALANCE

CHECK BOOK BALANCE
REGULAR CHECKING SUBTRACT EXCHANGE AND
SUBTRACT SERVICE CHARGE
HERE, AND IN YOUR CHECK BOOK

ADJUSTED CHECK BOOK BALANCE

ADJUSTED STATEMENT BALANCE AND ADJUSTED CHECK BOOK BALANCE SHOULD AGREE

Monthly Record-keeping Responsibilities—A Summary

Your record-keeping responsibilities, then, include these steps:

1. For payments received:
   a. Write a receipt for every payment made.
   b. Enter the payment on the patient's account record.
2. For services to patients:
   a. Enter on the day sheet the name of each patient for whom service is performed and the service and charge.
   b. Check to see whether the dentist has entered the information on the patient's service record. See that it is entered.
   c. Enter the charges for this service on the patient's account record.
3. For money disbursed:
   a. Collect a receipt and write an entry in the petty cash fund book for every penny of cash which is spent through your office.
   b. Write any disbursements other than petty cash in the disbursement record. (If you are writing a check to reimburse petty cash, as must be done once a month or as needed, enter that check on the disbursement record and properly disburse the money so spent.)
   c. Once a month check the statements from firms against the invoices received during that month and pay the bills.
4. Once a month put your totals on the yearly summary sheet.
5. Check all invoices as they come to your attention.
6. Reconcile the checkbook once a month.
7. Make deposits on a daily, biweekly, or weekly basis, or as your dentist directs.
8. Prepare and send statements to patients for services rendered.

The Write-It-Once or Pegboard Bookkeeping Systems

If you work in an office which employs a mechanized system, you will be given specific instructions about its operation and your responsibilities for that system. However, a brief résumé may be helpful. This system is modern —it is referred to as "instant bookkeeping." It is so designed that one writing of information by the assistant enters the information everywhere it is needed. It records all necessary

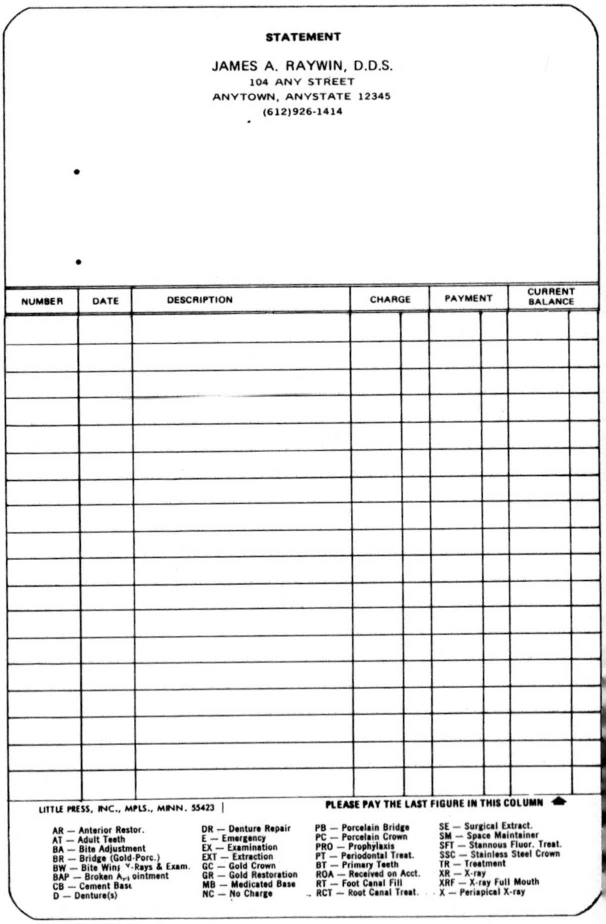

STATEMENT

JAMES A. RAYWIN, D.D.S.
104 ANY STREET
ANYTOWN, ANYSTATE 12345
(612)926-1414

NUMBER	DATE	DESCRIPTION	CHARGE	PAYMENT	CURRENT BALANCE

LITTLE PRESS, INC., MPLS., MINN. 55423

PLEASE PAY THE LAST FIGURE IN THIS COLUMN

AR — Anterior Restor.
AT — Adult Teeth
BA — Bite Adjustment
BR — Bridge (Gold-Porc.)
BW — Bite Wing X-Rays & Exam.
BAP — Broken Appointment
CB — Cement Base
D — Denture(s)
DR — Denture Repair
E — Emergency
EX — Examination
EXT — Extraction
GC — Gold Crown
GR — Gold Restoration
MB — Medicated Base
NC — No Charge
PB — Porcelain Bridge
PC — Porcelain Crown
PRO — Prophylaxis
PT — Periodontal Treat.
BT — Primary Teeth
ROA — Received on Acct.
RT — Foot Canal Fill
RCT — Root Canal Treat.
SE — Surgical Extract.
SM — Space Maintainer
SFT — Stannous Fluor. Treat.
SSC — Stainless Steel Crown
TR — Treatment
XR — X-ray
XRF — X-ray Full Mouth
X — Periapical X-ray

Courtesy Little Press, Inc.

Fig. 17.15. Pegboard patient account card

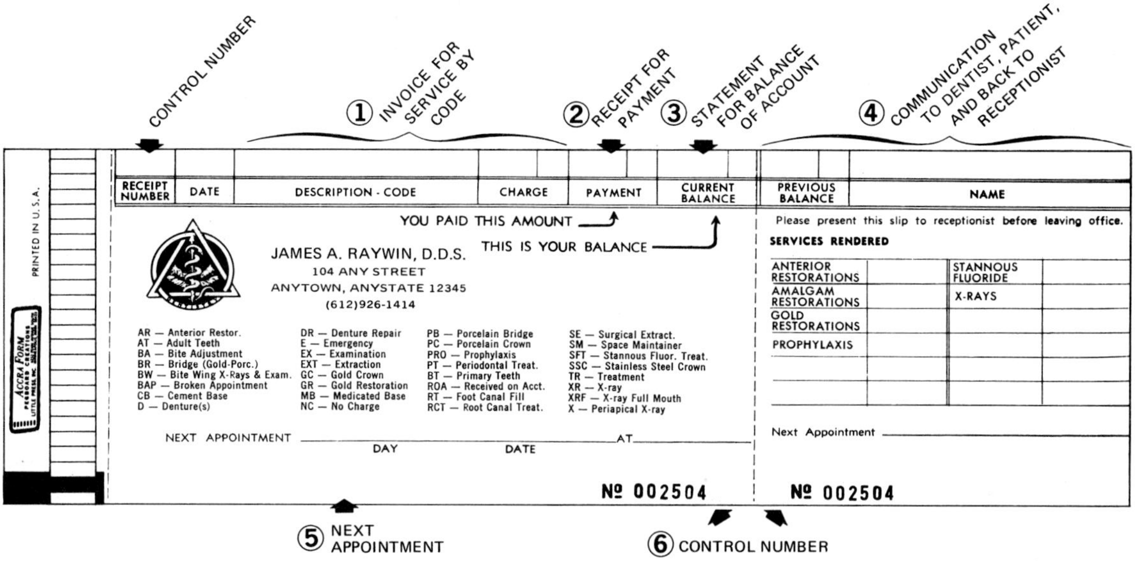

Fig. 17.16. Pegboard charge/receipt slip

Courtesy Little Press, Inc.

records with proof of accuracy (because they are all written at the same time). There can be no transposing of figures or miscopying of names or services. You simply write it once. It records all these records at once: patient's receipt-statement (record of today's charge), patient's monthly statement, patient's financial card, record of charges and receipts (daily log), and the bank deposit record.

A pegboard system of record keeping differs in the following ways from the explanation of the basics of record keeping.

1. The patient account card is a special form. As in other systems, all the charges and payments must be entered on this card. It may be a *family* card, that is, the responsible adult has a card, and all the charges for dentistry for his family are entered on his card. It may be an individual card if the person is responsible for only his own dentistry.

Type at the top of the card the name and address of the person responsible for the account. These cards are kept in a tray, alphabetically arranged.

At the time chosen by your dentist for sending out statements, the account cards are run through a copying machine, and the copy is sent to the patient as his statement.

2. The day sheet is mounted on the pegboard. It is a special sheet furnished by the company that manufactures the pegboard system used in your office. The pegboard is a flat board usually made of some kind of composition board. It has a row of pegs on the left side designed to hold two or three papers in a certain position. The day sheet is on the bottom and a carbon is placed over it. A slip called by various names, such as charge/receipt, is placed over the first open line for writing on the day sheet. (Fig. 17.16 is a sample charge/receipt.) This charge/receipt slip has carbon on the back of it for the top line only. Anything written on that top line makes a carbon copy.

DAILY JOURNAL WITH DISTRIBUTION OF CHARGES AND RECEIPTS

DATE________ SHEET NO.________ PREPARED BY________

	RECEIPT NUMBER	DATE	DESCRIPTION · CODE	CHARGE	PAYMENT	BALANCE	PREVIOUS BALANCE	NAME				
1												1
2												2
3												3
4												4
5												5
6												6
7												7
8												8
9												9
10												10
11												11
12												12
13												13
14												14
15												15
16												16
17												17
18												18
19												19
20												20
21												21
22												22
23												23
24												24
25												25
26												26
27												27
28												28
29												29
30												30
31												31
32												32
33												33
34												34
	♠ ALL RECEIPTS MUST BE IN NUMERICAL ORDER			Column A	Column B	Column C	Column D	TOTALS				35

FORM NO. 110-3

ACCRAFORM PEGBOARD SYSTEMS

PRINTED IN U.S.A.
LITTLE PRESS, INC., MPLS., MINN.

PROOF OF POSTING

COLUMN D TOTAL $______
"PLUS" COLUMN A TOTAL $______
SUB TOTAL $______
COL. B TOTAL $______
COL. B-1 TOTAL $______
"MINUS" B & B-1 SUB TOTAL $______
EQUALS COLUMN C TOTAL $______

ACCOUNTS RECEIVABLE CONTROL

PREVIOUS BALANCE $______
"PLUS" COLUMN A $______
SUB TOTAL $______
"MINUS" COL. B TOTAL $______
COL. B-1 TOTAL $______
"MINUS" B & B-1 SUB TOTAL $______
PRESENT ACC'TS REC. BALANCE $______

DAILY CASH SUMMARY

OPENING CASH ON HAND AT BEGINNING OF DAY $______
CASH RECEIVED DURING DAY $______
TOTAL $______
CASH LONG $______
TOTAL $______

CASH PAID OUT $______
BANK DEPOSITS $______
CLOSING CASH ON HAND $______
TOTAL $______
CASH SHORT $______
TOTAL $______

Courtesy Little Press, Inc.

Fig. 17.17. Pegboard day sheet

The information which is written on the charge/receipt also appears on the patient's account card and on the day sheet through the use of the carbons.

The charge/receipt slip may be used as a receipt or a statement for the patient. The stub of the charge/receipt slip becomes a communication channel between the dentist, receptionist, and patient.

Pegboard systems differ somewhat depending on the arrangements offered by the several manufacturers. Basically, the record-keeping duties are the same regardless of the system used. The day sheet of the pegboard

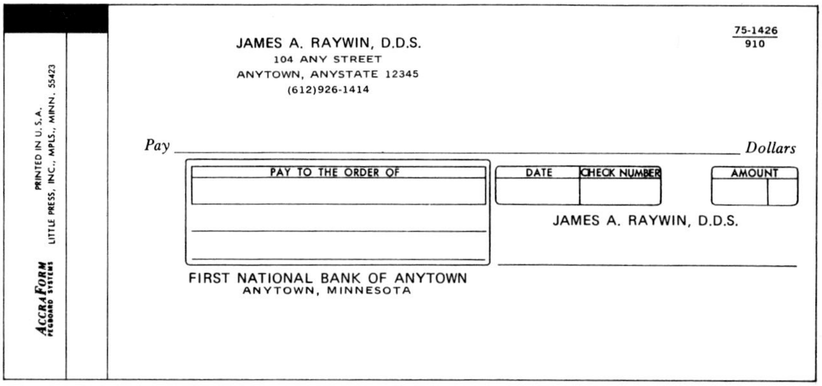

Fig. 17.18. Pegboard check form—often used with pegboard accounting.

JAMES A. RAYWIN, D.D.S.
104 ANY STREET
ANYTOWN, ANYSTATE 12345
(612)926-1414

75-1426
910

Pay _____ *Dollars*

| PAY TO THE ORDER OF | DATE | CHECK NUMBER | AMOUNT |

JAMES A. RAYWIN, D.D.S.

FIRST NATIONAL BANK OF ANYTOWN
ANYTOWN, MINNESOTA

PRINTED IN U.S.A.
LITTLE PRESS, INC., MPLS., MINN. 55423

AccraForm
PEGBOARD SYSTEMS

Courtesy Little Press, Inc.

systems usually supplies the dentist with desirable information concerning his financial status. (Fig. 17.17 is a sample day sheet.)

Figure 17.18 is a check form often used with a pegboard system. The check is placed over the check register, and the information transfers to the register by carbon as the check is written.

Additional Banking Services

There are many services offered by banks, and an assistant should be familiar with them. One such service is a *safe deposit box* which may be rented for an annual fee. This box is in a vault, assuring protection against theft, fire, or almost any type of catastrophe, and usually valuable papers are kept here. Only the person or persons whose names are recorded at the Safe Deposit Registry are permitted to use the box, and each time the box is used, the user must sign a request to enter the box and write his key number on the slip. This slip is then verified by a clerk to be sure it compares with the information recorded when the box was rented. The person is given permission to enter the vault area where a uniformed attendant takes the registration slip and the person's key to the box. He unlocks the safe deposit box, using two keys: his own and the key of the box renter. The box is given to the renter who then goes to a private booth and conducts his business—puts in or takes out papers or valuables. The renter then returns the box to the attendant, and the attendant again uses the two keys to relock the box.

Loans are made by banks for a number of purposes. The bank investigates the individual who applies for a loan. If he meets certain standards, the bank will loan the individual a designated amount of money to be repaid on a specified schedule for a certain percentage of interest plus the charges for the paper work of making out the loan. These standards mean the borrower has something of value for collateral (something the bank could take from him and sell if he doesn't pay the money he owes as agreed) or the bank administrators decide he is a good risk for repayment for some other reason.

Loans are made for small amounts of money, some under a hundred dollars, and also are made for large sums, hundreds of thousands of dollars, depending on the purpose of the loan, the reputation of the borrower, and the risk involved. To begin to practice dentistry, a dentist may find it necessary to borrow several thousand dollars, which he repays with interest from the income he earns practicing dentistry.

As a dentist acquires more patients and his income increases, he not only pays off his loan, but he may be in a position to begin saving money. A dentist, since he works for himself without the protection of a large firm to provide a retirement fund for him, must build a retirement fund. He must also set aside money for the education of his children, if he has any.

It becomes necessary for him to handle his investments wisely. (Investments are those business transactions in which an individual puts money into some venture which he believes will increase his money or will at least pay him for the use of it.) Perhaps the dentist invests in the stock market in some "blue chip" stocks (those which are considered very safe investments). These stocks pay him a dividend (interest for the use of his money). He has become a lender, in a sense, like the bank that loaned him money to start his practice. He may also discover that these investments become so good—increase in value, both from the fact that he kept adding money to his investment account over the years and that the stocks themselves increased in value—that he decides to establish a trust fund.

A *trust* is the setting up of an arrangement whereby someone, usually a bank, holds your investments for you, and when you reach the age you have specified, they begin to pay you a monthly income from these investments. Should a dentist die prematurely, the trust may begin to pay his widow an income immediately and provide for his children's education. Trusts have many advantages and are very complicated. There are numerous choices which one can make when he sets out to arrange a trust. It has some definite inheritance tax advantages.

You may find yourself writing checks for deposit in a trust fund.

The bank also issues *cashier's* and *certified checks.* These checks are important for you to understand. If a patient presents you with one of these checks, you know the bill is paid. This check cannot be returned marked "insufficient funds" because the person drawing the check must go to the bank and pay the money before the bank makes out the check. The funds are then held in reserve by the bank until the check is cashed. These checks are sometimes necessary to use when you wish to pay a bill in some distant city. Some firms insist that all out-of-town accounts be paid by cashier's or certified checks.

Possibly the most familiar area of banking service for the dental assistant is the checking account. A checking account is simply a way of transferring money to other people for the things you wish to buy. A check cannot be cashed except by the person to whom it is drawn (made out). This means that it is safe to send a check through the mail. No one can steal it.

Basically, the checking account simply means that the owner has gone to the bank, signed a card with his signature, deposited some money, and has been given some checks to use. In today's mechanized banking world, almost all checks have an account number printed on each check. The owner of a checking account has his own account number. All his banking transactions (deposits and withdrawals by means of check writing) are performed on checks and deposit slips which have his number printed on them. These numbers are usually sensitized, and a machine automatically enters the transaction on the correct account.

The checking account balance does not earn interest as a savings account does. If the owner keeps enough money in the checking account (an amount specified by the bank), the account costs him little or nothing to operate. However, if his balance falls below this specified amount, he is charged for each check he writes. This is called a *service charge.*

Power of Attorney

A *power of attorney* is a legal device by which a person authorizes someone else to act for him in legal matters. If a patient is to undergo surgery, for example, and expects to be incapacitated for a period of time, he may decide to have someone he trusts handle his legal affairs for him. It would mean that someone else could pay his bills, and so on. Many husbands and wives have power of attorney drawn for each other so they can take care of each other's business as the occasion arises. Sometimes an elderly person will have someone younger help him in this way.

As you know, the only person who can request a disclosure of a patient record is the patient himself. If he is incapacitated and the information is necessary for his welfare, someone who has power of attorney can make the request in his name, or even pay a bill for him with the person's funds.

Whenever you see a request with a power of attorney attached (a letter properly signed and notarized), consult the attorney of your dentist to be certain that you do have the legal privilege of conforming with the request.

Notary Public

A notary public is an individual who has been given power by the courts to legalize certain documents. If a person has to sign certain papers witnessed by a notary, the seal of the notary and his signature must be on the document. Since frequently it is necessary for documents in the dental office to be notarized, a dentist may request that one of his employees be a notary public. A fee is paid for this privilege. Usually a charge is made when you use the services of a notary public outside your office.

Summary

Financial records are as important to the dentist and his patients as the clinical records are. The record keeper should maintain careful records of that which the office owes others, that which others owe the office, all money which is received, and all money which is spent.

Basic bookkeeping requirements include:

1. *Source documents* (records of proof of billing or proof of payment which must be permanently filed).
2. *Records of receipts* issued by the office. (A receipt must be written for each payment received.)
3. An *office change fund* (necessary to make change for patients who pay cash).
4. A *patient's service record* (to show the dentistry performed).
5. A *patient's account record* (to show the financial transactions for the services performed).
6. The *day sheet* (to show all the activity in dentistry and finance for a single day).
7. *Discounts* (must be shown as discounts on the records).
8. *Statements* (must be sent to patients and should indicate the dentistry performed and the charges to be paid. These statements should be mailed on the same date each month).
9. *Checks received* (should be endorsed immediately with the words "For deposit only" or should be endorsed with a bank stamp).
10. *Third-party payment records* (must be maintained as required by the third party whether it be a government agency or an

insurance firm or any other organization. It is important to follow the regulations of the particular agency to assure payment for the services performed).

11. An *accounts receivable control* (to permit verification of the outstanding accounts so the record keeper knows whether or not the correct number of statements are being sent to patients).

Records about money spent include:

1. A *petty cash fund* for minor office expenditures.
2. *Invoices* for dental office charge accounts which are verified as correct at the time of delivery of the supplies ordered and are then filed in "Current Invoices."
3. *Statements* for dental office charge accounts which are verified against the invoices prior to payment of the statement. Invoices and lower half of the statement are then filed by firm name.
4. A *disbursement record* shows the classification of purchases during the month.
5. A *yearly summary* shows the income and expenditures for an entire year.

All money received is deposited in the office checking account.

Deposit slips are made in duplicate.

The business checking account is used *only* for business.

A *check* is an authorization to the bank to pay a specified amount of money to the person named on the check from the account of the person who signs the check.

A *check stub* or *check register* is a record retained in the office and gives information found on the check as well as the bank balance.

Checkbook reconciliation is a procedure to ascertain that the bank records and the office records agree about the amount of money in the checking account.

Write-It-Once or pegboard bookkeeping systems offer a method of record keeping which avoids errors in copying figures because items are written only once.

Banks offer services including safe deposit boxes, loans, trusts, certified and cashier's checks, as well as savings accounts and checking accounts.

A *power of attorney* is a legal device which permits an adult to allow someone else to act for him in legal matters.

A *notary public* is a person who has been given power by the courts to legalize certain documents. Sometimes it is necessary to use a notary public in preparing papers.

Study Questions

1. Describe the records which are essential for operating the dental office effectively.

2. Explain these terms:

source document	patient's account record
day sheet	accounts receivable control
discount	third-party payment
statement	patient's service record
receipt	disbursement record
invoice	yearly summary

3. Distinguish between an office change fund and a petty cash fund.

4. Describe a checkbook reconciliation procedure. Why is it important?

18 | *Tax Records*

Complete Records for Taxes

It is to your dentist's advantage that complete, accurate records be kept of *all* transactions involving money. It is also wise to use the services of a CPA in the preparation of tax returns. The Internal Revenue Service is more likely to accept his statement of earnings because his business record is built on training and knowledge in such matters and in accurate record keeping.

If your office uses the services of a CPA or management consultant, the area of record keeping for tax purposes will be designed for you, and it will be necessary for you to keep only such records as the service directs.

If you are expected to keep records for the state and federal taxes, you should be familiar with the material in this chapter.

Every employee in the office must have social security tax, federal income tax, and, in some states, state income tax withheld from his salary. In addition, some states have a state unemployment compensation tax. If the office employs more than four auxiliary personnel, there is a federal unemployment tax.

Most of these taxes are paid quarterly, and special forms are required. Some forms are mailed to the office, but in certain states it is necessary to send for the unemployment compensation forms.

Records must be kept of the total salary of each employee and the amount withheld for

SALARY AND TAX RECORDS

Employee's Name: Smith, Mary   Number of Exemptions: 0

Address: 215 Elm Street   Social Security Number: 123-11-2345

Anytown, Anystate 12345

DATE	TOTAL EARNINGS	FEDERAL WITHHOLDING TAX	O. A. B. (SOCIAL SECURITY)	STATE WITHHOLD-ING TAX	OTHER ITEMS	NET PAID
6 1	175.00	31.70	10 24	5 25		128 01
6 15	175.00	31.70	10 24	5 25		128 01

Fig. 18.1. Office salary and tax record

each individual tax, and must specify the purpose for which other amounts are withheld. At the end of the year, special forms which list all taxes withheld and the total salary paid must be completed.

Any inaccuracies or omissions in these reports can lead to a penalty payment of six percent of the amount not reported, so take care that you prepare them accurately and *on time.* If your dentist has not made tax reports (perhaps you are his first employee), you must secure the forms from your nearest federal and state offices. If he has previously submitted tax reports, the forms will be sent directly to your office each quarter.

Tax Forms

The most commonly used federal government tax forms are illustrated in the sections which follow. If you can understand how to prepare these forms, you will be able to master the state forms required in your state. Since most states have withholding taxes and some form of unemployment insurance compensation, it is wise to investigate *before* you are penalized for nonpayment.

Because most reports are filed on a quarterly basis, it is easier to complete reports if you keep regular bookkeeping records from which you can summarize the quarterly information.

Office Salary and Tax Record

The first form is a summary which you maintain each time you write out a paycheck. There is one sheet for each office employee (fig. 18.1).

Since no employee is able to take home his entire earnings, records must be kept of the taxes and amounts withheld from the take-home pay. The example shows federal withholding tax, F.I.C.A. (also referred to as social security or old age benefits (O.A.B.) on some forms), state withholding taxes, and net paid.

Some states have other taxes which are also withheld. In most states unemployment compensation is not withheld from an employee's wages. It is a tax paid by the employer only. For every item which is to be withheld in your particular locality, there should be a column so listed on the Salary and Tax Record sheet for each employee.

Employer's Quarterly Federal Tax Return and Quarterly Report of Wages

Social security or old age benefits (O.A.B.) and withheld taxes are paid on a quarterly basis unless the amount exceeds $100 per month, in which case the money must be paid more frequently. (See "Federal Depositary Receipt," p. 221.) Figure 18.2, Form 941, is

Fig. 18.2. U. S. Tax Form No. 941, Employer's Quarterly Federal Tax Return.

Please remove this strip at perforation before mailing.

E.I. 56-0690964

Form **941**
(Rev. July 1972)
Department of the Treasury
Internal Revenue Service

Employer's Quarterly Federal Tax Return

SCHEDULE A—Quarterly Report of Wages Taxable under the Federal Insurance Contributions Act—FOR SOCIAL SECURITY
IF WAGES WERE NOT TAXABLE UNDER THE FICA MAKE NO ENTRIES IN ITEMS 1 THROUGH 9 AND 14 THROUGH 18

1. (First quarter only) Number of employees (except household) employed in the pay period including March 12th ▶
2. Total pages of this return including this page and any pages of Form 941a ▶
3. Total number of employees listed ▶

List for each nonagricultural employee the WAGES taxable under the FICA which were paid during the quarter. If you pay an employee more than $9,000 in a calendar year report only the first $9,000 of such wages. In the case of "Tip Income" see instructions on page 4.

Please report each employee's name and number exactly as shown on his Social Security card.

4. EMPLOYEE'S SOCIAL SECURITY NUMBER (000 00 0000)	5. NAME OF EMPLOYEE (Please type or print)	6. TAXABLE FICA WAGES Paid to Employee in Quarter (Before deductions) Dollars Cents	7. TAXABLE TIPS REPORTED (See page 4) If amounts in this column are not tips, check here ☐ Dollars Cents

If you need more space for listing employees, use Schedule A continuation sheets, Form 941a.

Totals for this page—Wage total in column 6 and tip total in column 7 →

8. TOTAL WAGES TAXABLE UNDER FICA PAID DURING QUARTER. (Total of column 6 on this page and continuation sheets.) Enter here and in Item 14 below . . . . . . $..........

9. TOTAL TAXABLE TIPS REPORTED UNDER FICA DURING QUARTER. (If no tips reported, write "None.") (Total of column 7 on this page and continuation sheets.) Enter here and in Item 15 below . . . . → $

Employer's name, address, employer identification number, and calendar quarter. (If not correct, please change)

Name (as distinguished from trade name) — Date quarter ended

▶ Trade name, if any — Employer Identification No.

Address and ZIP code

............Entries must be made both above and below this line; if address different from previous return, check here ☐ ....

Name (as distinguished from trade name) — Date quarter ended

▶ Trade name, if any — Employer Identification No.

Address and ZIP code

T | FP
FF | I
FD | TOT

10. TOTAL WAGES AND TIPS SUBJECT TO WITHHOLDING PLUS OTHER COMPENSATION . . . . →
11. AMOUNT OF INCOME TAX WITHHELD FROM WAGES, TIPS, ANNUITIES, etc. (See instructions) . . . .
12. ADJUSTMENT FOR PRECEDING QUARTERS OF CALENDAR YEAR . . . .
13. ADJUSTED TOTAL OF INCOME TAX WITHHELD . . . . →
14. TAXABLE FICA WAGES PAID (Item 8) . . . . $.......... multiplied by 10.4%=TAX
15. TAXABLE TIPS REPORTED (Item 9) . . . . $.......... multiplied by 5.2%=TAX
16. TOTAL FICA TAXES (Item 14 plus Item 15) . . . . →
17. ADJUSTMENT (See instructions) . . . .
18. ADJUSTED TOTAL OF FICA TAXES . . . . →
19. TOTAL TAXES (Item 13 plus Item 18) . . . .
20. TOTAL DEPOSITS FOR QUARTER (INCLUDING FINAL DEPOSIT MADE FOR QUARTER) AND OVERPAYMENT FROM PREVIOUS QUARTER LIST IN SCHEDULE B. (See instructions on page 4) . . . .

Note: If undeposited taxes at the end of the quarter are $200 or more, the full amount must be deposited with an authorized commercial bank or a Federal Reserve Bank. This deposit must be entered in Schedule B and included in item 20.

21. UNDEPOSITED TAXES DUE (ITEM 19 LESS ITEM 20—THIS SHOULD BE LESS THAN $200). PAY TO INTERNAL REVENUE SERVICE AND ENTER HERE . . . . →
22. IF ITEM 20 IS MORE THAN ITEM 19, ENTER EXCESS HERE ▶ $ AND CHECK IF YOU WANT IT ☐ APPLIED TO NEXT RETURN, OR ☐ REFUNDED.
23. If not liable for returns in succeeding quarters write "FINAL" here ▶ and enter date of final payment of taxable wages here ▶

Under penalties of perjury, I declare that I have examined this return, including accompanying schedules and statements, and to the best of my knowledge and belief it is true, correct and complete.

Date .... Signature .... Title (Owner, etc.) ....

Please remove this strip at perforation before mailing.

the report which must be filed. This form actually has two pages, the second being a copy for your files.

Check for Internal Revenue Service

A check made payable to the Internal Revenue Service must be sent with these forms. The check and the two forms should be sent in the same envelope on or before the last day of the first month following the close of the quarter.

Withholding Tax Statement, Form W-2

At the close of the year it is necessary to fill out and file two annual tax forms, W-2 and W-3. Form W-2 has four copies, each labeled for a specific purpose: *A* is for the district director, *B* is for the employee to be filed with his tax return, *C* is for the employee's personal records, and *D* is for the employer's records.

Transmittal of Wage and Tax Statements, Form W-3

Form W-3 (fig. 18.4) is furnished in duplicate—one copy for the district director and one for the employer.

Type information requested across the top. Answer item A. Items B-E depend on size of office; answer as necessary. Complete item 1; omit item 2; item 3 is the total of 1 and 2. Item 4 is not applicable to the dental office. Date the form and have your dentist sign his name and title.

File the district director's copy at the same time you file your Employer's Quarterly Federal Tax Return, Form 941, for the fourth quarter of the year.

Instructions are printed on the back.

Federal Depositary Receipt

If your office pays more than $100 per month in combined social security and with-

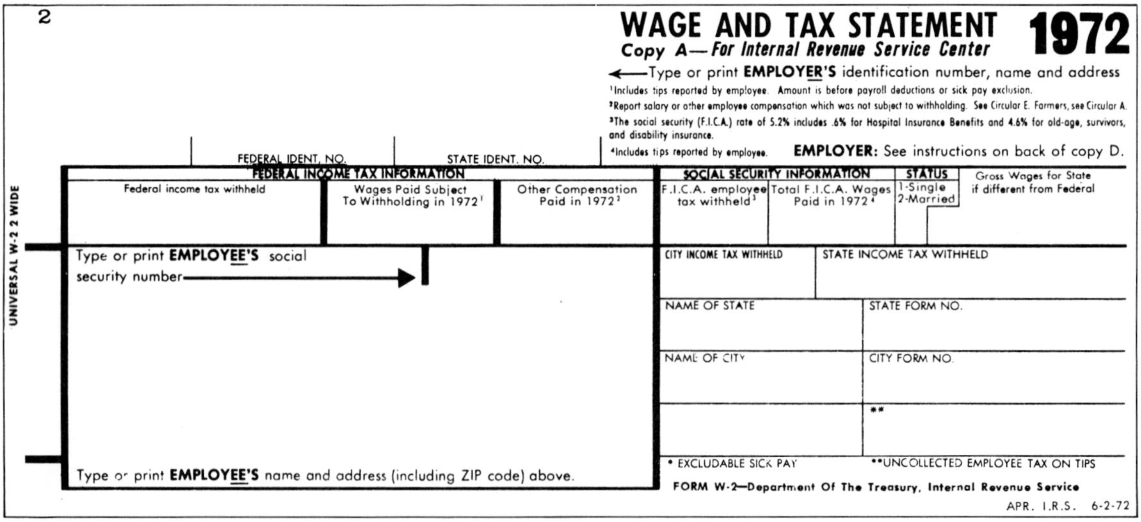

2

WAGE AND TAX STATEMENT 1972
Copy A—*For Internal Revenue Service Center*
←Type or print **EMPLOYER'S** identification number, name and address
[1]Includes tips reported by employee. Amount is before payroll deductions or sick pay exclusion.
[2]Report salary or other employee compensation which was not subject to withholding. See Circular E. Farmers, see Circular A.
[3]The social security (F.I.C.A.) rate of 5.2% includes .6% for Hospital Insurance Benefits and 4.6% for old-age, survivors, and disability insurance.
[4]Includes tips reported by employee. **EMPLOYER:** See instructions on back of copy D.

FEDERAL IDENT. NO. | STATE IDENT. NO.

FEDERAL INCOME TAX INFORMATION: Federal income tax withheld | Wages Paid Subject To Withholding in 1972[1] | Other Compensation Paid in 1972[2]

SOCIAL SECURITY INFORMATION: F.I.C.A. employee tax withheld[3] | Total F.I.C.A. Wages Paid in 1972[4]

STATUS: 1-Single 2-Married

Gross Wages for State if different from Federal

UNIVERSAL W-2 2 WIDE

Type or print **EMPLOYEE'S** social security number→

CITY INCOME TAX WITHHELD | STATE INCOME TAX WITHHELD

NAME OF STATE | STATE FORM NO.

NAME OF CITY | CITY FORM NO.

**

Type or print **EMPLOYEE'S** name and address (including ZIP code) above.

* EXCLUDABLE SICK PAY | **UNCOLLECTED EMPLOYEE TAX ON TIPS

FORM W-2—Department Of The Treasury, Internal Revenue Service

APR. I.R.S. 6-2-72

Fig. 18.3. U. S. Tax Form W-2, Withholding Tax Statement holding taxes, it is necessary to deposit money in a Federal Reserve Bank each month. You will receive a Federal Depositary Receipt (fig. 18.5) when the bank receives your money. This receipt is very important.

Form for Correcting Errors

If you discover an error on a report after it has been forwarded, ask for Form 941C, which is the form for correcting such errors. Fill it out and mail it promptly.

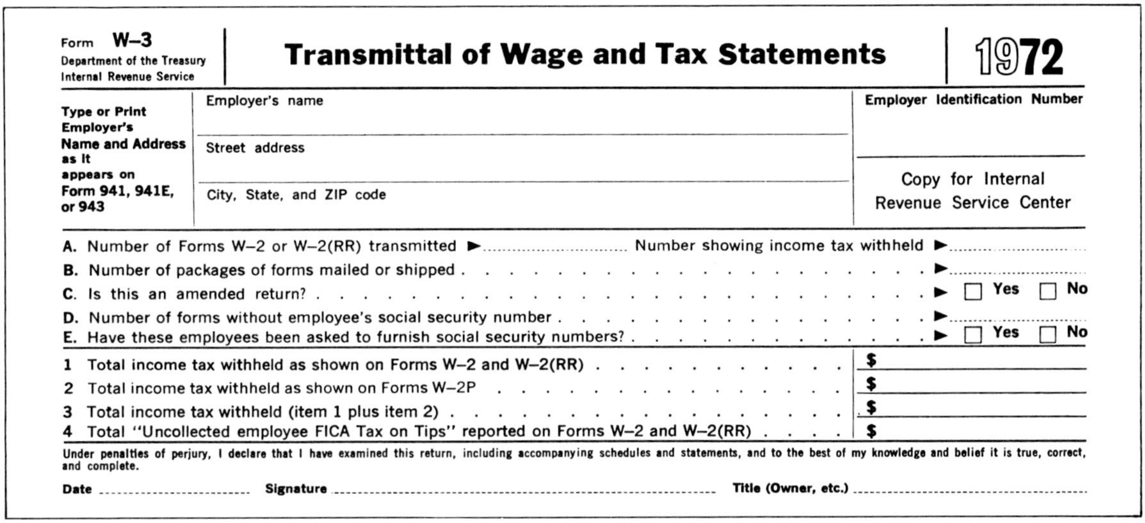

Form W–3
Department of the Treasury
Internal Revenue Service

Transmittal of Wage and Tax Statements **1972**

Type or Print Employer's Name and Address as it appears on Form 941, 941E, or 943

Employer's name
Street address
City, State, and ZIP code

Employer Identification Number

Copy for Internal Revenue Service Center

A. Number of Forms W–2 or W–2(RR) transmitted ►........ Number showing income tax withheld ►........
B. Number of packages of forms mailed or shipped . . . . ►........
C. Is this an amended return? . . . . ► ☐ Yes ☐ No
D. Number of forms without employee's social security number . . . . ►........
E. Have these employees been asked to furnish social security numbers? . . . . ► ☐ Yes ☐ No

1 Total income tax withheld as shown on Forms W–2 and W–2(RR) . . . . $
2 Total income tax withheld as shown on Forms W–2P . . . . $
3 Total income tax withheld (item 1 plus item 2) . . . . $
4 Total "Uncollected employee FICA Tax on Tips" reported on Forms W–2 and W–2(RR) . . . . $

Under penalties of perjury, I declare that I have examined this return, including accompanying schedules and statements, and to the best of my knowledge and belief it is true, correct, and complete.

Date .... Signature .... Title (Owner, etc.) ....

Fig. 18.4. U. S. Tax Form W-3, Transmittal of Wage and Tax Statements

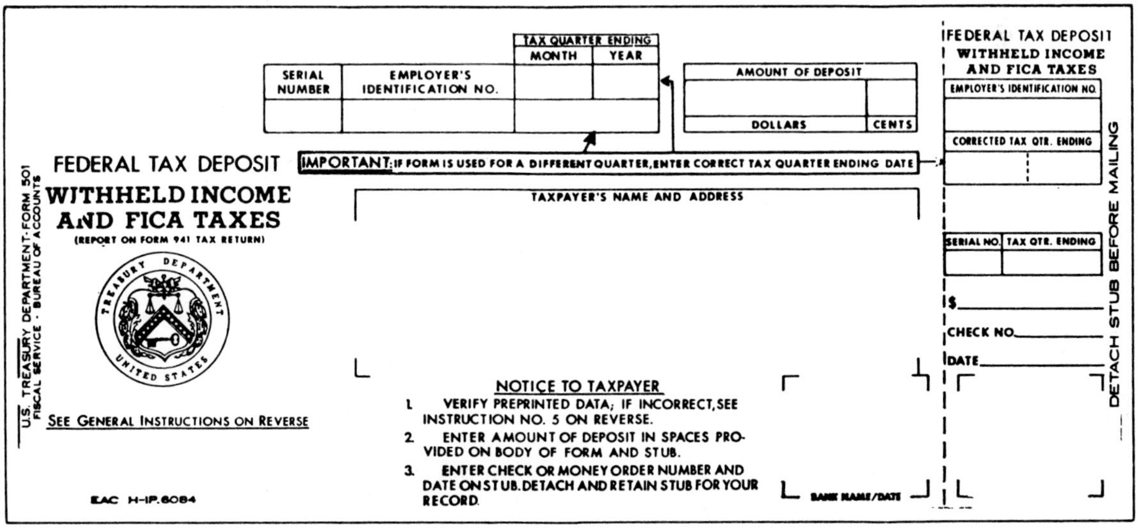

SERIAL NUMBER	EMPLOYER'S IDENTIFICATION NO.	TAX QUARTER ENDING MONTH	TAX QUARTER ENDING YEAR	AMOUNT OF DEPOSIT DOLLARS	CENTS

FEDERAL TAX DEPOSIT
WITHHELD INCOME AND FICA TAXES
(REPORT ON FORM 941 TAX RETURN)

IMPORTANT: IF FORM IS USED FOR A DIFFERENT QUARTER, ENTER CORRECT TAX QUARTER ENDING DATE

TAXPAYER'S NAME AND ADDRESS

U.S. TREASURY DEPARTMENT-FORM 501
FISCAL SERVICE · BUREAU OF ACCOUNTS

SEE GENERAL INSTRUCTIONS ON REVERSE

NOTICE TO TAXPAYER
1. VERIFY PREPRINTED DATA; IF INCORRECT, SEE INSTRUCTION NO. 5 ON REVERSE.
2. ENTER AMOUNT OF DEPOSIT IN SPACES PROVIDED ON BODY OF FORM AND STUB.
3. ENTER CHECK OR MONEY ORDER NUMBER AND DATE ON STUB. DETACH AND RETAIN STUB FOR YOUR RECORD.

BANK NAME/DATE

EAC H-IP.6084

FEDERAL TAX DEPOSIT
WITHHELD INCOME AND FICA TAXES
EMPLOYER'S IDENTIFICATION NO.
CORRECTED TAX QTR. ENDING
SERIAL NO. | TAX QTR. ENDING
$
CHECK NO.
DATE
DETACH STUB BEFORE MAILING

Fig. 18.5. Federal Depositary Receipt

Form **W-4** (Rev. Dec. 1971)	Department of the Treasury—Internal Revenue Service **Employee's Withholding Exemption Certificate**

Type or print full name

Social security number

Home address (Number and street or rural route)

City or town, State and ZIP code

Marital status—check one (if married but legally separated, or spouse is a nonresident alien, check "Single"): ☐ Single   ☐ Married

If you expect to owe more tax than will be withheld, you may either claim fewer or zero exemptions or ask for additional withholding on line 8.

1 Personal exemption for yourself. Write "1" if claimed . . . .

2 If married, personal exemption for your wife (or husband) if not separately claimed by her (or him). Write "1" if claimed . . . .

3 Special withholding allowance.¹ (See instruction 2.) Write "1" if claimed . . . .

4 Exemptions for age and blindness (applicable only to you and your wife but not to dependents):

   (a) If you or your wife will be 65 years of age or older at the end of the year, and you claim this exemption, write "1"; if both will be 65 or older, and you claim both of these exemptions, write "2" . . . .

   (b) If you or your wife are blind and you claim this exemption, write "1"; if both are blind, and you claim both exemptions, write "2" . . .

5 Exemptions for dependents. (Do not claim an exemption for a dependent unless you are qualified under instruction 5.) . . . .

6 Additional withholding allowances for itemized deductions. See table on reverse . . . .

7 Add the exemptions and allowances (if any) which you have claimed above and enter total . . . .

8 Additional withholding per pay period under agreement with employer . . . . $

Under the penalties of perjury, I certify that the number of withholding exemptions and allowances claimed on this certificate does not exceed the number to which I am entitled.

(Date) ...., 19...... (Signed) ....

Fig. 18.6. Employee's Withholding Exemption Certificate

Employees' Withholding Exemption Certificate

When a new employee joins your staff, it is necessary for her to complete a form W-4, Employee's Withholding Exemption Certificate, illustrated in figure 18.6. This form is kept on file as long as the person is employed in the office.

The federal unemployment tax, should your office employ more than four persons, is filed the same as social security, listing the amount your office owes and enclosing a check for this amount with the form.

State Unemployment Tax Form

The state unemployment form will also require a check sent with it for the entire amount owed by your office. Usually a percentage is determined by the use your office has made of the state unemployment insurance funds.

If, for example, no one has filed a claim against your office for unemployment compensation (in other words, your dentist has never fired an employee), the rate may be the lowest the state collects. If, however, the office has had one or two claims filed against it, the rate is immediately higher. As the number of claims increases, the rate of the tax increases. If a period of time, such as three years, has elapsed and no claims have been filed, the tax rate may again drop to its lowest point.

The form which your office receives from the unemployment compensation fund will state the rate which your office is required to pay.

Summary

Tax records must be kept for the state and federal taxes which every business must pay.

Fig. 18.7. U. S. Tax Form 940, Employers' Annual Federal Unemployment Tax Report.

Form **940**
Department of the Treasury
Internal Revenue Service

Employer's Annual Federal Unemployment Tax Return

1972

SCHEDULE A—Computation of Credit Against Federal Unemployment Tax

Name of State (1)	State reporting number as shown on employer's State contribution returns (2)	Taxable payroll (As defined in State act) (3)	Experience rate period (4) From—	To—	Experience rate (5)	Contributions had rate been 2.7% (col. 3 × 2.7%) (6)	Contributions payable at experience rate (col. 3 × col. 5) (7)	Additional credit (col. 6 minus col. 7) (8)	Contributions actually paid to State (9)

Totals ▶

10. Total tentative credit (Column 8 plus column 9) . . . .
11. Enter 2.7% of the amount of wages shown in Item 13 below . . . .
12. Credit allowable (Item 10 or 11 whichever is smaller). Enter here and in Item 15 . . . . . .

EMPLOYERS—Do Not Use This Space—CONTINUE BELOW

State reporting number as shown on employer's State contribution returns	Taxable payroll (As defined in State act)	Experience rate period From— To—	Experience rate	Dates and amounts of contributions actually paid to State after January 31	Contributions actually paid to State before February 1

To the Internal Revenue Service:

I hereby certify that, except as noted above, the records of this office agree with the entries made by the employer in columns (2), (3), (4), (5), and (9) of Schedule A, and that all contributions were paid before February 1.

Signature of State Officer ▶

Name of State ▶

Name (as distinguished from trade name)

Calendar Year
1972

Identification No.

Employer's name, address, identification number and calendar year. (If not correct please change.) ▶

Trade name, if any

Address and ZIP code

------------------ Entries must be made both above and below this line ------------------

Name (as distinguished from trade name)

Calendar Year
1972

Identification No.

Trade name, if any

Address and ZIP code

T	FP
FF	I
FD	TOT

13. Total taxable wages paid during calendar year (From Schedule B, on other side) . . . .
14. Gross Federal tax (3.2% of Item 13) . . . .
15. Less: Credit from Item 12, Schedule A . . . .
16. Item 14 less Item 15 . . . .
17. Total tax deposited (From Schedule C, on other side) . . . .
18. Balance Due (Item 16 less Item 17). Pay to "Internal Revenue Service" . . . . ▶
19. If no longer in business at end of year, write "FINAL" here ▶

Under penalties of perjury, I declare that I have examined this return, including accompanying schedules and statements, and to the best of my knowledge and belief it is true, correct, and complete, and that no part of any payment made to a State unemployment fund which is claimed as a credit in Item 15 above, was or is to be deducted from the remuneration of employees.

Date

Signature

Title (Owner, etc.)

Form **940** (1972)

Records to keep include office salary and tax record, employer's quarterly federal tax return and quarterly report of wages taxable under the federal insurance contributions act (FICA), withholding tax statements, transmittal of wage and tax statements, federal depositary receipt, and the federal unemployment tax record should the office employ more than four persons. If an error in the report is made, a special form should be mailed promptly.

Study Questions

1. Why is it important for a dental office to have complete and accurate records of all income and outgo?
2. Why is it advisable to employ a CPA?
3. What taxes must be withheld from each employee's pay?
4. What happens if your office is late in paying the taxes withheld?
5. Describe an office salary and tax record.
6. When and for what reason is a federal depositary receipt issued?

19 | *Insurance and Health Care Plans*

The Principle of Insurance

Insurance was developed a long time ago based on the idea that a group can better manage catastrophe than an individual. When all the neighbors would try to help put out a fire on someone's farm, this was a form of insurance. "We help each other." When the neighbors formed a crew to help harvest the crops of a sick farmer, this was insurance. Gradually the idea grew that it would be possible to use the same principle to handle many catastrophes which could occur. A hail storm or a tornado might wreck a house. Who would rebuild it? For a time the immediate neighbors would cooperate, lending their skills and services in the rebuilding. Gradually it became popular to take out an insurance policy. If 100 persons bought a tornado insurance policy and one home was devastated by a tornado, the premiums (amount of money paid in by the subscribers) were used to pay the bills to reconstruct the demolished house. Each family which had been spared the demolishing would be grateful that their house had been spared.

This principle, that we can all pay a little something to insure ourselves against a catastrophic major loss, is the idea which gave rise to the hundreds of insurance companies in existence today. First it was life insurance. Later, health and accident insurance became very popular. Today we have hundreds of programs —Blue Cross, Blue Shield, Delta Dental Plan, Medicare, government-sponsored insurance, nonprofit dental care, prepaid dental care, health and accident insurance, workmen's compensation insurance, and group prepaid dental insurance plans.

Insurance is based on the law of probability which is figured carefully by actuaries (persons who figure the necessary premium needed to provide the coverage in insurance offered to any group of persons). Life insurance premiums are based on the life expectancy table prepared by actuaries. Insurance is so much a part of our lives today that groups of persons are insured who have some common factor in their lives (it may be religion or the same employer). For example, Blue Cross and Blue Shield contracts are offered to groups of persons working for the same employer. The premium (amount necessary to pay each year) depends on the size of the group and the conditions which the actuaries have determined about that group. The rates are the lowest possible for persons working at that occupation, in that particular office or area of the country. Dentists and physicians have special group insurance policies to which they can subscribe. This is true of almost every profession and every business.

Increasingly, dental bills are being paid by insurance and dental care programs. Some of these are group insurance programs, some private, and some government. This type of dental care requires special handling of billing procedures because insurance companies have special forms which must be completed before they will pay any dental bill. The procedure can become very complex since some types of insurance pay all the expenses, some pay part, and some pay part depending on certain circumstances. It is important that you understand exactly what is expected of the office and the patient for each insurance form which must be completed. It is helpful if you understand what part of the bill the insurance company will pay. It may save confusion and irritation on the part of the patient.

Your patient registration information form should contain all information which you may eventually need in preparing insurance papers. Name of the insurance company, type of benefits, the patient's insurance policy number, the type of insurance carried, and the employer's name and group number (if it is group insurance) should all be in the file for each patient.

When you have an insurance form to complete, attempt to have your dentist complete the dental part of the report at the time of the examination. Dental terminology is very important on the insurance form, and you must be certain you know what you are writing. If there is any question, ask your dentist.

It will be your duty to check the fee schedules issued by the insurance companies to be certain that you list on an itemized statement all the items for which charges are acceptable under the insurance plan. (For example, the insurance firm may break down the charges for services in the office so that it is necessary to list two or three items.)

You can see why this is complicated. Each insurance firm may handle claims differently and may pay for different services. It is your responsibility to see that the correct information reaches the insurance firm so that you will receive full payment from the insurance company. Read the fine print on each form you must complete!

Types of Insurances

Health insurances vary from nonprofit organizations to commercial insurance companies, from individual policies to group policies, from prepaid dental care to care only when qualified by the terms of the insurance policy. In prepaid policies, the insurance firm has an arrangement with a dentist so that all the patients carrying the insurance receive their care without paying the dentist. They simply pay the insurance firm an annual premium. The dentist is paid by the insurance company.

The insurance companies state in their policies the fee regulations by which the dentist is to be paid, the method of paying him (that is, whether they pay him direct or whether they pay the patient and the patient pays the dentist), and any exclusions or special provisions. Policies must be read carefully.

The assistant to a dentist who is affiliated with any prepaid dental plan must be very certain that she understands the terms of the insurance and that each patient who claims membership in such a group is actually enrolled at the time of the dental care. (The membership card may have expired.)

Delta Dental Plans

The nonprofit Delta Dental Plan has been developed as a result of the growing interest in prepaid dental care. The national association of Delta Dental Plan has its office in the headquarters building of the American Dental Association in Chicago and is approved by the A.D.A. as well as the forty-five states in which the plan operates.

The purpose of this type of insurance is to provide basic dental care. Options allow partial payment of other, more extensive dentistry. Firms and unions join. Their employees and/or members are then insured under the group plan. The families who are insured go to the dentist of their choice, and the bill is prepaid through their group. The family either pays a monthly premium or the union or employer furnishes this care as a fringe benefit.

Figure 19.1 shows the Delta Dental Plan of Minnesota Examination and Treatment Plan Form and the code to be used with it.

Other Plans

There are other plans whereby a family may receive complete care by belonging to a group which employs a clinic of dentists to care for them. Almost all their dental care is covered by their annual premium payment. There are many plans of this nature throughout the United States, including some established by unions. The dentist is paid a definite amount annually for each person who places himself in the dentist's care. The dentist must then provide complete service with certain listed exclusions.

If the patient has a private insurance policy —not a group policy—it is usually one in which the insurance company pays the patient and the patient pays the dentist.

Procedures for Managing Insurance Cases

It is very important that you keep *all* the necessary records. Be alert to educating patients to just how much their insurance covers and what their responsibilities are. See that you send accurate reports to the insurance firms on time.

There are two ways in which dentists are paid by insurance. If they agree to participate, they agree to serve for a minimum fee for families whose income falls below a set amount established in the Schedule of Allowances. If the income of the family is above that amount, the dentist is free to charge his usual fee. The patient pays everything above the Blue Shield basic amount. It is important for the secretary to be certain that the patient who uses such an insurance plan understands exactly his financial obligations to the office. Some people are very confused by insurance terms.

Have necessary information about patient's insurance records on his acquaintance card.

A nice way to approach the patient is to say, "Mr. Jones, if you care to, you may sign this

RETAIN LAST COPY FOR YOUR FILES. MAIL ALL OTHER COPIES TO DELTA DENTAL PLAN OF MINNESOTA. STAPLE X-RAYS (NOT REQUIRED FOR AMALGAMS, PLASTICS, SILICATES) TO TOP RIGHT CORNER OF FORMS.

PRINT OR TYPE
YOU ARE PREPARING
MULTIPLE COPIES

FORM APPROVED BY THE
MINNESOTA AND AMERICAN
DENTAL ASSOCIATIONS

20061

CHECK ONE: PRESTATEMENT OF COSTS ☐ OR ALL SERVICE COMPLETE ☐

IF PRESTATEMENT, DELTA MN. WILL COMPLETE DATES "FROM" AND "THRU" IMMEDIATELY BELOW. IF SERVICE WILL EXTEND BEYOND "THRU" DATE YOU MUST INQUIRE TO DELTA MN. FOR CONFIRMATION OF CONTINUED ELIGIBILITY.

APPROVED FOR BENEFITS
FROM   BY

USE THIS NUMBER
FOR ANY INQUIRY ↓

DELTA DENTAL PLAN of MINNESOTA
P.O. BOX 24105
MINNEAPOLIS, MINNESOTA 55424

▶ THRU

1. EMPLOYEES NAME
2. SOCIAL SECURITY NO.
3. NAME OF GROUP DENTAL PLAN

4. MAILING ADDRESS
5. GROUP NUMBER
6. LOCATION

FOR DELTA MN. USE ONLY

7. CITY   STATE   ZIP
8. EMPLOYERS NAME

PARTICIPATING
FEE SCHEDULE
NON-PARTICIPATING

9. PATIENT NAME
10. PATIENT RELATIONSHIP TO EMPLOYEE-MEMBER
11. PATIENTS SEX ☐ M ☐ F
12. PATIENT BIRTHDATE MO. DAY YEAR
13. DATE PATIENT FIRST VISIT (CURRENT SERIES)

14. DENTIST NAME
15. SOCIAL SECURITY NO.
17. IS PATIENT COVERED BY OTHER PLAN? (NAME OTHER PLAN)   YES   NO

JAN	FEB	MAR	APR
MAY	JUN	JUL	AUG
SEP	OCT	NOV	DEC

16. LICENSE NO.
18. DENTIST MAILING ADDRESS
19. PHONE NO.
20. IS ANY OF TREATMENT FOR ORTHODONTIC PURPOSES?

21. CITY   STATE   ZIP
22. TREATMENT RESULT OF ACCIDENT?

ELIG.   DATE   INITIALS

23. RESULT OF OCCUPATIONAL INJURY?

AUTH.

24. IF PROSTHESIS, IS THIS INITIAL PLACEMENT?   YES   NO (IF NO, REASON FOR REPLACEMENT)
25. DATE OF PRIOR PLACEMENT
26. ARE X-RAYS ENCLOSED? (REQUIRED FOR ALL SERVICES OTHER THAN AMALGAMS, PLASTICS, SILICOTES) HOW MANY?

27. EXAMINATION AND TREATMENT RECORD - LIST IN ORDER FROM TOOTH NO. 1 THROUGH TOOTH NO. 32

TOOTH # OR LETTER	SURFACES	DESCRIPTION OF SERVICE (INCLUDING X-RAYS, PROPHYLAXIS, MATERIALS USED, ETC.)	DATE SERVICE PERFORMED MO. DAY YEAR	PROCEDURE NUMBER	FEE

FOR DELTA MN. USE ONLY

28. REMARKS FOR UNUSUAL SERVICES

FOR DELTA MN. USE ONLY
AUTHORIZED FOR DENTAL CARE

FROM _____ THROUGH _____
IF TREATMENT EXTENDS BEYOND THIS DATE YOU MUST REQUEST FURTHER ELIGIBILITY FROM DELTA MN.

WE HAVE REVIEWED THIS TREATMENT PLAN. THE COMPUTATIONS AND ANY ADJUSTMENTS MADE BY DELTA MN. AND HAVE APPROVED SAME.

_____ _____
DENTIST   PATIENT (EMPLOYEE)

DELTA MN. 201 8-71 TREATMENT FORM

I HEREBY ACCEPT THE FOREGOING TREATMENT PLAN AND AUTHORIZE RELEASE OF ANY INFORMATION RELATING TO THIS CLAIM.

PATIENT (PARENT OR EMPLOYEE-MEMBER) SIGNATURE   X

I HEREBY CERTIFY THAT THE SERVICES LISTED ABOVE HAVE BEEN PERFORMED AND TO THE BEST OF MY KNOWLEDGE ARE WITHIN THE PROVISIONS OF THE GROUP DENTAL PLAN PAYMENT IS THEREFORE DUE.

DENTIST SIGNATURE   X   DATE _____

(A) TOTAL FEE

PATIENT PAYS   (B)
DEDUCTIBLE
% of $

DDPM PAYS   (C)
100 % of $
% of $

(B + C = A)

OK TO PAY _____ _____
INITIAL   DATE

EXAMINATION AND TREATMENT PLAN FORM
(SEE BACK OF THIS PAGE)

Fig. 19.1. Delta Dental Plan of Minnesota Examination and Treatment Plan Form

form from your insurance company, and then we can collect your bill directly from them."

Be sure to add, "You know they may not pay the entire bill, but when we have received the payment from them, we shall send you a statement showing what they paid and what you still owe us."

If he agrees to this method, he signs the form and your office assumes the responsibility for completing and mailing the form to the office which processes these claims for your city or state.

If the patient refuses to permit the payment to be made directly to the dentist, a receipted itemized bill for services rendered must be attached to the form.

The information which the insurance company needs in this case includes:

Dentist's name.

Patient's name.

Each date services were provided.

Place services were provided.

Description of the services provided on each occasion.

(It is important to document special circumstances which would explain a higher-than-normal charge for a specific service.)

Charges for each service.

Amount the patient has paid.

Determination of Reasonable Charge

Payment for service of dentist is made on the basis of "reasonable charges." The reasonable charge is determined by (1) the customary charges for similar services generally made by the dentist and (2) the prevailing charges in the locality for similar services.

A *customary charge* is one which a dentist most frequently charges his patients for that particular service.

A *prevailing charge* is a range of charges most frequently and widely charged in a specific community. In one community the prevailing charge for a crown might range from $100 to $130. In another community the range might be from $50 to $100.

Population density, economic levels, and other major differences in communities will affect the determination of prevailing charges.

It is important for you and your patients to understand what portion of the total charges will be paid by insurance.

For example, the prevailing charge for a specific service in your community is $30 to $75. Dr. Jones charges $25 in this case although he usually charges $35. Dr. Knudson charges $50, his usual charge. Dr. Lawson charges his customary $100, and Dr. Myers charges $75, although he usually charges $50 and there are no unusual circumstances involved.

The reasonable charge for Dr. Jones is $25 because the law states that the reasonable charge cannot exceed the actual charge.

The reasonable charge for Dr. Knudson is $50 because it is his customary charge.

Dr. Lawson cannot receive more than $75 because that is the top of the prevailing charge for this service in this community.

Dr. Myers cannot receive more than $50, his *usual* charge, since no unusual circumstances exist and he usually charges $50.

If the dentist does not wish to be bound by the prevailing fees, he must have the patient pay him in full and have the patient collect from the insurance company whatever part of the charge the insurance company will pay.

Summary

Insurance and dental care programs are paying an increasingly large share of dental bills. When you have an insurance form to complete, be sure that it is accurately prepared. Have your dentist prepare the dental report.

Insurances vary in coverages and types of policies.

Insurances similar to Blue Cross and Blue Shield are common throughout the country. They provide prepaid insurance, with certain exclusions. It is necessary for the assistant to be certain she knows the basic data for collecting fees from the insurance companies.

It is important to collect the necessary insurance information from the patient at the time of registration.

Payment for dentistry performed is made on the basis of a "reasonable charge" which is determined by customary and prevailing fees.

Study Questions

1. Why is it necessary to be certain that the insurance reports are accurately prepared?
2. What is prepaid insurance?
3. What information should the dental assistant record on the patient's Acquaintance Form?
4. Discuss reasonable charge.

Bibliography

Insurance Billing Procedure Handbook. Downey, Calif.: E. & S. Publishing Co., 1967.

20

Credit and Collections

Collecting Remuneration

"You give something and you get something." You perform dental service for a patient, and you receive money for the service— or do you? With most people the answer is yes, but there are a few who do not part with money unless coerced. Many more people are inclined to pay the doctor last, while others intend to pay, but unless reminded to do so, they just forget.

Years ago it was considered "too commercial" to discuss fees for dental and medical services. Today this is no longer true. Society recognizes that dentists and their staffs deserve remuneration for their services. Dentists recognize that patients need to understand exactly what service they are paying for and how much that service will cost. It is also true that patients frequently need to arrange for payments extended over a period of time.

Thus it is recognized that both the dentist and the patient have need for a clear understanding of the financial arrangements for dental service.

Credit and collections are a significant part of a dental practice. They involve important work for the dental assistant because she is the

Permission granted by the International Consumer Credit Association to include material supplied by them with modifications and additions by the authors.

individual who must complete all records of services rendered and payments received. She must also be certain that amounts are actually paid.

Some patients pay cash for the services, and some use budget payments of one kind or another. The dentist determines the credit policies for his office. The assistant follows his instructions accurately about extending credit and collecting all accounts due. It may be that the patient will not pay his bill personally. A third party—the company for which he works, his union, or an insurance firm—may pay the bill for him. It is necessary for the dental assistant to know about each patient's method of payment.

Since not all dentists have been able or willing to carry large accounts over long periods of time, a relatively recent addition to the credit area in dentistry is the *bank plan* discussed in this chapter.

An understanding of credit and collections will enable the dental assistant to do an excellent job in a very important area in the dental office.

Credit

Exactly what is *credit* ? The word *credit* comes from the Latin *credere,* meaning "to believe." In the sense in which we use the word, it means a trust in an individual's business integrity and in his financial capacity to meet all obligations when they become due.

There are many kinds of credit. Credit for professional services is classified under the general heading "Consumer Credit," and this is the area dental assistants must understand thoroughly.

Consumer Credit

Credit has become a tool for modern and better living. Gone are the days when only a few socially prominent persons could get cred-

it. Today most people are not only able to purchase things on credit, but are eagerly urged by moneylenders to buy "on time." In fact, some firms are so aware of the interest they can earn by selling goods on credit that they discourage cash customers.

Consumer credit has developed largely since World War I, with greater emphasis occurring since World War II.

At least ninety percent of all business transactions today are based entirely or partly on the use of credit. Readily available consumer credit has had much to do with the development of the high standard of living we enjoy in America. If all forms of consumer credit were suddenly to be abolished, our entire economy would slow down very markedly, if not collapse.

In spite of the tremendous growth in the use of consumer credit, traces of the old idea that it is not right to owe anyone are occasionally seen. Many adults were taught in childhood that it is best to pay cash; that only those who do not properly prepare for the future make purchases on credit. This attitude is far less in evidence in the United States than elsewhere, although in very recent years Europe has been slowly increasing its use of consumer credit in much the same manner.

Credit is not merely and only a substitute for money; credit multiplies the effective value of money. Credit, therefore, is creative. When a seller of either merchandise or professional services invites his customers or patients to use credit facilities, he is merely employing a business principle, advantageous to buyer and seller alike when rightly used, *but a principle which could be a detriment to them both if abused.*

Consumer credit in the retail field has for many years been managed on a relatively sound basis. Of department store sales, more than one-half are credit sales; about one-third of the total retail sales volume is on a credit basis. Yet nationwide credit losses average one percent of total sales. Monthly collection percentages in charge accounts generally range from forty to sixty-five percent. The dental office should be able to reach the same level of performance.

Dental Credit

Dental and medical credit has lagged behind other consumer credit in the degree to which it is used and in the public regard. Exact figures are not available (as they are in other business classifications) concerning the losses sustained by dentists and physicians through the slow payment and nonpayment of accounts. All available evidence shows that the losses are considerable. The attitude of "pay the doctor last" still lingers enough to cause the professional man troublesome financial problems. While this attitude *is* being slowly overcome, there is still a long road to travel. Good management of credit in the professional office can do much to change this attitude more rapidly. It is up to the dental assistant to provide this management.

The biggest asset of the professional man is his personal earning power, his ability to provide services. When losses due to credit abuse cause substantial inroads on that ability, the matter becomes a concern not only to the professional man himself, but to *all* credit granters in general. Weak spots in the total credit pattern make good credit management more difficult for everyone. There is general agreement that professional credit is one such weak spot.

The attitude of "pay the doctor last" is perhaps helped along by the fact that most dentists have not had business experience and frequently little business training, due, at least partly, to the many years of education required for a dental degree. From a business standpoint, there is no reason for the dentist's collection losses to be any greater than is normal in the broader credit field. Good management of credit and collections in the dental office is just as possible and just as ethical as good management of any phase of dental treatment itself.

Credit in the dental office is a business arrangement based on the ability and willingness of the patient to pay bills according to a predetermined agreement. Credit granting in the dental office, therefore, should follow correct procedures. These procedures have been well worked out and have long been used to achieve good credit management. They can be stated in three short points: (1) have a complete registration record of your patient, (2) tell the patient what the charges will be, and (3) make a definite arrangement for payment before services are performed. It is unimportant whether the payment plan is one lump sum, one-half down and the balance on a certain date, or budget payments of a certain amount on or before a specified date each month.

Truth-in-Lending Laws

Normally, dentists do not charge interest for carrying patients' accounts over a period of months. However, the national truth-in-lending laws pose a problem. Any account carried over three months is *assumed* by the Internal Revenue Service to carry interest, regardless of whether or not an interest charge is stated. It may surprise some dental assistants and dentists to discover that this law applies to dentists as well as to retail business.

The dentist is apt to exclaim, "But I have never charged interest! That is my fee for the work done." The Internal Revenue Service will assume that there is hidden interest *unless* a written statement appears that there is no interest charged. Any dentist who wishes to carry patients' accounts for three months or longer may do so, therefore, by posting a written statement that there are no interest charges.

Once this statement is made, the office credit arrangements can proceed as before.

Bank Plans

Increasingly, today, dentists are aware that it is difficult, if not impossible, to carry many patients' accounts over long periods of time. To alleviate the conflict between immediate remuneration for the dentist and a payment schedule which the patient can manage, dental societies and banks have developed *the dental bank plan*. It is an arrangement between a local dental society and a community bank.

Minor variations in the collection procedures and arrangements about payments exist, but essentially the procedure is as follows:

1. The dentist and the bank sign an agreement to participate in the plan.
2. The patient signs a written agreement with the dentist determining the dentistry to be performed.
3. The patient signs a contract with the bank for the payment of the fee.
4. The bank pays the dentist.
5. The patient pays the bank, with interest.

One such plan is illustrated in figure 20.1.

Good Management of Credit and Collections

The professional aspect of the office should be separated from the business aspect of the office, if possible. The dentist should be encouraged to give the full benefit of his skill and knowledge in providing dental services for his patients, up to and including the determination of the cost of those services. Originally he determines the policies for credit and collections for his office. Once the dentist has indicated the cost for an individual patient's dentistry, the financial arrangements from this point on are best handled entirely by his secretary or financial assistant. If you have the good fortune to work in an office where this division of duties and responsibilities has already been established, be sure that you are fully informed of the manner in which you are to carry out the established policies. If this division of duties has not been set up in the office in which you are employed, discuss the matter frankly and fully with your dentist and arrive at a general credit and collection policy for the office. It would be a good idea to set down in writing just what that policy is to be, what is to be done, how, and by whom. Make sure that there are no misunderstandings. It is also generally true that it is best if there are no exceptions in applying the agreed-upon policy to the office accounts. You will then be ready to apply the three tested procedures to achieve good management of credit. What is important is that the patient is told about the charges, that the arrangement for payment is made *before* work is done, and that accurate records are kept—and *used*.

Patient Registration

Taking a complete registration record on a new patient is the first step in good management of credit and collections. The education of the patient begins, therefore, *with the patient's first visit to the dental office.*

The Acquaintance Form is illustrated in chapter sixteen. We shall discuss the information requested on this form.[1]

Name: First name, middle initial, and last name. If the patient is a married woman, it is correct to register her as "Johnson, Mrs. George W. (Grace)." A woman separated from her husband, divorced, or a widow is correctly registered as "Johnson, Mrs. Grace L." When an office has thousands of records on file, a completely detailed name helps identify the patient more easily. Several patients may have names very similar, if not identical, and

1. Courtesy Dr. James Kershaw, with modification by the authors.

DENTAL SERVICES TIME PAYMENT CONTRACT

——————————————————————————————————— , 19 ————

In consideration of dental work to be performed by ——————————————————————————————— (the "dentist") at the request of the undersigned, the undersigned, and each of them if more than one, hereby agrees to pay for such dental work on a time basis and not on a cash basis and to pay the Deferred Payment Price (item 6 below) which is computed as follows:

1. Cash Price $ —————————

2. Less: Cash Downpayment, if any $ —————————

3. Unpaid Balance of Cash Price—Amount Financed (item 1 minus item 2) $ —————————

4. FINANCE CHARGE (time price differential) $ —————————

5. Total of Payments (item 3 plus item 4) $ —————————

6. Deferred Payment Price (item 1 plus item 4) $ —————————

7. ANNUAL PERCENTAGE RATE   ————————— %

Undersigned jointly and severally agree to pay to the order of the dentist at the office of ————————————————————

——————————————————————————— the Total of Payments set out as item 5 above in ———— equal consecutive monthly installments of $ —————— each on the 5 - 10 - 15 - 20 - 25 - 30 day of each month commencing with ———————— , 19————
(CIRCLE DUE DATE)
except that last payment will be the unpaid balance thereof.

In the event of default in the payment of any installment hereunder, all unpaid installments shall at the option of the holder hereof become immediately due and payable without notice and the undersigned, and each of them, agrees to pay all costs of collection, including reasonable attorneys' fees. Any installment not paid when due hereunder shall thereafter bear interest at the rate of 8% per annum.

The unpaid balance hereunder may be paid in full at any time and a partial refund of the Finance Charge, based on the rule of 78's, will be made.

Undersigned acknowledge receipt of a completed copy of this contract.

Signed ————————————————————————————

Signed ————————————————————————————

MINNEAPOLIS DISTRICT DENTAL SOCIETY • DENTAL TIME PAYMENT PLAN
in cooperation with
PARTICIPATING BANKS

APPLICANT ————————————————— WIFE'S OR HUSBAND'S NAME ———————————————

AGE ———————— MARITAL STATUS ☐ SINGLE ☐ DIVORCED ☐ MARRIED ☐ SEPARATED ☐ WIDOWED   NUMBER OF DEPENDENTS ——————————

ADDRESS ——————————————————— ZIP ———— HOW LONG ———— MO. YRS. ☐ RENT ☐ OWN

PHONE NO. ——————— PREVIOUS ADDRESS ——————————— HOW LONG ———— MO. YRS.

EMPLOYER ——————————— POSITION ——————— HOW LONG ———— MO. YRS.

EMPLOYER'S ADDRESS ——————————— PREVIOUS EMPLOYER ——————— HOW LONG ———— MO. YRS.

WIFE'S EMPLOYER ——————————— BANK ——————— ☐ CHECKING ☐ SAVINGS ☐ LOAN

CURRENT CREDIT REFERENCES: 1. ——————— 2. ——————— 3. ———————

AUTO (YEAR AND MAKE) ——————————— FINANCED WITH ———————

AMOUNT TO BE FINANCED $ ———— FOR ———— MOS.   SERVICES PERFORMED FOR ☐ HUSBAND ☐ CHILDREN ☐ WIFE ☐ OTHER

(DENTIST)

F 36-248NS 6-69   USE REVERSE SIDE FOR ADDITIONAL INFORMATION

Fig. 20.1. A bank plan application form

then the address must be checked to completely identify the individual.

Date of Birth: Correct diagnosis of conditions in the mouth and decisions about the best method of treatment are often affected by the age of the patient. The amount of wear and the relationship of the mandible (lower jaw) to the maxilla (upper jaw) will also vary with age. Age is sometimes important in indicating possible psychological complications in undertaking certain types of treatment.

Person Responsible for Account: Naturally you and your dentist are interested in who is going to pay the bill for the dental services which your office performs. All statements must be sent to the person who is *legally* responsible for the services rendered. It is wise for the dental staff to be alert to all the unintentional indicators which may reveal invaluable information about patients and their abilities and intentions concerning the payment of fees for services rendered.

An account is usually billed to the head of the family, but there are situations which require different arrangements:

1. A woman may have a divorce pending. She may name herself as the person responsible and thereby cause you to discover why she names herself for billing. There is also the possibility that she may have a large amount of necessary dental work performed so that her about-to-be-divorced husband receives the bill. He may or may not be responsible.
2. An employed minor may name himself as the person responsible for the account although he is still living at his parents' home. Should he cease working, there could be difficulties in collecting the account.
3. An unmarried woman patient might undertake a considerable amount of dental treatment, then quit her job and marry. Is she still responsible? Is the account collectible?

These and other difficulties concerning the person legally responsible for the account should be consciously considered as you study a patient's registration information.

Investigate the legal aspects of various typical situations under the laws of the state in which you are employed so that you are better equipped to protect the investment which your dentist and his staff will make in providing dental treatment to patients.

Residence Address and Telephone: Obviously a necessity.

Business Address and Telephone: There may be times when the residence address may change while the individual is still working at the same place of employment. Your office may or may not be notified of the change of residence. If you are not notified, this will give you a place with which to check. In other words, if you are registering the wife, the place of employment of the husband should be given. In the event of difficulty with the account at a later date, a means of following up the collection of the account is available. It also may provide a means of appointment notification in an emergency, when no one is available at the residence address. If this place of employment is with a firm of considerable size, you should secure information as to which department employs the individual.

Occupation: There are many occupational diseases which may be demonstrated in the mouth. Lead poisoning may be developing in a painter or lead worker. Some occupations may be more inclined to develop tensions than others, which may affect the choice of materials for a dental procedure, the design of a dental replacement, or the method of dental treatment. Knowing the occupation is also helpful in judging the acceptability of the patient as a credit risk.

How Long in Present Place of Employment: This information is helpful in its relationship to the previous item insofar as possible dental complications are concerned. It is also one of the most important individual factors in relation to the extension of credit. A person who has been with the same firm for six years is obviously a better risk than one who started with a company last week and has not worked with one firm or on one job for any length of time. Previous length of employment should be determined if the present employment period has been short. In addition, if employment and working hours have been established for some time, it is easier for you to plan appointment time with the patient, and generally it is easier for the patient to arrange to keep appointments.

Physician: Many systemic diseases have effects which are apparent in the mouth. Cancer occurs with frequency in the area under the dentist's observation. Dentists often check with the patient's physician before making a definite diagnosis and plan of treatment. Frequently the dentist and physician work together to solve a patient's difficulties.

Referred By: Your office should be sure to send a note of appreciation, preferably handwritten by the dentist, to every individual who refers a patient to your office. It is frequently true that patients refer others who are quite like themselves in socioeconomic status and dependability.

Relative or Close Friend: Should your office have to change an appointment suddenly for reasons beyond your control, or should you wish to call the patient to change an appointment, you may not be able to reach him. A relative or close friend can sometimes take the message or tell you where the patient may be reached. Should a patient leave town before paying his bill, having the name of a relative or friend gives you a means of locating the patient. Sometimes it is possible to obtain this information in casual conversation with the patient; however, if there is the least doubt in your mind about the patient's ability to pay his

bills, be certain to obtain the name of a relative or close friend.

Former Dentist: It may be desirable to contact the former dentist, if the patient gives his permission, to discover the exact treatment of a given condition. If the patient does not wish you to contact his previous dentist, carefully ascertain his dependability. Quite likely he may only be embarrassed about telling his former dentist he is leaving him, but this reluctance can also indicate trouble—and perhaps it was collection trouble.

Convenient Time for Appointments: For the convenience of the patient and for insurance against broken appointments, records for each patient should be made, and *used*, of the best time for his appointment. The record should include the time of the week (early part or latter part); morning or afternoon; early or latter part of the morning or early or latter part of the afternoon. In some cases, it could be extended to include the preferred time during a given month.

Insurance Firm and Number of Policy: This information is very important when the insurance forms are to be completed. Having it on the registration is helpful in your work.

Acquiring Patient Registration Information

Whether the patient is given a registration form to fill out or whether you ask the questions is not important. *How* it is done, in either case, *is* important. All consideration must be given to the patient's self-respect. Securing the desired information should not be made an obvious process.

If the patient is filling out the registration and does not fill in certain answers, you can quietly, gently, and with a smile explain why you wish such information on the record. If patients are approached with an attitude of genuine liking for people and a real desire to be of service to them, plus an indication that the process is one which is routinely performed with everyone who enters your practice, you usually will find that everything you wish to know is given freely. Those occasions in which the opposite is true deserve further investigation on your part to establish a good relationship.

It is possible for a patient to develop a lasting dislike for a dental office simply due to seemingly unfriendly, discourteous, or snobbish attitudes on the part of the office assistant. Clumsy and thoughtless handling of the business details can be damaging to the dentist, no matter how excellent his professional services may be.

It is important for you to develop the ability to pick up impressions—of sensing the reaction of a patient to your conversation or questions. At times patients will, consciously or unconsciously, withhold certain essential information. Behavior, mannerisms, nervous gestures, and other characteristics will often give an alert, sensitive interviewer clues to possible financial or domestic irregularities. Such clues mean that you should keep gently probing until either the irregularities prove groundless or the true facts are brought out.

Very often difficulties in collections, when they occur, can be traced to the purchase of a new car, a new television set, or some other outlay rather than the dental payment itself, even though something about the dental service may be picked out by the patient as being the cause—too high a fee, the denture doesn't fit, etc. This can be the reason a longtime, regular patient suddenly develops trouble in paying his account.

Avoid developing a generally suspicious attitude, however, looking for hidden things that probably do not exist. The vast majority of people are honest. What is more, practically everyone *wants to be honest*. Patients are people.

In registering a new patient, you should aim for the following objectives:

1. Obtain complete details of name and address, sufficient for positive identification.
2. Secure as much personal history as is necessary to establish credit responsibility.
3. Make the registration a pleasant and agreeable experience for the patient.
4. "Sell" the office and its service.
5. Leave the patient with a friendly attitude toward the office so he will feel free to discuss personal financial problems at any time.

Credit Control

Patients desire most to know what is to be accomplished in the dental treatment, how much it will cost, and exactly what is expected of them in paying for the service. Misunderstanding any one of these points is frequently the cause of difficulty with an outstanding account. Remember that patients on every level of income often prefer to arrange payment for large fees on a time basis, not necessarily due to poverty but for convenience.

We have suggested that you, as the dental assistant, take charge of a specific method of handling accounts in your office, with the method in writing and completely understood by both yourself and your dentist. You must develop your own skill and judgment. After you have earned your dentist's confidence, he will gladly leave financial matters largely to you and be pleased to have them off his mind.

We have also emphasized the need for patients to be educated to regard bills for dental services in the same light as other consumer credit obligations—to be paid promptly as arranged. This begins with the patient's first visit to your office—with the complete registration of information about that patient. The fact that your office is so thorough gives the patient the impression that your office is businesslike, in the best sense of the word, and will stimulate him to regard his obligations to your office as important.

The third factor in good management of credit and collections is bookkeeping. Adequate bookkeeping or accounting records should be kept by every professional office. The keeping of dependable records is a long step toward increasing office income and preventing avoidable losses. The basis for any effective collection of overdue accounts is complete, dependable records. Inability to substantiate by date and detail the various charges and credits, when required, weakens a claim against a patient. Minimum bookkeeping requirements are discussed elsewhere. Complete names, accurate dates, accurate data on the services rendered, and accurate figures are a basic requisite.

Accuracy is of major importance in building good dentist-patient relationships. The name of the person to be billed should be recorded exactly. Few things cause greater annoyance to a person than to have his or her name mispronounced or misspelled. Accuracy in the address, including the zip code, leads to prompt delivery of statements. The amounts billed should be correct. Errors are embarrassing to both the patient and the dentist. Patients are somewhat inclined to believe that if you can make an error in billing their account, your office can also make an error in their treatment.

Whatever bookkeeping or accounting system is used in your office, it should provide for the quick and accurate determination of the amount owed by each patient at any given time. It should also yield detailed information about all those accounts, for example the "age," which we shall discuss later.

Now we come to the fourth essential point in good credit control: a systematic and regular collection follow-up of those who delay payment unduly.

Collection Follow-up Procedures

Whenever credit is given, there will always be some collection problems. *Train yourself to accept the responsibility for following up accounts promptly when necessary.* The sooner you learn to do so, the easier your work will be in this phase of dental practice.

While collection problems are relatively few in number, they are important. Slow accounts lead to bad debts, and bad debts reduce office earnings. Fortunately, most patients are both able and willing to pay their bills promptly. They want to justify the confidence shown in them. Good professional collections depend, first, on the ability and willingness of the patient to pay promptly and, second, on the follow-up procedures used in that dental office.

The *ability* of the patient to pay can be fairly well determined when an accurate registration has been secured, aided often by familiarity with the individual's personal situation in the locality or, in larger areas, by a credit report from the local Retail Credit Association. Except for unforeseen financial complications (with which your office can be cooperative), payments should be expected as promised.

The *willingness* to pay is more difficult to pinpoint. The patient must be given the best possible service and attention in both the professional and the business functions of the dental office. That is to say, he must feel that his needs have been sympathetically and competently met. If the patient likes the dentist and his staff—has found them to be cooperative, friendly, and pleasant—he will be more willing to pay his bill promptly as agreed.

On the other hand, if he is dissatisfied or if he feels that the services in the office are inadequate in any area—business, professional, or public relations—he will lack willingness to pay. Your dentist must assume the responsibility for the professional service given and be certain unwarranted promises are not made.

The staff must provide an interested, friendly, cooperative, and competent atmosphere for the patient. If the patient is dissatisfied, he may become a collection problem. That is why good public relations are important. The atmosphere of the office and the attitudes of the staff have much to do with success in gaining confidence, in winning cooperation, and in bringing about prompt payment of accounts.

Every effort should be made to get monthly statements out promptly on the same date. When this is not done, patients are inclined to treat their payments in the same haphazard manner. Set a definite date for mailing statements; make sure they go out on that date. Arrange your schedule of work so that this highly important task of billing your patients is accomplished. Double-check for accuracy. *Promptness* and *accuracy.* You are two-thirds on the way to good collections by following these two rules.

Age Analysis

In a small office, it is possible to do an age analysis of the accounts receivable on the cards used as the individual patient's account record. In the larger office, it may be more practical to make up a separate "Age Analysis" form. In either case, this analysis should be done during the first week of each month. An age analysis is simply a summary form which shows who has or has not been paying his bills. It is a preliminary step in recommended collection follow-up, and it also gives a comprehensive and easily understood analysis of all money owing. Age analysis is an essential tool of sound credit management. Make up a sheet with space for the name of the patient first, then seven vertical columns, such as on a seven-column journal sheet. On the first line write the name of the patient who owes the office money.

In the first column place the figure of the total present balance.

In the second column place that part of the total present balance which has been owing thirty days or less.

In the third column place that part which has been owing over one month.

In the fourth column place that part which has been owing over two months, etc.

Room should be available beyond column seven for notes on collection follow-up procedures used so that none will be accidentally repeated. The total of all columns, other than the first, should equal the total of the first or "Present Balance" column. Notes of promises or other comments regarding an account should be recorded on this form. The age analysis forms are your collection work sheets.

The age analysis figures can also be used as indications of collection trends. The various totals in the separate columns can be compared with totals for different periods (more accurate when taken as percentages of the whole total). These comparisons give a good picture of whether payments are being held to a previous level, are improving, or are getting worse. By keeping this analysis, you will also begin to see a definite pattern of pay habits for individual patients.

Collection Percentage

The collection percentage is obtained by dividing the amount outstanding on the first of the month (the total of accounts receivable owing your office) into the amount collected during that same month on those accounts. Noting in a separate record the monthly collection percentage builds up a valuable record of payment trends. The collection percentage each month can be an indication of the soundness of your entire collection procedures.

This brings up a parallel point: How much should your dental office have in accounts receivable (money due the office for professional services) at any given time? This is not a question which can be answered broadly for all dental offices, but a good general rule can be given. An office which operates on "open accounts" completely, that is, with no "budgeting" of accounts, should preferably not have more than three to four months' gross production outstanding. That is, if the total amount of work produced by the office in one month is $10,000, the total accounts receivable should preferably be between $30,000 and $40,000. An office which operates on a well-developed budget plan should preferably not have over four or five months' gross production outstanding, or in the case of our example, this second office should have accounts receivable between $40,000 and $50,000. If we put these figures into *collection percentage* for each office, the first office should be in the range of twenty-four to thirty percent, the second between twenty and twenty-five percent to be considered equally healthy from a collections' standpoint.

Depreciation of Accounts Receivable

Lend a friend $5.00 for six months. At the end of that time he is to pay you, but instead of giving you $5.00, he pays you $3.35 because that is all it is worth now. You would feel quite upset, wouldn't you? Perhaps you would demand the other $1.65.

Accounts receivable depreciate in value. The United States Department of Commerce states that after specified periods of time, each accounts-receivable dollar is worth the following amounts:

After 6 months	67 cents
After 1 year	45 cents
After 2 years	23 cents
After 3 years	15 cents
After 5 years	1 cent

Surely this should convince you and your dentist—if convincing is needed—of the necessity for systematic and regular collection follow-up of accounts. The rapid depreciation of

professional accounts is even more marked because services, not tangible goods such as a car or television set, are involved. The gratitude felt by the patient on being restored to good oral health soon evaporates. Try to collect as near to the peak of gratitude as possible. It takes a surprisingly short time to drop from the "peak" of gratitude to the "valley" of cost-consciousness and irritation at having to pay.

Routine for Follow-up Procedures

What is a program of collection follow-up? The first statement for amounts due should be mailed to the patient on the date which you have chosen as your mailing date, following the service for which a charge is being made. It can be expected that many patients will remit sometime during that month. These are the "prompt pay" people. Collection follow-up routine *may* begin with the second billing, with the third billing, or with whatever billing your dentist decides is appropriate for all accounts. *That is where care must be taken to make sure that the routine does begin.* And, having begun, it must be followed, step by step.

For example, let us say that we have decided to begin follow-up procedures with the third month's billing. To all those statements for professional service remaining unpaid at the time the third billing is prepared, unless specific arrangements have been made or extension of time granted, a *reminder* notice should be attached. (It is recommended that "impersonal" types, such as a printed sticker or a rubber stamp, be used for the first 120 days if begun at the second billing; for the first 90 days if begun at the third billing.) A set series to be used should be selected for your office. The first might be simply a large *PLEASE*. The following month this account, if still unpaid, would receive the second in the series—perhaps, *This account is overdue. May we hear from you?* Since our example begins to use an impersonal reminder on the third billing, it is continued for one more billing (90 days). The third reminder used routinely might be, *Unless this account is paid within ten days we shall be required to take further action.*

Each office should decide when to start the series on all accounts, which "reminders" to use, the order in which they are to be used, and how many are to be used. When the final sticker or stamp is placed on an account, that account should be given to a reputable collection agency, without fail, at the expiration of the promised number of days—as, in our example, after ten days.

You select your charities; don't let charities select your office for free dental work.

Collection Agencies

The collection agency you select to work on your accounts should be selected with the same care you use when you select your bank. Both handle your money. Some local credit bureaus associated with the International Consumer Credit Association have collection departments. Dentists who are members will find many advantages in using these services.

You may be approached by smooth-talking salesmen for certain collection agencies seeking your collection accounts. Some of these, unfortunately, are unreliable. Do not sign a contract with a collection salesman before you have taken every precaution to establish the trustworthiness and responsibility of the agency he represents.

After an account has been turned over to the collection agency, all further dealings with the patient should be left entirely in their hands. Professional collectors specialize in collecting accounts, and best results are gained when they have a free hand. Patients will often contact the office when they receive the first letter from the agency and will attempt to make arrangements or plead for an extension of time. The position of the office assistant in such cases is to tell the patient that the account is now being handled by the agency and that all discussion must be with that agency.

Give the agency the full information needed: complete name and address and an itemized statement of amounts owing, together with dates of all payments or other transactions. Do not send the patient any more monthly statements or write him any letters. Should he call you, patiently refer him to the agency.

If the agency asks you to accept payments if offered, report them promptly. If any information comes to you that you believe would assist in effecting collection, report it to the agency immediately.

One common problem in collection work involves debtors who have moved and have neglected to give the office their forwarding addresses. These careless people are known by the descriptive title of "skips."

The first idea that a patient has become a skip usually occurs with the return of mail addressed to him at the last known address. Such returned mail is cause for immediate action.

Reference should be made to the original registration blank. Now the value of the information secured is recognized. Telephoning to the personal references sometimes brings results. The place of employment as given should be called and inquiry made as to current employment or if the personnel office has any knowledge of where the person has moved. The locating of skips can be a fascinating game —it brings into play the qualities of the amateur detective.

Should your own efforts to locate the skip fail, you then turn to the credit bureau. Many bureaus have "locating" facilities.

Of course, it is always possible that the patient has innocently failed to tell the office about his change of address. In such cases, certainly, he is entitled to the benefit of the doubt and every cooperation in arrangements for payment. Usually, however, skips mean collection problems, and it is wise to allow the professional collector to handle them.

The collection system outlined will suffice for most of your accounts. It will bring money in without loss of goodwill. Success of the system will depend on regularity in carrying it out.

It is dangerous to think, for example, that for one reason or another collection work can be suspended without mattering too much. Once patients come to know that your office expects prompt payment, you will gain respect for your businesslike attitude.

It is unnecessary to employ hard-boiled tactics or be rude at any time. On the contrary, it is important to retain a good-tempered approach and not allow angry feelings or annoyance to get the best of you. The stubborn and selfish attitudes of many people will exasperate you, but do not allow your feelings to be revealed. *Patience, persistence, courtesy* are the qualities that lead to success in collections.

Procedures Without Collection Agencies

If your office so chooses, instead of going to the collection-agency step after a certain number of billings have been made without result, you may end the impersonal sticker or stamp type of prodding and start a more personal phase of attention. No stated routine can be set forth. The problem is to discover why the bill has not been paid. In most cases there will have been some reaction from the patient to the collection reminders. From what is known about the patient and from what has been elicited by the collection procedure, the office assistant should be in a good position to decide the next step.

The Telephone

The telephone is a valuable collection tool. Of course, do your telephoning at times when patients are not in the office, or at least not within hearing distance. When you are positive that you are talking with the patient, or the person responsible for the account, make no apology for calling, and in a friendly but emphatic manner say that you would like to have an understanding about the account. Before you complete the conversation try to secure a definite promise for payment. Note the date carefully on the age analysis form. Exactly on the date promised, call the patient if the payment has not been received. If the patient realizes that you are following promises closely, he will regard the matter with greater respect.

Your office has a hard-and-fast policy about collections; you talk it over frankly with the patient and establish a payment plan in the beginning, if cash isn't possible by the time the work is finished. The plan is established, and all you have asked is cooperation. When unexpected problems arise—Johnny breaks his leg; Daddy is ill and hasn't been able to work for three weeks—adjustments can be made, of course, to help the family over a hard financial period. However, the alert dental assistant, keeping constant watch over the accounts, allows no one to miss a payment without calling to find out why the payment has not been made and to arrange to have it made up. The constant "jacking up" of slow payers, or those who slip, often turns them into patients who pay their bills promptly. Handling them otherwise can just as well turn them into patients who never pay their bills until forced to—even when they are personal friends of the dentist!

Remember that no matter how much the patient may not like being called about an overdue account, you, the bookkeeper, are doing it *as part of your job*. There will be no feeling of resentment directed at the dentist, and this is important. The patient may feel sorry for the dentist who has such an employee, but he doesn't resent the dentist. Be a third party to the situation to absorb such feelings as a protection to your dentist's practice.

One value of telephoning is that the patient is almost obliged to say something, even if only to offer a vague assurance that the matter will be looked into. Patients may ignore notices and letters, and perhaps even say they were never received. The telephone offers no such easy escape. Always be courteous. Consider the patient. The telephone often rings in the home at most inconvenient times. Experienced telephone collectors, after having first made sure they have the right person on the line (an important point), ask if it is convenient for the patient to talk about the account. Should the patient indicate that it is not, ask when it would be convenient to call back. It is both smart and courteous, after announcing who is calling, to let the patient talk. Some grievances or details of unexpected circumstances may be discovered. Listen attentively and courteously to such stories, but toward the end of the conversation try for some definite assurance of specific payment. Even when calling a "problem" patient, who perhaps has made several promises and failed to keep them or ignored your polite collection reminders, remember that your job is to *sell* payment rather than to force it. Control your feelings, pause before you call the patient, study the best approach to make, and above all, retain your poise and charm.

The Letter

Instead of going to the telephone after using collection reminders on the specified number of billings or statements, your office may prefer to use a personal letter to the patient.

There is no place in professional collections for the "form" letter as used in collection and other correspondence by business firms. Such form letters are often inaccurately and poorly filled in. Where a rubber stamp or printed facsimile signature is used, the effect is still less impressive.

Effective composition of letters is discussed in "Written Communications." The sample letters in that chapter are just that—samples. Write your own letters based on the personal patients in your office. The basic ideas to remember in writing a collection letter are these:

1. Remember the patient. Write something which appeals to him. Talk his language. Use the *you* approach.
2. Use some idea to motivate him—to make him want to pay his bill. Show how he will be benefited by doing so.
3. Be sure the patient knows exactly what you expect him to do. Give him a choice of two ways of paying, for example, but never give him the idea he does not need to pay the bill.

No more than two such letters should be written to any patient. Other means of collection must follow the second letter, either a personal interview or a collection agency.

The Personal Interview

Perhaps you will prefer to use a personal interview with a delinquent account. Possibly you will wait until you have contacted the patient by mail and/or telephone. When the time comes for this personal interview, remember that it is an interview—an appointment with *you*, the assistant, not with the dentist.

Make an appointment with the patient and arrange to confer in private.

Your attitude is most important in this interview. It should be pleasant—one of sympathy and understanding. If you are sympathetic and ask for clarification of reasons why the account has not been paid, the patient is more likely to feel like confiding.

Your conduct following his explanation is determined by the factors involved. If he has had an illness, an accident, or is unable to pay for some other reason, be sure that the arrangement you make with him for monthly payments is one he can meet. Remember that if he is unable to pay, you will have this same problem again in a month or two.

It is wise to verify his statement that he cannot pay. He may have some assets which could be used, but he either doesn't recognize them or doesn't want to recognize them as assets to be used. A lending agency, such as a bank, may loan money, provided the borrower has something the bank can hold until the loan is paid. This "something" is called *collateral*. For example, a person may have stock which he does not wish to sell but which he could give the bank to keep for him while he is repaying the loan. He uses the stock as collateral to secure the loan to pay his dental bill, and it is the bank who extends credit—not the dentist.

Collection Advice from the American Collectors Association

The American Collectors Association has some words of advice about the collection accounts. When to seek help and what to look for in selecting a collection agency are quoted from one of their brochures.

When to Seek Help

Remember, time is the safest refuge of any delinquent debtor. The more he gets of it, the less likely he is to pay.

It can be stated, with near categorical certainty, that the time has arrived for professional assistance:

1. When the new patient does not respond to your letters or telephone calls.
2. When payment terms fail for no valid reason.
3. When repetitious unfounded complaints occur.
4. When there is a denial of responsibility.
5. When repeated delinquencies are concurrent with repeated changes of address and/or occupation.

6. When a delinquency co-exists with serious marital difficulties.
7. When an obvious financial irresponsibility is exposed.
8. When a patient is a skip.
9. When any delinquent patient fails to sustain communication.

Other situations of equal urgency may occur, but when any of your past-due accounts meets any of these points, it is time to recognize that your further efforts on these claims will produce fewer positive results than the amount of effort expended in the professional side of your practice.

In summary, it can be said that you need the assistance of a professional collector "when you have lost effective contact with your patient." To ignore his delinquency is to encourage him to continue bad paying habits. It also means that it is highly unlikely that he or any member of his family will return to you for further services. Every credit grantor has an obligation to insure that every patient who is financially able to pay does so.

What to Look for in Selecting a Collection Agency

Selecting someone to work with you in collecting your past-due accounts is like selecting one's physician or dentist, or any business association. One does it by reputation and by recommendation.

However, in selecting a collection agency a few other guideposts should be followed:

1. The owner will, in almost all cases, be a local, well-established businessman.
2. You will know him from his membership in civic and business clubs and activities.
3. He will be a member of a recognized national trade association, such as the American Collectors Association. This assures you that he has met a rigid set of membership requirements and that he is able to offer complete collection service not only locally but through his 2,400 fellow members throughout this part of the world.
4. He will seldom use a written contract. Most agencies work on a "contingent fee basis" which means they get paid a percentage of what they collect. There is no charge for listing accounts with the agency for collection, and they make no charge for work on any claim they are not able to collect.

If a collector wishes to have you sign a contract, have it checked carefully by your attorney before signing.

5. And finally, visit the collector's office and become familiar with the procedures he uses.

Once this working relationship is established, you have confidence in him to represent you in the way you want, and to recover for you as high a percentage as possible of your past-due accounts.

Summary

Patients need to understand the financial arrangements for their dental service. It is important for both the dentist and his patient to understand what the fee is and how it is to be paid. Careful control of credit is essential to any good dental practice.

Credit in the dental office is a business arrangement based on the ability and willingness of the patient to pay bills according to an arranged agreement. Procedures to achieve good credit management are (1) have a complete registration of the patient, (2) tell the patient what the charges will be, (3) make a definite arrangement for payment *before* services are performed, and (4) follow up on patients who do not pay promptly.

Patients need to be educated to regard bills for dental services in the same light as other consumer credit obligations—to be paid promptly, as arranged.

Good bookkeeping is necessary to manage credit and collections.

Following up accounts of patients who fail to keep their agreement to pay at a certain time must be done promptly and with unvarying routine. An age analysis of accounts receivable shows the pattern of pay habits for individual patients.

The collection percentage for dental offices should range between twenty-four and thirty percent, depending on the practice.

A routine for following up slow accounts should be established and then followed. One such method advises an impersonal reminder on the statement beginning with the third month of billing and continuing for three months. After this length of time, the account should be turned over to a reliable collection agency. If you do not wish to use a collection agency, follow-up may be accomplished by telephone, letter, or personal interview.

Study Questions
1. What is credit?
2. Credit in the dental office is a business arrangement. What are three procedures which are effective in managing credit?
3. Discuss the items important to good patient registration and explain why they are important.
4. State the objectives in registering a new patient.
5. Discuss the ability and willingness of the patient to pay.
6. Discuss age analysis of accounts.
7. What is a collection percentage and how do you determine it?
8. After six months, how much is each accounts-receivable dollar worth? After five years how much is it worth?
9. Discuss follow-up procedures.
10. What procedures for collection are available if you do not use a collection agency?
11. Why should the dental office refuse to work with the patient on collection after the account has been given to a collection agency?

Bibliography
Checkup for Collection Problems, American Collectors Association, Inc., A.C.A. Center, 4040 West 70th St., Minneapolis, Minn. 55435. Free.
INTERNATIONAL CONSUMER CREDIT ASSOCIATION. *Health Care Credit and Collection Practices.* St. Louis: International Consumer Credit Association, 1964.
————. *How to Use Consumer Credit Wisely.* St. Louis: International Consumer Credit Association, 1962.

PART FIVE | # ELEMENTARY
DENTAL KNOWLEDGE

Basic information which the good dental assistant knows as part of her cultural background will be found in this section of your text:

History—for the satisfaction it gives you to know something about the background of your profession.

Nomenclature—for a working knowledge of the terminology of your chosen work.

And the basics—anatomy, anesthesia, annotating teeth, diet, microbiology and sterilization, oral pathology, caries, drugs, first aid and emergency care, oral hygiene, and some of the dental specialties with which you may be associated are discussed in succeeding chapters.

This section gives you an opportunity to saturate your mind with technical knowledge which will be invaluable to you in your work.

21 | *History*

Dentistry is usually thought of as a relatively young profession. Certainly the advances since World War II encourage such an attitude about both medicine and dentistry. The farther we probe into the past, the less separation there was between these branches of the healing arts. Specialization was reported among the Egyptians centuries ago, but in general, no real division existed as we know it today. When we look at the historical records, therefore, we are looking at the history of the healing arts as a whole. Even the highlights of medico-dental history impress one with the tremendous amount of work which many investigative, curious, analytical minds have accomplished over thousands of years.

In very early recorded history, the practice of the healing arts was intermixed and confused with religious activities, incantations as often as not being a method of treatment. As records gradually accumulated, the effectiveness of certain methods or materials in the treatment of specific diseases became evident. As information was passed on to succeeding religious leaders, treatments became more and more specific and eventually were separated from the religious element, until such work was carried on entirely by individuals trained for it. Dentistry may be considered as having become a separate entity around A.D. 1500, although specialization was reported among the Egyptians many centuries before.

The American Dental Association was of assistance in supporting the most complete compilation of dental history ever made—the work of Vincenzo Guerini.[1] Most dental libraries have copies of the history. Another recommended book in this field is *Dental Chronology*.[2] Any student of dentistry will spend a most fascinating time reading these books. He will find that much that is believed to be "new" is not new; and much that is accepted as "old" is not really old.

As mentioned in chapter one, Prinz has reported that the earliest written information concerning dentistry appeared on one of several clay tablets made about 7,000 years ago—giving a treatment for painful teeth! These tablets were found in the valley of the Euphrates river, in what is now known as Iraq.

Egyptian records, too, go back far beyond the Christian era. Circumstantial proof dates some information as early as 3700 B.C. Since the development of the healing arts depends on the development of civilization as a whole, we can see why these early records go back to the areas which were known to have a high degree of learning in all fields—the centers of civilizations.

When a person became ill, it was usually assumed that it was a punishment visited upon him because the gods were displeased. Considering that nothing was known about causative factors in disease, this association with the supernatural was to be expected. The priests, therefore, were the first to be associated with treatment for disease. Treatment consisted of incantations and sacrifices, and occasionally the application of some type of remedy which over the years had been helpful either in fact or in fancy. The learning thus acquired by the priests through generations of such observation

was improved upon and passed along successively to following generations. It is from records of this kind that much of the very earliest history of medico-dental treatment is secured.

The replacement of missing teeth by means of bands of metal or ligatures wrapped around artificial substitutes of one kind or another, and thence around natural teeth in the mouth, was probably performed by both the Egyptians and Phoenicians. The Etruscans, or Toschi, perhaps learned their dental art from the Egyptians and Phoenicians with whom they traded. The Etruscans lived in what is presently Tuscany in middle Italy. Tombs in that area which date prior to the founding of Rome (753 B.C.) have supplied evidence of such appliances for the replacement of teeth. Sufficient evidence is available to indicate that the Etruscans developed their skill in dental work to a higher level than either the Egyptian or Phoenician artisans.

The removal of teeth in earliest times consisted simply of knocking them out—sometimes by placing a stick against the offending tooth, then hammering on the stick until the desired result was obtained. The use of some type of forceps has been mentioned in Greek writings dating around 330 B.C. to 250 B.C. Removal of a tooth was considered the last resort, however, and was usually a case of removing an already loosened tooth.

Galen, born in Asia Minor A.D. 129, was second only to Hippocrates as one of the great physicians of early times. He spoke of nerves in the teeth, of removing caries with files, and of using other dental treatments. Galen also performed successful operations on harelips.

Marco Polo, famous traveler to the Orient, related in his *Travels* (1295) that both men and women in the province of Karbandan in southern China practiced the custom of covering teeth with thin plates of gold. Leonardo da Vinci (1452-1519), famous artist, engineer, and general genius, described and pictured the

1. Vincenzo Guerini, *History of Dentistry.*
2. Herman Printz, *Dental Chronology.*

maxillary sinus—a space existing within the bone directly above the bicuspid and molar area in the head—more than one hundred years before Nathanial Highmore's description gave it the name of Antrum of Highmore. Benvenuto Cellini (1500-1571), Italian sculptor and worker in gold, invented a method of casting gold into molds. Transplantation of teeth and the first known prosthetic appliance to replace a large part of the tongue were described by Ambroise Paré, a French surgeon (1510-1590). Endodontic treatment, including method and the materials to be used, was described by Pieter van Foreest, a professor in Leyden, Holland, in 1602.

Paul Revere (of "The Midnight Ride" fame) was a practicing dentist, as well as an excellent silversmith, in Boston, Massachusetts, in 1775.

With the turning of the year 1800, many of the notable names and discoveries seem much closer to us, although some may not be as familiar as others. Norman W. Kingsley (1829-1913) was one of the earlier pioneers in the field of orthodontics, although Edward Hartley Angle (1855-1930) is perhaps more widely known because he systematized the practice of orthodontics, founded the first postgraduate school of orthodontics, the first society, and the first journal of orthodontics.

Greene Vardiman Black (1836-1915) probably did more to foster preventive dentistry than any other man, standardizing cavity preparations and designing dental instruments, while contributing to the advancement of every form of dentistry to such a degree that he really revolutionized its practice.

In 1833 two Frenchmen, the Crawcour brothers, came to New York to establish their dental practice. They introduced in this country an amalgam filling material consisting of filed French five-franc pieces (silver), mixing the filings with mercury, under the name of "Royal Mineral Succedaneum." Apparently their minds were more on returning to France with a fortune, which they eventually did, than on service to their patients. Their rather careless use of amalgam was the cause of the "amalgam war," a dissension among the American dentists of the times which lasted about fifteen years, from 1835 to 1850. The dental profession as a whole took sides in the argument over their filling material—was it or was it not a safe material to use? Prior to this time, various combinations of metals were used as amalgam filling materials. It remained for G. V. Black to do the necessary research to determine the ideal components of a good amalgam filling material. His results still bear much influence in the manufacture and use of our present-day silver amalgam filling materials.

In the year 1839 the first dental school, the Baltimore College of Dental Surgery, was founded; the first dental magazine, the *American Journal of Dental Science*, was begun; and the first dental society in the United States, the American Society of Dental Surgeons, was organized. The original dental college is now a part of the University of Maryland.

The relief of pain during surgical and dental operations began to make progress with the introduction of ether anesthesia between 1842 and 1846 by two American physicians, Crawford W. Long and Charles T. Jackson, and two American dentists, Horace Wells and William T. G. Morton. In 1844 Horace Wells, who practiced dentistry in Hartford, Connecticut, first demonstrated (with himself as patient) the use of nitrous oxide to prevent pain.

Plaster of Paris was introduced this same year for the taking of impressions.

Dr. Samuel Stockton White founded the S. S. White Dental Manufacturing Company in Philadelphia in 1844. The firm of Claudius Ash, Sons, and Company, Limited, had been founded in London in 1820 and is still one of the most widely known dental supply houses in the world.

Queen Victoria's dentist, Edwin Truman, introduced gutta-percha as a base material for artificial dentures. At this same time, it had become necessary to re-cover the Atlantic Cable, its original cover having been seriously corroded by the action of saltwater. Truman suggested the use of gutta-percha for this purpose, for which it was admirably suited. As a result, he enjoyed an annuity of 1,000 British pounds per year for fifty years as a reward.

In 1848 Thomas W. Evans, of Paris, began using vulcanized rubber as a base for artificial dentures. In 1854 he constructed a vulcanite denture for Charles Goodyear, Sr., and in 1855 Charles Goodyear, Jr., obtained a patent on the use of this material for denture bases in this country for the Goodyear Dental Vulcanite Company. A fee was charged for license to use the material. Dr. Samuel Stockton White did much to get the Goodyear Dental Vulcanite Company to cease this practice.

Robert Arthur, M.D., D.D.S., of Philadelphia, introduced in 1852 a method of dental prophylaxis known as "Arthurizing," which consisted of separating the teeth and filing away portions of the approximal surfaces of the crowns to prevent and arrest incipient caries. Further work about caries was published in 1890 by Willoughby D. Miller, an American dentist who for many years was professor of operative dentistry at the dental institute of the University of Berlin. Dr. Miller first demonstrated the essential relationship between mouth bacteria and the decay of teeth.

Joseph Lister introduced the idea of antiseptic procedures in 1867. Cocaine, derived from the leaves of the cocoa plant, was the first local anesthetic to be used. It was isolated by Niemann in 1860 in Germany. Koller introduced it as a topical anesthetic in 1884. It was first used as an injection anesthetic in dentistry by Hall and Halstead in 1885 and 1886.

In 1871 the dental foot-engine was introduced, operated with a treadle. The same basic mechanism was used throughout most of the armed services overseas in World War II, although it was replaced where feasible before the termination of that war.

In 1896 C. Edmund Kells (1856-1928), of New Orleans, began the practical application of the X rays (or roentgen rays) discovered by W. K. Roentgen in 1895. Kells used them as a means of revealing anatomical and pathological conditions of the teeth and jaws, including stereoscopic radiography. Dr. Kells died from overexposure to X rays.

William H. Taggart, of Chicago, is generally credited with developing inlay casting as we know it today. However, B. F. Philbrook, of Denison, Iowa, presented a paper before his fellow dentists of that city in 1897 in which he described the use of a disappearing wax pattern in the casting of inlays. Dr. Taggart's efforts to patent his process in 1907 were refused, largely because Philbrook's paper had been given ten years previously.

Dentistry required four years of college in the year 1917. This was lengthened to a total of five years in 1927 and to six years in 1942. The explosion of knowledge in basic science and dental technology has been such that students today spend seven or more academic years in preparation for the practice of dentistry or any of its specialties.

Einhorn synthesized procaine in 1905. It was introduced as "Novocaine," a product of the Novol Chemical Company. Braun and Bieberfeld introduced its use in combination with adrenalin, which is still one of the commonly used forms of local anesthesia today.

In 1906 Hopkins demonstrated the presence of what we call vitamins in foodstuffs.

Alexander Fleming, in London, discovered the bacteriostatic influence of penicillin in 1929, but a German botanist, Link, had isolated and studied the mold in 1824. Domagh demonstrated the action of sulfanilamide in 1932, and Long and Bliss introduced it into this country in 1936. Work in the field of antibiotics has advanced rapidly ever since, aureomycin appearing in 1948 as a product of Lederle Laboratories, with many newer derivatives.

Polymerized acrylic resin (methyl methacrylate) as a base material for artificial dentures made its appearance in 1935, following many other efforts to improve on vulcanite as a denture base material. At the present time, resins of various types have replaced vulcanite for this purpose.

The search to improve the old and to discover the new goes on constantly.

Major Developments Since 1945

Growth of Preventive Dentistry

Following World War II, a greater social consciousness of public and individual health care needs developed. During that war, young men and women in the armed services were exposed to health care as many of them had never experienced it before, and they developed an appreciation for it.

At the same time within the health professions, the idea of total health care delivery resulted in the development of the team concept with emphasis on prevention of disease. Within the specialized health area of dentistry, the result has been education of the patients and advocacy of certain measures which affect the well-being of the entire population. For example, fluoridation of public water supplies has progressed, resulting in a well-documented decrease in the incidence of caries. Many states have laws which require fluoridation of all communal water supplies.

To assist the patient in his *Personal Oral Hygiene* (POH) today, dentists and their oral health care delivery teams are teaching home care and utilizing such recent developments

as oral irrigating devices, disclosing tablets, dental flossing aids, anticariogenic toothpastes, and improved brushes and brushing techniques.

Advances in clinical dentistry, especially endodontics and periodontics, have greatly reduced the number of teeth extracted and the number of prosthetic appliances prescribed.

Equipment Advances

Dentists in 1872 used a foot-engine to rotate their drills. In 1910 the electric engine was added as the power source and continued to be used without challenge until 1956 when the air turbine was developed. Since 1956 much refinement of cutting instruments has occurred.

The air turbine is superior to older methods of instrumentation for tooth reduction. It is more efficient, offers far greater control of the cutting instrument, and results in much less pulp damage through trauma and the heat of cutting. It also provides more comfort for the patient because it reduces to a negligible degree the vibrations the patient feels through the bones of the skull.[3]

In 1878 diamond instruments were invented to help reduce tooth structure. Rough chunks of diamonds were pounded into the steel blank shaped like a dental bur or cutting disc. In 1932 modern diamond instruments were perfected, resulting in precision diamonds with accurate sizes, shapes, and grits. The fine diamond pieces were evenly plated on the blanks.

In 1949 tungsten carbide burs were developed to replace the less efficient steel burs.

The danger of exposure to radiation has been greatly reduced by changes in X-ray equipment. Exposure time has been shortened by the use of high-speed films and improved X-ray equipment. The area of exposure is re-

3. James R. Jensen, "New Instrumentation in the Surgery of Hard Tooth Tissues," *ADA Journal* 60 (May 1960): 591-594.

duced by filtering and restricting the useful beam.

Cross-contamination in patients is now avoided by the use of disposable needles and carpules. (See chap. 26, "Microbiology and Sterilization.") Other disposable items, such as saliva ejectors, have been introduced for the convenience, comfort, and safety of the patient. An item which is used for only one patient cannot contaminate (infect) the next patient should there be some failure in the complete sterilization process.

Development of ultrasonic cleaners has simplified the process of cleansing instruments in preparation for sterilization, resulting in more efficiency with greater ease for the assistant.

Prophylaxis units have been developed which simplify work and increase efficiency.

Prefabricated and prewelded orthodontic bands have increased the efficiency of orthodontic treatment.

Organizational Developments

As a result of the total health care concept, the organization of dental practice is changing. There is a trend toward more group practices and an incorporation of group and individual practices.

Extended duties personnel free the dentist from certain routine operations which auxiliaries can be trained to perform. Today the dentist is likely to be a supervisor of several team members as well as an operator contributing his skill and knowledge to the overall production of the oral health care delivery team.

Fee payments for dental services are more frequently included in government health programs, insurance programs, and other third-party payment systems.

Summary

Dentistry is a relatively young profession, although dental treatment was recorded in very early history—7,000 years ago.

Skills, processes, and materials necessary in dentistry have been developed by many people throughout the world.

The knowledge explosion in basic science and dental technology since World War II has increased the academic study of dentists to seven or more years.

Significant developments have occurred since 1945 in preventive dentistry, equipment design, and organization of practice. Some of these developments are

1. fluoridation of water supplies,
2. POH education of patients, including the use of disclosing tablets, flossing, irrigating devices, improved brushes and brushing techniques,
3. improved techniques in endodontics and periodontics which help patients retain their teeth,
4. improved instruments including the air turbine, diamond instruments, and tungsten burs,
5. improved X-ray equipment with accompanying reduction in exposure of patients and staff,
6. disposable supplies to avoid cross-contamination,
7. ultrasonic cleaners and prophylaxis units,
8. prefabricated and prewelded orthodontic bands,
9. new philosophy of group practice and use of the oral health care delivery team, and
10. third-party payment for dental services.

Study Questions
1. When was the earliest record of dental treatment and where did the treatment occur?
2. What significant factors have changed the type of dental treatment offered in the last twenty-five years?
3. Name five equipment changes which have greatly affected dentistry since World War II.
4. What preventive dentistry measures have been developed?

Bibliography

FLEMING, WILLARD C. "An Inventory of Dentistry." *Caementum* 21 (January 1964): 3-10. Portland, Oreg.: University of Oregon Dental School.

GUERINI, VINCENZO. *History of Dentistry*. Philadelphia: Lea & Febiger, 1909.

PRINZ, HERMAN. *Dental Chronology*. Philadelphia: Lea & Febiger, 1945.

22 | *Dental-Medical Terminology (Nomenclature)*

Technical versus Colloquial Language

Technical language has been developed for most professions. It is difficult, if not impossible, to understand and be understood without learning the technical words and their meanings. Any member of the oral health care delivery team should acquire the necessary technical vocabulary to converse intelligently with members of the dental profession.

A dental assistant must further be able to translate discreetly the patient's use of layman's language. The layman is Mr. Public, the man you and I meet on the street, who may not possess the technical vocabulary. He uses other words often referred to as *colloquial terms.* Following are some common examples:

Correct Terms	Colloquial Term
orthodontics	straightening teeth
dentures	plates or false teeth
upper cuspids	eye teeth
lower cuspids	stomach teeth
gingivae	gums
six-year molars	first molars
twelve-year molars	second molars
deciduous teeth	milk teeth or baby teeth
granulation tissue	proud flesh
cleft upper lip	harelip
restricted tongue movement	tongue-tied

Please remember that there is nothing wrong with these terms, but they are colloquial terms and not the proper professional terminology. Often the oral health care delivery team members explain technical terms to patients. Many dentists consider it important to teach the patients the correct terminology, rather than use the layman's terms when conversing with them.

Aids for Developing a Dental-Medical Vocabulary

A large dental-medical vocabulary must be mastered by anyone who wishes to be an effective member of an oral health care delivery team. Some of the terms look frighteningly difficult, but with the proper approach to visualizing them, you will find you can master all the vocabulary you desire to learn.

Occasionally the vocabulary contains a proper name. Usually an anatomical part of the body or some specific disease has been given the name of the man who first described it. For example, Salk vaccine is so named to recognize the man who developed it. In dentistry an example is Stenson's duct, named for the man who described the parotid duct. These names may be easier to remember than the dental-medical vocabulary.

Study the next few paragraphs before turning to the Glossary at the back of the text. It is hoped that you will have some better insights into the problem of building your vocabulary and will find it much easier to do than you expected.

The English language is composed of many words, some of them similar to each other because they belong to the same family. When words belong to the same family, they usually come from the same "root" or "stem" word. The root, stem, or basic part of the word expresses its primary or essential meaning. Prefixes and suffixes may be added.

Prefixes are letters or syllables placed before the word. A prefix modifies or qualifies the meaning of the root word.

Suffixes are syllables or letters placed at the end of the word. A suffix also modifies or qualifies the meaning of the word.

Affixes are both prefixes and suffixes. For example, the root word *part* comes from the Latin word *pars* or *partis*. It means "something less than the whole." Add a prefix, *de,* to make the word *depart,* which means "to go away." Add a suffix, *ment,* and we have *department,* meaning "a separate division." Or if you wish to add just a suffix and drop the prefix *de,* you may use *parting* which means "taking leave."

Words in dental terminology can also be classified as root words, root words with prefixes, root words with suffixes, and root words with affixes. If you will learn the meaning of certain dental prefixes, stem words, and suffixes, your understanding of a dental vocabulary will be acquired much sooner than if you try to memorize each word individually.

Since it is not really essential to know whether the terminology is a prefix, a suffix, or a stem word, an alphabetical list of word elements follows. These are word elements which you should know for your work with the profession of dentistry. Careful study of this list will help you learn vocabulary much faster.

Important Word Elements for a Dental-Medical Vocabulary

a, an	without; not; lacking
ab abs	} from; away
ad	to; toward
aden	gland
aer	air
aesth	perceive, feel
aesthesio	sensation
agog ag ig	} lead, drive, make

al	of; like; pertaining to (example: palatal—pertaining to the palate)
alg	pain
algia	pain
ambi	both
ana	again; back; up
anim	life; mind
ant / anti	counter; against, in return; opposed to; instead
ante	before; preceding; in front of
anthrop	man; mankind
auto	self
bi / bin	two
bio / bi	relation to life or living organisms
blast	sprout, put forth
cale / calor	heat
cardi	heart
cata	down; lower; under
cau	burn
centi	1/100
cephal	head
cheil	lips
chemo	relating to chemistry
chrom	color
chron	time
cid / cis	kill; cut; fall
circum / circu	around
clud / clus	close; shut
co / com / con	together; with; very
contra	against; counter
corp	body
crani	skull
cresc / creas / cret / cru	grow
cyt / cyto	cell
de	down; from; very
denti / dento	tooth; dental
derm / derma	skin
di	two
di / dia	through; between; apart; across
digit	finger; toe
dis	apart; not
dynia	pain
dys	bad
e	without; as dentulous means with teeth, edentulous means without teeth
ec	out of
ecto	outside
ectomy	surgical removal of
en	in
end / endo	within, inside
epi	upon
esthesia	sensation
ex	beyond; out of; without; from; off
er	one who belongs to or is connected with, such as a lawyer, bookkeeper
exo	beyond; out of; without; from; off; outward; outside
flu / flux	flow
form	shape
fus / fund	pour
fy / fic / feit	make; do
gastr / gastro	stomach
gen / genesis	origin; birth; race; kind; be born; produce
genetic	producing; origin
genous	kind
gingivo	gum
glossia	tongue
gnos	know
grad / gress / gred	go; step; walk; degree

gram	tracing; picture
graph	write; record; describe
hem	
hema	
em	} blood
hemo	
haemo	
hemi	half
homo	} same; similar
homeo	
hydr	} water or defining a relation to water, as a disease which indicates an accumulation of water or other fluids in some part of the body. In chemistry the meaning refers to hydrogen.
hydro	
hyp	under, less than
hyper	excessive
hypo	insufficient or defective; under; deficient
iatr	heal; treatment
ics	(1) study of, practice, skill: *pedodontics* (2) characteristic actions: *acrobatics* (3) characteristic qualities: *numeric* (file)
in	in; not; on; very
inter	between
intr	} within
intra	
intro	into
iso	equal
itis	forms the names of inflammatory diseases, means inflammation of. Example: *gingivitis*, inflammation of the gingivae (gums).
ject	throw, cast
junct	} join; hook
jug	
juxta	near; nearby
kilo	thousand
labi	lip
lact	milk
laryng	larynx
later	} side; wide
lati	
leuc	} white
leuk	

liter	1.0567 liquid quarts
lith	stone
logy	study of. Example: *periodontology, pharmacology, psychology, pathology.*
lysis	decomposition; destruction; dissolution
macro	large
mal	ill or bad; poor; evil
meter	a measuring unit
mia	pertaining to blood
micro	small
mille	1/1000
mini	} less; least
minu	
mit	let go; send
mon	} one
mono	
morph	form
multi	many; much
my	muscle
myo	muscle
narc	numb; drug; sleep
nat	born; birth
necr	dead
neur	nerve; pertaining to the nerves
neuro	pertaining to the nerves
noct	night
nom	law; rule
ob	over; to; against
odont	tooth
odot	tooth
oid	resemblance; form
olig	} few, less than normal
oligo	
oma	tumor; usually tumorlike nodule or swelling
op	
ops	} vision; view; eye
opt	
ortho	normal; straight
osis	degeneration or loss of; diseased condition
osteo	bone
ostomy	opening
otomy	incision

pan	all; every
para	beside; beyond; near; abnormal
par	bear
path	disease; feeling; suffer
pathia	disease of; feeling
patho	disease
pathy	disease of; feeling
pedo	child
per	throughout; also; very; by
peri	about; enclosing; around
phag	eat
phan, phas, phen	show; image
phil	love
phobia	fear of
phon	sound
phot	light
phylac	guard, defense
plasia	biological cellular growth, formation
plast	mold
ple, plex, plic, ply, plect	fold; twist
plegia	paralysis
pneum, pnea, pnoe	lung; air
poly	many
pond	weigh
post	behind; after
pre	before
pro	forward; forth; before; fore; for; in front of
pros	toward
psych	mind
puls, pel	drive; force; beat
py, pyo	pus formation
pyr	fire
pyre	fever
quadr	four
radio	radium referral
re	again
retro	backward; back of
rhin	nose
rrh	flow
rrhagia	sudden flow
rrhea	flow
rube, rubi	red
rupt	break
sacchar	sugar
sangui	blood
sarc	flesh
scler	hard
scop	examine; view
sect	cut
semi	half
sens, sent	feel
sep	rot
septic, sepsis	putrefaction
septo	(septicemia) disease produced by microorganisms and their poisonous products in the bloodstream
sequ, secu, sue	follow
son	sound
spect, spic, spis	look
steno	contracted; narrow
stereo	firm; solid
sthen	strength
stom	mouth
sub	under; below; deficient
super, supr	above
syn, sym, sys	with; together
tain, ten, tin, tang	hold; touch
tax	arrangement; order

tens	stretch
tend	
therap	treatment; cure
therm	heat
tom	cut
toxi	poison
tract	draw
trans	through; across
tri	three
trud	thrust
uni	one
ultra	beyond; excess
vers	turn
vert	
zoo	animal

Become familiar with these word parts. They will help you discover the meaning of many words quickly because you have learned the meaning of part of the new word. For example, by using the word parts in this chapter, you can be quite sure you know the meaning of *odontoma* and *odontalgia*. If you are unable to figure it out, look in the Glossary.

Sound-alike, Look-alike Words

Some word parts look alike and sound alike. They may even be exactly alike but have different meanings. For example, *os* means "mouth" or "opening" and also "bone." Other words are spelled differently but sound much the same. Sometimes only one vowel makes the difference in spelling. For example:

Hema refers to blood.
Hemi means half.

Para means beyond, near, or beside.
Peri means about or around, especially, enclosing a part.

Stoma means mouth.
Stomach means the most dilated part of the alimentary canal in which part of the digestive process occurs.

Cocci is the plural form of *coccus*, a bacterium.
Coxa means hip joint or hip.

Make your own list of such similar looking words. Listen carefully to be certain that you understand the terminology used.

Word Study

Knowledge of word parts is only the beginning of building a technical vocabulary. The second step is to study the words used in your profession. Turn to the Glossary, page 640, and read it. These are the more commonly used words in dentistry.

You will find the vocabulary is given in layman's language—for you to understand more easily than you can grasp the technical language of a medical dictionary. When you understand the definitions given in the Glossary, you can then read any of the medical dictionaries listed and better understand the technical language used therein. One book which you may wish to study is *Current Clinical Dental Terminology*, edited by Carl O. Boucher, D.D.S.—a most excellent work in the field of dentistry.

The chapters which follow contain much technical language. Apply your knowledge of word construction and similarity in building your vocabulary—and then *memorize* to aid in retaining the new words.

Summary

Understanding the technical language associated with the practice of dentistry is a necessary part of the education of a member of the oral health care delivery team.

Parts of words, prefixes, suffixes, and root or stem words are used to form many of the words in a dental vocabulary. Familiarity with some of these word parts is a great aid in developing an understanding of the language of dentistry.

The dental assistant is encouraged to study this chapter intensively, as well as the Glossary.

Study Questions

1. Why is it important to study the word parts in this chapter?
2. List the meanings of these word parts:

algia	anti	bin	bio
cheil	circu	corp	crani
denti	derma	di	dento
e	en	endo	esthesia
gingivo	hyper	hypo	itis
labi	micro	narc	odont
oma	ortho	para	patho
pedo	peri	plegia	poly
post	pre	pyo	pyre
rupt	sepsis	stom	sub

3. Find five of the above word parts used in words in your Glossary. Write the words here.
4. What difference would it make if someone wrote *hema* instead of *hemi*?
5. Find and define five words containing the suffix, *itis*. (Use your Glossary.)

Bibliography

AGARD, WALTER R., and HOWE, HERBERT M. *Medical Greek and Latin at a Glance.* New York: Hoeber-Harper, 1955.

Blakiston's New Gould Medical Dictionary. 2nd ed. New York: McGraw-Hill, Blakiston Division, 1956.

BOUCHER, CARL O., ed. *Current Clinical Dental Terminology.* St. Louis, Mo.: C. V. Mosby Co., 1963.

BURRISS, ELI E., and CASSON, LIONEL. *Latin and Greek in Current Use.* New York: Prentice-Hall, 1939.

Dorland's Illustrated Medical Dictionary. Philadelphia: W. B. Saunders Co., 1957.

FRENAY, SISTER MARY AGNES CLARE. *Understanding Medical Terminology.* St. Louis, Mo.: Catholic Hospital Association, 1964.

MEYER, MAURICE W., and HALL, A. B. "A Partial Vocabulary for Dental Students." Unpublished paper. Minneapolis, Minn.: University of Minnesota School of Dentistry, 1962.

23 | *Anatomy of the Head and Anesthesia*

Anatomy of the Head

Anatomy is the science of the form, structure, and parts of animal organisms. The anatomy of the head has, of course, an obvious and direct connection with the practice of dentistry, a science concerned in general with the treatment of teeth and their surrounding structures.

Since the dental assistant is not required to possess the same knowledge of the anatomy of the head as the dentist must have, we shall give a broad sketch of the very basic, but useful, general information in this field. There are several excellent books concerned specifically with the anatomy of the head and neck for that assistant who wishes to broaden her knowledge in this field. This can be a complicated study, but the basic essentials necessary for beginning dental assisting are quite easily learned.

Bones

The head is made up of twenty-three different bones. All but two of these bones, the *mandible* and *hyoid*, are connected by sutures, which are bony unions. The mandible and hyoid bones are connected to the rest of the head by muscles and ligaments. Only three bones, the *mandible*, or lower jaw, and the

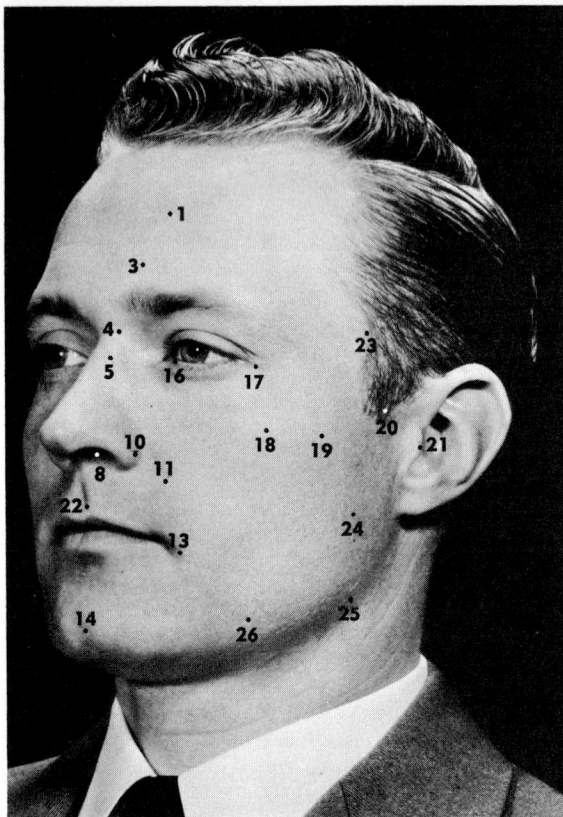

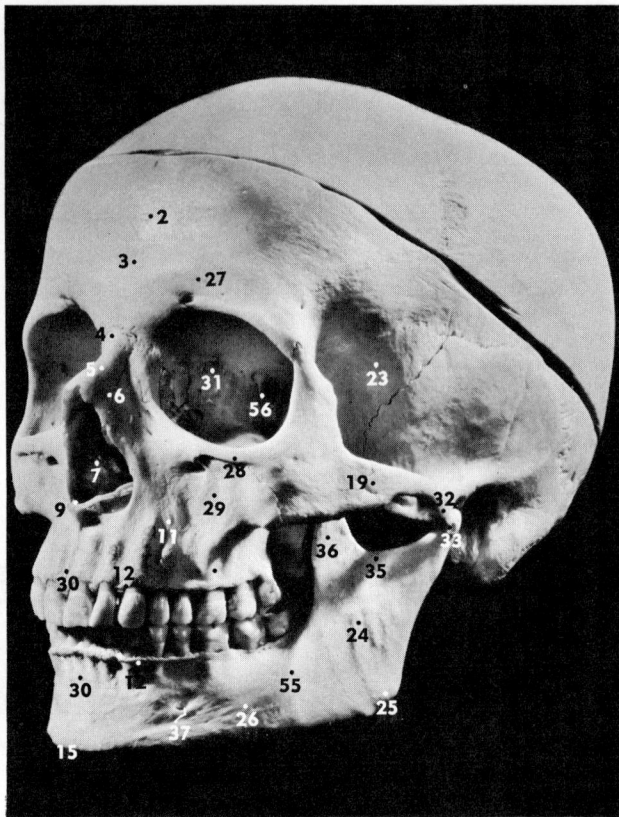

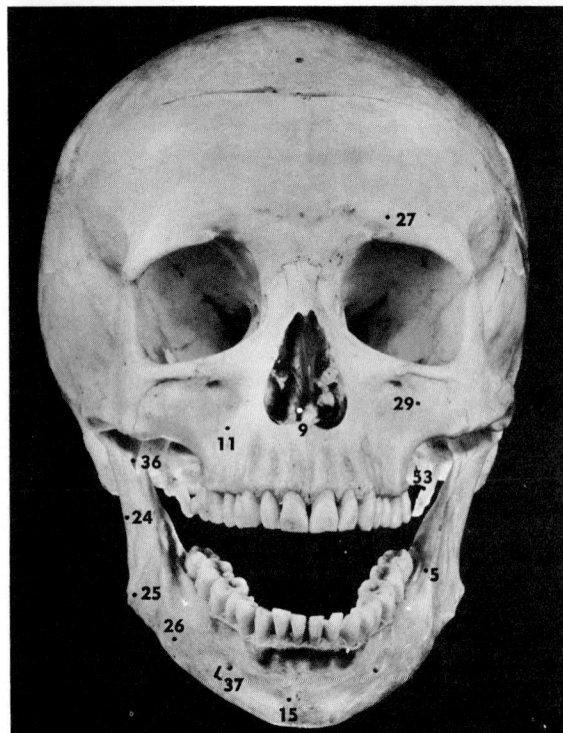

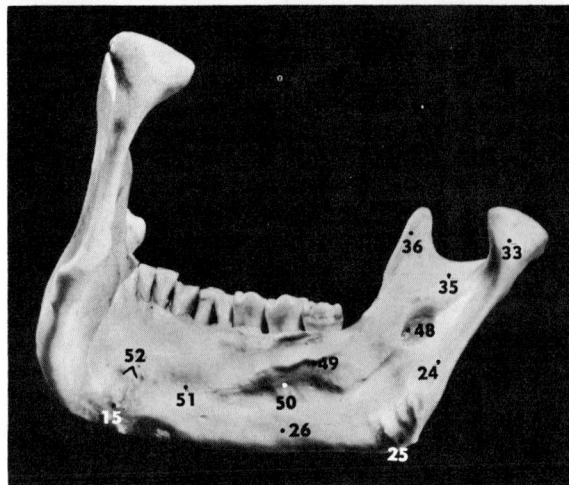

(top left) **Fig. 23.1** Facial landmarks

(top right) **Fig. 23.2.** Three-quarter anterior (front) view of skull.

(left) **Fig. 23.3.** Anterior (front) view of skull

(above) **Fig.23.4.** Inner aspect of mandible

Legend for figures 23.1 through 23.6.

1. Forehead
2. Frontal bone
3. Glabella
4. Frontal suture (nasion)
5. Bridge of nose
6. Nasal bone
7. Nasal cavity
8. Nostrils
9. Anterior nasal spine
10. Ala of nose
11. Canine fossa
12. Alveolar ridges
13. Labial commissure
14. Chin
15. Mental symphysis
16. Inner canthus of eye
17. Outer canthus of eye
18. Cheekbone (zygomatic bone)
19. Zygomatic arch
20. Temporomandibular articulation
21. Tragus
22. Philtrum
23. Temple: Temporal fossa
24. Ramus of mandible
25. Angle of mandible
26. Body of mandible
27. Supraorbital ridge
28. Infraorbital ridge
29. Superior maxilla
30. Alveolar process
31. Orbit
32. Articular eminence
33. Mandibular condyle
34. Mandibular fossa
35. Mandibular notch
36. Coronoid process
37. Mental foramen
38. Median palatine suture
39. Palatine process
40. Transverse palatine suture
41. Posterior palatine foramen
42. Anterior palatine foramen
43. Nasal septum
44. Posterior nasal spine
45. Vomer
46. Lateral pterygoid plate
47. Medial pterygoid plate
48. Mandibular foramen
49. Internal oblique ridge
50. Submaxillary depression
51. Sublingual depression
52. Genial tubercles
53. Styloid process
54. External acoustic meatus
55. External oblique ridge
56. Optic foramen
57. Pars tympanica

Courtesy Eastman Kodak Co., Rochester, N. Y.

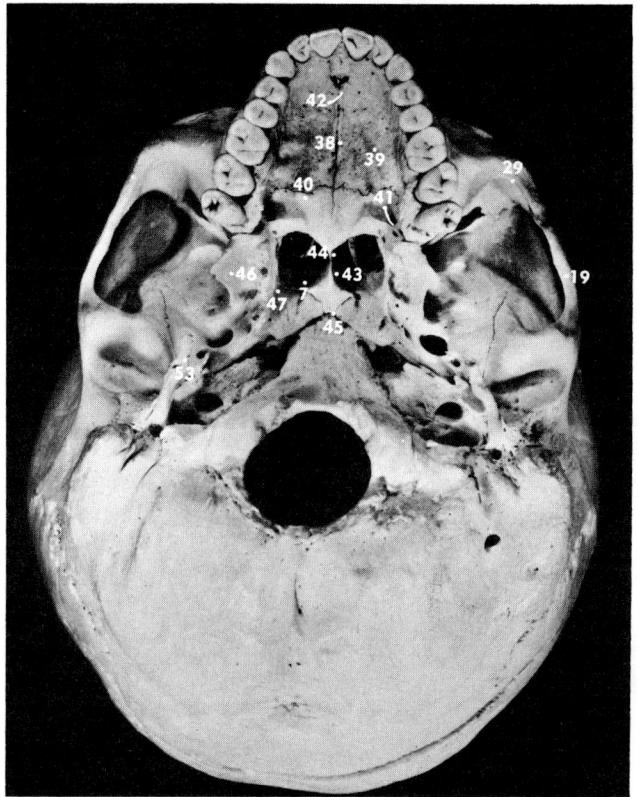

Fig. 23.5. Inferior (from underneath) view of skull

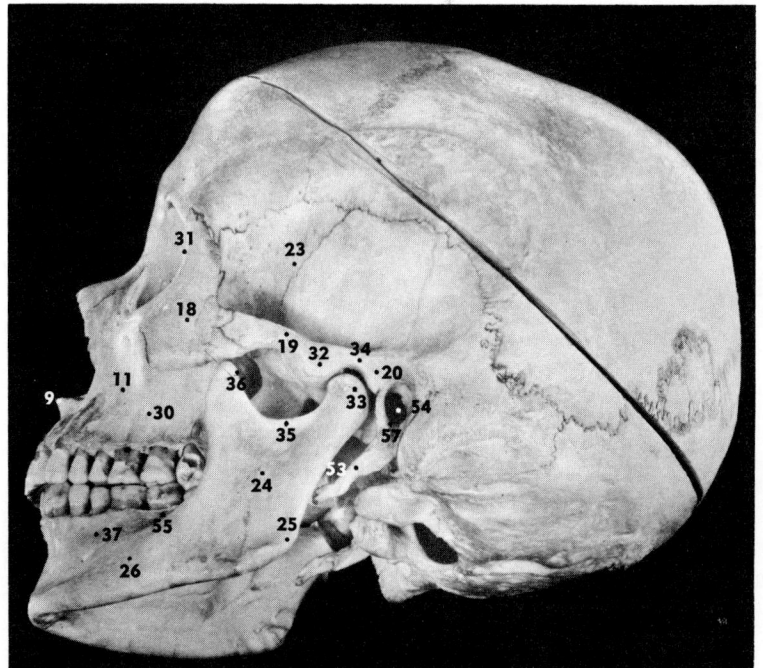

Fig. 23.6. Lateral view of skull

two *maxillary* bones, or upper jaw, will be discussed in this text.

The Mandible

Run your finger downward from just behind the ear on one side of your head and follow the shape of the bone you will feel as it turns forward, around the point of the chin, then backward, until it turns upward again and seems to disappear just behind the other ear. The bone which you have followed forms the lower jaw and is called the *mandible*. It is a bone with a horseshoe-shaped body and five *processes,* or extensions. The curved alveolar process extends upward and surrounds the roots of the mandibular teeth, providing their support. It also provides places for the attachment of the various muscles which make it possible for us to chew. That portion of the mandible which extends on each side from near the ear downward to the angle is called the *ramus,* pronounced ray′-muss. That portion which runs from one angle around the point of the chin to the other angle is called the *body* of the mandible. Each ramus has two processes, the anterior, or *coronoid process,*

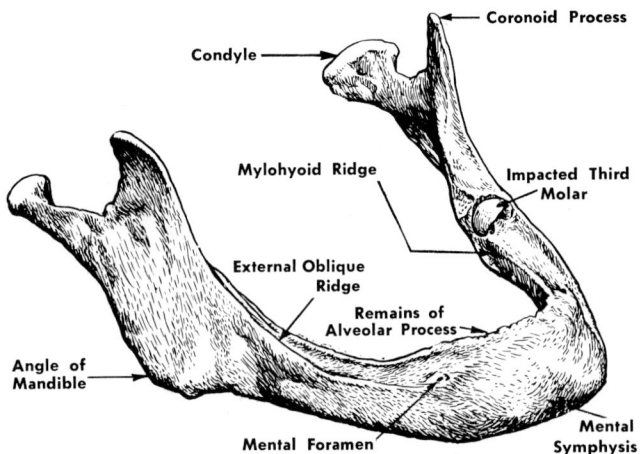

Courtesy Densco, Inc., Denver

Fig. 23.7.   An edentulous mandible

and the posterior, or *condylar process.* They are separated by a notch called the mandibular notch.

The condylar process *articulates* (joins) with the temporal bone to form the *temporomandibular joint.* Contraction and relaxation of the muscles of mastication cause movement of the mandible at the temporomandibular joint and thus permit speech and mastication of food.

There are four openings, or *foramina,* in the mandible. The two mandibular foramina are located on the inner *aspect* of the mandible, and the two mental foramina are on the outer *aspect.* (Aspect, in this usage, means the side or position from which the object is viewed.) The nerves and blood supply for the teeth and surrounding tissues pass through these foramina.

The Maxilla

Only the mandible moves as you open and close your mouth. The upper jaw is continuous with the rest of the skull and does not move. That portion of the upper jaw which corresponds to the mandible in providing the support for the upper teeth is made up of two bones joined in a suture at the midline (the median palatine suture) called the *maxillae.* By pressing firmly with your fingers, starting under the nose and following backward just under the cheekbones, you can feel the maxillae. The maxilla consists of a central body and four *processes,* or extensions. The frontal process extends upward to connect with the frontal bone. The *zygomatic process* (cheekbone) begins just in front of the ear, arches slightly outward, forward, and then curves slightly inward to an area just below the outer corner of the eye. The *arch* portion of this bone is just above the ramus of the mandible. You can't get your fingers under the *arch* because it is blocked by muscles. The *hard palate* is formed by the horizontal palatine process and the process from the other maxillary bone. The curved alveolar process, extending downward, surrounds and supports the roots of the maxillary teeth.

The central body of the maxilla has a hollow area called the *maxillary sinus.* The maxillary sinus has a direct connection with the nasal passage, and infections of this area commonly cause maxillary teeth to ache.

There are several openings, or *foramina,* in the maxilla through which blood vessels and nerves pass. The *infraorbital foramina* are located below the eye socket. The anterior and posterior palatine foramina are located in the hard palate.

The Temporomandibular Joint

While you face a good light source, examine your own mouth very carefully, using a large, clear hand mirror. As you open and close your mouth, you will notice that the lower jaw swings on two joints, one just ahead of each ear. These two joints are called the *temporomandibular joints* which are the connections of the mandible and temporal bones. They are considered as one joint because they function together.

The rounded condyle of the mandible fits in a depression of the temporal bone called the *glenoid fossa.* The joint is surrounded by a *fibrous capsule* and is separated by a *fibrous articular disc.* The disc divides the joint space into an upper and a lower compartment. The disc allows the mandibular condyle to both rotate and slide during jaw movements.

The Muscles of Mastication

Four pairs of powerful muscles control the movement of the mandible and are called the *muscles of mastication.* Three of these pairs, the *masseter,* the *temporal,* and the *internal pterygoid,* act to close the mandible. The

fourth, the *external pterygoid,* acts to open the mandible. Because the muscles act in pairs, they can also cause movement of the mandible from side to side.

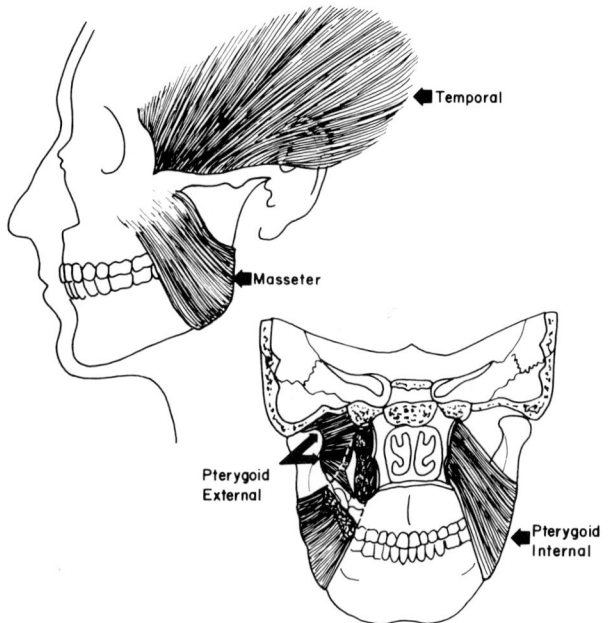

Fig. 23.8. The muscles of mastication

The Masseter Muscle

The masseter is the most superficial of the muscles and extends from the zygomatic arch downward and backward to the outer surface of the mandibular ramus and angle (fig. 23.8). Place your fingers just below the zygomatic arch as you hold your teeth very lightly together, then clench them, then very lightly together, then clench again. You will feel the *masseter muscle* in action.

The Temporal Muscle

The temporal muscle is a fan-shaped muscle extending from a large area on the side of the skull downward and forward to the coronoid process and anterior border of the mandibular ramus (fig. 23.8). Hold your fingers firmly against the side of your head, just above the zygomatic arch, as you open and close your mouth. You will feel the *temporal muscle* in action.

The Internal Pterygoid

The internal pterygoid is similar to the masseter but is located on the inner surface of the mandible. It extends from the pterygoid fossa of the sphenoid bone downward and backward to the inner surface of the mandibular ramus and angle (fig. 23.8).

The External Pterygoid

The external pterygoid extends in a horizontal direction backward from the sphenoid bone to the mandibular neck and condyle (fig. 23.8).

Exploration of Anatomical Landmarks

Now examine your lips. They are composed of muscles and glands and are covered by skin on the outside and by *mucous membrane* on the inside. The area between these two, the *vermilion border,* is found only in human beings. The thin connecting fold at the corners of the lips is called the *labial commissure,* an area which is quite tender. During dental operations, it is wise to protect this area with a very light coating of vaseline to prevent soreness.

You will notice a groove which runs from the *ala* or *wing* of the nose (the nostril) downward and outward beyond the corners of the mouth. This is the *nasolabial groove,* the deepening of which occurs with advancing age. When artificial dentures are constructed for a patient, the depth of this groove can be controlled to a great degree, and thus the appearance of aging can be influenced.

The little shallow, vertical groove which runs from the area between the nostrils of the nose down to the vermilion border of the lip is called the *philtrum.* Running parallel to the lower lip, and slightly below it, is the *labio-mental groove.*

You will notice when you barely part your lips that the edges of the upper front teeth are just visible below your upper lip. This is true in the large majority of people and is often used as a guide in making artificial dentures when no previous record of the natural teeth is available.

Look inside your mouth. The *oral cavity* is the space which is enclosed by the lips in front, the cheeks on either side, the *palate* above, and the floor of the mouth below. In a more restricted sense, the *oral cavity* might also refer to the space enclosed by the teeth, when closed together, with the palate above and the floor of the mouth below.

Place your finger on the outer (toward the cheek) surface of the last lower tooth in your mouth, moving it downward as far as it will go. Your finger is in a trough between the *gingivae,* or *gums,* and the inner surface of the cheek. As you slide your finger forward toward the front teeth, it is sliding along the *oral vestibule* or *mucobuccal fold.* If you pull your lower lip strongly forward and outward with your other hand as your finger follows the vestibule around, you will feel your finger bump across a weblike structure almost exactly in the midline. This is the *frenum* of the lower lip. The upper lip has its *frenum* on the midline also, and it is usually more prominent, or larger, than the lower frenum. The *frena* contain no muscle tissue.

As your finger continues around the lower vestibule, this time follow around behind the last tooth (assuming that you have a full complement of teeth). Just behind and in line with the last tooth you will feel a little rounded hump. This is called the *retromolar pad or area.* There will be one on each side. The same area, behind the *upper* tooth on each side, is called the *maxillary tuberosity*. These areas will be of importance to you when pouring casts in impressions which the dentist has taken for any reason. They should be included in the cast and not lost.

The pale pink tissue you see lining the mouth is called the *mucous membrane*. It is so named because it contains many tiny glands which secrete *mucus*, a viscid, watery secretion. That part of the mucous membrane which is located between the vestibule and the necks of the teeth is divided into two areas, that closer to the teeth being called the *gingiva* or *gum* (as in sugarless chewing *gum*). The area toward the vestibule is called the *alveolar mucosa*. That portion lining the cheeks is called the *buccal mucosa*.

The gum, or gingiva, is a pale pink color when in healthy condition and, when wiped dry, appears to be finely stippled, somewhat like a very fine sandpaper. The mucosa lining the cheeks, lips, vestibule, and up to the area of the gums is usually a deeper pink color with a smooth surface.

Around the base of each tooth the gum is not attached, forming a very shallow groove, actually, much like the cuff on a man's shirt except that the *free gum margin* is very snug around the tooth. The free portion, or the depth of the groove in that area alongside the base of the tooth, is very shallow. The depth normally does not exceed approximately one-sixteenth of an inch. The broad, thin end of a toothpick placed against a tooth, then gently moved downward into this groove, will demonstrate the free gum margin to you.

Now place the pad of your index finger on the palate just behind your upper front teeth. In the area exactly centered between the two *central incisors*, the two largest front teeth, you will feel a small hump. This is the *incisal papilla* or *palatine papilla*. Applying a firm pressure with your index finger, slide slowly from the incisal papilla backward toward the

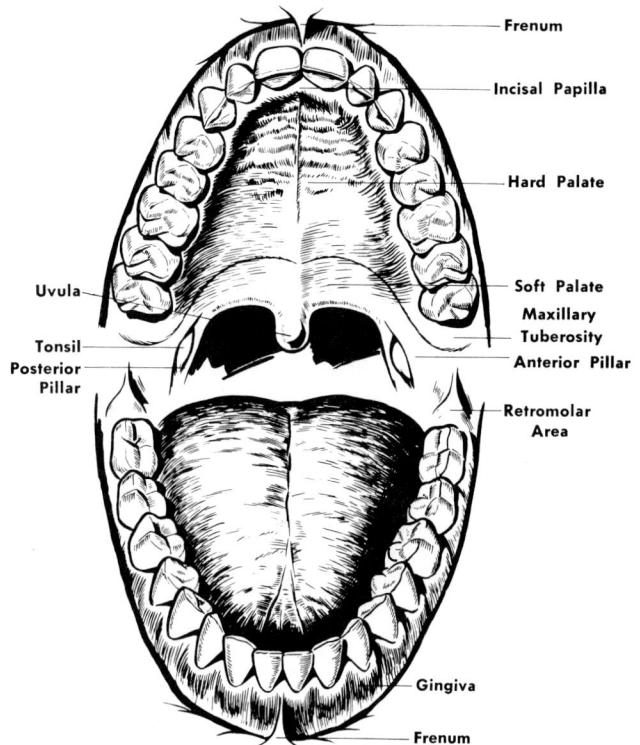

Fig. 23.9. The mouth

throat. You first feel a very firm section of the palate which extends as far back as the last teeth, if you have them all. This is called the *hard palate*, an area which has bony support and also forms the floor of the nasal passages.

At the end of the hard palate, the firm pressure will cause a slight amount of pain. Beyond this you will feel a soft area. This is the *soft palate*, also called the palatine velum. As you look at this area with the mirror say, *ah-h-h-h-h*, and repeat it several times. You will notice the rise and fall of the soft palate. That little fingerlike projection hanging downward from the center rear edge of the soft palate is called the *uvula*. The soft palate and uvula close off the nasal passages when swallowing and are also used in speech. The soft palate and uvula are very muscular.

Looking at the area on either side of the uvula, you will notice two arched folds on each side, arching from the soft palate and disappearing beyond the edges of the tongue. Another heavier arch appears to run from behind the last upper tooth to the retromolar pad behind the last lower tooth. This latter archlike fold is called the *pterygomandibular fold*. The foremost of the next two arches is called the *palatoglossal arch* or *anterior pillar,* and the farthest back is the *palatopharyngeal arch* or *posterior pillar.* Your tonsils, if you still have them, lie between these two last-named arches, a softly rounded, irregular mass of tissue, the *palatine tonsils.*

While examining this area, slightly close your mouth and with your free hand pull the cheek firmly away from the sides of the last upper teeth. If you look carefully, and think of eating something which you like very much, you may notice a small point jutting out from the inside surface of the cheek, just about opposite the next to the last tooth. This is the opening of the *parotid duct,* also called *Stensen's duct,* which leads to the *parotid gland.* The parotid gland is located in the soft tissue mostly ahead of and below the ear and produces saliva. The salivary glands will be discussed later.

Now look underneath the tongue. As you hold the tip of your tongue up behind the upper front teeth, with your mouth open wide, you will notice two little humps, one on either side of the *lingual frenum,* just behind the lower front teeth. These are the openings of the salivary ducts, called the *submaxillary caruncle.* The lingual frenum extends from the undersurface of the tongue to the floor of the mouth near the lower front teeth, along the midline. In some individuals it is more apparent than in others.

Now look at your lower teeth. Since they are arranged in a **U**, the entire group is often called the *lower arch*; the upper group is the *upper arch.* The teeth themselves are in pairs in each arch, starting at the midline. In the adult mouth having a full complement of teeth thirty-two teeth are present. In the child, a complete *deciduous dentition* is twenty teeth. Very frequently the last tooth on each side in the adult mouth is not visible because it does not have room to come into the mouth and is *impacted.*

As you close your teeth together, they are *occluding,* and when closed are in *occlusion.* If you relax your muscles, you will notice that the teeth drop apart just a very small distance. This position of the lower jaw is called the *rest position.* When you close your teeth together (as though you are biting on the back teeth), your jaws are said to be in *centric occlusion.* Just what *centric* position is, with respect to the proper relationship of mandible to maxilla, and with respect to the proper relationship of the parts in the temporomandibular joints, is the subject of much discussion among dentists. The definition given is technically loose: "that position of the mandible in relation to the maxilla when the teeth are closed in the 'normal' position."

Salivary Glands

Saliva has several functions: (1) It moistens and lubricates food which we eat, (2) It contains enzymes which aid in the digestion of food; and (3) It acts to cleanse the oral cavity of food particles which contribute to caries and periodontal disease.

There are three major salivary glands: (1) sublingual, (2) submandibular (or submaxillary), and (3) parotid. There are also smaller glands which are close to the surface and open with numerous narrow ducts on the surface of the oral mucosa.

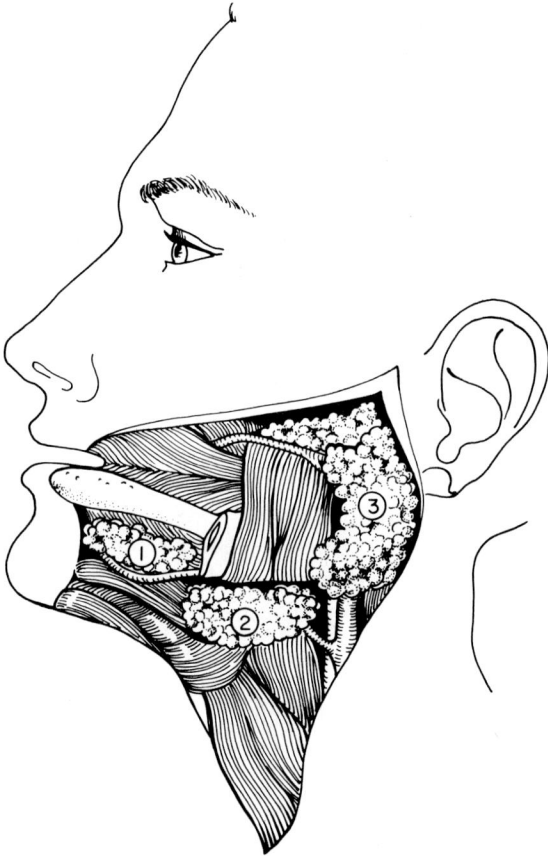

Fig. 23.10. The salivary glands: (1) sublingual, (2) submandibular (submaxillary), (3) parotid.

Sublingual Gland

The sublingual gland (fig. 23.10) is also located in the floor of the mouth near the mandible, and its secretion, primarily mucus, enters the mouth through Bartholin's duct which also opens on the sublingual caruncle. Bartholin's and Wharton's ducts may enter the mouth together, rather than individually.

Occasional patients have such an excessive flow of saliva (sialorrhea) that certain dental procedures are very difficult to perform. Sialorrhea may be involved in several physical disorders. The amount of secretions of all kinds in the body can be reduced by the use of one of the drugs classed as an *anti-sialogogue*. A substance which increases the flow of saliva is a *sialogogue*. Salivary glands or ducts can become blocked by calcareous deposits, one of the diagnostic symptoms being the swelling of the gland at mealtimes. The removal of such deposits is a surgical procedure known as a *sialolithotomy*.

Submandibular Gland

The submandibular gland is located on the inner surface of the mandible and extends downward toward the hyoid bone (fig. 23.10). It is also called the *submaxillary* gland, which you can explain from your knowledge of dental terminology. This gland opens into the mouth through Wharton's duct, in a prominence called the *submaxillary caruncle*, which is located on the forward midline of the floor of the mouth near the lingual frenum. The submandibular gland produces both serous and mucous secretions and therefore is called a mixed gland.

Parotid Glands

The parotid glands are located in front and a little below the ear (fig. 23.10). The opening into the mouth is Stensen's duct, easily visible in the cheek just about opposite the upper second molar, as mentioned before. The parotid gland produces mostly a serous secretion (clear, almost watery) which is ptyalin. It is this gland which is involved in the disease you know as mumps—properly called parotitis.

Teeth and Their Supporting Structures

Teeth

Every individual has two sets of teeth—primary and secondary. *Eruption* is the name given the process of a new tooth entering the mouth. It applies to the primary dentition as well as the permanent dentition.

Primary Teeth

There are twenty primary teeth, ten in the maxilla and ten in the mandible. These erupt at varying times from individual to individual, but generally between six months of age and two years. They are usually lost or "shed" between ages six and twelve and are replaced by the secondary teeth.

Secondary Teeth

The secondary teeth generally erupt between ages six and twelve with the exception of the third molars, or "wisdom" teeth, which erupt sometime around age eighteen. There is a total of thirty-two secondary teeth in most individuals. Table 23.1 shows the *approximate* ages when teeth erupt. Note that the mandibular teeth usually precede the maxillary teeth.

Anatomy of the Teeth

A tooth is made of several kinds of material. That part which is visible in the mouth, under normal circumstances, is called the *crown.* The surface of the crown is *enamel,* the hardest material in the body. The enamel is in the form of a shell, covering the crown or *coronal* portion of the tooth. It varies in thickness, being heaviest on the chewing or biting surface of the tooth, and becoming thin toward that part of the crown which is farthest from the chewing or biting surface. The enamel consists of microscopic *rods,* which point generally in the same direction as the lines drawn across the enamel in figure 23.11.

Calcium and phosphorus make up approximately ninety percent of the enamel. The rest is made up of other minerals, plus a small amount of organic matter.

Inside the enamel shell, forming the main body of the tooth, is the dentin. The dentin has innumerable tiny canals and many nerve fibers which make the junction of the enamel with the dentin a very sensitive area. Dentin is slightly elastic, although not visibly so, and is very strong. It is approximately sixty-seven percent calcium and phosphorus, about five

TABLE 23.1

ERUPTION TABLE FOR PRIMARY AND PERMANENT DENTITION

Primary	Age in Months	Permanent	Age in Years
Lower central incisor	6	Upper and lower first molars	6-7
Upper central incisor	7½	Lower central incisor	6-7
Lower lateral incisor	7	Upper central incisor	7-8
Upper lateral incisor	9	Lower lateral incisor	7-8
Lower cuspid	16	Upper lateral incisor	8-9
Upper cuspid	18	Lower cuspid	9-10
Lower first molar	12	Upper cuspid	11-12
Upper first molar	14	Lower first premolar (bicuspid)	10-12
Lower second molar	20	Upper first premolar (bicuspid)	10-11
Upper second molar	24	Lower second premolar (bicuspid)	11-12
		Upper second premolar (bicuspid)	10-12
		Lower second molar	11-13
		Upper second molar	12-13
		Upper and lower third molars	17-70

Apical Foramina (Nerves and blood vessels enter here)

Cementum

Peridental Membrane

Bone

Gum, or Gingiva

Gingival Crevice, or Free Gum Margin

Pulp Tissue in Pulp Chamber

Dentin

Enamel

Enamel Fissure

Cusp

Enamel

Crown, or Coronal Portion of Tooth

Pulp Horn

Pulp Chamber

Dentin

Cemento-Enamel Junction

Pulp Canal

Cementum

Root Bifurcation

Root Portion of Tooth

Root Apices, with Apical Foramina

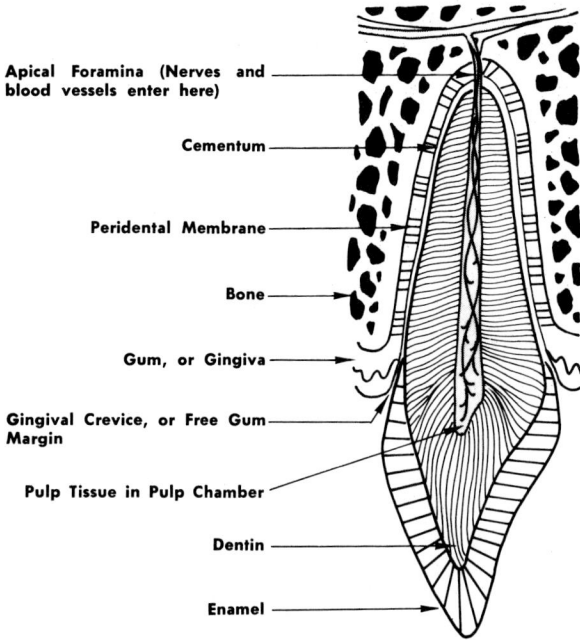

Fig. 23.11. Schematic drawing of a tooth and its supporting tissues.

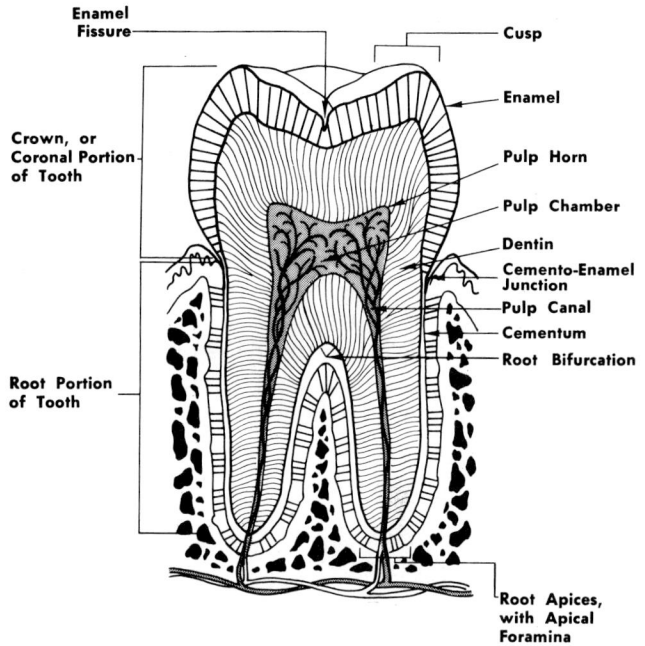

Fig. 23.12. Schematic drawing of a cross section of a posterior tooth.

percent other minerals, and about twenty-eight percent organic matter.

In the central area of the tooth is a chamber which is filled with many different kinds of tissue—blood vessels, the main nerve supply of the tooth, connective tissue, and others. This central chamber (*pulp chamber*) has *canals* which form a passageway for the blood vessels and nerve fibers to the tip of the root (the *apex*). These vessels and fibers pass through the apical foramen (*foramina*, pl.), and thence to the circulatory and nerve structures of the rest of the body.

That portion of the dentin which lies beyond the enamel-covered coronal part of each tooth forms the root. The root, however, is covered by a thin, dense, sensitive material called *cementum*. The line at which the cementum meets the enamel is called the *cemento-*

enamel junction and locates the *cervical* portion of the tooth or the *gingival* portion, since the gingiva is attached to the tooth near this junction.

Thousands of tiny fibers run from the cementum to the tooth socket, the *peridental membrane*, supporting the tooth in the socket. Note that a tooth is not directly in touch with the bone of the jaw in which it is located. A slow, steady pressure on a tooth can move the tooth a noticeable amount in its socket. These supporting tissues of the teeth are extremely sensitive to pressure.

The words used here as the basic "terminology" the dental assistant should learn are not used by all schools and, therefore, are not used by all dentists. The differences, generally, are minor, but the dental assistant should be aware that differences do exist.

Functions of Teeth

The incisor teeth, four in the upper arch and four in the lower arch, are chisel-shaped. Their primary function is to "incise" food—to cut the food placed between them. When these teeth are recently erupted in a child's mouth, the biting edge has a lumpy appearance due to three small bulges or lobes. These teeth are formed in three sections, around three *centers of calcification* which fuse together as the tooth develops. This gives the biting edges the characteristic three-lobed appearance when they first erupt in the mouth. The biting edge wears to a more or less flat edge very quickly when the tooth begins to be used for incising food.

The incisor teeth normally erupt (at the proper time) just inside the mouth from the primary teeth, which often will still be in position in the child's mouth when the incisor of the permanent dentition erupts into view. It is a rare mother, indeed, who does not call the dental office in alarm at this appearance of the permanent incisors in the mouth of her first child.

The next tooth distally in each quadrant of the adult mouth is the cuspid tooth. A cusp is a notably pointed or rounded eminence on or near the masticating surface of a tooth. The *cuspid* tooth is so named because it has a prominent, heavy cusp shaping the tooth to a relatively sharp point. Since the tooth also has a strong and very long root, it is ideal for its purpose—that of tearing food.

The premolars (bicuspids) are the next two teeth in each dental arch. As the name implies, the premolars have two cusps. Some premolars, particularly the lower first premolars, may not seem to comply with this description because of a poorly developed cusp (the lingual cusp, in this case) or because of other minor variations in development. The upper first premolar generally has two roots; the

others usually have one. The premolars begin the grinding or milling of food after the incisors and cuspids have performed their work. They cannot do the heavy-duty milling which is required of the group of teeth farthest back in the mouth.

The molars are the heavy-duty grinders of the dentition. With the advantage of position in relation to the temporomandibular joint, these teeth can be used to apply a tremendous pressure to food which the tongue and cheeks place on their masticating surfaces. To support these stresses, the lower molars generally have two broad, heavy roots—one under the mesial half of the crown, the other under the distal half of the crown. The upper molars generally have three roots—one longer heavy root toward the palate, and two somewhat shorter toward the buccal side of the tooth. The maxillary sinus can be seen (on a full-mouth X-ray series) dipping down between the lingual and buccal roots of the upper first and second molars.

The Blood Supply to the Dental Area

The blood supply to the head and neck is an amazing network of large arteries, smaller arteries, branches to every structure and area, and branches which anastomose (a-nas'-tu-moz)—intermix—with branches from other supplying arteries. To be exactly detailed in describing the circulation which supports the dental structures would be beyond the necessary scope of the dental assistant. Textbooks on the subject of oral anatomy are recommended reading for the inquiring student or for the advanced student of dental assisting and are generally available in every dental office and every school which endeavors to teach students of dental assisting.

The direct course of blood which supplies the teeth is more properly within the scope of the dental assistant and can be illustrated sche-

Fig. 23.13. Course of blood supply for dental area.

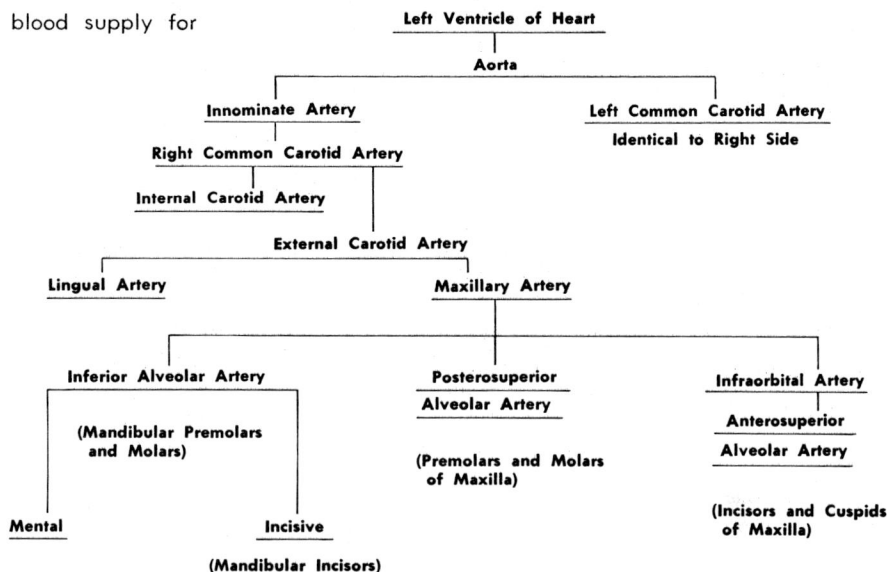

```
                                    Left Ventricle of Heart
                                              |
                                            Aorta
                    ┌─────────────────────────┴─────────────────────────┐
            Innominate Artery                                  Left Common Carotid Artery
                    |                                          Identical to Right Side
        Right Common Carotid Artery
                    |
            Internal Carotid Artery
                    |
                              External Carotid Artery
                    ┌─────────────────────────┴─────────────────────────┐
            Lingual Artery                                      Maxillary Artery
                                          ┌───────────────────────┼───────────────────────┐
                                  Inferior Alveolar Artery    Posterosuperior       Infraorbital Artery
                                                              Alveolar Artery
                                      (Mandibular Premolars                         Anterosuperior
                                          and Molars)                               Alveolar Artery
                                                              (Premolars and Molars
                                                                  of Maxilla)
                                                                                   (Incisors and Cuspids
                              Mental              Incisive                             of Maxilla)

                                  (Mandibular Incisors)
```

matically. It is this limited blood supply which will be discussed here, with the reminder that it is a relatively small percentage of the total blood supply to the head and neck areas.

When oxygenated blood leaves the left ventricle of the heart, it passes into a large, arched vessel called the aorta, from which successive branches take off for various areas of the body. The first branch from the aorta is the innominate artery, from which the right common carotid artery branches. The second branch from the aorta is the left common carotid. From this point, both the right and left common carotid arteries are similar; that is, each gives off the same branches and supplies the same areas in its particular side of the body.

Each common carotid artery divides, forming an internal carotid artery and an external carotid artery.

The external carotid arteries supply the lingual arteries (to the tongue) and the internal maxillary arteries.

From the maxillary arteries branch the inferior alveolar arteries which supply the mandibular premolar (bicuspid) teeth and the molar teeth. The inferior alveolar arteries branch again into the mental arteries (which supply the chin area) and the incisive arteries which supply the incisors and cuspids of the mandible.

The internal maxillary arteries also give rise to two other branches (on each side), the posterosuperior alveolar (dental) arteries, which supply the premolars (bicuspids) and molars of the maxillae, and the infraorbital arteries, which supply the incisors and cuspids of the maxillae.

If the course of the foregoing blood supply is illustrated schematically, it may be comprehended more easily (fig. 23.13).

The Nerve Supply in the Dental Area

Nerves may be thought of as telephone wires, in a very good analogy. If you were to think of them as telephone wires between two computers, the analogy might be more correct, because the nerves carry impulses rather than conversation. In general, those nerves which tell a muscle what to do are called *motor* nerves. Those nerves which carry a message back to the brain from an outlying area or organ are called *sensory* nerves.

There are twelve cranial nerves which, as the name implies, branch off from the brain (within the cranium). As with many other structures of the body, remember that we are again speaking of something in the singular sense, when actually the structures occur as a symmetrical pair, usually a left and a right.

The first nerve to branch off the brain is the olfactory, a sensory nerve which provides our nasal mucosa with the sense of smell.

The second cranial nerve is the optic, again a sensory nerve, this time bringing impulses from the retina, giving us our vision.

The third cranial nerve is the oculomotor, a motor nerve involving control of many of the muscles which regulate the movement of the eye.

The fourth cranial nerve is the trochlear, again a motor nerve. Its function is the control of the muscle fibers which move the eyeball in an outward and downward rotation.

The fifth cranial nerve is the one most important dentally. It is both sensory and motor in its functions—the motor root is the minor portion sometimes called the masticator nerve. The trigeminal (try-gem'-in-al) nerve (a more common name for the fifth cranial nerve) is the largest of the cranial nerves with the exception of the optic.

As the fibers of the fifth cranial nerve approach the brainstem, there is found a kidney-like shape called the Gasserian, or semilunar, ganglion. From the convex portion, the root of the nerve enters the brainstem. From the concave portion (which is directed forward), three divisions of the trigeminal are given off. These branches are the ophthalmic, maxillary, and mandibular. Each of these is purely sensory, although the mandibular nerve is joined by the fibers of the masticator nerve (which is motor) and serves to innervate some of the muscles of mastication.

The ophthalmic nerve is the smallest of the three branches of the trigeminal. The ophthalmic again divides into three terminal branches which are involved with the cornea, iris, tear gland, eyelid, eyebrow, and skin of the forehead, among other areas, through further branches.

The maxillary nerve is the second division of the trigeminal and is also intermediate in size—larger than the ophthalmic but smaller than the mandibular nerve (the third division).

The branches of the maxillary nerve are many, but the first to be specifically involved

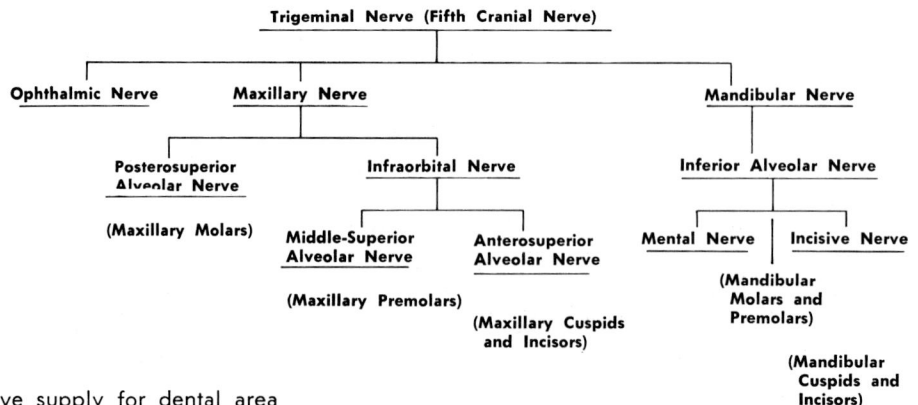

Fig. 23.14. The nerve supply for dental area

in the innervation of teeth are the postero-superior alveolar nerves which are usually two in number. These give off branches to the gums and the posterior portion of the mouth, then pass on to enter the posterior alveolar canals and join with the other alveolar branches to form the superior dental plexus, through which they give innervation to the upper molar teeth.

The branches of the maxillary nerve given off in the infraorbital area are the middle-superior and anterosuperior alveolar nerves.

The middle-superior alveolar nerve gives off branches which again join with other alveolar branches to form the superior dental plexus, and through this it supplies the bicuspid teeth as well as the mucous membrane of the maxillary sinus and the gums.

The anterosuperior alveolar nerve is given off by the infraorbital nerve, unites with other alveolar nerves to form the superior dental plexus, and supplies the cuspid and incisor teeth, and again supplies an area of the mucous membrane of the maxillary sinus and the gums, plus another small branch to part of the nasal cavity.

As has been said, these branches are but part of the many divisions of the maxillary or second division of the trigeminal nerve.

The superior dental plexus is a network formed in the alveolar canals by the three superior alveolar nerves: the posterosuperior alveolar nerve, the middle-superior alveolar nerve, and the anterosuperior alveolar nerve. This network makes connection across the midline with the corresponding network on the other side. It is because of this that the dentist, in anesthetizing a central incisor, lateral incisor, or cuspid on one side of the arch, will also add some anesthetic to an area over the apex of the opposite central incisor.

The third division of the trigeminal nerve is the mandibular nerve, the largest of the three divisions. It is commonly described as formed by the union of two distinct nerves: the entire masticator nerve (motor in function) and the large bundle of sensory fibers from the Gasserian ganglion which is actually the third division of the trigeminal. The single trunk divides into the anterior portion and the posterior portion.

The anterior portion is smaller than the posterior and is composed mainly of motor fibers of the masticator nerve which supply the muscles of mastication (temporal, masseter, and external pterygoid). The balance of this anterior division is sensory and forms (mainly) the long buccal nerve, innervating the cheek as far forward as the angle of the mouth.

The posterior part of the mandibular nerve forms into three branches. Two, the lingual and the auriculotemporal, are sensory; the third contains some motor fibers from the masticator nerve for the innervation of the mylohyoid muscle.

This third branch of the posterior portion of the mandibular nerve is directly concerned with innervation of the mandibular teeth. It is the largest of the three branches and is called the inferior alveolar nerve. Shortly after its formation it enters the ramus of the mandible at the mandibular foramen, (No. 48 on the illustration of the mandible).

The inferior alveolar nerve branches to form the inferior dental plexus and the mental nerve. (A bundle of motor fibers to the mylohyoid muscle is given off before the interior alveolar nerve enters the mandibular foramen.)

The inferior dental plexus is a series of fine branches intermingling within the bone, giving off two definite sets: the inferior dental branches which go to the mandibular molars and bicuspids (entering through the single—or multiple—foramina at the tip of each root) and the inferior gingival branches which supply the gums. (See fig. 23.15.)

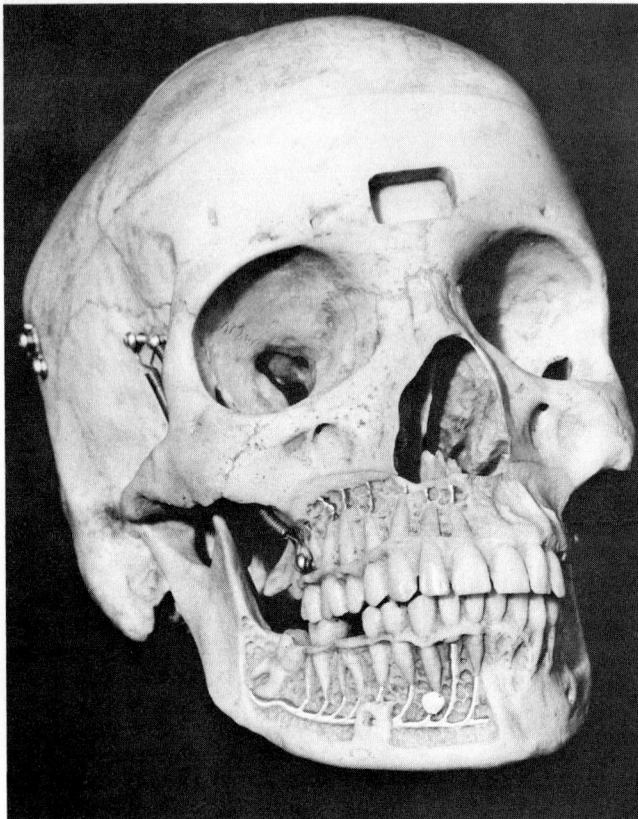

Courtesy Medical Plastics Lab., Gatesville, Tex.

Fig. 23.15. A skull reproduction illustrating the nerve supply to the teeth.

Motor and Sensory Nerves

There are two types of nerves: motor and sensory. The motor nerves control the function of muscle fibers; the sensory nerves carry "messages" to the brain from their "sensory endings."

The message which cries "Pain!" to the brain must be "received" or "perceived" before the person is aware of pain. If the perception of this message is interfered with by some chemical means, the individual is *anesthetized.* If the message is not permitted to leave the area of origin, the anesthesia is *local.* If the

message is sent but not perceived by the brain, the anesthesia is *general.*

Anesthesia

How We Sense Pain

The function of the nerves is to carry a message from the sense organ (for example, in your fingertip) to the central nervous system, and also from the central nervous system back to muscles or glands which in turn translate the return message into action. The nerves act exactly like the telephone wire which connects your telephone to the central office—they conduct an impulse, or message. Nerves can be seen. They appear as long cords of whitish, translucent material. Large nerve "trunks" may be half an inch in width and at their terminal distribution have end branches so tiny as to be almost invisible. The messages, or impulses, which these nerves transmit or carry are actually tiny electrical impulses, which, on an "incoming" message, are "read" in the spinal cord and brain. The brain and spinal cord again make up the answering message, or signal, and send it out along the nerve trunk to the proper place for action.

Let's take an example. Imagine that your finger is touching a hot stove. The sense organs in the deeper layers of the skin "feel" the excessive heat and are stimulated or "excited," and electrical impulses leave the sense organ to travel along the nerve to the spinal cord and brain. There the message is interpreted to indicate that your finger has been placed in contact with a hot stove. Immediately another message is relayed from the brain and spinal cord as a series of impulses along a nerve trunk, finally reaching the muscles which move your finger, hand, and arm. The muscles accept the order and promptly remove your finger from the hot stove—and have most likely been told to take it to your mouth so that you could have another set of muscles squeeze air out of your lungs to blow on the hot finger!

The word *pain* is derived from the Latin *poena*, meaning "penalty." Mankind has been trying since the earliest of times to eliminate pain from his sensations, and perhaps thought of pain as a penalty for misbehavior in much the same way that disease or injury also was thought to be a penalty.

Pain is a very personal and individual experience. What one person considers pain may not be considered pain by another person. A pain which is intolerable to one person may be quite tolerable to someone else. Our response is conditioned by practice, by general health, by mental conditions, and by environment, and many of these can change from day to day or hour to hour.

Anesthesia, from the Greek *an+aisthēsia* meaning "not feeling," is the word given to the state or condition which exists, whether involving the entire body or only a part, when man has succeeded in his efforts to eliminate his sensation of pain. More correctly, the word is used to indicate a lack of sensibility to impressions of any kind which originate from outside the area concerned (again, whether it be the entire body or a part of the body).

An *anesthetic* is an agent which is capable of producing anesthesia.

General Anesthesia

In *general* anesthesia, the brain and spinal cord are no longer able to read messages or to send out messages, except for a few which are set on "automatic," such as breathing and heartbeat. While under general anesthesia, therefore, the patient will feel no pain since the general anesthesia produces unconsciousness, and as a result, the message or impulses cannot be "read" by the spinal cord and brain.

Ether was one of the earliest agents used to produce anesthesia, as was nitrous oxide. While the arguments about names and dates still do occur, it should be remembered that there have been instances when various men have actually made numerous discoveries but have not publicized them. Sometimes a later worker in the same field of research repeated the identical discovery and, because he made it known, became the man credited with the original discovery. This has been the case with early work with general anesthesia (anesthesia which results in a loss of sensation in the entire body). Oxygen and nitrous oxide, the gases, were discovered by Joseph Priestley in 1772, but their use as an anesthetic agent was not known. It wasn't until December 1844 that Horace Wells, a dentist, had nitrous oxide used as an anesthetic on himself for the removal of a tooth. William T. G. Morton first demonstrated in public in October 1846 the use of ether to stop pain in surgery.

The use of nitrous oxide requires a "gas machine," a mechanism for mixing nitrous oxide gas with oxygen, and with carbon dioxide when indicated, in the proper proportion to produce and maintain anesthesia. The mechanism provides a support for the various cylinders of gases which are attached to mixing valves, pressure gauges, hoses, mask, and breathing bag for the patient.

While nitrous oxide with oxygen continues to be administered as an inhalant anesthetic, there are also other combinations and other inhalant anesthetics. One of the combinations is nitrous oxide-oxygen-trichlorethylene. Ether with oxygen continues in use, especially in hospitals in more rural areas of the country. Chloroform was first used by James Simpson in 1847 but was never as popular for general anesthesia in this country as it was in Europe.

One of the well-liked combinations in hospital use is nitrous oxide with oxygen as an inhalant anesthetic, used together with thiopental sodium, which is an injected anesthetic. Other inhalation anesthetics are ethylene, ethyl chloride, and cyclopropane.

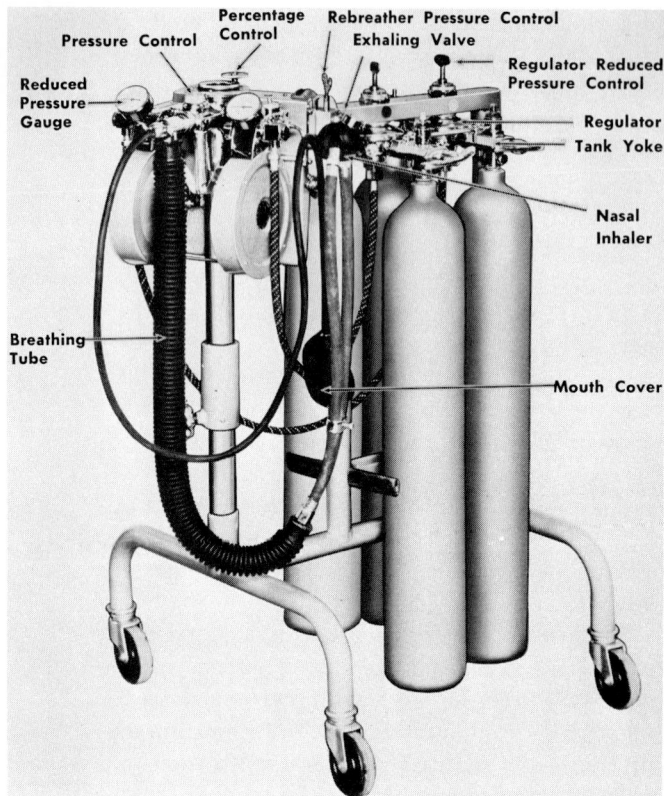

Fig. 23.16. Unit for the administration of nitrous oxide and oxygen.

There are other methods by which general anesthesia (affecting the entire body—loss of consciousness) can be achieved, but only one, thiopental sodium (pentothal sodium), has achieved much use in dentistry. Pentothal sodium is prepared as a liquid solution which is injected into a large vein in the forearm. The injection is made at a certain rate to produce general anesthesia, and certain amounts are periodically added during the operation to maintain anesthesia.

Analgesia

Analgesia is the loss of the ability to feel pain without loss of consciousness. This in-

sensibility to pain is "general" as it is in general anesthesia. Often the same anesthetic agent is used to produce analgesia when inhaled in smaller quantity as is used to produce anesthesia when higher concentrations or greater quantities are inhaled. This is true of nitrous oxide and oxygen and also of trichlorethylene, for example.

Generally, the patient himself controls the amount of the gas inhaled for analgesia. If the patient begins to pass from analgesia into anesthesia, he also loses control of the equipment, which is generally made to automatically reduce or completely stop providing anesthetic gas if the patient is unable to squeeze a bulb or hold a slide against the pressure of a spring.

As a dental assistant, you will not be required to give general anesthesia. It is given by a person thoroughly trained in anesthesia, under conditions which provide the patient with every safeguard possible. While there are dental offices which are able to meet these requirements, they are not common.

If analgesia is used in the office in which you are employed, you will be expected to learn the proper use and care of the equipment concerned. This should be carefully and thoroughly studied, because there are dangers present whenever an anesthetic agent is used, whether for analgesia or for anesthesia, whether it is a local or a general anesthetic.

Local Anesthesia

In *local* anesthesia, the manner in which the patient is relieved of the sensation of pain is somewhat different from the manner in which general anesthesia relieves pain.

Local anesthesia is by far the most common form of anesthesia for dentistry and is produced by using a syringe to inject the anesthetic agent into an area which is as close as possible to the nerve the dentist desires to anesthetize.

The local anesthetic agent is particularly attracted to the actual nerve fibres which make up the "telephone line." When a quantity of this agent is placed where it will "soak into" (infiltrate) the area through which a nerve passes, it seems to particularly soak into the nerve fibres—and puts the nerve itself "out of business." Impulses or messages will no longer be able to pass the point at which the local anesthetic agent has been absorbed by the nerve until the agent has been carried away by the blood circulation in the area.

There is an additional peculiarity in this situation. The feeling of numbness which occurs when a local anesthetic is blocking a nerve at a given spot seems to extend from the spot at which it actually is soaking into the nerve all the way to the end of the nerve at the sensory organs. If, for example, all the nerve trunks at your elbow were penetrated with local anesthetic solution, your arm from the elbow to the fingertips would feel numb, or "asleep."

To help maintain this condition of local anesthesia, the anesthetic agents are commonly used with another chemical which acts as a *vasoconstrictor,* a chemical or drug which shrinks or constricts the blood vessels in the injected area to retard or slow down the rate at which the bloodstream can circulate so that it cannot carry away the local anesthetic solution as rapidly.

The original local anesthetic was *procaine hydrochloride,* which was made in a laboratory by Einhorn in 1905. It was introduced as *Novocaine,* a product of the Novol Chemical Company, and this name is used by the public today for all local anesthetic agents, whether or not they are procaine hydrochloride. Others used are metycaine, nupercaine, pontocaine, and lidocaine hydrochloride; almost all have trade names by which they are known and sold by dental supply houses.

Local anesthetic solutions as discussed above are designed to produce anesthesia when injected close to a nerve or nerve trunk. Few of these solutions will produce any anesthetic action when applied on the surface of the mucous membrane (the lining of the mouth) or on the surface of the skin.

Topical Anesthetics

There are anesthetic agents, however, which are designed to work when applied to the surface of the mucous membrane. They are called *topical* anesthetics and can be found as liquids or as pastes. Many dentists use a topical anesthetic on the mucous membrane before injecting a local anesthetic solution, since most of the discomfort of an injection is caused at the surface of the mucous membrane by the act of puncture with the hypodermic syringe.

Summary

Anatomy is the science of the form, structure, and parts of animal organisms. The anatomy of the head is of particular interest in dentistry.

Three bones are important to dentistry: the mandible (lower jaw) and the two maxillae which form the upper jaw.

There are four openings, called foramina, in the mandible.

The maxilla consists of a central body and four processes or extensions. The zygomatic process (one of them) is the cheekbone. Several foramina are in the maxilla.

The two temporomandibular joints permit the mandible to move. They are treated as one joint because they function together.

Muscles of mastication are the masseter, temporal, and internal and external pterygoid.

Other terms to identify include *vermilion border, ala, wing of the nose, labial commissure, oral cavity, gingivae, frenum, retromolar pad, maxillary tuberosity, soft and hard palate, and mucosa.*

Teeth are occluding when the mouth is closing and are in occlusion when the mouth is closed and the upper and lower arches are touching.

Three salivary glands are important: sublingual, submandibular, and parotid.

Each individual has two sets of teeth: primary and secondary.

Table 23.1 indicates the approximate ages when teeth first appear in the mouth.

A tooth is composed of enamel, dentin, pulp chamber, and cementum.

Incisors incise (cut) food, cuspids tear food, premolars grind food, and molars mill food.

A blood supply is directed to each area of the mouth.

Nerves may be compared to wires between two computers. The fifth cranial nerve supplies the dental area. Motor nerves control the function of muscle fibers. Sensory nerves carry the messages to the brain.

Anesthetics are capable of blocking feeling. General anesthesia makes it impossible for the brain and spinal cord to recall or send messages. Analgesia is loss of ability to feel pain without loss of consciousness. Local anesthesia temporarily blocks the ability of a particular nerve to transmit messages. Topical anesthetic temporarily blocks the nerves in the surface of the mucous membranes.

Study Questions

1. Describe the bones, joints, muscles, glands, and anatomical landmarks important to dentistry.
2. Describe the structure of a tooth.
3. What is meant by *erupt*? When do teeth erupt?
4. Detail the functions of the various teeth.
5. Describe the blood and nerve supplies to the teeth.
6. Differentiate between sensory and motor nerves.
7. Explain how we sense pain and differentiate between general anesthesia, analgesia, local anesthesia, and topical anesthetics.

Bibliography

SICHER, HARRY. *Oral Anatomy.* 4th ed. St. Louis, Mo.: C. V. Mosby Co., 1965.

24 | *Identification of Teeth and Cavity Classification*

Names for Teeth

Individual teeth have been given specific names (for verbal) and specific systems of annotation (for written) identification in order that we can discuss them intelligently. These names are important to know in order that you can recognize the specific tooth and area involved in a planned dental operation, and with this knowledge can be better prepared to assist the dentist.

Assuming we are discussing a mouth which has a complete set of teeth, we have an upper and a lower arch of teeth. Each arch we can imagine as being divided into two halves—the left half and the right half. Since each half-arch is one-quarter of the full set of teeth, we call each half-arch a quadrant. Thus, four quadrants make a complete set of teeth.

Left and *right* are always noted from the patient's point of view. That is, the teeth on the patient's left are annotated as *left* in referring to position. The four quadrants are called the upper left quadrant, the lower left quadrant, the upper right quadrant, and the lower right quadrant. (See fig. 24.1.)

A complete adult mouth contains thirty-two teeth—eight teeth in each quadrant. The teeth in *each* quadrant, starting from front to back, have the same names, in the same sequence, as the teeth in any other quadrant:

> central incisor
> lateral incisor
> cuspid (canine)
> first premolar (first bicuspid)
> second premolar (second bicuspid)
> first molar
> second molar
> third molar ("wisdom" tooth)

Since this means that in a complete set of teeth we have four teeth with the same name (one in each quadrant), we also add to the name of each tooth the location of the quadrant. (See fig. 24.1.)

The teeth in the upper left quadrant, for example, are labeled as follows:

upper left central incisor
upper left lateral incisor
upper left cuspid
upper left first premolar (bicuspid)
upper left second premolar (bicuspid)
upper left first molar
upper left second molar
upper left third molar

Each quadrant is similarly labeled—upper right incisor, lower left incisor, and lower right incisor—throughout the entire quadrant.

Written Identification

If we wished to quickly write a list of various teeth, this would be a cumbersome way to write an identification of each tooth; there-

PERMANENT TEETH

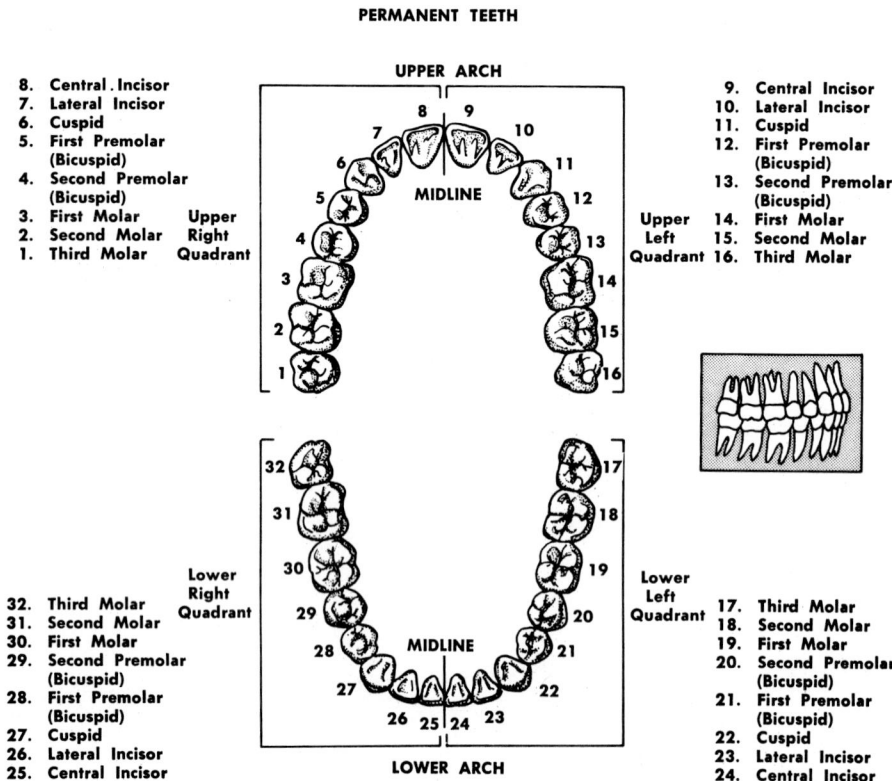

8. Central Incisor
7. Lateral Incisor
6. Cuspid
5. First Premolar (Bicuspid)
4. Second Premolar (Bicuspid)
3. First Molar   Upper
2. Second Molar   Right
1. Third Molar   Quadrant

9. Central Incisor
10. Lateral Incisor
11. Cuspid
12. First Premolar (Bicuspid)
13. Second Premolar (Bicuspid)
14. First Molar
15. Second Molar
16. Third Molar

Upper Left Quadrant

UPPER ARCH

32. Third Molar
31. Second Molar
30. First Molar
29. Second Premolar (Bicuspid)
28. First Premolar (Bicuspid)
27. Cuspid
26. Lateral Incisor
25. Central Incisor

Lower Right Quadrant

17. Third Molar
18. Second Molar
19. First Molar
20. Second Premolar (Bicuspid)
21. First Premolar (Bicuspid)
22. Cuspid
23. Lateral Incisor
24. Central Incisor

Lower Left Quadrant

LOWER ARCH

Fig. 24.1. Schematic drawing showing quadrants, names, and numbers of teeth in both upper and lower arches as you face the patient's mouth.

fore, various shortcuts have been devised to make it easier to write such an indication of a particular tooth. Several methods are used, but each dentist uses only one method routinely in his office.

Method "A"

The upper teeth are numbered in sequence from right to left and the lower teeth in a continuing sequence from left to right. Thus, the upper right third molar is tooth number 1; the upper left third molar is tooth number 16; the lower left third molar is tooth number 17; and the lower right third molar is tooth number 32. This is the most widely used method of tooth identification.

Method "B"

Number the teeth in the upper quadrants from one to eight, beginning with the front tooth in each quadrant, as follows:

1—central incisor
2—lateral incisor
3—cuspid
4—first premolar (bicuspid)
5—second premolar (bicuspid)
6—first molar
7—second molar
8—third molar

In the lower arch, number the teeth in each quadrant from nine to sixteen, beginning with the front tooth in each quadrant, as follows:

9—central incisor
10—lateral incisor
11—cuspid
12—first premolar (bicuspid)
13—second premolar (bicuspid)
14—first molar
15—second molar
16—third molar

In this method we can tell by the number alone whether the tooth is an upper or a lower tooth.

To indicate which side the particular tooth is on, all we need to add is the letter L for left side or R for right side. Thus, an upper left first molar would be written as "L6," a lower left cuspid as "L11," or a lower right second molar as "R15."

Method "C"

This method was adopted as official by the American Dental Association, Committee on Nomenclature, in 1947.

There are eight teeth in a quadrant, in the same sequence and with the same names as the eight teeth in each of the other quadrants. We can simply number the teeth in each quadrant from one to eight, beginning with the front tooth, as follows:

1—central incisor
2—lateral incisor
3—cuspid
4—first premolar (bicuspid)
5—second premolar (bicuspid)
6—first molar
7—second molar
8—third molar

Even in conversation, dentists commonly use the tooth number instead of its proper name and say, for example, "upper right six" instead of upper right first molar, or "lower left four" instead of lower left first bicuspid. However, the main reason for using numbers is to simplify indicating a particular tooth in writing.

To this numbering system, then, is added a simpler and shorter method of indicating which quadrant the tooth is in, to replace writing "upper left," "upper right," "lower left," or "lower right." First write the number of the tooth you wish to indicate, for example, a *first* molar: 6. Then if the 6 is an *upper* first molar, let the number be placed *above* a short line, thus: 6̲. If it is an upper *right* first molar, add a vertical line to the *right* side of the number, thus: 6⌋ If the 6 is a *lower* first molar, let the number be placed *below* a short line, thus: 6̄. If it is a lower *left first molar,* add a vertical line to the left side of the number, thus: ⌈6̄. An upper left first molar would be ⌊6, and a lower right first molar would be 6̄⌋.

Ask your dentist which method he uses. Practice until you can write the correct identification for any tooth easily and quickly.

To help yourself learn this more quickly, first make up a list of the teeth in each quadrant as they are listed in figure 24.1. After each tooth indicate the number and position by the method your dentist uses. Follow this with a fully written list of all thirty-two teeth in a mixed-up order and do the same. Show this listing to your dentist to be checked for error.

Tooth Terminology

Each tooth has five sides (called surfaces) that have names for identification either in speech or in writing. The six upper front teeth and six lower front teeth actually have four surfaces and a biting edge, while the back teeth have four sides and the chewing surface. On the six upper and six lower front teeth, these five surfaces are named as follows:

incisal	biting edge
labial (or facial)	surface toward the lip
lingual	surface toward the tongue
mesial	side toward the midline of the arch
distal	side away from the midline of the arch

As a group, the six upper and the six lower front teeth are referred to as the *anterior* teeth, *upper anteriors* and *lower anteriors.*

For the back or *posterior* teeth, the five surfaces are named as follows:

occlusal	chewing surface
buccal	surface toward the cheek
lingual	surface toward the tongue
mesial	surface toward the midline of the arch
distal	surface away from the midline of the arch

A tooth touches its neighbor toward the front with its *mesial* surface and its neighbor toward the back with its *distal* surface. Of course the last tooth in each quadrant has no tooth behind it, so its distal surface does not touch another tooth. The two central incisors in each arch are the first teeth in their respective quadrants, and their two mesial surfaces touch each other. Their mesial surfaces both touch the imaginary midline of the dental arches. The portion of a tooth which touches the tooth next to it is called the *contact area.*

You will notice that only the first two surface names differ for anterior and posterior teeth, as listed. The *incisal* edge of the anterior teeth becomes the *occlusal* surface of the posterior teeth, and the *labial* surface of the anterior teeth becomes the *buccal* surface of the posterior teeth. All teeth have a lingual, mesial, and distal surface.

You may be required to write the location of surfaces named by the dentist during an oral examination. There are abbreviations of the surface names. The abbreviations, when written as single surfaces, are:

incisal	Inc
occlusal	Occ
labial	Lab
buccal	Bu
distal	D
lingual	Li
mesial	M

Very frequently you will hear references to surfaces in groups of two or three. The surface names take on a uniform change when combined into such groups: mesial and occlusal become mesio-occlusal; distal and occlusal change to disto-occlusal; and mesial, occlusal, and distal become mesio-occluso-distal.

In writing *groups* of surfaces, the following abbreviations are used:

mesio-occlusal	MO
disto-occlusal	DO
mesio-occluso-distal	MOD
mesio-incisal	MI
occluso-lingual	OL
disto-buccal	DB
mesio-buccal	MB
disto-lingual	DL
mesio-lingual	ML

This same pattern, using just the first letter of each word, is used with all the group abbreviations.

Identification of Children's Teeth

The *primary* teeth are the first set of teeth. They are also properly called the *deciduous* teeth, although this term is not often used. You will hear parents refer to them as "milk" teeth or "baby" teeth.

The child has a complete set of twenty teeth in his mouth at approximately two years of age. Their replacement by the permanent teeth begins at about six years of age and is completed at about twelve to thirteen years of age. From the age of six to the age of twelve or thirteen, both primary and permanent teeth usually will be found in the mouth—not all the primary teeth have been shed, and not all the permanent teeth have come into position. This period is referred to as the period of "mixed dentition."

There are five primary teeth—central incisor, lateral incisor, cuspid, first molar, and second molar—in each quadrant. The first three are eventually replaced with their identically named permanent teeth, while the last two

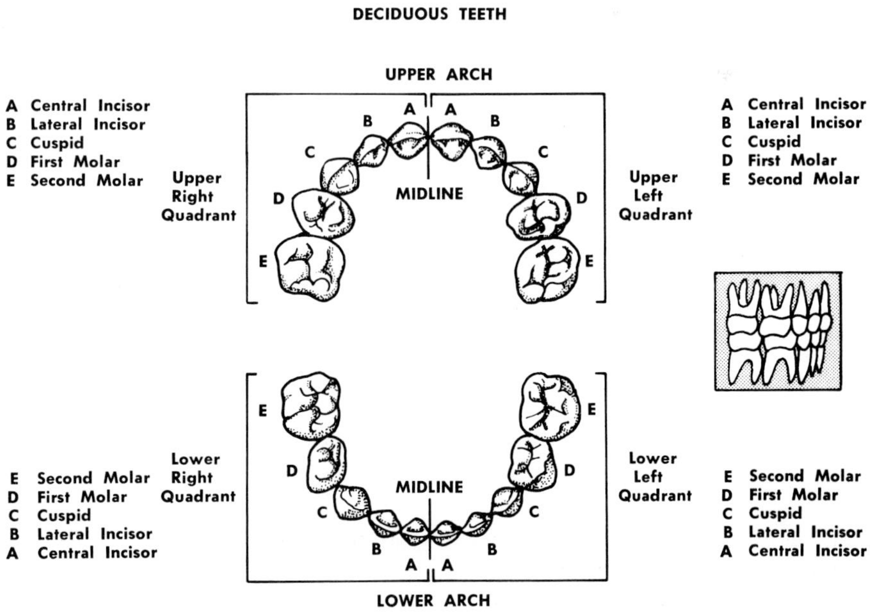

DECIDUOUS TEETH

UPPER ARCH

A Central Incisor
B Lateral Incisor
C Cuspid
D First Molar
E Second Molar
Upper Right Quadrant

MIDLINE

Upper Left Quadrant
A Central Incisor
B Lateral Incisor
C Cuspid
D First Molar
E Second Molar

Lower Right Quadrant
E Second Molar
D First Molar
C Cuspid
B Lateral Incisor
A Central Incisor

MIDLINE

Lower Left Quadrant
E Second Molar
D First Molar
C Cuspid
B Lateral Incisor
A Central Incisor

LOWER ARCH

Fig. 24.2. Schematic drawing of upper and lower deciduous arches (children's teeth).

are replaced by the first and second permanent bicuspids.

The American Dental Association official method of annotating primary teeth uses the letters A, B, C, D, and E from mesial to distal in each quadrant, then indicating the proper quadrant by Method "A."

Another method of annotating these primary teeth substitutes the Roman numerals I, II, III, IV, and V for the foregoing letters, still using the quadrant indication as in Method "A."

Thus, the lower left primary central incisor would be indicated by I͟. An upper right primary first molar would be indicated by IV͟.

Cavity Classification for Restoration

Your dentist may indicate the cavity classification for the carious lesion he has discovered in examining the patient's mouth as it relates to the preparation necessary for the restoration.

Class I.   Pit and fissure cavities.
   a. In the occlusal surfaces of bicuspids and molars.
   b. In the occlusal two-thirds of the buccal surfaces of lower molars.
   c. In lingual surfaces of upper incisors.
   d. In the occlusal one-third of the lingual surfaces of upper molars.

Class II.   Cavities which occur in the proximal surfaces of bicuspids and molars and necessitate the involvement of the occlusal surface for restoration.

Class III.   Cavities which occur in the proximal surfaces of incisors and cuspids and *do not* involve the removal and restoration of the incisal angles.

Class IV.   Cavities which occur in the proximal surfaces of incisors and cuspids and *do* involve the removal and restoration of the incisal angles.

Class V.   Cavities which occur in the gingival third of labial, buccal, or lingual surfaces of any teeth.

Class VI.   Incisal edges of anterior teeth.

In addition, a cavity may be referred to as a "simple" cavity or a "compound" cavity. A

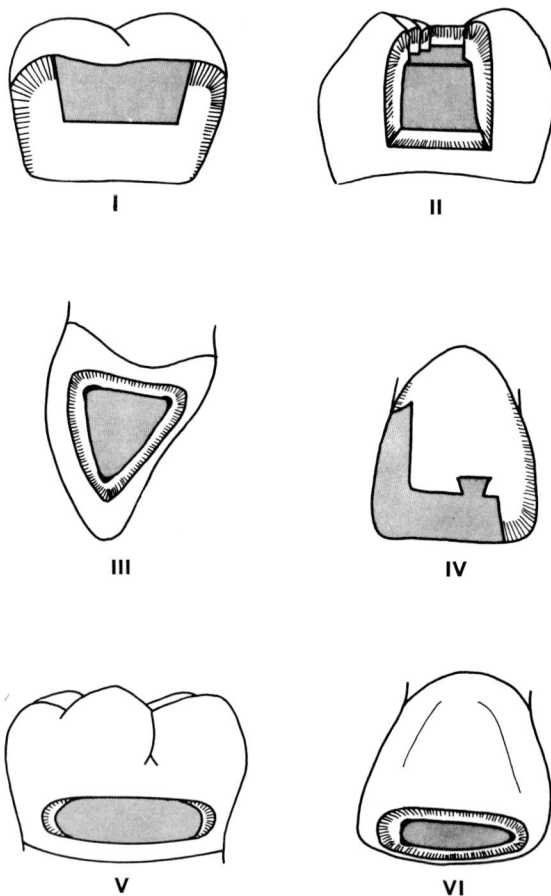

Fig. 24.3. Cavity classification: I. Pit and fissures; II. Proximals of bicuspids and molars; III. Proximals of incisors and cuspids not involving incisal angles; IV. Proximals of incisors and cuspids involving incisal angles; V. Gingival third of labial, buccal, or lingual surfaces of any teeth; VI. Incisal edges of anterior teeth.

simple cavity involves but one surface of a given tooth; a compound cavity involves two or more surfaces of a given tooth.

Charting

Dentists vary in the type of information they wish recorded in an oral examination. If the patient is new to the dental office, it is well to record all previous work present in the patient's mouth (including the material used for each restoration), the areas which need restoration because of visible caries activity, the restorations which need replacement because they are no longer serviceable, missing teeth, drifting of teeth, information in detail on all oral structures, condition of the gums, presence and depth of periodontal pockets, teeth with questionable prognosis, marginal ridge discrepancies, overhangs, poor or open contacts, mobility, and perhaps other details. On recall examinations, only areas of new caries or new pathological conditions are generally noted.

Charting of the dental restorations already present in the patient's mouth, and the material of which they are constructed, is usually done in detail and must be done accurately if it is to be useful to the dentist. Colored pencils may be used to indicate different materials. On the tooth outlined on the patient's chart, color the restored area with the correct color for that type of restoration.

Regardless of the form or amount of detail required for examinations in your dental office, be very certain *to write legibly and accurately.* If for any reason you do not get one notation written before the next is given, immediately ask your dentist to slow down. Do not expect to remember. There may be so many items that you will be hopelessly confused, and the examination will have to be started over again. You will gradually develop speed in writing these notes as you become more familiar with

them. Your dentist will be glad to dictate at a speed at which you can notate accurately if you will ask him to do so. He does not usually realize how rapidly he gives these notes.

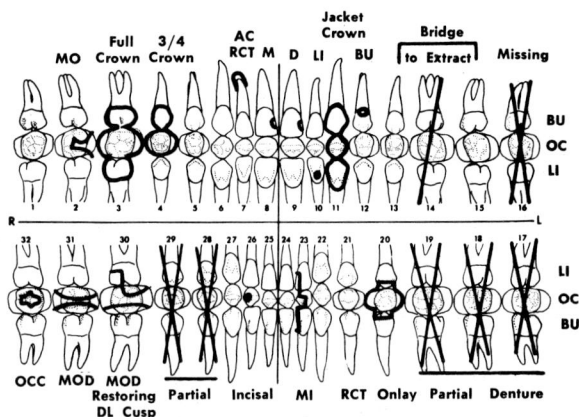

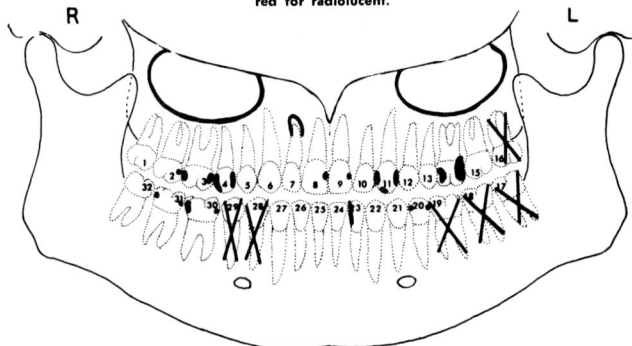

Fig. 24.4. One method of charting. (Used by the University of Minnesota School of Dentistry.)

It is preferable to write out fully any terms with which you are not familiar. When you have learned the terms well, then proceed to use the proper abbreviations. Your dentist undoubtedly has or can get for you one of the basic dental textbooks which will help you familiarize yourself with the terminology of dentistry in a more complete way than is possible in this text.

Summary

Identification of teeth requires a fundamental use of technical terms. The dental assistant must learn to use these terms with ease and facility because their use will save time through efficiency and will prevent error through accuracy. The basic technical terms provide the dental assistant with tools with which to work. Practice in their use is essential. Proficiency in their use is very desirable.

Study Questions

1. Name the teeth in each quadrant of the mouth.
2. Identify the teeth by Method "A," or the method used by your dentist.
3. Name the five surfaces of the anterior teeth.
4. Name the five surfaces of the posterior teeth.
5. Write the abbreviations of the surface names.
6. Write the abbreviations for groups of surfaces.
7. Describe identification of children's teeth.
8. Describe the cavity classifications in terms of classes.
9. Distinguish between a simple cavity and a compound cavity.
10. Discuss charting of teeth and practice the methods.

25 | *Diet and Nutrition*

Food and You

What did you eat for lunch today? a malt? a coke? a hot dog? an ice cream bar?

Did you have breakfast? Did you eat an egg? cereal? fruit? . . . or did you just have a cup of coffee?

What you eat determines your vitality, your enthusiasm, and your health—sometimes not immediately, but always eventually! It is a rare person who understands enough about diet and nutrition—or who uses the knowledge to establish the very best diet possible for excellent nutrition. Most of us are inclined to eat for reasons other than health.

We find that present-day psychiatrists are relating eating habits to events in the early stages of a baby's life—whether he received enough milk, whether he received it when he needed it, and whether he received enough love and cuddling. Many children learn to use food as a weapon in defying their parents. Parents often unwittingly, and sometimes consciously, use food as a reward or punishment. In some homes the parents refer to a food as "good" and to be eaten, yet they don't eat it themselves. Other foods or beverages are called "bad," yet parents indulge themselves in front of their children. Our eating habits are therefore developed emotionally, and we eat to satisfy emotional cravings more frequently than to satisfy our hunger or nourish our bodies.

Diet and nutrition are not one and the same thing. Diet refers to everything we eat as food or medication to satisfy a need or an appetite. Nutrition refers to how these foods and medications are used by our bodies after we put them in our mouths—their use after assimilation. (Assimilation is the process of the absorbing of food by the digestive organs and turning it into living tissue.)

Food serves three purposes:

1. It provides energy.
2. It regulates body functions.
3. It promotes growth.

A well-balanced diet includes foods which supply all the elements the body needs. If an adequate amount of any one of these elements is not included in the diet *regularly*, your health suffers—your vitality is lowered, your resistance to fatigue and disease is lowered, your teeth may show more decay, and anemia may develop. Prolonged lack of certain food elements brings on the deficiency diseases—scurvy, rickets, pellagra, beriberi.

Your appetite is your pleasant emotional desire for food, and quite probably for specific foods, especially chocolate cake or coconut cream pie. Your appetite may be providing the food elements necessary for good nutrition.

A nutrient is a food element which provides material the body cells can use. The essential food elements which must be present in your diet are:

1. carbohydrates
2. fats
3. proteins
4. minerals
5. vitamins
6. water
7. bulk or roughage

If you see to it that these essential food elements are in your diet, it really does make a difference in your health. Studies show that mental performance may be measurably inferior due to depleted energy, inability to concentrate, and fatigue.[1]

One study of teen-age boys with and without breakfast showed a need for an adequate breakfast if the boys were to be attentive and achieve scholastically in the latter morning hours.[2]

Nervous stability is also affected by malnutrition. Tests show undernourished humans are more irritable and restless.[3] The ability to work physically—strength, speed endurance, and the amount of work accomplished—is adversely affected by poor nutrition. Illness, resulting in absenteeism from the job, is also found more frequently if an individual has a nutritionally poor diet.[4] It is also reported that resistance to infectious diseases is lowered by poor nutrition[5] and that the body (bony framework and soft tissue) is directly affected by nutrition.

Good nutrition produces larger, stronger bodies. During World War II the diet of children in Norway was changed due to food rationing. They received less sugar and refined carbohydrates and more whole grains and milk. There was a marked improvement in their teeth—less caries. Following the war, the Norwegians returned to a free choice of diet. The caries rate began to increase.[6]

1. A. Keys et al., *The Biology of Human Starvation,* p. 36.
2. W. W. Tuttle et al., "Effect on School Boys of Omitting Breakfast," pp. 674-77.
3. A. Keys et al., p. 36.
4. R. M. Peel and M. L. Dodds, "Nutritive Intake of Women Factory Employees," pp. 1150-53.
5. N. S. Scrimshaw et al., "Interactions of Nutrition and Infection," pp. 367-403.
6. G. Toverud, "The Influence of War and Post-War Conditions on the Teeth of Norwegian School Children," pp. 354-430; "Caries in the Permanent Teeth of Children Aged 7-8 and 12-13," pp. 127-96; "Discussion of Food Supply and Dental Condition in Norway and Other European Countries," pp. 373-459.

Whether we wish to face up to the facts or not, it remains that nutrition determines the health of our bodies, and eating can no longer be considered just our pleasure. We must feed our bodies for their own good if we wish to live long and feel enthusiastic about doing so.

Diet

We must have the food elements given on page 292 to meet the nutritional demands of our bodies. Home economists have recently regrouped the Basic Seven Foods (so labeled during World War II) into the Basic Four. If you see that your diet includes the proper number of foods from each of these four groups every day, you can be *reasonably* certain that your diet is providing the nutrients which you need. Beyond that it is important to realize that other foods—those "snack" or "treat" foods not included in the Basic Four —usually are actually harmful for you to eat if you are considering your longevity and health.

The foundation food groups, then, are:

1. Dairy Foods. Milk, including cheese, ice cream, and other milk products. Milk supplies proteins, calcium, minerals, vitamins, and fat. Sometimes it is called nature's most nearly perfect food. Vitamin A is already in the cream, and vitamin D can be added to milk since milk is considered one of the most suitable carriers for vitamin D. Milk provides energy and promotes growth. Drink one to two glasses daily as the minimum requirement for an adult. There are differences of opinion about the quantity of milk needed in the diet. A pint is recommended for everyone, and for some people a larger quantity. Some pediatricians have shown that more than a pint per day may increase the caries rate in the teeth of some children. When this is discovered to be true for a child, his milk intake should be restricted to no more than a pint per day.

2. Meat, Poultry, Fish, and Eggs. This group may be called the protein group—the tissue-building and tissue-repairing foods. Some of these foods contain iron and other minerals as well as protein. Two or more servings are needed. The servings should be approximately three ounces of cooked meat. Preferably, eat one egg per day in addition to the servings of meat. At least three or four eggs per week are necessary for health.

3. Vegetable-Fruit Foods. Four or more servings are needed per day. A dark green or deep yellow vegetable is to be eaten at least every other day and citrus fruit or other rich vitamin C source used daily. Other fruits and vegetables are added to make up the four servings.

Green and yellow vegetables have a high vitamin A value. They contain carotenes which our bodies are capable of using to form vitamin A. Certain of the leafy vegetables also have iron and calcium in a form which can be used by the body. Some leafy vegetables contain riboflavin and ascorbic acid. Careful preparation is necessary to keep these food values. This group provides vitamins, minerals (iron and calcium), some proteins, and roughage.

Citrus fruits and tomatoes provide vitamin C or ascorbic acid as well as vitamin A and minerals. The vitamin C is so important that one should always have his orange juice or *equivalent* each day.

Potatoes are included each day for their high energy value as well as for the thiamin and iron they add to the diet. Primarily they are a carbohydrate. Other vegetables help the mechanical action of the digestive tract.

4. Bread or Cereal Foods. Four or more servings are suggested, with one slice of bread, two-thirds cup of cooked cereal, or one cup of ready-to-eat cereal constituting a serving.

These, of course, should be the enriched, whole grain, or "restored" foods.

Some of our energy foods (carbohydrates) are found in this group. There are vitamins in whole grain foods also, especially the B complex. Of course, if you are overweight, your physician may reduce your carbohydrate intake.

Other foods which are to be added to increase the calorie limit to the required amount per day include fats, sweets, unenriched cereals, and flavorings. (See p. 303 for calorie limits.)

Your daily diet, then, should include:

4 servings of vegetables and fruit, including
  2 leafy green or yellow vegetables
  1 orange, or grapefruit or tomato equivalent of the C content of an orange
  1 serving of other vegetables or fruit
2 servings of meat, fish, or poultry (3-ounce servings)
2 glasses of milk
1 egg or a minimum of 3 per week
4 servings of bread or cereal
8 glasses of water per day

Coffee and tea do not count as water intake because they contain caffeine which has a strong diuretic action and causes the elimination of the same quantity of liquid as the coffee or tea which you drink.

The other foods providing interest and energy which are not listed in the Basic Group should be eaten only after you have had the proper amounts of food from each group of the Basic Four.

Nutrition

Now that you understand the Basic Four, you should learn something about "nutrients." Most commonly mentioned as nutrients are foods which can be classified as carbohydrates, fats, proteins, minerals, and vitamins. Some nutritionists mention water as a nutrient; others mention it only as essential to life.

Nutrients are taken into the body in the foods you eat. Then they must be sorted, separated, and simplified so that your body can put them to work. The processes which make these foods part of you are *digestion, absorption,* and *assimilation.* You cannot expect to have a well-nourished body unless the nutrients your body needs are present in adequate amounts in the foods you eat.

Digestion means the processes by which nutrients are changed into their simplest forms and become liquids ready for absorption in the lower part of the digestive tract. The solid foods are broken down by digestive juices and by the mechanical action of the digestive muscles which contract and push the food along the intestines, mixing and churning the food mass. Absorption occurs when the foods have become liquid and are in their simpler form. Most of the absorption occurs in the linings of the small intestines. The blood carries the digested foods to all parts of the body.

Metabolism is the chemical process which releases energy or builds tissue in the body. If the nutrients are lacking, the energy or tissue-building process is affected.

Proteins, Carbohydrates and Fats— The Energy Foods

We are concerned first with the energy foods.

Energy is the power for doing work. Our bodies need energy for two kinds of work— that which goes on inside us twenty-four hours a day, the action of the heart, lungs, digestion, etc., and that which we do ourselves externally like working, playing, swimming, etc.

The amount of energy required varies with the activity of the individual and with his age. The energy which the body uses is largely in the form of heat. In nutrition, therefore, we use the heat unit—the calorie—to measure the energy which our bodies use.

A calorie is the amount of heat necessary to raise the temperature of one kilogram of water 1° centigrade.

The body's daily requirement for energy is met by three types of nutrients: carbohydrates, fats, and proteins. These nutrients are found in varying amounts in different foods. Some foods are primarily composed of one of these nutrients and will be so listed in any table of foods as the Basic Four.

Carbohydrates

Chemically, carbohydrates are made up of carbon, hydrogen, and oxygen. They contain twice as much hydrogen as oxygen.

Sugars and starches are carbohydrates. Sugar is found dissolved in fruits and vegetables as well as in a package of cane or beet sugar. Starch must be changed to sugar before the body can make use of this nutrient.

One gram of carbohydrate contains four calories. For practical purposes, consider 30 grams equal to one ounce.

The body changes carbohydrates to glucose which then passes to the liver and is used by the body as needed. The glucose not needed immediately is changed to glycogen and is stored in the liver and in the muscles. If more carbohydrates are consumed than the body can use and store as glycogen, they are stored as *fat*.

Fats

Chemically, fats are made up of carbon, hydrogen, and oxygen. They are arranged in different proportions from carbohydrates. Fats are low in oxygen and, therefore, can absorb oxygen in large quantities. Fat burns quickly and gives more than twice as many calories as carbohydrates or proteins. One gram of fat contains nine calories; thus, amounts of fats have high caloric value.

Fats stay with us because they require more time to digest, which is the reason that a bit of bacon with breakfast makes breakfast seem to last longer. Four of the important jobs which fats do for our bodies are (1) carry phosphorus, (2) carry fat-soluble vitamins, (3) conserve body heat, and (4) spare protein since the body will not use protein for energy if there is fat or carbohydrate present in the body.

For digestion, absorption, and assimilation, fat must be broken down into glycerol and fatty acids. Essential fatty acids cannot be synthesized by the body; they must be eaten. However, any excess fat—that which is not utilized by some part of the body during absorption—is stored in the body as *fat*. Since only a small quantity of fat is needed each day,[7] it follows that only a very small amount should be eaten by one who is not *overweight*. When one is overweight, fat, as such, can be eliminated from the diet. If the only fat being eaten is that which cannot be separated from the simple foods consumed on a reducing diet, this lack of fat intake will cause the body to draw on its reserve fatty tissue. Since protein foods and carbohydrates also become fat when eaten in excess, overfed Americans need to watch their fat intake most carefully.

Proteins

Proteins are the nutrients which build the body, repair worn parts, and supply heat and energy. The word *protein* comes from the Greek *prōteios* which means "primary or hold-

7. The Food and Nutrition Board of the National Academy of Sciences–National Research Council stated in their 1968 report that while research has been insufficient to set up maximum and minimum amounts of fat necessary to humans, it has been found that 1 to 3 percent of the total calories as linoleic acid fulfills the daily infant requirement and probably adult needs essential for growth and dermal integrity. (See p. 304.) On a 2000 calorie diet this means 20 to 60 calories in food fat is sufficient. One teaspoon of butter or margarine equals 35 calories!

ing first place." Protein is essential to all living plant and animal tissue. Milk, milk products, meat, and eggs are protein foods.

Chemically, the same three elements of carbon, hydrogen, and oxygen are present in protein as in carbohydrates and fats. There are also the elements nitrogen, sulphur, and sometimes phosphorus and iron. Proteins are made of amino acids, the materials with which our body can build or rebuild tissue. They are the final products of digestion of protein. In a watery solution, the amino acids are absorbed through the walls of the small intestine into the bloodstream. They are carried to the liver and then to the tissues and organs of the body. The tissues and organs select the amino acids they need. What acids are not used by the body are returned to the liver. The nitrogen in them is removed and excreted. Then the remaining carbon, hydrogen, and oxygen can be used for energy—or if not needed immediately, stored as *fat*.

One of the important points to remember about the difference between amino acids and the final products of carbohydrate and fat digestion is that amino acids provide nitrogen in addition to carbon, hydrogen, and oxygen. Nitrogen is essential to every cell of the body and thus to life itself. But if you eat more protein than you need for building, repairing, and maintaining the cells of your body, the excess is stored as fat, just like the carbohydrate and fat excesses you may eat as cookies or sweets.

Minerals

The body is made up of cells, tissues, and organs. They in turn are composed of different chemical elements. Chemical elements are the building stones of the body. Carbon, oxygen, and hydrogen are the chief elements of the body. Nitrogen is a fourth important element. These four elements make up ninety-six percent of the body weight and are supplied by carbohydrates, fats, and proteins in our food. These, the energy foods, we have just discussed. Let us turn our attention to the other elements.

Four percent of the total body weight is composed of mineral elements. They are small but exceedingly important to life.

Elements	Percentage of Total Body Weight
Calcium and phosphorus	2.3-3.4%
Potassium, sulfur, chlorine, sodium, and magnesium	0.95%
Iron	0.004%
Manganese	0.0003%
Copper	0.00015%
Iodine	0.00004%

Other minerals present in trace amounts, considered to be essential to health, are cobalt, fluorine, molybdenum, silicon, and zinc.

Although they may only be needed in minute amounts, mineral elements are essential and must be present in the diet to maintain life. It is not possible to say that because calcium and phosphorus are required in larger quantities, they are therefore more important to the body. Iron is one of the most vital elements for the well-being of the body. However, only a few thousandths of a gram is needed daily. (Iron is needed for making hemoglobin. Copper is necessary to the making of hemoglobin, but it is not present in hemoglobin.)

Most of the metallic elements needed in trace amounts seem to be useful as part of the enzymes, hormones, or vitamins necessary to create some essential chemical reaction in the tissues. *Cobalt* is known to be an essential component in vitamin B_{12} (the vitamin which helps form new red blood corpuscles). *Iodine* is a necessary part of the hormone *thyroxine,* made by the thyroid gland. *Zinc* is used as part of the pancreatic hormone *insulin. Magnesium* has been linked to some enzymes that are necessary to body oxidation.

Most of the trace elements are found in so many foods that they are usually found in a normal diet. One exception is iodine. There are sections of the country where a lack of iodine in the water causes a greater incidence of thyroid problems.

Fluorine is not considered an essential nutrient, but it is an element which is very important to dental health. Water containing one part fluorine per million parts water is considered safe. Large amounts of fluorine have caused stiffening of the backbone and mottling of teeth. Test studies have shown that dental caries is reduced or arrested in young children when they drink water which has up to one part per million of fluorine.

The need for mineral elements is summarized in table 25.1. From this table we see that bones and teeth need calcium and phosphorus. There are two to three times as much calcium and phosphorus in the body as the other elements, most of it in the bones and teeth. However, *calcium* is present in blood plasma, also. *Calcium* is needed for blood clotting. It is also needed for muscle tone, for proper regulation of the heart (with *sodium, postassium,* and *magnesium*). The *parathyroid gland* regulates the blood calcium level through its hormone. *Vitamin D* is required for the utilization of calcium.

Phosphorus has more uses in the body than any other element: tooth development; skele-

TABLE 25.1

BODY'S NEED FOR MINERALS

Minerals Needed	Purpose	Penalty If Lacking
Calcium Phosphorus	Build bones and teeth; regulate body processes, especially clotting of blood	Rickets Malformed teeth Caries Stunted growth Soft or weak bones

All salts
  potassium
  sulfur
  chlorine
  phosphorus
	Build soft tissues including muscles	

Phosphorus & all salts	Nervous tissue	
Iron, calcium, phosphorus, sodium, and chlorine	Blood	Nutritional anemia
Sulfur	Skin, nails, hair	
Iodine	Thyroid secretion needs iodine	Enlargement of thyroid gland
Iron and iodine	Allow oxidation in digestion	
All salts	Maintain normal exchange of body fluids	

tal growth; carbohydrate, fat, and protein metabolism; and brain and nerve metabolism—all are affected by phosphorus. It is vital to the functions of the cells of the body's soft tissues as well as the bones and teeth. Whole blood contains phosphorus.

Iron is concentrated in the blood, specifically in the red corpuscles. It is also found in the liver, spleen, and bone marrow. Iron has a special ability to be alternately oxidized and reduced, that is, to take on oxygen and later give it up. It is precious to the body, but it is difficult for the body to absorb it from food. However, the body stores this element and uses it over and over again. The best sources for humans are liver, eggs, lean meats, legumes, nuts, dried fruits, whole grains, and all green, leafy vegetables. Milk is poor in iron value.

Copper is necessary for the production of red corpuscles, although copper will not be found in the blood.

Iodine is most essential to the body. Each cell has traces of iodine in it. About three-fifths of the iodine in the body is in the thyroid gland, located in the neck. This gland selects iodine from the blood, stores it, and uses it to make thyroxine, the hormone so necessary for metabolism. The thyroid gland mixes iodine and an amino acid called tyrosine to obtain thyroxine. *Thyroxine* regulates the rate of body metabolism. *Metabolism* refers to the chemical changes which occur in the body. Physical changes go on in the body whereby the chemical energy in food is changed to heat which the body can use for its work.

Minerals are equally important with energy foods and proteins as nutrients. Minerals are tissue builders, repairers, and aids to digestion. Calcium, iron, and iodine are very important. Calcium and phosphorus (usually considered together) build strong bones, sound teeth, and regulate the body processes. Calcium and phosphorus are found in large quantities in milk and milk products. Some nutrients which our bodies need are found in food in a form our bodies cannot use—cannot assimilate. The calcium and phosphorus must be in a usable form. Iron builds rich, red blood and is needed for carrying oxygen to all parts of the body. Iodine is usually found in saltwater fish and shellfish. It is also found in water, but certain parts of the country (around the Great Lakes) have a low iodine content in the soil and water. In these parts of the country, people should use salt which has been iodized.

Mineral elements are not used up nor do they provide energy. When they are no longer needed, they are discarded. A regular supply is needed to keep up with the body's process of using and discarding them.

Most mineral salts are water-soluble.

Vitamins

Vitamins are body regulators. They are defined as organic compounds different from any food materials, needed only in small amounts, but necessary for normal growth, regulation of the body functions, and the protection and maintenance of health. Vitamins must be supplied in food. They are either fat-soluble or water-soluble. They have been named and numbered. The fat-soluble vitamins are A, D, E, K; the water-soluble vitamins are the B complexes and vitamin C. Fat-soluble means "stored in fats in the bloodstream." Water-soluble means "carried by water." These vitamins are much harder to control because they can escape from a leafy vegetable into the water in which it is cooked.

Vitamins promote growth, the ability to produce healthy offspring, normal functioning of the digestive tract, nutrition, and central nervous system stability. They also regulate health of the body tissues and resistance to bacterial infections.

Vitamin deficiency causes illnesses. A multiple vitamin deficiency refers to a lack of several vitamins in the body. Symptoms of chronic illness will usually be present. An acute deficiency is more likely to be severe and recognizable.

The Fat-Soluble Vitamins

VITAMIN A This vitamin may either be present in the body as vitamin A or is formed in the body from carotene. When vitamin A is present in foods as vitamin A, it is called *preformed vitamin A*. Some of the carotene in foods is converted into vitamin A in the intestinal wall during digestion. Carotene is called *provitamin A*. Carotene is found in both animal and vegetable foods, but preformed vitamin A is present only in animal foods.

Vitamin A is essential to growth, is important for resistance to infection, is necessary for vision (functional night blindness is due to an insufficient supply of vitamin A), prevents certain eye diseases, increases longevity, delays senility, and aids bodily functions.

Sources of vitamin A are liver, spinach, carrots, and sweet potatoes. (A two-ounce serving of liver provides three times as much vitamin A as the next most importance source. Liver is the body organ which stores vitamin A, thus its high content.)

The most important sources of vitamin A and the number of international units of vitamin A these foods contain are the following:

Food	Measure	International Units of Vitamin A
liver, beef	2 oz.	30,330
spinach	½ cup	10,600
carrots	½ cup	9,000
sweet potato	one, medium	9,000
cantaloupe	½ melon	6,600
squash, winter yellow	½ cup	6,350
broccoli	½ cup	2,550
apricots, dried, cooked	½ cup	2,290
tomato juice, canned	½ cup	1,270

The National Academy of Sciences, Food and Nutrition Board, has listed the vitamin A requirements for adults at 5000 international units per day.[8] (See Recommended Dietary Allowances chart, p. 304.)

The United States Department of Agriculture reports that sixty percent of the available vitamin A value in the United States is in fruits and vegetables. (About half this amount comes from leafy green and yellow vegetables.) The remaining forty percent comes from four sources:

14% from dairy products excluding butter
8% from fats
8% from eggs
10% from meats.

Thus, vegetables are a more quantitatively important source of vitamin A than animal foods in the American diet. Vitamin intake depends on what the people actually eat, however. Simply knowing where the vitamins are in the food will not put vitamins into your diet.

Since vitamin A and carotene are insoluble in water and resist destruction by ordinary cooking temperatures, they are not lost by boiling, canning, or freezing. Vegetables may lose much vitamin A when dried in the air; those dried in a vacuum retain much vitamin A. Fats become rancid when exposed to warm air. Rancidity destroys vitamin A and carotene, so meat must be kept cold.

It is possible to have too much vitamin A in your diet. The Council on Foods and Nutrition of the American Medical Association has warned that taking vitamin A in excess of 50,000 international units over a prolonged period of time can result in loss of appetite, irritability, and bone and joint pains.

8. *Recommended Dietary Allowances, Revised 1968,* Publication 1694 National Academy of Sciences National Research Council, Washington, D.C.

VITAMIN D There are two forms of this vitamin found in the body: preformed and provitamin. Vitamin D is needed for the utilization of calcium and phosphorus in the normal nourishment of bones and teeth. It helps make and keep a satisfactory balance between calcium and phosphorus in the body. A serious shortage of this vitamin produces a disease called rickets. Bones bend easily and sometimes are malformed. Teeth erupt early and decay readily.

Vitamin D is found in its most concentrated form in an oil which contains ergosterol. The ergosterol (from yeast) is irradiated and then dissolved in the oil. It is used by the *drop* because it is so powerful. It is regularly added to milk. Other sources are butter, egg yolk, beef liver, salmon, sardines, cod liver oil, and halibut liver oil. Another excellent source is sunlight. The recommended dietary allowance for vitamin D is 400 international units per day for all ages.

Vitamin D is stored in the liver. It is stable and does not disappear with normal cooking temperatures. Excesses of this vitamin can cause toxicity, illness, nausea, diarrhea, and loss of appetite. Usually an overdose is unintentional. No figure is given for an overdose since this varies with individuals and how much sunlight they receive.

VITAMIN E This vitamin is important because it can unite with oxygen and protect red blood cells from being destroyed by such substances as hydrogen peroxide. It also prevents the destruction of vitamin A and carotene by oxidation in the body and in foods. It is stored in the body in muscles and fat deposits. It is not affected by ordinary cooking temperatures. Since it is fat-soluble, it is not dissolved in cooking water. It isn't likely that anyone will be short of vitamin E. It is present in wheat germ, leafy vegetables, legumes, whole grains, vegetables, oils, liver, butter, milk, and eggs.

The adult requirement will vary from 10 to 30 mg. per day. *Recommended Dietary Allowances* of the National Academy of Sciences states, "The average daily adult consumption of Vitamin E has been calculated to be about 14 mg. of d-alpha-tocopherol."

VITAMIN K Vitamin K is essential to normal clotting of the blood and normal functioning of the liver. It has not been possible to determine a dietary allowance since the natural sources of vitamin K vary with the individual human. Vitamin K_1 is found in common foods: green, leafy vegetables, egg yolk, and organ meats. Vitamin K_2 is produced by intestinal bacteria and varies from individual to individual.

The Water-Soluble Vitamins

The water-soluble vitamins are the larger group. All of the B vitamins and vitamin C, or ascorbic acid, are water-soluble. They generally are not stored in the body. This means that the possibility of toxicity from an overdose is not possible as with the fat-soluble vitamins.

Three of the B complex are better known vitamins, and dietary allowances have been established for them. We will consider them first.

THIAMINE OR B_1 Thiamine is one of the first three B vitamins which function together to make it possible for carbohydrate to "burn" at body temperature. It is known as the appetite vitamin. In addition, its uses include helping the nervous system to function normally and helping carbohydrate metabolism. Deficiency in thiamine hydrochloride or B_1 results in beriberi.

Some of its best sources are whole grains, enriched flours and breads, lean pork, peas, liver, milk, vegetables, and fruits. It is difficult to find a very rich source. One must eat several foods to maintain the minimum daily requirement—0.4 mg. per 1,000 calories for all ages. If your dietary allowance is 2,000 calories per day, your daily thiamine requirement is 0.8 mg. per day. Three cups of milk and a half cup of peas will give you about *half* your day's requirements.

RIBOFLAVIN, B_2 Also known as riboflavin and sometimes as G, vitamin B_2 is necessary for growth of all tissues of the body and for maintenance of healthy skin. Deficiency in this vitamin produces cheilosis. Lesions are present on the lips, the tongue is sore and purplish, and the skin of the nose is rough and scaly.

The major sources of riboflavin are in three groups: milk, meats, and grains. Eighty percent of consumption in the United States is in these three food groups. It is also part of the enrichment program. The recommended dietary allowance for this vitamin is 0.6 mg. per 1,000 calories.

Riboflavin can be lost in discarded cooking water and meat drippings. It is unstable when exposed to direct sunlight, daylight, or artificial light. It is best to store milk in paper or dark-brown glass containers.

NIACIN The third vitamin of the B complex, niacin is concerned with the problems of translating sources of energy into energy that the body can burn and is also helpful in cellular respiration. Lack of niacin (or nicotinic acid) produces a disease called pellagra. It is known as the disease of the three *d's*—dermatitis, diarrhea, and dementia. If the disease is not treated, dementia eventually occurs and death follows.

Niacin is available to the body in two forms, niacin and proniacin. Proniacin is tryptophan —one of the amino acids. The human body can make 1 mg. of niacin from 50 to 60 mg. of tryptophan. The recommended dietary allowance is 6.6 mg. niacin equivalents per 1,000 calories. Nearly half the niacin is supplied by meat, poultry, and fish. About one-fourth is supplied by flour and cereals.

Niacin is relatively stable to heat but can be poured off in water used for cooking foods.

THE OTHER MEMBERS OF THE B COMPLEX Four of these are nutritionally important, but dietary allowances have not been ascertained specifically. Some recommendations have been made, but much needs to be learned about them. They include B_6 (*pyridoxine, pyridoxal,* and *pyridoxamine*). All three must be present for the breakdown of amino acids in body tissues, for building body proteins, and for converting tryptophan to niacin. *Pantothenic acid* is essential to utilizing carbohydrates, fatty acids, and other nutrients, in the body. *Biotin* is synthesized by intestinal bacteria and is believed to participate in the activity of several enzyme systems. *Folic acid,* or *folacin,* stimulates the formation of blood cells in certain anemias. There seems to be a relationship between ascorbic acid and folacin. Green leaves, liver, legumes, muscle meats, whole grains, and other vegetables are sources of folacin. B_{12}, originally obtained from liver, is sometimes called the antipernicious anemia vitamin. The requirement for normal adults is unknown, but best food sources are liver, milk, kidney, muscle meats, cheese, and eggs. *Choline* can be made in the body from methionine, an amino acid. Its chief function is the utilization of fat.

These vitamins of the B complex, then, are important in the diet for their contribution to the digestive process, even though exact allowances have not been discovered. The vitamins are B_6 (pyridoxine, pyridoxal, and pyridoxamine), pantothenic acid, biotin, folic acid, B_{12}, and choline.

VITAMIN C, ASCORBIC ACID Ascorbic acid, or vitamin C, is very important in our diet. It prevents scurvy. It is used to help make a substance which binds cells together. If this material is weak, the walls of small blood vessels will hemorrhage. Hemorrhage commonly occurs in the gums. Ascorbic acid also helps build body resistance to bacterial infection and helps heal wounds. It is an unstable vitamin and must be supplied daily. Health can be poor if the intake of C is low, even though it is high enough to prevent scurvy. People can be irritable, have minor illnesses, and be generally listless.

Ascorbic acid is found in greatest concentration in citrus fruits, especially oranges. Since ascorbic acid is unstable and can be destroyed by oxidation, care must be used in handling foods high in ascorbic acid. The recommended dietary allowance for ascorbic acid is 70 mg. daily. To be safe, for daily use it is advisable to choose a very rich source of vitamin C, such as an orange.

We are now ready to look at excerpts from *Recommended Dietary Allowances,* published by the Food and Nutrition Board of the National Academy of Sciences—National Research Council. The summary which they have made of the nutrients is also included.

Recommended Dietary Allowances*

. . . The levels of intake recommended by many nutrition authorities allow for a margin of sufficiency above average physiological requirements to cover variations among essentially all healthy individuals in the United States under present living conditions. The RDA are intended "to serve as goals toward which to aim in planning food supplies and as guides for the interpretation of food consumption records of groups of people. Actual nutritional status of *groups* of people or individuals must be judged on the basis of physical, biochemical, and clinical observations combined with observations on food or nutrient intake."

*Reproduced in part from the National Dairy Council *Digest.*

Discussion of Tabulated Nutrients

Calories. The recommended adult calorie allowances are for a reference man and woman, both age 22, weighing 154 and 128 lbs. (70 and 58 kg.) respectively, living in an environment with a mean temperature of 20°C. They are considered to be moderately active physically, being neither sedentary nor engaged in hard physical labor as a major occupation. . . . [The daily calorie allowances for the reference man and woman are at present 2800 and 2000 respectively.] Adjustments should be made for individuals differing from the reference in age, body size, climate, and activity. . . . Special energy demands of pregnancy and lactation also require consideration. . . .

Age. Because there is a decrease in resting metabolic rate as well as lessened physical activity, energy requirements decline progressively after early adulthood. The decline of resting metabolic rate is known to be 2 percent per decade in adults. However, it is difficult to estimate the reduction in physical activity as a person advances in age. The recommendations have been made that calorie allowances be reduced by 5 percent between ages 22 and 35, 3 percent per decade between 35 and 55, 5 percent between 75, and 7 percent after age 75. If an individual remains physically active after 22, he should not reduce his calorie intake as much as this recommendation indicates. . . .

Body Size. Calorie allowances must also be adjusted for variation in energy requirements which are caused by differences in body size. The larger allowances are for individuals whose body size is greater than the reference man or woman; the smaller allowances for those of smaller size. Table 25.2 gives the adjustment of calorie allowances for adult individuals of various body weights and ages.

Table 25.3 gives the suggested weights for various heights of men and women. . . .

Activity. Although physical activity is the major variable affecting energy requirements, no simple procedure is available for estimating the extent of adjustment required. In general, individuals who are physically active increase caloric intake to cover energy expenditure; but inactive persons tend not to reduce intakes sufficiently to remain in energy balance. The proper calorie allowance for an individual is that on which he maintains body weight and health at a level most conducive to his well-being. . . .

TABLE 25.2

ADJUSTMENT OF CALORIE (KCAL) ALLOWANCES[a]
FOR ADULT INDIVIDUALS OF VARIOUS
BODY WEIGHTS AND AGES
[at a mean environmental temperature of 20°C
(68°F), assuming light physical activity]

Body Weight		RMR[b] at Age 22	Age[c]		
kg	lb		22	45	65

MEN

kg	lb		22	45	65
50	110	1540	2,200	2,000	1,850
55	121	1620	2,350	2,150	1,950
60	132	1720	2,500	2,300	2,100
65	143	1820	2,650	2,400	2,200
70[d]	154	1880	2,800	2,600	2,400
75	165	1970	2,950	2,700	2,500
80	176	2020	3,050	2,800	2,600
85	187	2110	3,200	2,950	2,700
90	198	2210	3,350	3,100	2,800
95	209	2290	3,500	3,200	2,900
100	220	2380	3,700	3,400	3,100

WOMEN

kg	lb		22	45	65
40	88	1280	1,550	1,450	1,300
45	99	1380	1,700	1,550	1,450
50	110	1460	1,800	1,650	1,500
55	121	1560	1,950	1,800	1,650
58[d]	128	1620	2,000	1,850	1,700
60	132	1640	2,050	1,900	1,700
65	143	1740	2,200	2,000	1,850
70	154	1830	2,300	2,100	1,950

[a]Kcal allowance (males) = (RMR + 13w) × (percent adjustment for age) kcal allowance (females) = (RMR + 7w) × (percent adjustment for age); w = wt in kg. Values are rounded to the nearest 50 kcal.
[b]RMR = resting metabolic rate, approximately 10 percent above the metabolic rate measured under basal conditions.

[c]Age adjustments:

	Age	Adjustment (percent of Kcal allowance at age 22)
	22-35	100-95
	35-45	95-92
	45-55	92-89
	55-65	89-84
	65-75	84-79
	75-85	72

[d]Reference man and woman.

TABLE 25.3

SUGGESTED WEIGHTS FOR HEIGHTS[a]

Height		Median Weight			
		Men		Women	
in.	cm	lb	kg	lb	kg
60	152			109 ± 9	49.5 ± 4
62	158			115 ± 9	52.2 ± 4
64	163	133 ± 11	60.5 ± 5	122 ± 10	55.5 ± 5
66	168	142 ± 12	64.5 ± 5	129 ± 10	58.6 ± 5
68	173	151 ± 14	68.6 ± 6	136 ± 10	61.8 ± 5
70	178	159 ± 14	72.3 ± 6	144 ± 11	65.5 ± 5
72	183	167 ± 15	75.9 ± 7	152 ± 12	69.0 ± 5
74	188	175 ± 15	79.5 ± 7		
76	193	182 ± 16	82.7 ± 7		

[a]Modified from Table 80, Hathaway and Ford, 1960. "Heights and Weights of Adults in the U.S.," *Home Economics Research Report No. 10*, ARS, USDA. Weights were based on those of college men and women. Measurements were made without shoes or other clothing. ± refers to weight range between the 25th and 75th percentile of each height category.

A careful study of table 25.4, the recommended dietary allowances, will indicate the adequate amounts of nutrients in a proper diet for peoples of all ages. . . .

Opinions about diet have changed. It has been decided Americans need less calories per day because we are not as active as the day laborer of years ago, or our life is more sedentary. Each individual's daily calorie intake is determined by his height, ideal weight, size of build, age, and physical activity. The calorie table gives the calorie intake necessary to maintain the desirable weight. It is recognized now that the weight reached by twenty-five to thirty years of age should be maintained throughout life. Thus we see that the average man weighing 154 pounds is allowed 2,800 calories a day, and the average woman weighing 128 pounds is allowed 2,000 calories—an important change to note in overfed America.

TABLE 25.4

FOOD AND NUTRITION BOARD, NATIONAL ACADEMY OF SCIENCES—NATIONAL RESEARCH COUNCIL RECOMMENDED DAILY DIETARY ALLOWANCES,[a] REVISED 1968
Designed for the maintenance of good nutrition of practically all healthy people in the U.S.A.

	AGE[b] (years) From – Up to	WEIGHT (kg)	WEIGHT (lbs)	HEIGHT cm	HEIGHT (in.)	kcal	PROTEIN (gm)	FAT-SOLUBLE VITAMINS — VITAMIN A ACTIVITY (IU)	VITAMIN D (IU)	VITAMIN E ACTIVITY (IU)	WATER-SOLUBLE VITAMINS — ASCORBIC ACID (mg)	FOLACIN[c] (mg)	NIACIN[d] (mg equiv)	RIBOFLAVIN (mg)	THIAMIN (mg)	VITAMIN B_6 (mg)	VITAMIN B_{12} (µg)	MINERALS — CALCIUM (g)	PHOSPHORUS (g)	IODINE (µg)	IRON (mg)	MAGNESIUM (mg)
Infants	0 – 1/6	4	9	55	22	kg × 120	kg × 2.2[e]	1,500	400	5	35	0.05	5	0.4	0.2	0.2	1.0	0.4	0.2	25	6	40
	1/6 – 1/2	7	15	63	25	kg × 110	kg × 2.0[e]	1,500	400	5	35	0.05	7	0.5	0.4	0.3	1.5	0.5	0.4	40	10	60
	1/2 – 1	9	20	72	28	kg × 100	kg × 1.8[e]	1,500	400	5	35	0.1	8	0.6	0.5	0.4	2.0	0.6	0.5	45	15	70
Children	1 – 2	12	26	81	32	1,100	25	2,000	400	10	40	0.1	8	0.6	0.6	0.5	2.0	0.7	0.7	55	15	100
	2 – 3	14	31	91	36	1,250	25	2,000	400	10	40	0.2	8	0.7	0.6	0.6	2.5	0.8	0.8	60	15	150
	3 – 4	16	35	100	39	1,400	30	2,500	400	10	40	0.2	9	0.8	0.7	0.7	3	0.8	0.8	70	10	200
	4 – 6	19	42	110	43	1,600	30	2,500	400	10	40	0.2	11	0.9	0.8	0.9	4	0.8	0.8	80	10	200
	6 – 8	23	51	121	48	2,000	35	3,500	400	15	40	0.2	13	1.1	1.0	1.0	4	0.9	0.9	100	10	250
	8 – 10	28	62	131	52	2,200	40	3,500	400	15	40	0.3	15	1.2	1.1	1.2	5	1.0	1.0	110	10	250
Males	10 – 12	35	77	140	55	2,500	45	4,500	400	20	40	0.4	17	1.3	1.3	1.4	5	1.2	1.2	125	10	300
	12 – 14	43	95	151	59	2,700	50	5,000	400	20	45	0.4	18	1.4	1.4	1.6	5	1.4	1.4	135	18	350
	14 – 18	59	130	170	67	3,000	60	5,000	400	25	55	0.4	20	1.5	1.5	1.8	5	1.4	1.4	150	18	400
	18 – 22	67	147	175	69	2,800	60	5,000	400	30	60	0.4	18	1.6	1.4	2.0	5	0.8	0.8	140	10	400
	22 – 35	70	154	175	69	2,800	65	5,000	—	30	60	0.4	18	1.7	1.4	2.0	5	0.8	0.8	140	10	350
	35 – 55	70	154	173	68	2,600	65	5,000	—	30	60	0.4	17	1.7	1.3	2.0	5	0.8	0.8	125	10	350
	55 – 75+	70	154	171	67	2,400	65	5,000	—	30	60	0.4	14	1.7	1.2	2.0	6	0.8	0.8	110	10	350
Females	10 – 12	35	77	142	56	2,250	50	4,500	400	20	40	0.4	15	1.3	1.1	1.4	5	1.2	1.2	110	18	300
	12 – 14	44	97	154	61	2,300	50	5,000	400	20	45	0.4	15	1.4	1.2	1.6	5	1.3	1.3	115	18	350
	14 – 16	52	114	157	62	2,400	55	5,000	400	25	50	0.4	16	1.4	1.2	1.8	5	1.3	1.3	120	18	350
	16 – 18	54	119	160	63	2,300	55	5,000	400	25	50	0.4	15	1.5	1.2	2.0	5	1.3	1.3	115	18	350
	18 – 22	58	128	163	64	2,000	55	5,000	400	25	55	0.4	13	1.5	1.0	2.0	5	0.8	0.8	100	18	350
	22 – 35	58	128	163	64	2,000	55	5,000	—	25	55	0.4	13	1.5	1.0	2.0	5	0.8	0.8	100	18	300
	35 – 55	58	128	160	63	1,850	55	5,000	—	25	55	0.4	13	1.5	1.0	2.0	5	0.8	0.8	90	18	300
	55 – 75+	58	128	157	62	1,700	55	5,000	—	25	55	0.4	13	1.5	1.0	2.0	6	0.8	0.8	80	10	300
Pregnancy						+200	65	6,000	400	30	60	0.8	15	1.8	+0.1	2.5	8	+0.4	+0.4	125	18	450
Lactation						+1,000	75	8,000	400	30	60	0.5	20	2.0	+0.5	2.5	6	+0.5	+0.5	150	18	450

[a] The allowance levels are intended to cover individual variations among most normal persons as they live in the United States under usual environmental stresses. The recommended allowances can be attained with a variety of common foods, providing other nutrients for which human requirements have been less well defined. See text for more-detailed discussion of allowances and of nutrients not tabulated.

[b] Entries on lines for age range 22–35 years represent the reference man and woman at age 22. All other entries represent allowances for the midpoint of the specified age range.

[c] The folacin allowances refer to dietary sources as determined by *Lactobacillus casei* assay. Pure forms of folacin may be effective in doses less than ¼ of the RDA.

[d] Niacin equivalents include dietary sources of the vitamin itself plus 1 mg equivalent for each 60 mg of dietary tryptophan.

[e] Assumes protein equivalent to human milk. For proteins not 100 percent utilized factors should be increased proportionately.

It becomes increasingly evident that in planning meals and re-forming one's eating habits, it is necessary to recognize that certain foods must be eaten for adequate body nourishment. After the food plan has included all the necessary items for nutrition, it is possible to build to the total caloric consumption allowed for that day with foods which you eat strictly for pleasure. Not only is it necessary to eat the foods listed on page 294 each day, but also to select the *type* of meat, the individual vegetables, fruits, and other foods which *together* provide you with the correct amount of vitamins, minerals, carbohydrates, proteins, and fats needed for complete nourishment of your body. Emphasis was formerly on providing *enough* food elements, with no thought of harm from overproviding. We now face the recognition that it may be just as harmful to overeat, to provide too many nutrients. It isn't enough to say that you will eat two servings of meat, four of vegetables and fruits, two servings of milk, and four servings of breadstuffs. It is necessary to check these food items for their nutrient content as well as for their caloric content.

Eating to keep our bodies healthy rather than satisfying emotional needs may take severe self-discipline. Habits formed even beginning in early childhood influence our reaction to food subconsciously. Food becomes a symbol of many different things as we grow up. It may become a reward or a punishment symbol with some families. It may have been used by the child to control his parents (by eating, refusing to eat, creating a scene). In some homes the food is not nutritious, and food habits are built around a poor diet—and habit sets in. Many adults eat as they do because they acquired the habit of eating in such a fashion from long exposure to certain foods. A "finicky" eater—one who doesn't like certain foods and makes his dislikes known to all around him—conditions little children to such eating patterns. A child learns to eat by example, and parents need to eat well-balanced, nutritionally excellent meals if they expect their children to do likewise.

It is wise to remember that appetite is our desire for food and the pleasure we remember from eating. Hunger is our need for food. Few of us are ever really hungry. The sensations we experience which we think of as hunger are usually tied emotionally to the rest of our lives.

It can be a very satisfying experience to learn about good nutrition and change our eating habits to give us the opportunity to have better health, disposition, and longevity.

Diet AND Nutrition

We have said that food serves three purposes: to provide energy, to regulate body functions, and to promote growth.

The essential food elements which serve the first purpose are carbohydrates, fats, and proteins. They are high in calories. They furnish heat and energy. If you eat more carbohydrates and fat than you need, the excess is stored in your body as *fat*. If you have a tendency to overweight, watch out for that cinnamon roll or candy bar!

The essential food elements which serve the second purpose, regulating body functions, are the following:

Proteins	Build and repair body tissue (except body fat).
Some Minerals	Regulate body functions. Example, iodine regulates the rate at which the body uses other energy foods.
Water	Aids in regulation of body functions such as digestion and elimination of body waste. Controls temperature.

Vitamins	Promote growth and help the body remain healthy and vigorous.
Roughage	Aids in the elimination of body waste.

The third purpose of food, promoting growth, is accomplished by these elements:

Proteins	Build and rebuild tissue.
Minerals	For calcification. They build teeth, build and repair bones, and build blood.
Water	The structure of all body tissue is composed of cells. Cells need water to maintain life.

It is possible to plan an adequate diet to satisfy all these nutritional needs of the body. The best way for the average person to be certain that he is nourishing his body as well as satisfying his appetite for food is to use the Basic Four as a daily plan of diet, checking carefully, at least for a time, to be certain that the menus so planned do include the necessary daily food nutrients in the amounts specified in table 25.4.

Diet and the Oral Cavity

Certain diseases and mouth conditions result from insufficient nutrients. (See "Oral Pathology" for further discussion of this topic.)

The supporting tissue of the teeth will not be healthy without an adequate vitamin C intake. Sometimes the deficiency shows in bleeding gums. If the deficiency continues over a long period of time, scurvy results.

Vitamin B is important in preventing a breakdown of the capillary wall. Milk in proper quantities will prevent this breakdown.

The effect of carbohydrate (especially the refined carbohydrates—sugar, candy, gum) on the oral cavity is particularly important. The use of too much sugar, especially in children, is responsible for much dental caries. The time of day that sugar is used is also important. Snacks should not be of high sugar content and should be followed by careful cleansing. Use raw apples, celery, or carrot straws to cleanse teeth at the close of a meal or snack. (See the section on "Dental Caries" for a diet specifically arranged for the control of dental caries.)

An important factor to remember about sugar and sweets in connection with diet for caries control is that it isn't the quantity—it is the fact that caries-producing materials are in the mouth. If sweets are used, follow them with a thorough cleansing, including brushing —*immediately*. The sooner the residue is removed from the teeth and oral tissues, the less damage will occur.

It has also been suggested that if one insists on eating sticky rolls, he should eat them at a meal with other foods which will help remove the gummy caramel from the teeth as he eats. As a separate snack, they create a caries-inviting environment.

Nutrition is important, then, for your teeth and mouth because what you eat as a child influences largely the calcification of your permanent dentition. The prenatal diet of the mother influences largely the calcification of the deciduous teeth of the baby.

There is no way to separate the health of one part of the body from the rest of the body. All the parts are interdependent, and a good, well-balanced diet with sufficient nutrients in a form which can be utilized by the body is the best way to preserve the health of the dental organs—or any other organ.

The diet of the late teen-age period is usually poor—unbalanced—overloaded with refined carbohydrates. The nutritionists believe that the diet during these years directly affects the ability of the young woman to carry a baby effectively during the young adult years when she is likely to be pregnant. What you eat as a late teen-ager affects your health and the health of any children you may have in the early adult years!

Diet, health, and longevity have been associated in a strikingly clear statement by a well-known authority in nutrition and public health, H. W. Sebrell. He says, "Diet is one of the most important factors in determining how long an individual lives . . . even though you never suffer from acute malnutrition, years and years of improper eating will add up to various kinds of damages to your body that will eventually shorten your life. . . . While a good diet can't guarantee that you will be in good health, you can't be in the best of health unless you live on a good diet."

Now to return to your lunch:

What will you have tomorrow? a coke? a hot dog? a malt? . . .

. . . or a meat sandwich, milk, and carrot straws?

How about breakfast? The milk, fruit, egg, and toast or cereal which you need? . . .

. . . or a cup of coffee?

Summary

Diet refers to everything we eat to satisfy a need or an appetite. *Nutrition* refers to how the foods and medications are used after assimilation.

Food serves three purposes: provides energy, regulates body functions, and promotes growth. The essential elements needed in the diet are carbohydrates, fats, proteins, minerals, vitamins, water, and bulk or roughage.

Nutrients must be changed into simplified forms for absorption by the cells. *Energy foods* are proteins, carbohydrates, and fats. We measure energy by the *calorie*, a unit of heat.

Chemical elements form the tissues of the body. *Vitamins* are body regulators. The recommended dietary allowances are based on research findings and should be used as a guide in planning the food intake of each individual.

Eating is closely related to emotions. *Appetite* is the desire for food. *Hunger* is the need for food. Most of us eat to satisfy emotional needs. We need to consider nutrition in planning our diets to properly nourish our bodies so we can enjoy a healthier and longer life.

Diet also affects oral health. Certain diseases and mouth conditions result from insufficient nutrients. *When* snacks are eaten, as well as what food is used for the snack, is important when considering the effect of snacks on teeth. *Adequate care of the oral cavity after eating is essential.*

Study Questions

1. Differentiate between diet and nutrition.
2. Name the energy foods.
3. What are the three purposes of food?
4. Why should we limit our fat intake?
5. Discuss the Basic Four food groups.
6. Discuss vitamins.
7. Discuss essential elements for nutrition.
8. Why do we have a conflict between diet and proper nutrition?
9. Discuss the effect of diet on the oral cavity.
10. Discuss proper care of the oral cavity following eating.

Bibliography

LEVERTON, RUTH M. *Food Becomes You*. Ames, Ia.: Iowa State University Press, 1960.

MARTIN, ETHEL A. *Nutrition in Action*. New York: Holt, Rinehart & Winston, 1963.

NIZEL, ABRAHAM E. *Nutrition in Preventive Dentistry: Science and Practice*. Philadelphia: W. B. Saunders Co., 1972.

WRENN, C. G., and SCHWARZROCK, SHIRLEY. *Food as a Crutch*. Circle Pines, Minn.: American Guidance Service, 1971.

Additional References Used in Preparation of this Chapter

BECK, MARY E. *Nutrition and Dietetics for Nurses*. London: Livingstone Ltd., 1962.

BOGERT, L. J. *Nutrition and Physical Fitness*. Philadelphia: W. B. Saunders Co., 1954.

GOLDSMITH, G. A. "Vitamins of the B Complex," *Food—The Yearbook of Agriculture*. Washington, D. C.: U. S. Dept. of Agriculture, 1959.

KEYS, A.; BROZEK, J.; HENSCHEL, A.; MICKELSEN, O.; and TAYLOR, H. L. *The Biology of Human Starvation*. Vols. I and II. Minneapolis: University of Minnesota Press, 1950.

MOTTRAM, V. H. *Human Nutrition*. London: Edward Arnold Ltd., 1963.

PEEL, R. M., and DODDS, M. L. "Nutritive Intake of Women Factory Employees." *J. Am. Dietet. Assoc.* 33 (November 1957): 1150-53.

SCRIMSHAW, N. S.; TAYLOR, C. E.; and GORDON, J. E. "Interactions of Nutrition and Infection." *Am. J. Medical Sciences* 237 (March 1959): 367-403.

TOVERUD, G. "The Influence of War and Post-War Conditions on the Teeth of Norwegian School Children—Eruption of Permanent Teeth and Status of Deciduous Dentition." *The Milbank Memorial Fund Quarterly* 34 (October 1956): 354-430; II. "Caries in the Permanent Teeth of Children Aged 7-8 and 12-13" 35 (April 1957): 127-96; III. "Discussion of Food Supply and Dental Condition in Norway and Other European Countries" 35 (October 1957): 373-459.

TUTTLE, W. W.; DAUM, K.; LARSEN, R.; SALZANO, J.; and ROLOFF, L. "Effect on School Boys of Omitting Breakfast." *J. Am. Dietet. Assoc.* 30 (July 1954): 674-77.

WALDO, MYRA. *The Slenderella Cook Book*. New York: Putnam's Sons, 1957.

26 *Microbiology and Sterilization*

Microbiology

Microbiology is the science of the nature, life, and actions of microorganisms—those organisms visible only through a microscope. These microscopic organisms are either animal or plant. Bacteria, protozoa, fungi, rickettsiae, and viruses make up the microorganisms (although some viruses differ from true microorganisms in some respects).

While each group has some members which are pathogenic (cause disease) in man, not all are by any means harmful to man. This is a common misconception of the importance of microorganisms in everyday life. The truth is that without bacteria there could be no other living thing in the world. All plant and animal life is dependent upon the fertility of the soil. Soil fertility depends, in turn, upon the activity of the microorganisms which inhabit the soil in almost inconceivable numbers.

Knowledge of the existence of a world of small creatures was noted in the early part of the seventeenth century. The major advancements came at a much later date and were the product of the labors of many men, but notably of the three mentioned here.

Louis Pasteur, 1822-1895, was a French chemist. His earliest work in the field of bacteriology was concerned with diseases of beer and wine, the process of fermentation, then diseases of silkworms. His later work was concerned with isolating the causative bacteria in other diseases, some affecting man. You may be familiar with his name as used in the "pasteurization" of milk.

Joseph Lister, 1827-1912, was an English surgeon, considered to be the founder of antiseptic surgery but whose work involved many other aspects of surgical procedures.

Robert Koch, 1843-1910, a German bacteriologist—one of the greatest—was awarded the Nobel prize for medicine in 1905. Koch developed the conditions which he felt must be met to prove a given bacterium was the cause of a given disease. Known as Koch's law, the conditions are these: The microorganism must be present in every case of the disease; It must be capable of cultivation in pure culture; It must, when inoculated in pure culture, produce the disease in susceptible animals. To this has been added a fourth condition: The organism must be recovered and again grown in pure culture.

Bacteriology

Bacteriology is the science and study of bacteria, a very large group of one-celled, vegetable microorganisms. They do not contain chlorophyll. In structure and form (morphologically) these microorganisms exist as oval or spherical cells called *cocci*; as rods, *bacilli*; as spiral shapes, *spirilla*; and also a small group usually included in the spirilla which are comma-shaped and are called *vibrios*.

The three general morphologic types of bacteria—bacilli (rod-shaped), cocci (spherical), and spirilla (spiral-shaped)—also may have many variations. Some bacilli are slender with parallel sides, others are short and fat with rounded sides, some have pointed or tapered ends, others are flat-ended. Some bacilli occur singly, others lie end to end in pairs or chains, or they may be stacked.

Cocci are named by size and arrangement, rather than by variations in shape. Occurring singly, after division, they are called *micrococci*; if they remain in pairs, *diplococci*; in chains, *streptococci*; in sheets or clusters, *staphylococci*; in cubes or packets of eight, *sarcinae*.

Spirilla also may occur in many forms. They may have a single curve, may be coiled, may have many curves, or may be coiled and curved at the same time.

Bacteria are *aerobic*, requiring free oxygen in order to survive, or *anaerobic*, able to live without oxygen. Some can live under either condition and are called *facultative* aerobes or anaerobes. The cells are either *motile*, able to move under their own power, or *nonmotile*, unable to move by themselves. If they exist on living hosts, they are *parasites*; if they exist on dead hosts, *saprophytes*. Again, some bacteria can do either and are called facultative parasites, while others are true parasites. These, the parasites, are the pathogenic types of bacteria.

In cell structure, it is evident that the bacterial cell is extremely complex. It is known that a definite cell wall exists, surrounding the protoplasm[1] of the cell. In addition to the cell wall, all bacteria have a slime layer which, when enlarged or thickened, is called a *capsule*. The capsule is a defensive structure for the protection of the bacteria and is usually present on only a pathogenic organism. This is one type of cell structure.

Bacteria may also have organs of locomotion, called *flagella*. If the organism is flagellated, it is motile; otherwise it is nonmotile. Special stains are required to show the flagella. This is a second type of cell structure.

Bacterial cells reproduce by division. The material of the cell itself increases in volume;

---

1. Protoplasm (*protos* = first, *plasma* = form, in Greek) is the physical basis of all life and is found in all cells.

spherical forms become oval, and rod forms become nearly double their original length. The cell becomes constricted at the middle, and eventually the cell contents are held in two compartments separated by a wall formed at the place of constriction. Sooner or later the separation is complete—two new individuals, or daughter cells, have been formed which are exactly the same as the mother cell and identical to each other.

Some species of bacteria also are capable of a third form, called a *spore.* This is considered a form of hibernation. Spores generally are formed when conditions for reproducing by division have become unsatisfactory for any reason, such as dryness, heat, cold, or through the presence of a chemical substance which is poisonous. In some cases, spores are formed in the normal life cycle of the bacteria. The spore form of the organism is most difficult to destroy. Some sporulating organisms have been known to remain alive for more than ten years; the organisms capable of multiplication only by cell division usually are dead in twelve months or less. However, when conditions are right for the sporulating organism, the spore becomes a cell again. Either the spore wall softens, thins, becomes plastic, and the cell appears to be the ordinary type, or the wall of the spore thins and breaks down either at one end or the middle of the cell, permitting the cell contents to emerge and assume the typical form, leaving the empty spore shell behind. The spore form is a third type of cell structure.

Spores are by nature of their structure extremely resistant to the usual types of sterilization. They will survive hours of boiling and dry heat of more than 100°. No method of sterilization can be considered satisfactory and entirely safe if it ignores the sporogenic types of bacteria.

Microorganisms are so tiny that a small dot could cover as many as 250,000 bacteria of average size. The unit of measurement used for such tiny sizes is the micron μ, which is 1/1000 of a millimeter, or roughly 1/25,000 of an inch. An average bacillus may measure about 2 microns in length and 1/2 micron in width; but there is a considerable variation in size. Lengths of 40 microns may occur; others are as short as 0.4 of a micron. The cocci, or round forms, may be between 0.8 and 1.3 of a micron in diameter. Bacilli are shorter, generally, than spirilla.

Bacteria are identified in various ways. In cultivating growths or colonies of the unknown bacteria in a laboratory, the addition of certain chemicals to the *media,* or material on which the bacteria can grow, might stimulate certain species to grow more rapidly, while the growth of others might be slowed. The media may be either a broth (liquid) or agar-agar (a gel-like solid). When various dyes are placed in the media, some species will absorb the color, others will not. If blood is added to the media, some pathogens may destroy the red blood cells; others will not. All these tests give a basis for determining the particular bacteria under examination.

One of the most common staining techniques used in identifying bacteria is called the Gram stain. Some bacteria will withstand decolorizing agents such as alcohol and acetone, while others will not. In applying this test, a prepared sample of the organism (usually on a glass slide) is first washed with a purple stain, then decolorized; then a red counterstain is applied. The organisms which resist the decolorization remain purple in color and are said to be *gram positive.* Those which do not resist the decolorization lose the purple dye and take on the red color of the counterstain. These organisms are called *gram negative.* This test is widely used to tell the difference between organisms that frequently appear identical.

Many types of stain tests are used in bacteriology, but it is not necessary to investigate further. If the office in which you are employed has special reason to use tests of this nature, it will also be prepared to teach you the required techniques.

Protozoa

The protozoa are the simplest form of animal life, essentially one-celled animals. However, because the protozoa are one-celled does not mean that the function of that cell is simple. Each single protozoon performs all the functions of life as the higher animals do with their multiplicity of cells grouped into special types for special purposes. Since the complete functions of life are carried on within a single cell, these functions can be very complicated beyond our experience with higher forms of animal life simply by reason of being carried on within a single cell.

Protozoa generally require a fluid environment for active life. They are found in pools and puddles, oceans, lakes, in bodies of higher animals and plants, as well as in soil—wherever moisture is present. In a dormant state, they may exist in dry conditions. Up to 1945, only about 20,000 species had been described, although it seems likely that there are more kinds of protozoa than other animal forms.

At times no definite line can be drawn at this primitive level between animal and plant kingdoms. For example, some of the flagellated protozoa contain chlorophyll. Under certain conditions they may synthesize food as do green plants; under other conditions they are able to engulf and digest solid food. The majority of protozoa are aerobic.

Protozoa reproduce mainly by binary fission, budding, and sporulation. Sporulation is especially characteristic of the parasitic forms which have been most intensively studied because of the diseases they produce in man. Of these, the most well known are the malarial organisms.

Fungi

The fungi are a low form of plant life. They are a division of the Thallophytes without chlorophyll. The four classes are Phycomycetes, Ascomycetes, Basidiomycetes, and Fungi Imperfecti. Most of the pathogenic fungi belong to the Fungi Imperfecti.

Fungi reproduce by spores, which may consist of one or many cells.

Since fungi do not have chlorophyll, they are dependent on other plants or animals for food. When the food is obtained from living organisms, the fungi are parasitic; when (as is more common) it is obtained from dead remains, the fungi are termed saprophytes. The number of species is probably in excess of 100,000.

The yeasts and molds are fungi. The drug penicillin is a product of the fungus *Penicillium notatum*. Another fungus, the common mushroom, *Psalliota campestris*, is a wholesome food. *Candida albicans* is the fungi responsible for the disease we know as thrush. Thus, fungi provide man with medicine, food, and disease.

Rickettsiae

These microorganisms are smaller than bacteria but larger than the filterable viruses. They are usually found in ticks, fleas, and lice (the arthropods) and are difficult to grow under laboratory conditions. The life cycle involves the arthropods as well as certain small animals.

R. rickettsii is that species which is the causative agent of Rocky Mountain spotted fever. Others are the causative agents of American Q fever and several forms of typhus.

Viruses

The virus (Latin: poison) organism is even smaller than the rickettsiae. In fact, most viruses are impossible to see in an ordinary microscope. They usually will pass through a filter which would catch bacterial forms.

Viruses cannot be cultivated on inanimate media such as the broth which can be used in agar to cultivate bacteria. They must be cultivated on surviving cells or proliferating embryonic cells (or chorioallantois of the developing chick).

The ultraviruses, those of smallest particle size, are about 10 millimicrons. The larger sizes range up to 200 millimicrons.

The better-known virus diseases are rabies, encephalitis lethargica, poliomyelitis, herpes facialis, herpes zoster, smallpox, chickenpox, the common cold, yellow fever, influenza of various types, mumps, and infectious and serum hepatitis.

In the case of the two types of hepatitis, and other diseases caused by the viruses, the low "dosage" required to produce infection is amazing. As little as 0.0004 ml of contaminated blood or serum will produce infection.[2]

Sterilization

Why Do We Sterilize?

Proper sterilization of instruments, materials, and equipment in the dental office is one of the greatest responsibilities of the dental assistant toward the patients who come for treatment. Unless you have had training in hospital surgical procedures, be assured that you will confuse cleanliness with sterility. You can care for instruments, for example, with a high degree of cleanliness, and yet not have sterile instruments. Conversely, you will not have sterile instruments without a habit of cleanliness in their care and handling. In many cases, in the dental office particularly, it is not always possible to sterilize everything in the true sense of the word. The effort should be

2. *Accepted Dental Therapeutics* (Chicago: American Dental Association, 1971-72), p. 55.

made, however, to approach sterility as much as possible.

Foremost in importance is self-cleanliness, or personal hygiene. You cannot possibly have clean instruments and equipment if your own hands and clothing are not clean. Uniforms or other clothing worn in the dental office must be clean at all times. Hands and arms should be washed thoroughly with a good soap and scrubbed with a hand brush before touching instruments and before assisting with each patient.

In the "Microbiology" section we discussed the general groups of microorganisms which concern us: bacteria, protozoa, fungi, rickettsiae, and viruses. To do our best to properly prepare instruments, materials, and equipment for the dental patient, we must proceed as though the most difficult organisms, the bacterial spore forms and certain of the viruses, were to be constantly encountered in routine preparations.

For example, how resistant are the causative viruses of hepatitis? Experiments have established that they will withstand an *indefinite exposure* to 0.25 percent phenol, 2 percent tricresol, 1:2000 merthiolate, 70 percent alcohol or ether U.S.P. They will withstand for one month or longer exposure to any of the quaternary ammonium disinfectants in *any commonly used concentration*. The viruses are destroyed by twenty minutes' boiling; but autoclaving or exposure to dry heat at 160° C. (320° F.) or higher for one hour are the best methods of destroying them.

How resistant are bacterial spores in some cases? They have been known to withstand boiling water for sixteen hours.

It has been suggested that disease-producing spore-forming types of bacteria are rarely encountered in dental practice. As long as infectious and serum hepatitis maintain their present high incidence, in addition to the fact that an individual, though apparently healthy, may have hepatitis and be a "carrier," there can be no acceptance of a sterilization procedure which does not adequately consider the destruction of the viruses. The state of Minnesota in 1931 first had reports of five cases of hepatitis with three deaths; in 1955 there were 1,287 cases with seven deaths. Contaminated needles used in syringe injections are a very suspect cause of these increases. A 1956 study in one city traced seventeen out of twenty-two cases of serum hepatitis to dental offices. The further depressing facts are that twenty-three percent of those over the age of forty who contract the disease will die from it. Of those infected after the age of fifty, four out of ten will die. Currently, 900,000 unknowing carriers of serum hepatitis will indirectly cause the infection of 15,000 to 100,000 fellow Americans, but the majority of these victims would never contract the disease if their physician or dentist would employ sterile procedures.[3]

Proper preparation of syringe needles is so easily accomplished in a modern dental office with modern equipment that no question of their sterility need arise. The current development and availability of the presterilized disposable needle is a tremendous aid in the elimination of one source of infection, although the needle does *not* eliminate the problem.

In order to better understand the various methods of preparation and what each can accomplish, it is desirable to define the commonly used terms.

Sterilization is the removal or destruction of all forms of life.[4] Therefore, an object is either sterile or it is not sterile. All forms, including spores and viruses, are destroyed.

A *germicide* is an agent that destroys germs.[5] Thus anything which is not a germ, such as a spore or virus, may not be destroyed.

A *disinfectant* is an agent, usually a chemical substance, which destroys or inhibits the microorganisms causing disease. Ordinarily, spores are not destroyed. Usually this refers to an agent which is used, for example, in cleaning a hospital room.

An *antiseptic*, one of a large group of compounds, stops or inhibits the growth of bacteria without necessarily killing them. Alcohol, mercuric chloride, and phenol are examples.

Various methods of disinfection or sterilization are available to the modern dental office. The choice of method is determined largely by the instruments, equipment, or surgical materials, by their ability to withstand various methods of preparation, and by the necessity to sterilize or merely to disinfect.

Methods of Sterilization

Sterilization can be accomplished by autoclaving or by dry heat. However, dry heat takes so long to accomplish sterilization that it is less frequently used. Heat transfer media are also used by endodontists for certain very specific operations during surgery.

Be aware of sterilization—what it means and how it is accomplished. *Never substitute a lesser process where sterilization is required.* Be certain that you *have* sterilized.

Autoclave

Autoclaving is the method of choice. Steam under pressure rises in temperature. It is this rise in temperature, together with the moisture necessarily present, which makes autoclaving so desirable. Corrosion of sharp-edged instruments is considerably less than when boiling water is used. Packaging and loading must be done correctly. Syringes with needles can be

3. Nils U. Bang, Paul Ruegsegger, Allyn B. Ley, and John S. Ladne, "Detection of Hepatitis Carriers by Serum Glutamic Oxalacetic Transaminase Activity," *A.M.A.J.* 171 (December 26, 1959): 2303.
4. *Accepted Dental Remedies* (Chicago: American Dental Association, 1964), p. 93.
5. Ibid., p. 106.

autoclaved with a cotton roll, the roll later placed over the needle for storage until the syringe is used.

You should periodically test your method of loading the autoclave by means of the Diack control pellet available at your dealers. Since the coolest part of any autoclave chamber is at the bottom, a Diack control pellet should be placed in the center of the largest and densest pack in the load. This pack should be placed in the bottom of the autoclave. Immediately after sterilization, examine the Diack control pellet. If the pellet inside the hermetically sealed glass tube has fused and changed to a crimson color, proper sterilizing temperature has been attained. Do this about once a week, or oftener if you prefer, to check your procedures. Check an unusual load in this manner.

An autoclave must be operated correctly to achieve its purpose. When it is operated correctly, no living thing can survive ten minutes

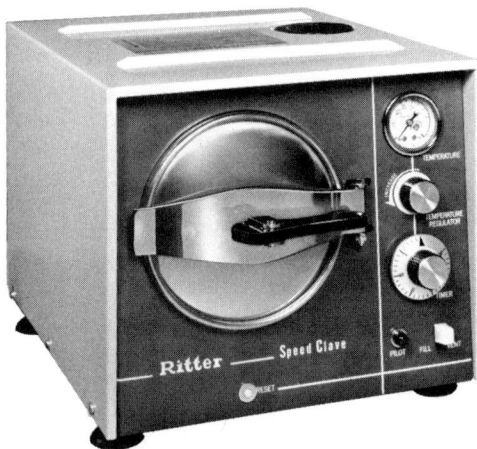

1. Check water reservoir daily. Fill tank to "full" indicator with distilled or demineralized water when necessary.
2. Press "Fill-Vent" lever. Water will flow into Speed Clave chamber. Hold lever down until water rises to within one-half inch of rim.
3. Load Speed Clave and close door.
4. Set timer, which is the "on-off" switch, for approximately fifteen minutes.
5. When desired temperature is reached, reset timer for sterilizing time.
6. Automatic timer will shut off heater and energize buzzer when sterilizing cycle is complete.
7. Press "Fill-Vent" lever. Hold lever down until all exhaust noise ceases.
8. Swing door handle straight out. When chamber pressure is sufficiently reduced, door "pops."
9. Allow three to five minutes for drying before opening door and removing load.

Recommended Times and Temperatures

Article	Temperature	Time
Unwrapped instruments	270°F	3 minutes
Wrapped instruments	270°F	5 minutes
Cotton dressing and bandages	250°F	20 minutes
Syringes	250°F	20 minutes
Rubber goods and gloves	250°F	15 minutes

Suggested Loading Procedures:

Do not overload. Steam penetrates loosely packed loads best.
Place absorbent paper or linen towel in bottom of tray.
Jointed instruments should be opened.
Instruments should be cleaned and dried before sterilizing.
Tray and container covers must be left ajar.
Place jars and containers tipped onto sides so steam will enter and sterilize contents. Contents can be retained by cloth cover over open end of jars, etc.

Courtesy Ritter Equip. Co., Rochester, N. Y.

Fig. 26.1. Ritter Model 7 Speed Clave

Steam Sterilizing

FILL. Open safety door by exerting upward and inward pressure on the handle. Slide bolt to right. Turn lower knob counterclockwise to FILL. Allow water to enter chamber until water covers fill plate. Turn lower knob to STERILIZE position which also stops flow of water.

LOAD. Load chamber. See paragraph on preparation of materials and loading of chamber. Close and lock door by moving bolt to left and pushing handle down.

SET. Turn middle knob to point where indicator is pointing straight up. When thermometer reaches desired temperature, rotate middle knob counterclockwise slowly until yellow light goes off. Once set, this step may be eliminated unless it is desired to sterilize at a different pressure and temperature. Turning middle knob clockwise increases temperature and pressure. Turning knob counterclockwise decreases temperature and pressure. Set timer knob to prescribed time period. See chart for proper temperature-time relationship.

VENT. When bell rings, rotate lower knob to VENT position. Allow all steam to be discharged.

DRY. Open door about ½ inch to permit thorough drying of contents (3-5 minutes). Leave lower knob in VENT position during drying and standby periods. Omniclave will be ready for immediate reuse by repeating above steps.

Helpful Hints

1. Always rotate upper knob (timer) past 10 minutes before setting time.
2. Always rotate lower knob (valve) counterclockwise.
3. Standby periods—leave door closed and leave lower knob in VENT position.
4. Add water to reservoir **only** when lower knob is in VENT or POWER OFF position. It is advisable to add water as needed to keep reservoir adequately filled.
5. At conclusion of all sterilizing for the day, turn lower knob to POWER OFF.
6. As soon as possible after bell rings at end of sterilizing cycle, turn to VENT position. This practice will prevent the autoclave from boiling dry.
7. Never attempt to turn lower knob from STERILIZE to FILL or from VENT to STERILIZE. Stops are incorporated to prevent knob from being turned in this manner.
8. Safety valve is set for 30 pounds.

Dry Heat Sterilization

LOAD. Load instruments on trays without cloth or paper coverings. Only two trays may be used. Insert Auxiliary thermometer door.

SET. Turn lower knob to VENT position. **Do not** turn through FILL position. Depress button beneath middle knob and turn knob clockwise into DRY STER

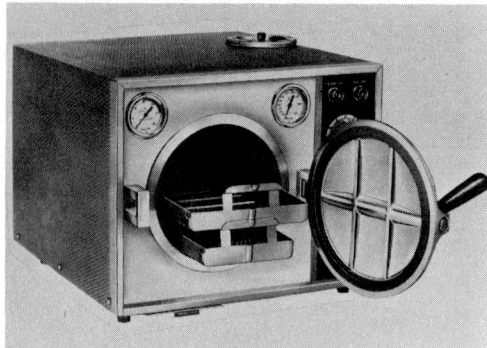

Fig. 26.2. Omniclave Sterilizer

section until it hits stop. This setting will give a temperature at approximately 350° (see Helpful Hints). Turn counterclockwise for a lower temperature. Set timer for 60 minutes as soon as thermometer reaches 320° F.

VENT. When bell rings, remove door and unload. If no additional dry heat sterilizing is desired, rotate middle knob into steam section. Button will pop out. Lower knob can **then** be turned to POWER OFF.

Helpful Hints

1. Middle knob cannot be turned to DRY STER section unless button is depressed. Button cannot be depressed unless lower knob is in VENT position.
2. When middle knob is in DRY STER section, lower knob cannot be turned from VENT position.
3. The density of the load will determine the time required to reach sterilizing temperature of 320°. Always distribute load loosely on trays.

Preparation of Materials—Steam Sterilization

INSTRUMENTS. **Clean thoroughly,** wrap in muslin and place on trays.

SYRINGES AND NEEDLES. Take syringe apart, wash thoroughly. Wrap each part separately in muslin. Cover entire tray with double thickness muslin cover.

FABRICS AND DRESSINGS. Fold into convenient packets. Always fold loosely. Avoid making many layers and never roll. Never use canvas as a covering. Wrap in muslin on tray. No not overload chamber.

UTENSILS AND GLASSWARE. Lay all jars or vessels on their sides. Fabrics may be sterilized in enamelware or glass jars; however, cover must fit very loosely, and container turned on its side.

SOLUTIONS. Fill flask no more than two-thirds full. Close end of flask with cotton or paper cups.

LOADING THE CHAMBER

1. Never overload or crowd chamber.
2. Do not let material come in contact with door.
3. Separate thick packs with loosely woven packs.

Recommended Periods of Exposure

Material to be Sterilized vs. Time in Minutes	PSI — F° — C°	15 — 250 — 121	20 — 260 — 127	25 — 267 — 131	DRY HEAT 320-355 160-180
Fabrics—Loosely woven—Wrapped in muslin		30	20	—	
Fabrics—Tightly woven		40	30	—	
Instruments—In Tray—Muslin cover		15	10	7	
Instruments—Individually wrapped in muslin		20	15	10	
Syringes & Needles		15	10	7	
Drums—Loosely woven contents		30	20	—	
Drums—Tightly woven contents		40	30	—	
Utensils—Loosely woven contents		30	20	10	
Rubber Gloves—In muslin packs		15	—	—	
Rubber Covers—In muslin packs		15	—	—	
Brushes & Miscellaneous Articles—Wrapped		15	—	—	
Solutions—1000 cc Flasks		30	25	—	

MINIMUM EXPOSURE PERIOD—60 MINUTES Do not sterilize fabrics, paper, or rubber at these temperatures. (See ADA **Accepted Dental Remedies,** Sterilization Section)

Courtesy Pelton and Crane, Charlotte, N. C.

Fig. 26.2. (Continued)

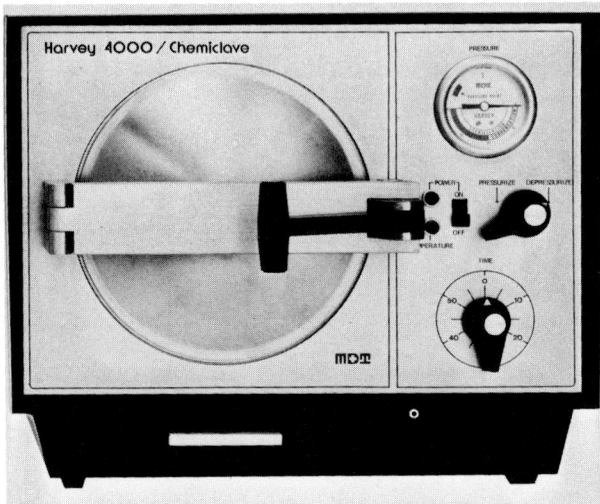

Courtesy Harvey Dental Specialty Co., Gardena, Calif.

Fig. 26.3. The Harvey Sterilizer. This is a vapor-type sterilizer, similar to an autoclave except that it uses a special alcohol-base solution called Vapo-steril.

of direct exposure to saturated steam at 121° C. (249.8° F.), the conditions in an autoclave (sea-level elevation) with fifteen pounds of pressure. It is the moist heat which kills.

Air must be completely removed from the sterilizing chamber. In most autoclaves this is accomplished automatically, except for the efforts of the operator to entrap air by placing such things as canisters or open jars (wrapped in muslin) in an upright position so that the air cannot be displaced. Items like these must be placed on their side so that air can be "poured" out by displacement with steam. Think of "air," in this case, as behaving like water—that is, always place items in such a way that if they contained water instead of air, the water would be able to run out of them. Space items out as much as possible. Hinged instruments, such as forceps, should be placed in the autoclave in an open or unlocked position so that steam can reach more of the surfaces.

Dry Heat

Dry heat sterilizers are available in very satisfactory designs for dental office use. A dry heat sterilizer is essentially an oven. Care in loading in order to aid proper circulation of air is important. Dry heat is especially satisfactory for cutting instruments, since corrosion is eliminated. Instruments must be thoroughly cleaned, as will be discussed under "Office Applications" later. Instruments or other materials to be sterilized should be spread out well either on gauze in racks or should be wrapped in aluminum foil. Excessively large loads should be avoided.

Temperature recommended for dry heat sterilizers range from 160° to 180° C. (320° to 355° F.) for at least one hour. When the load in the oven has reached this range, the temperature should be maintained for at least one hour—preferably longer.

Heat Transfer Media

A molten metal sterilizer is a device to melt and maintain in a molten state a small amount of low-fusing metal. This is accomplished by either a completely self-contained electrical unit or a simple device suspending a bowl of metal over the gas burner on the dental unit. The metal is melted and maintained at a temperature between 218° and 280° C. (424° to 536° F.).

The use of the molten metal sterilizer is limited largely to endodontics (root canal therapy). To allow a margin of safety, cotton points or tips of instruments are immersed in the molten metal for ten seconds immediately before the items are used in the mouth.

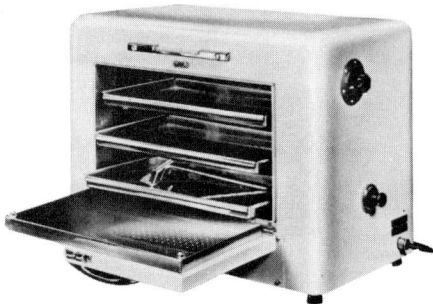

Fig. 26.4. Dri-Clave Model 180 with time and temperature chart (below).

Time and Temperature Chart*

Contents	Preparation	Temperature	Time (after reaching sterilizing temp)
Instruments	Thoroughly cleaned and rinsed and spread out on the trays or wrapped in aluminum foil.	350°F (180°C)	30 minutes
Sharps	Thoroughly cleaned and rinsed and spread out on gauze, or in racks, or wrapped in aluminum foil.	320°F (160°C)	40 minutes
Glass (Syringes, etc.)	Thoroughly cleaned with suitable detergent and rinsed in hot water; spread out (assembled or disassembled) on trays or wrapped in aluminum foil.	350°F (180°C)	30 minutes
Dressings	Loosely packed and well dispersed in container or wrapped in aluminum foil.	320°F (160°C)	60 minutes
Rubber Goods	Thoroughly cleaned and rinsed; well dispersed in a container or wrapped in aluminum foil.	248°F (120°C)	180 minutes

NOTE: Soft soldered instruments should be sterilized at 300°F for 60 minutes.
*These times and temperatures are adequate because of the small loads and the increased efficiency of the DRI-CLAVE. Verifying certified laboratory reports are available on request.

Courtesy Dri-Clave Co., Westbury, L. I., N. Y.

It is necessary to keep the surface of the molten metal as free as possible from *slag,* a collection of debris and impurities which floats on the surface. The slag is removed by collecting it on a small ball of loosely rolled cotton held with a cotton plier.

In some devices, the metal has been replaced with salt,[6] or with very small glass beads, to provide a means of sterilizing which eliminates the slag. Temperature in various parts of the media can vary considerably; use of an accessory thermometer is wise.

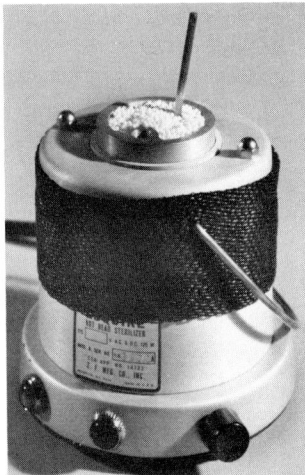

Fig. 26.6. Model A617 non-pressure office sanitizer (commonly called boiling-type sterilizers).

Courtesy American Sterilizer Co., S. S. White Co., Philadelphia

Fig. 26.5. Sterilizer for endodontics.

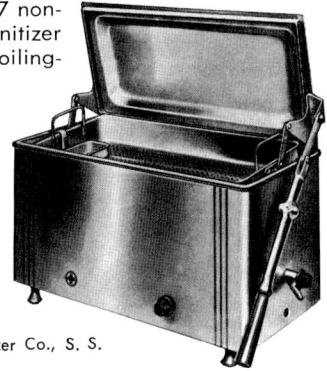

Sanitizing and Disinfecting

Disinfecting and sanitizing are processes used in the dental office, but they should in *no way* be confused with sterilizing.

Some commonly used methods of disinfecting or sanitizing instruments and equipment are discussed in this section.

Boiling Water

Many spores will survive hours of this treatment, but most vegetative forms of bacteria

6. L. I. Grossman, *Endodontic Practice,* pp. 170-173.

are destroyed in ten minutes. Tablets of alkalizing chemicals are available for use with boiling water to reduce corrosion of instruments. The water level should be such that the load is completely immersed at all times. Since the water is used at a brisk boil, the level needs to be checked periodically during the day. That this method is used widely in dental offices in no way alters the fact that its end result is not sterilization. It is not recommended for instruments which come in contact with the bloodstream of a patient or otherwise penetrate the oral mucosa, such as syringes and needles or surgical instruments.

Chemical Agents

There are many preparations available to the dental office which are used to make up a disinfecting solution by the addition of water. Many of these chemical disinfectants will not kill *Mycobacterium tuberculosis;* they do not destroy the causative agent of viral hepatitis.

The U. S. Department of Agriculture does not permit the designation "sterile" as the end result of a chemical action by a germicide. No chemical germicide on the market today can guarantee sterility; they are ineffective against spores, resistant bacteria, or the virus of serum hepatitis. The quaternary ammonium compounds (such as Zephiran) have soaplike properties. They kill ordinary vegetative bacteria but have no effect on the tubercle bacillus; in fact, they are used for the selective destruction of non-acid-fast bacteria in clinical specimens sent to the laboratory for diagnostic studies of tuberculosis!

Chemical disinfectants are capable of supporting bacterial life. Tetanus, serum hepatitis, and pyogenic (pus-forming) infections have been traced to storing autoclaved needles and syringes in chemical disinfectants.

The quaternary ammonium compounds are used most widely as cold disinfecting solutions. While they have the same limitations of effectiveness as other types of solutions, they have achieved wider use through their nonirritating qualities. Zephiran, Cetylcide, and Radiol are examples of these compounds. It is extremely important in using the quaternary ammonium compounds for disinfection of instruments that the instruments be carefully prepared, as discussed later ("Office Applications"). These compounds are incompatible with soap.

Chemical disinfectants should not be used for syringe needles because the effect is not one of sterilization, and in some cases any residual solution injected into tissue may cause swelling and edema. They should not be used to disinfect the end of an anesthetic cartridge for this same reason, as well as the fact that these solutions react with aluminum. Consequently, aluminum trays are best disinfected in some other manner.

Hot Oils and Silicone Fluids

Oil sterilizers are used in some dental offices for disinfecting contra-angles or some types of handpieces. To be as effective as boiling water, *Accepted Dental Therapeutics* suggests that the temperature of the oil or silicone fluid in one of these devices be maintained at 160°C. (320° F.). Hypodermic syringes and needles are never to be disinfected in this type of device. In addition to the lack of true sterility, the danger of injecting residual oil into a blood vessel and thereby causing an embolus (blockage of a blood vessel) is too great.

If the hot oil method of sterilization is to exceed the ability of boiling water to kill bacteria and spores, the instruments must be heated to at least 160° for one hour. To destroy bacteria in the vegetative form requires 150° for ten minutes or 125° for fifteen to twenty minutes. Care must be taken to start timing only after the load has reached the proper temperature. A common shortcoming in the use of the oil method lies in starting to time the load before this temperature has been reached.

The use of hot oil and silicone fluids originally designed to preclude corrosion of cutting edges and to provide a method of sterilizing the dental handpiece while providing for its lubrication. The lubrication provided under these circumstances is adequate for only the very low operating speeds. Equipment designed for high operating speeds is not designed for oil sterilization. Be sure that hot oil is used only as intended.

Two types of hot oil sterilizers are used, based on temperatures produced. Check the instructions for the one you use to be sure it is used as recommended. Hot oil can burn you very badly. Be extremely careful at all times. Instruments should be removed from the oil while still hot to facilitate draining. This can usually be accomplished by raising the tray containing the instruments and permitting the excess oil to drain into the main chamber.

If carbon tetrachloride is used to remove excess oil from the outer parts of contra-angles disinfected in this manner, remember carbon tetrachloride fumes are extremely poisonous. It should be used with extreme care in a room with good ventilation. Preferably, carbon tetrachloride should not be used at all.

Alcohol

Seventy percent isopropyl alcohol or seventy percent ethyl alcohol is recommended for the chemical disinfection of anesthetic cartridges. If syringes with attached needles are suspended for storage in either alcohol, they should be wiped with a sterile gauze to remove any excess alcohol, and the lumen of the needle should be flushed by ejecting some of the anesthetic solution prior to injection.

Seventy percent ethyl alcohol is an excellent germicide—but does not sterilize. When used undiluted, it is not nearly as effective. The greatest objection to its use is the heavy tax rate which applies when it is purchased. A permit is usually required to obtain ethyl alcohol.

Isopropyl alcohol is perhaps more effective than ethyl and is much lower in cost. It should not be used full strength but should be diluted with water to seventy percent, as should ethyl alcohol.

Flaming

Unless the instrument is held in the flame until it becomes red hot (which some dentists do with platinum syringe needles), sterilization is doubtful. Dipping into alcohol and lighting the excess solution achieves a questionable degree of disinfection.

Office Applications

The average adult mouth contains 160,-000,000,000,000,000,000,000,000,000 microorganisms. Your job is to limit their spread by using proper sterilization techniques.[7] The organisms may include hepatitis, syphilis, or tuberculosis. *Always prepare instruments and equipment as you would prepare them for use in your own mouth.*

7. N. B. Williams, "Microbial Ecology of the Oral Cavity," *J. Dent. Research* 42 (1963): 509-520. Supplement to No. 1.

Cleaning dirty instruments is a major menace to anyone working with them. It is extremely easy to prick a finger or hand. The dangers of cross-infection for patient, doctor, and staff exist in every operatory. Be careful as you handle these dirty instruments.

Regardless of the method of disinfecting or sterilizing used in your office, the first step is to start with instruments cleaned of all debris, blood, grease, and oil. Bulk-rinse the instruments in a commercial cleaning solvent to remove any possible grease or oil. After this rinsing, the instruments should be individually scrubbed with a brush and a very warm nonionizing detergent solution. Soaps are quite alkaline and not compatible with germicides; soap residues will prevent disinfection. Thoroughly rinse the detergent off the instruments and remove the excess moisture by rolling the group of instruments in a towel.

An alternative method for preparation of instruments for sterilization is to use an ultrasonic cleaner which can eliminate much of the danger of infection from working with dirty instruments and will insure thorough removal of the loosened dirt and cleaning solutions. The ultrasonic tank should be cleaned at periodic intervals; rubber gloves should be worn when removing any scum.

There are alternative methods for disinfecting instruments having a sharp or cutting edge. Your office may use chemical solutions, a dry heat oven, or the autoclave.

Several methods for sterilizing and disinfecting are acceptable in dental practice. Some offices use only the one method; others use several. Learn the methods of choice for your dentist. With these methods in mind, group the prepared instruments according to the type of sterilizing technique to be used with each group.

If a chemical solution is used, soap must not be present on the instruments. (It should not be in any case, but especially with the chemical agents.) Chemical disinfectants kill microorganisms by coagulating their protein. Dirty instruments coated with blood and tissue fluids placed in a chemical disinfectant would result in the coagulation of the surface protein and prevent further penetration of the chemical, thus protecting the microorganisms below the surface. All instruments going into disinfectants must be clean, free from grease, and dry. Even an autoclave cannot sterilize dirty instruments. Learn the proper minimum time of immersion for the solution used in your office, as well as the number of days or weeks the solution remains effective for use. The easiest way to remember when it is time to change the solution is to write the date of change on a piece of tape applied to the container.

The germicidal solution concentration is critical. A solution too strong will not kill organisms; each type of germicide has a killing range of concentration. Mix it exactly as directed; or use ready-to-use solution or premeasured concentrates.

Boiling-water sterilizers are not highly effective, but the office in which you are employed may use one. Instruments disinfected in this manner must be boiled for a minimum of ten minutes, completely immersed, and timed after the water is boiling vigorously. Check the water level frequently during the day. Use anti-rust tablets in the water. Dry instruments thoroughly with a sterile towel immediately after removal from the water. Deposits of lime in the boiler itself should be removed regularly, daily if necessary, by draining all the water and scrubbing the boiler with a stiff brush and cleanser. If you have a particularly difficult problem with deposits, you may find it worthwhile to use distilled water instead of tap water.

A third method of sterilizing instruments is autoclaving. Instruments which have a sharp cutting edge can be autoclaved without damage by dipping the operating end in an oil emulsion, prepared for this purpose, called I. S. L. Emulsion, Type A, made by the American Sterilizer Company. It is also useful for autoclaving hinged instruments such as forceps and scissors. Follow directions in its use. If anesthetic syringes are included in the load in an autoclave, sterilization at fifteen pounds' pressure and 250° is continued for fifteen minutes—after the temperature is reached. If loaded without syringes, most loads can be processed in ten minutes. Loads should not hang over the trays designed to hold them and should not be excessive. Make two separate loads rather than one very large load. Check results with a Diack control capsule occasionally to be sure that you are really sterilizing.

Instruments should not be touched with hands when removed from sterilizers. Instrument forceps, or transfer forceps, should be

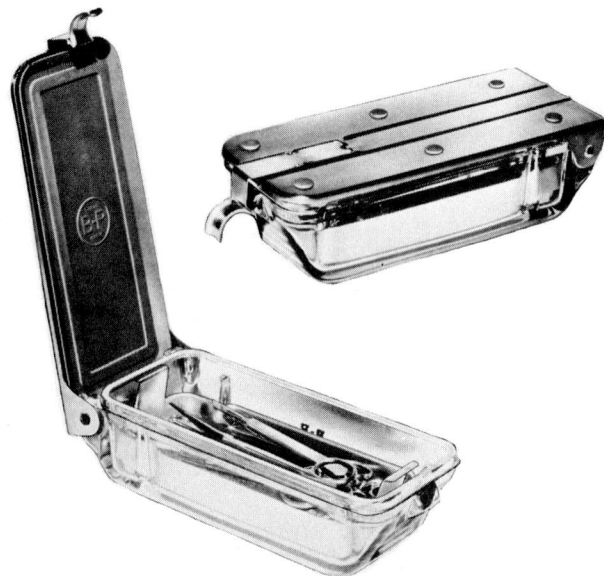

Courtesy Bard-Parker Co., Inc., Danbury, Conn.

Fig. 26.7. Instrument container No. 300

used. (See fig. 33.25.) If possible, the instruments can sometimes be tipped from the sterilizer tray into a sterile towel, the towel folded over the instrument and used to dry them, then used to place the instruments in their proper places. In this way the instruments will not be touched by your hands.

Rubber goods, such as bulbs of water syringes and chip blowers of the hand type, and the rubber tip on the saliva ejector hose into which the saliva ejector is placed, can be kept new-looking by wiping with a gauze moistened with benzene. This process merely refreshes the surface of the rubber and does not take the place of disinfection.

All operating levers on the chair, unit, lights, the bracket table itself, and any other item in the operating room which is touched in the course of treating a patient should be washed frequently with soap and water. Between patients they may be wiped with a gauze moistened with seventy percent isopropyl alcohol or sprayed with Bactine, a disinfecting spray.

The low-speed handpieces and contra-angles are preferably disinfected and lubricated after each use according to the method of choice. The increased speed types can sometimes be autoclaved (see the directions accompanying each), but often must only be wiped with seventy percent isopropyl alcohol.

Examining lamps may be wiped with seventy percent isopropyl alcohol, but the removable mirrors may be treated by other more effective methods, preferably autoclaving.

Hospitals find that five major sources of bacteria are important causes of cross-infection. These same sources may apply in the dental office:

1. Dust and dirt on floors are major sources. Floors should be carpeted or smooth-surfaced and easy to clean. Wet spots of blood, pus, or debris should be wiped up before they can dry and be carried into the air.

2. Ventilated air. Fans are taboo in operating rooms. Air conditioners should be mounted five feet above the floor to prevent stirring up of floor bacteria. Humidified air (about 50 percent relative humidity) helps settle airborne bacteria. Aerosols can be used effectively to settle air, but they are not effective if humidity is less than fifty percent.

3. Respiratory passages of personnel are a major source of cross-infection both for the individual himself and for others in the office.

4. Dirty linen and towels are a menace to all who handle them.

5. Dandruff and hair clippings from a fresh haircut are sources of cross-infection.

Hands can be washed with detergents containing three-fourths of one percent, or less, hexachlorophene, which will reduce the natural skin flora and eliminate the contaminating organisms.

The residue from bar soap left in a soap dish or the gummy deposits left around the opening on a liquid soap dispenser foster the growth of microorganisms. Be careful to remove these deposits frequently.

With the development of presterilized disposable needles for injection of local anesthetics, many offices may neglect proper care of the syringe itself. The syringe should be washed in a hot detergent solution, rinsed well, and autoclaved at 250° F. and with fifteen pounds' pressure for fifteen minutes. It requires sterilization, just as it always has, because the cartridge end of the needle must be inserted through the syringe tip with the possibility of contamination by touching the side wall on its way. The lumen of the syringe tip must be sterile.

Whatever is done to achieve asepsis in your office, be aware of the need to be constantly on your guard against habits or procedures which prevent the achievement of your primary responsibility: the protection of your patient, the protection of your doctor, and the protection of yourself.

Summary

Microbiology is the science of the nature, life, and actions of microorganisms which are either animal or plant. Bacteria, protozoa, fungi, rickettsiae, and viruses make up the microorganisms.

Sterilization is essential in the dental office to avoid cross-contamination of patients and to prevent infection. Sterilization and cleanliness are not the same. Autoclaving and dry heat are two methods of sterilization, which, if properly performed, will sterilize. Heat transfer media are also used for certain specific procedures in endodontics. Sanitizers and disinfectants are used in dental offices, but not for sterilizing.

Hospitals suggest five major sources of bacteria which are important causes of cross-infection. These five sources also apply to dental office problems in cross-infection.

Be aware of procedures which protect the patient, the dentist, and the assistant and establish them as your routines.

Study Questions

1. Discuss the three general morphologic types of bacteria.
2. Why is it important to understand spores?
3. Explain the differences between protozoa, fungi, rickettsiae, and viruses.
4. Why do we sterilize?
5. Describe the two best methods of sterilization.
6. Explain heat transfer media, flaming, chemical agents, hot oil and silicone fluids, and alcohol as used for cleansing, disinfecting, or sterilizing in the dental office.
7. What does boiling in water for twenty minutes do for an instrument?
8. What five major sources of bacteria are important causes of cross-infection?
9. How should you prepare instruments for use on patients?
10. Now that we have disposable presterilized needles for injection, what is the necessary minimum care for the syringe itself?

Bibliography

Accepted Dental Therapeutics. Chicago: American Dental Association, 1971-72.

BARTELS, H. A. "Relation of Bacteriology to Clinical Dentistry: Modern Methods of Sterilization in the Dental Office." *J. Dent. Educ.* 5 (1941): 312-327.

BURROWS, W. *Textbook of Microbiology.* 18th ed. Philadelphia: W. B. Saunders Co., 1963.

CROWLEY, M. C. "Obtaining and Maintaining Surgical Cleanliness." In *The Dental Clinics of North America,* p. 844. Philadelphia: W. B. Saunders Co., 1957.

EICHENWALD, MOSLEY. *Viral Hepatitis, Clinical and Public Health Aspects.* Public Health Publication No. 435. Rev. 1959.

FOLEY, GUTHEIM. "Serum Hepatitis Following Dental Procedures." Excerpts from *Annals of Internal Medicine,* September 1956.

GROSSMAN, L. I. *Endodontic Practice.* 7th ed. Philadelphia: Lea & Febiger, 1970.

HOLLAND, M. R. "A Review of Sterilization and Disinfection in Dentistry." *Oral Surgery, Oral Medicine and Oral Pathology* 8, no. 8 (August 1955): 788-795.

KNIGHTON, HOLMES T. "Significance of Tests for the Evaluation of Antiseptics and Germicides." *J.A.D.A.* 26 (December 1939): 2047-55.

————. "Value of Hot Oil as a Means of Disinfecting Instruments." *J.A.D.A.* 38 (March 1949): 309-313.

————. "Comparative Bactericidal Effects of Various Temperatures of Hot Oil." *J.A.D.A.* 48 (March 1954): 307-311.

SPAULDING, E. H., and EMMONS, E. K. "Chemical Disinfection." *American Journal of Nursing* 59 (September 1958): 1242.

27

Oral Pathology and Dental Caries

Oral Pathology

Pathology (from the Greek *pathos*, meaning "disease," and *log*, meaning "science of" is that branch of biological science which deals with the nature of disease through a study of its causes, how it proceeds, and its effects including changes in function and changes in structure. Pathologic changes in the tissues of the body may be caused by microorganisms, wounds or injuries, chemicals, cold or heat, or pressure. These may act individually or several may act together to produce pathologic results.

Oral pathology (diseases of the mouth) concerns the area of immediate interest to the dentist but also includes diseases which affect that area indirectly. Many systemic diseases (diseases of the body as a whole) produce visible effects in the mouth or cause accompanying changes which are apparent in the mouth. Many diseases of the mouth are not related to the teeth.

When we speak of diseases of the teeth themselves, such as dental caries (a localized, progressive disintegration of tooth structure) and the abnormal conditions which may follow dental caries, we use the general term *dental pathology*, which means diseases pertaining to or relating to the teeth.

The discussion of oral pathology in this volume will be very definitely limited to those

325

diseases which are most frequently of interest to the dental assistant, either as observations in the course of her normal duties or as diseases which require certain preparations on the part of the dental assistant in their treatment. Many books are available which will provide the necessary material for the advanced student of oral pathology.

Inflammation

The response of the tissues of the body to pathologic changes is called inflammation (from the Latin *inflammare*, "to set on fire"). It is the body's defense against injury and disease. The characteristics of inflammation are such basic responses that it is something every person who works in the health profession should know. For the dental assistant, knowledge of the inflammatory process is applied to conditions which commonly occur in the oral cavity.

If you should scratch the skin of your hand with a pin, you would notice a reaction to this injury within minutes. The skin around the scratch would be reddened due to increased blood flow in the area. If you ran your finger across the scratched area, you would feel an elevation of the tissue, indicating that the reddened area is also swollen. This is due to excess fluids from the bloodstream in the tissue diluting and attacking any toxins which may be present. You would also note increased sensitivity or pain when anything comes in contact with the scratch, causing you to favor the area and avoid further irritation. If you had a delicate thermal-sensitive instrument, you would be able to detect an increase in temperature in the area of the wound due to the increased blood flow. The *cardinal symptoms of inflammation* are *redness, swelling, heat, pain,* and *impairment of function*. If the area were to continue to show a more severe reaction, you would note an increased degree of

these cardinal symptoms and, perhaps, the formation of pus.

In the inflammatory reaction, the increase in blood supply (*hyperemia*) brings additional white blood cells (*leukocytes*) and fluids to the damaged area in an effort to fight invading bacteria and toxins. The cells phagocytize the bacteria by engulfing them and literally destroying them. The leukocytes die in the process, forming what you know as pus.

Immediately after the injury there is an initial constriction of the vessels, followed very closely by a dilation of the vessels which results in hyperemia. The total current of the blood through the area is slower due to the dilation of the vessels which permits the blood cells and fluid to penetrate the vessel wall and migrate into the injured or diseased area.

Inflammation of the tissue may be produced by microorganisms, wounds or injuries, chemicals, cold, heat, or pressure. One factor may act alone or several may act together. Some authorities, in discussing inflammation, also include the process of repair, which encompasses new capillary formation, the formation of granulation tissue, organization of the

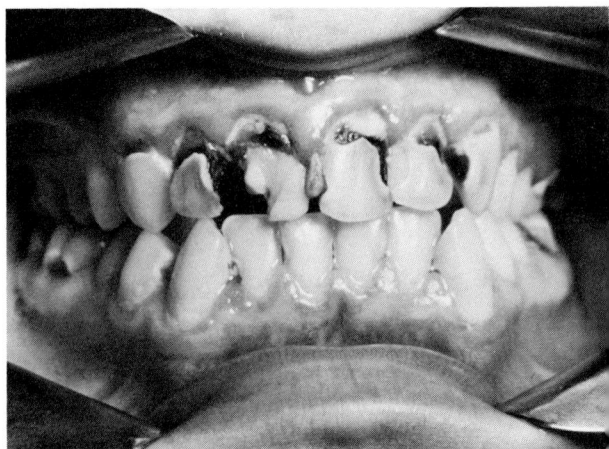

Fig. 27.1. Dental disease caused by oral neglect (caries, gingivitis).

wound, and finally, cicatrization (formation of scar tissue).

Inflammation is indicated in terminology by the suffix *itis*. If we say *gingivitis*, we indicate that the gingival tissues have an inflammatory reaction present. If we say *pulpitis*, we indicate that the pulp of the tooth is undergoing an inflammatory reaction. Inflammation, then, is a form of *body resistance to injury and disease*. It actually is a *helping process*.

Other Tissue Changes

If you were to look through a textbook of pathology, you would most likely think, "There are so many disorders and diseases how can anyone be healthy?" Even with reference to those diseases which most directly affect the oral cavity, the number seems overwhelming. In actual practice, however, most dentists will contact but a few pathologic conditions which are not directly associated with gingival, pulpal, or periapical changes in teeth. In dental schools the number will be greatly increased because practicing dentists tend to refer anything unusual for diagnosis and treatment to faculty in these areas.

The diagnosis of oral pathology is not always simple. A diagnosis may be made from recognition of the clinical symptoms of the disease alone; this is known as a *clinical diagnosis*. A *differential diagnosis* involves distinguishing between two or more diseases of similar character by comparing symptoms and any other known factors. A diagnosis can only be made after considering all the manifestations of the disease, visualizing the disorder in terms of its physiology and histochemistry, examining a biopsy of the lesion if indicated, conducting clinical tests, and finally, reasoning about the collected data.

Following is a brief list of the conditions which are most commonly observed in the dental office:

Abscess: An abscess is a localized area of pus. In the mouth this may be caused by infection: (*a*) inside the tooth, resulting in a periapical abscess; (*b*) alongside the root, resulting in a lateral or periodontal abscess (a periodontal pocket); or (*c*) around the crown of a partially erupted tooth, resulting in a pericoronal abscess.

Aphthous Ulcer (aphthastomatitis): This lesion is commonly called the canker sore. It is an ulcer of unknown origin which appears on the mucous membrane. It is similar to the herpes simplex lesion which occurs on the skin, but the aphthous ulcer is definitely not of viral origin whereas the herpes lesion is.

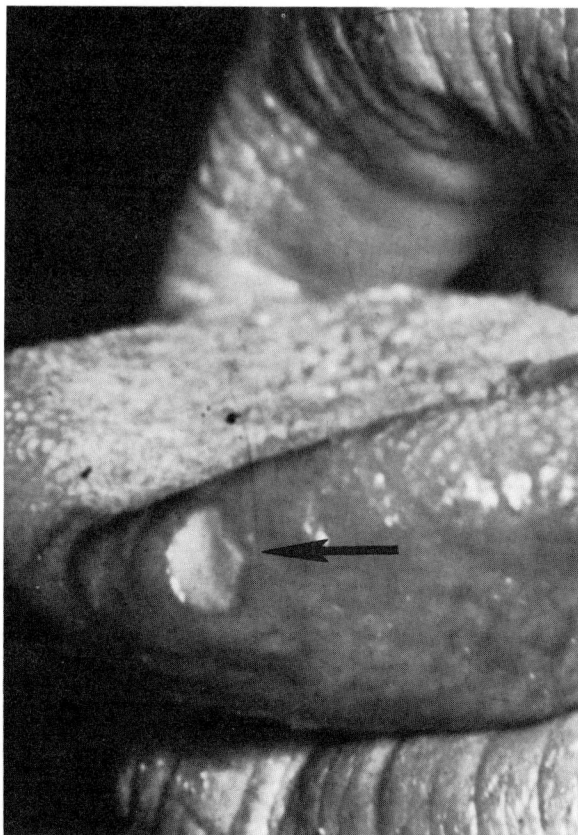

Fig. 27.2. Aphthous ulcer

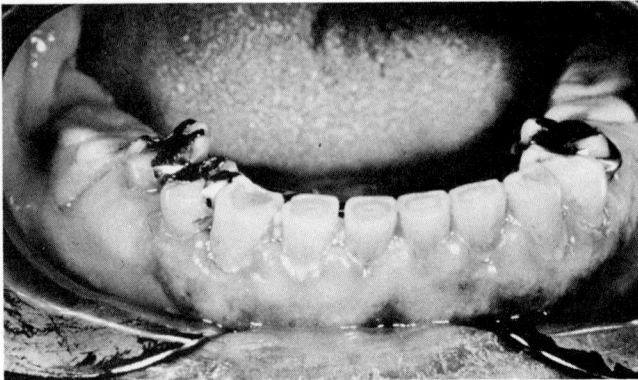

Fig. 27.3. Attrition-abrasion (anterior teeth worn down, posterior teeth missing).

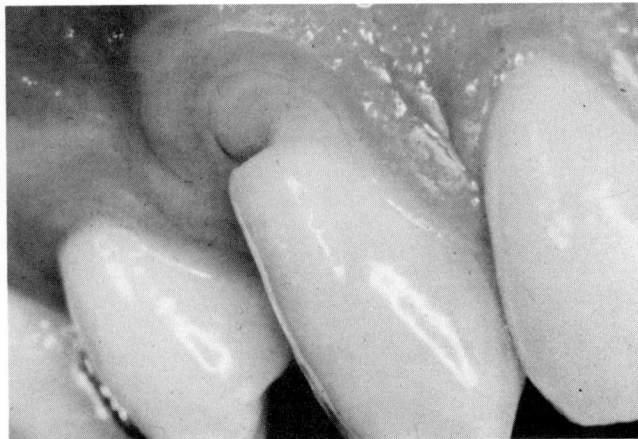

Fig. 27.4. Erosion

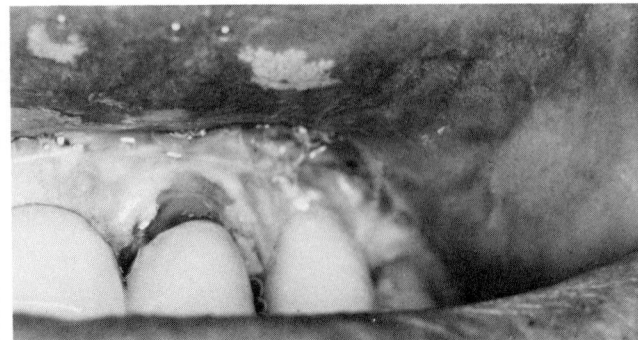

Fig. 27.5. Aspirin burn

Attrition, Erosion, and *Abrasion*: Pathologic wear from attrition, erosion, or abrasion can lead to pulpal injury, or even exposure, if secondary dentin does not deposit rapidly enough to protect the pulp.

Burns: On occasion, patients may attempt self-medication and place such drugs as aspirin directly on gingival tissues at the site of pain, producing a serious burn lesion.

Cheilitis: Inflammation of the lip. The lower lip is more often involved. Persons who are outdoors a great deal may have cheilitis occur as a swelling of the lip with a white, leathery covering sprinkled with red areas where erosion has occurred.

Cheilosis: A fissuring at the corners of the mouth due to vitamin B complex deficiency; or in the case of the patient who wears dentures, it may also develop because the vertical dimension (distance of the chin from the nose) is not great enough, resulting in a constant wetness of the corners of the mouth with cracks and fissures eventually forming.

Cleft Palate: A condition probably originating early in uterine life (congenital) characterized by the failure of the soft and hard tissues of the palate to join along the midline. When this condition extends through the lip, it is along the lines of the premaxillary region, so that the cleft (or harelip) is visible below the ala of the nose on one side (unilateral) or both sides (bilateral), since the premaxillary region is a pie-shaped segment extending its point back to the midline of the hard palate approximately in the region of a line drawn across the palate from first bicuspid to first bicuspid. While cleft palate is a failure of two halves to join properly during development, harelip is a failure of one side to join properly with the premaxillary segment on one or both sides.

Diabetes Mellitus: A disorder of carbohydrate metabolism. Dental involvement is characterized by multiple periodontal abscesses which also can be recurrent, changes in alveolar bone, lowered resistance to infection, and slow healing following any oral surgery.

Epulis: Any benign neoplasm of the gingiva, usually pedunculated and raised, like a small toadstool.

Exostosis: Overgrowth of bone projecting outward from the usual surface; the most common are the tori, bony protuberances occurring along the midline of the hard palate in about twenty percent of the population (this protuberance is called a torus palatinus), and

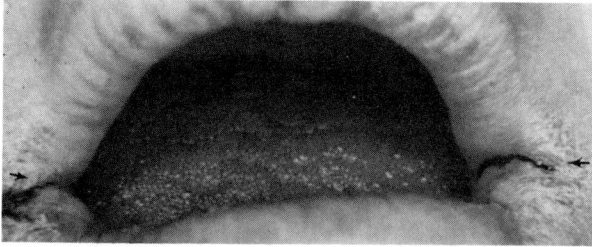

Fig. 27.6. Cheilosis

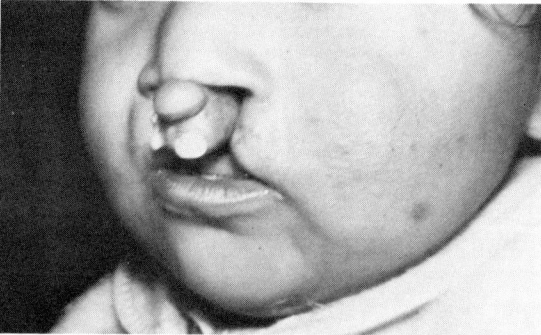

Fig. 27.7. Cleft lip and/or palate

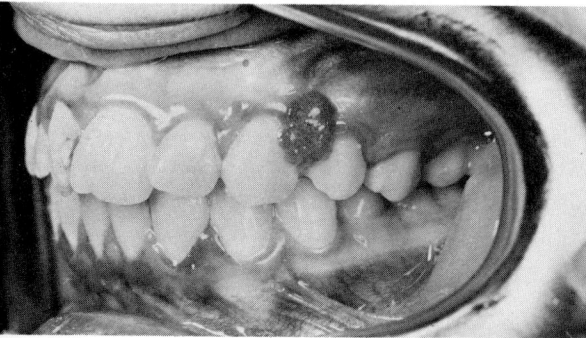

Fig. 27.8. Epulis

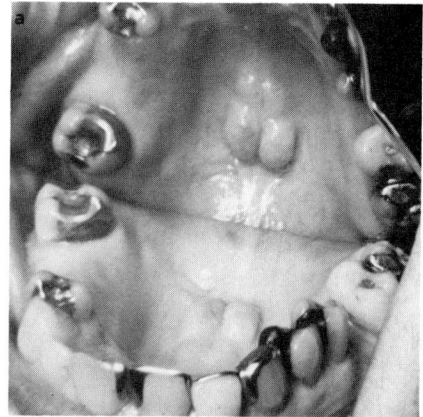

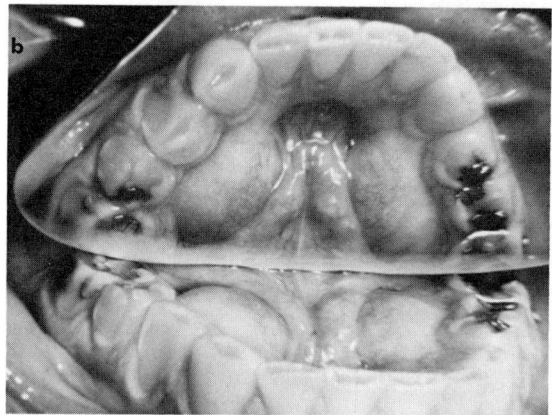

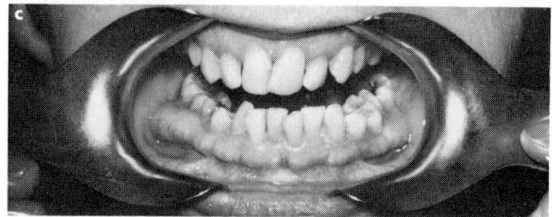

Fig. 27.9. Exostosis: (a) palatal, (b) lingual, (c) labial

the bilateral or unilateral protuberances occurring on the lingual surface of the mandible in the premolar region in about seven percent of the population (torus mandibularis).

Fibroma: A benign neoplasm of fibrous connective tissue.

Fistula: An oral fistula is usually an abnormal passage or communication from an abscess to the outer surface. It may be at the gingival tissue or may drain to the outer skin on the cheek or chin. This is a symptom of trouble which indicates that the body's defenses are unable to cope with some infection, such as that caused by infection within root canals and some periodontal pockets.

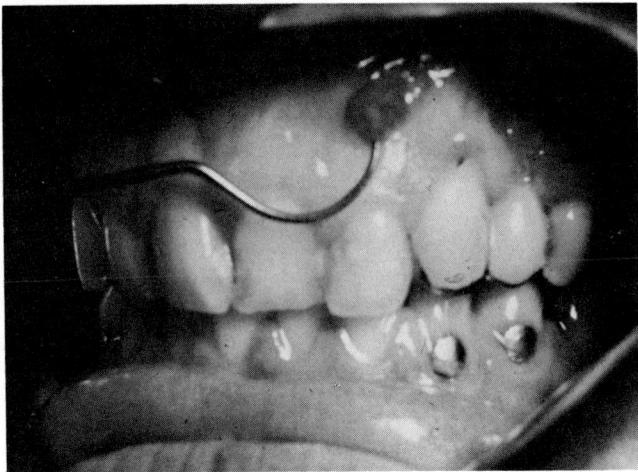

Fig. 27.11. Fordyce's spots

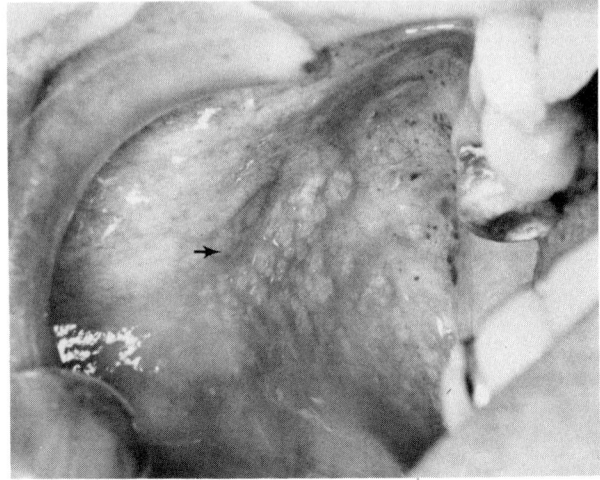

Fig. 27.10. Fistula

Fordyce's Spots: Harmless, brownish, slightly raised spots on the oral mucosa or lips, found in more than seventy percent of the population. Erroneously called Fordyce's disease.

Herpes Simplex: An infection caused by a virus of the same name. It usually occurs on the skin and rarely on the mucous membrane.

Hyperplasia: The abnormal increase in *number* of normal cells of a tissue, resulting in an enlargement or thickening of the tissue. One of the possible reactions of tissue to irritation, injury, or drugs; for example, continued long-term intake of Dilantin to control epileptic seizure may cause the formation of hyperplastic gingival tissue (Dilantin enlargement).

Hypertrophy: The abnormal increase in the *size* of the cells of a tissue, resulting in an enlargement or thickening of the tissue. True or physiologic hypertrophy results from excessive activity of muscle; for example, exercise makes a muscle larger.

Hypoplasia: Defective or incomplete development of any tissue; in dentistry, mostly associated with enamel hypoplasia: Pits or ringlike grooves left in enamel due to interference with the function of the ameloblasts (enamel-forming cells) at the particular time this area was being formed. Hypoplasia is often associated with a highly infectious illness with high temperature. The age at which this occurred can be estimated quite accurately by the position of the defect.

Internal Resorption: When the resorptive process involves the crown of a tooth and sufficient dentin is destroyed, the translucent enamel shows the pinkness of the vascular tissue underneath. This condition is verified by roentgenographic examination (Fig. 27.14*a* and *b*).

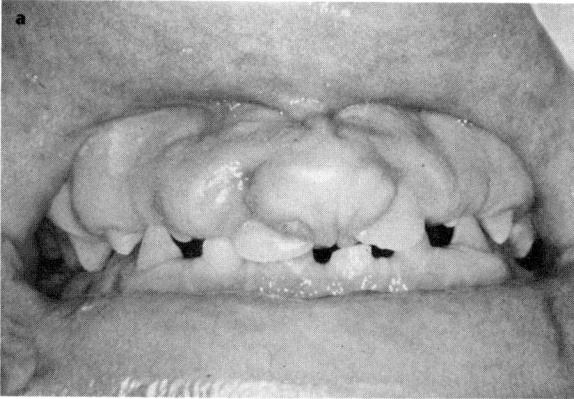

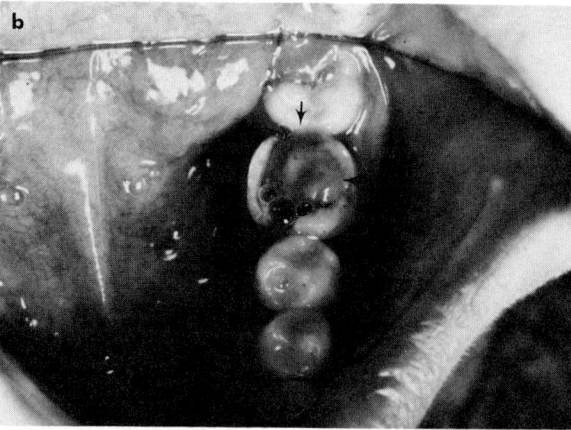

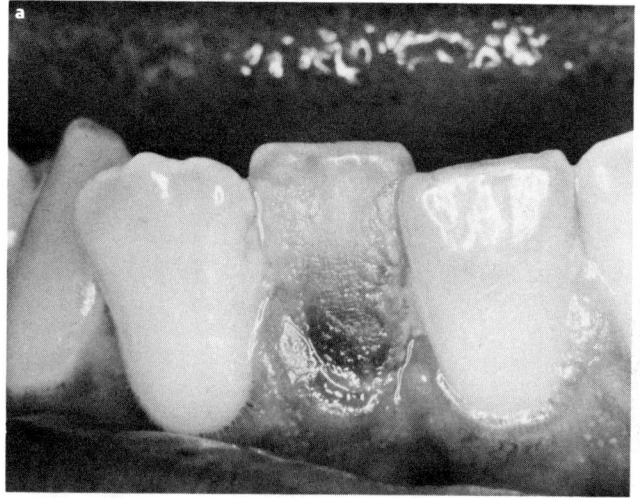

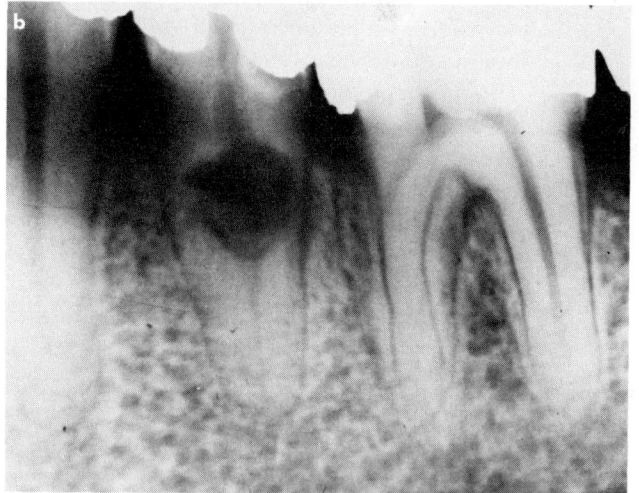

Fig. 27.12. Hyperplasia: (a) Dilantin hyperplasia, (b) Pulpal hyperplasia.

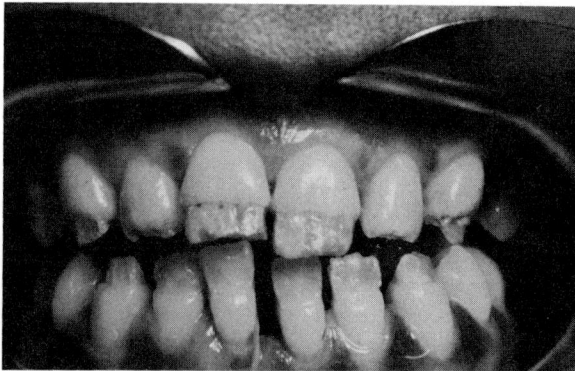

Fig. 27.13. Hypoplasia

Fig. 27.14. Internal resorption

Leukoplakia: A white, opaque, leathery plaque formed upon the oral mucous membrane. Considered premalignant. Resembles lichen planus in appearance; differentiated by biopsy.

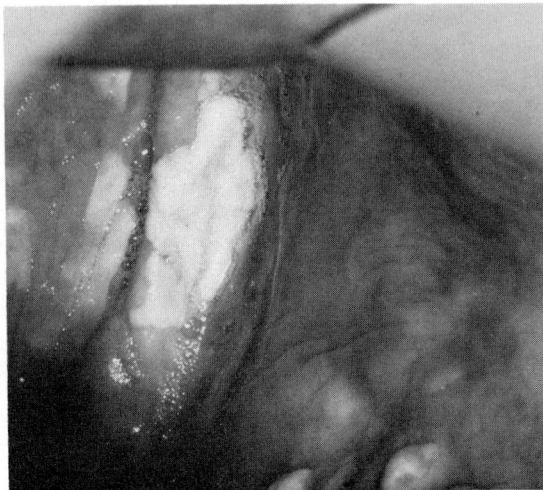

Fig. 27.15. Leukoplakia

Lichen Planus: A disease of unknown etiology affecting either skin or oral mucous membranes, sometimes both together. The oral lesion appears on the buccal mucous membrane most commonly, a lacy pattern of raised bluish-white or white porcelainlike fine lines or dots. Painless and harmless. Distinguished from leukoplakia by biopsy (the removal of a small tissue sample from the suspect area for the purpose of microscopic examination).

Malignant Neoplasms (cancer): Can occur in the mouth. Lesions suspected of being malignant are biopsied by the dentist and sent to a pathologist for microscopic examination.

Mottled Enamel: Due to excessive intake of fluoride during tooth development. See *fluorosis* in Glossary.

Mucocele: A dilated gland or duct filled with mucous secretion.

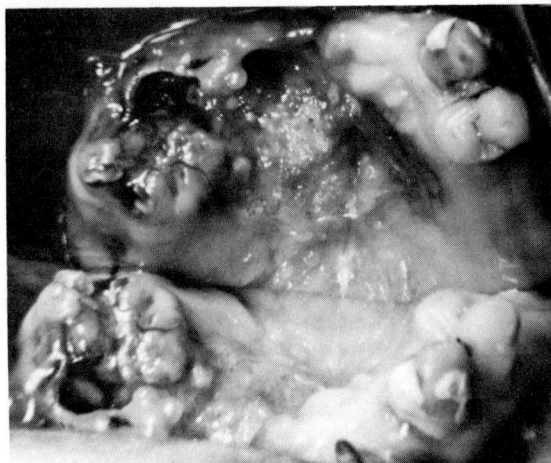

Fig. 27.16. Malignancy

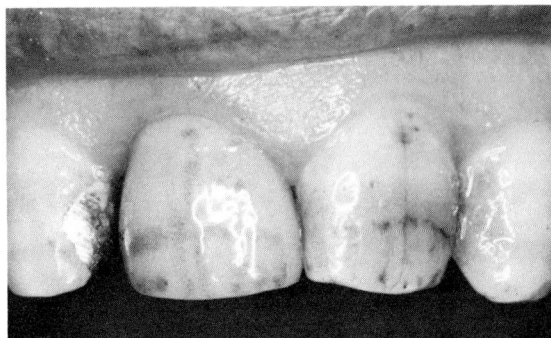

Fig. 27.17. Mottled enamel

Necrotizing Ulcerative Gingivitis: (Vincent's *gingivitis*): A periodontal disease. The gingival tissues are puffy, red, very painful, and bleed easily. The interdental papillae are gray, necrotic, and contribute to a very foul breath. The patient usually has an elevated temperature and feels sick.

Nevus: A congenital malformation seen occasionally on the oral mucosa; can be vascular (similar to a birthmark) or nonvascular with pigmentation. Some types can develop into malignancies.

Papuloma: A benign neoplasm made up of epithelial cells, warty in appearance.

Periodontitis: Inflammation of the tissues that surround and support the teeth—the gingivae, the cementum of the tooth, the periodontal membrane, and the alveolar and supporting bone.

Periodontosis (diffuse alveolar atrophy): A noninflammatory condition affecting the tissues listed under periodontitis in which the fibers of the periodontal membranes degenerate, alveolar bone is resorbed, and the epithelial attachment is proliferated along the root surfaces. The end result of the process is the loosening and moving of teeth.

Radiation Necrosis: Death of tissue caused by radiation. If treatment of carcinoma (cancer) of the throat, mouth, or lip is undertaken by means of X rays or cobalt, heavy destruction of bone and teeth with formation of a sequestrum (piece of dead bone, usually being expelled from the body) is generally one result. The destruction is apparently more easily controlled when teeth, if present in the area of treatment, are removed prior to exposure if possible.

Residual Cyst: An odontogenic cyst that remains within the jaw after the tooth with which it was associated has been removed.

Sialolithiasis: The formation of salivary calculi within the ducts of the salivary glands, or the condition or infection caused by such formation.

Stomatitis: A general term for inflammation of the oral cavity which may occur from bacterial, viral, mechanical, chemical, electrical, thermal, or radiation injury, from allergens, and as secondary (in sequence of time or development) manifestation of a systemic disease. May also occur as a reaction to medications or irritants, or systemic changes such as pregnancy. In the case of pregnancy it is often referred to as *pregnancy stomatitis,* and at this time a patient may also exhibit a gingivitis

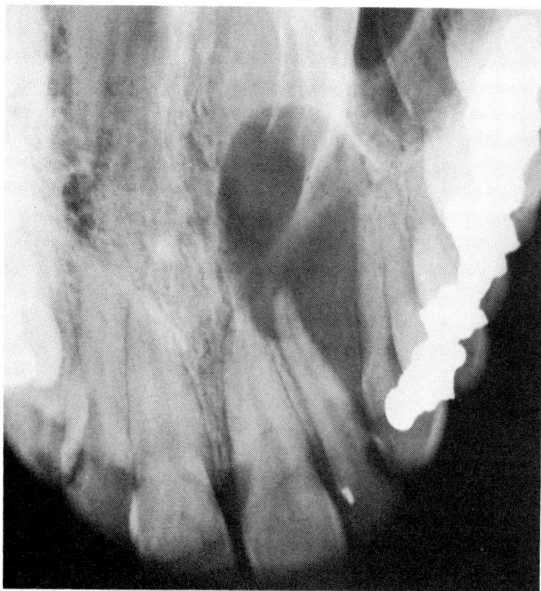

Fig. 27.18. Root-end cyst of maxilla

with hypertrophy of the gums, and occasionally develop a "pregnancy tumor" on the gingiva. Such pregnancy tumors are easily removed.

Thrush (moniliasis): A disease caused by the yeastlike *Candida albicans,* characterized by white, curdy, raised patches which can be scraped off, leaving a base which bleeds.

Trauma: Trauma to the oral cavity is manifested in a variety of ways; from lacerated, swollen, soft tissue damage through fractures of the teeth and supporting structures.

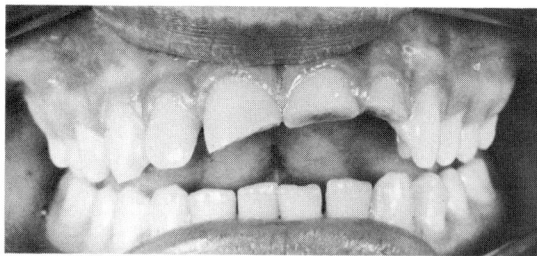

Fig. 27.19. Traumatic injury

Dental Caries

Dental caries, which you may have called "decay" until now, is a disease which is present in almost everyone's teeth at some time or other. It can begin at a very early age—as soon as the primary teeth begin to appear in the mouth. In some cases of an extremely active degree of dental caries, called "rampant" caries, the primary teeth have been destroyed by three or four years of age.

What is dental caries? It is a disease process which attacks the hard tissues of the teeth, demineralizing and eventually destroying these hard tissues through loss of both organic and inorganic elements. Its exact cause is not known.

In the process of eating we deposit a considerable amount of food debris in the nooks and crannies around our teeth, as well as over some of the flatter surfaces in certain areas. We also know that we do have bacteria in our mouths in considerable numbers. These bacteria cover various areas of the teeth in what is called a *bacterial plaque*, a filmlike cover-

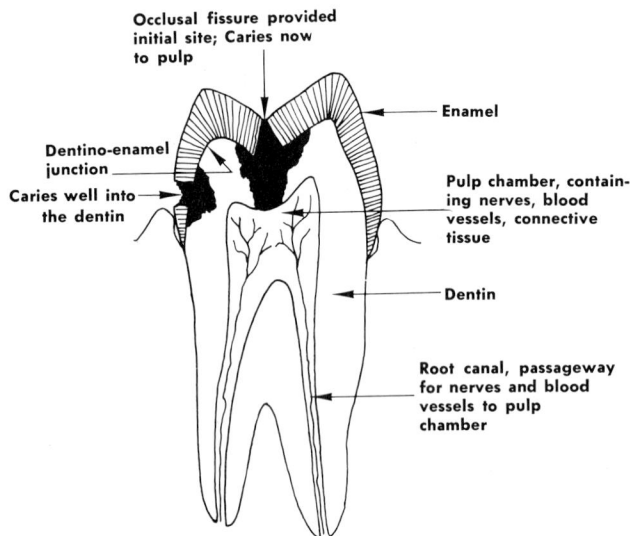

Fig. 27.20. Schematic illustration of the progress of dental caries.

ing which is often very difficult to see in a well-kept mouth. However, if we should paint the teeth with a dye, such as a five percent basic fuchsin or a one percent Mercurochrome solution, then rinse the mouth well with water, the bacterial plaques will become stained with dye and be easily visible.[1] An area of the tooth which is really clean and not covered with a bacterial plaque will not retain the dye. In the average well-kept mouth, even one which is scrupulously clean to all appearances, these bacterial plaques will be made visible most commonly in that area of each tooth which is close to the gum, tending to encircle the tooth and broadening in the area toward a neighboring tooth.

Most authorities think that the enzymes produced by the bacteria which provide the plaque cause an action on fermentable carbohydrate foods, forming relatively weak acids in the process, during and following eating. This production of acid proceeds rather quickly. Experimentally, it is apparent within ninety seconds after placing a ten percent solution of glucose (a simple sugar) in the mouth. It can reach its maximum formation within thirty minutes and may be hard to detect again after an hour.

When a certain level of acidity is reached, the acids are thought to cause a demineralization of the enamel, which produces an opaque white spot in the enamel substance. This acid-forming cycle is repeated whenever more fermentable material is brought into the plaque. The process is indicated first by this opaque white area, then by a loss in hardness of the enamel, then by the indication which everyone recognizes—cavitation, or the formation of a cavity in the tooth. This, if allowed to proceed

1. Sumter S. Arnim, "Dental Caries, October 1953," *Minneapolis Dist. Dent. J.* 37 (December 1953): 4; "The Present-Day Concept of Caries Based on Clinical Data and the Most Fruitful Approach to the Prevention and Control of the Condition," *Int'l. J. Orth. and Oral Surg.* 23 (October 1937): 1045.

farther, causes a discoloration of the surrounding area and eventually, although not always, results in pain.

Pain may occur when the advance of caries first reaches the dentino-enamel junction,

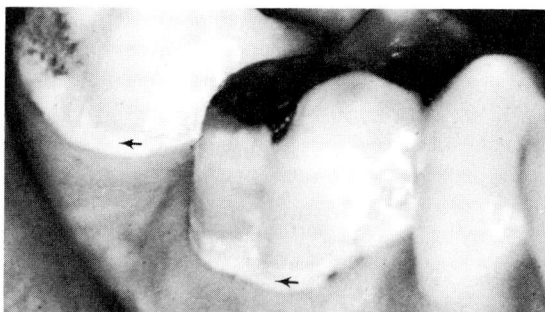

Fig. 27.21. Decalcification of enamel

where it usually is not severe, or when the advancing caries has affected the pulpal tissues at which time the pain is often most severe.

The *Atlas of the Mouth* groups ten stages in the progress of dental caries into four larger classifications:[2] (1) the formation of a small cavity in the enamel of the tooth, frequently detected by X ray; (2) the enlarged cavity beginning to make inroads in the dentin, usually with discoloration present; (3) penetration of the caries process into the pulp chamber, resulting in infection of the pulp; and (4) the formation of a periapical lesion, with the death of the pulp.

2. Maury Massler and Isaac Schour, *Atlas of the Mouth*, page facing plate 19.

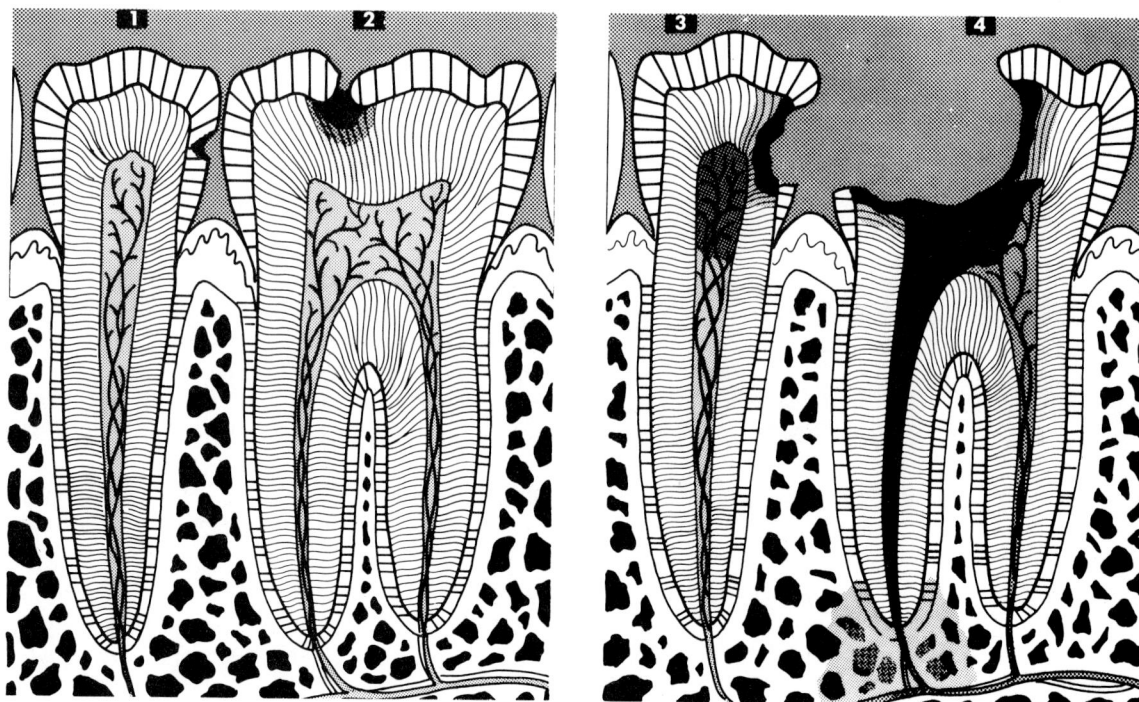

Fig. 27.22. Four stages of dental caries: (1) formation of a small cavity in enamel of the tooth, frequently detected by X ray; (2) enlarged cavity beginning to make inroads in the dentin; (3) penetration of the caries into the pulp chamber, resulting in infection of the pulp; (4) formation of a periapical lesion, with death of the pulp.

Pulp Reaction

If dental caries has penetrated a tooth to any degree, the pulp responds to the irritation so produced by showing certain inflammatory reactions, similar to those described in soft tissue. However, within the tooth secondary dentin forms to protect the pulp. As the caries progresses into the dentin, a mild hyperemia exists as white blood cells are carried to the area. If the caries is allowed to proceed without interruption, the inflammatory reactions become more severe.

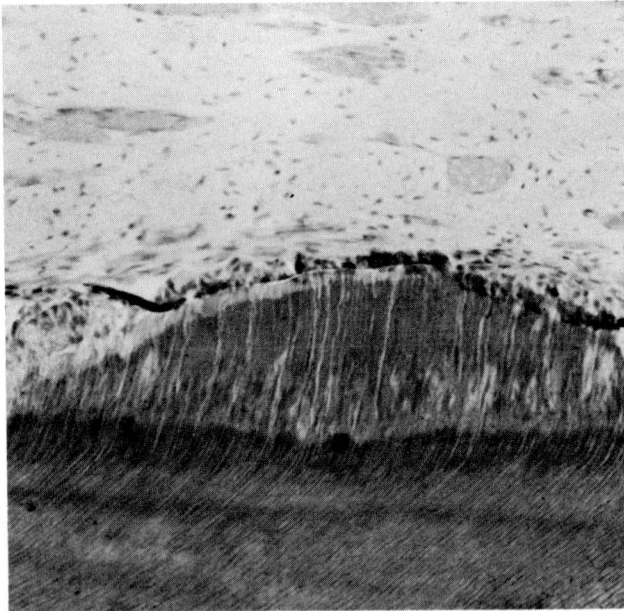

Fig. 27.23. Histological section of secondary dentin

There is one essential difference between the skin on your forearm and the pulp of the tooth in their inflammatory responses. In the case of your forearm, swelling can occur freely. The pulp of the tooth, however, is contained in a definite hard-walled chamber. The effort to swell merely produces pressure on nerves and blood vessels.

The pressure may cause certain reactions: mild toothache (if any toothache is mild to the person who is experiencing it); severe toothache; mild toothache progressing to severe toothache; or an intense toothache, followed by sudden cessation of the pain. First, the capillaries are contained within the hard walls of the canal and pulp chamber. A surge of increased blood pressure in the capillaries occurs. When the pressure created by the hyperemia and edema of the pulpal tissues has made the tooth more sensitive than normal, the pressure of the hyperemia (increase in blood supply) is sometimes sufficient to cause quite severe pain. This is *pulpitis* (toothache).

If the hyperemia proceeds slowly, the pain is usually less severe, often intermittent, as the invasion of bacteria progresses toward the pulp. If the invasion of bacteria and toxins is rapid, an intrapulpal abscess occurs before secondary dentin can form. Death of the pulp tissue progresses to the apex of the root(s). The patient will often give a history of a severe throbbing or pulsating pain which suddenly stopped (upon the death of the pulp). The severe stage is referred to as *acute pulpitis*, which is an advanced inflammatory involvement of the pulp of the tooth. Bacteria have invaded the pulp chambers in numbers. The battle with the white blood cells can extend to an area around the apex of the root, where the early stages of *periapical abscess* formation are now evident.

Periapical Abscess

As the pulpal infection proceeds through the apical foramen into the periapical area, the body defenses through the inflammatory process are usually more capable of containing the bacteria and preventing the spread of the disease.

A root canal containing necrotic, perhaps infected, material acts as a reservoir for toxins which may escape into the periapical area. In this situation, the inflammatory process is not capable of entering the minute apical foramen into the root canal to remove the toxic products and probable bacteria present. The best it can do is attempt to prevent the dissemination of the toxins by walling off the apical foramen with granulation tissue. This tissue will convert to normal periapical tissue or scar tissue when the source of irritation is removed from the root canal.

If the host's defenses are inadequate to counter the virulence of the invading micro-organisms, the pressure of pus and gas will cause increased redness, swelling, heat, and pain. The tooth will be extremely tender, and obviously its function will be impaired. An *acute abscess* exists. The patient seeks immediate relief from the dentist who will open into the pulp chamber and root canal to release the pressure and concomitantly the reason for the pain. On occasion, the swollen area is localized enough as evidenced by a palpable fluid mass in the gum, and relief may be obtained by lancing (fig. 27.25).

The dentist may decide to assist the patient in fighting the infection by prescribing systemic antibiotics. He may also prescribe a medication, such as Darvon or aspirin with codeine, to relieve the intense pain during the early stages of gaining control of the infection.

When infection invades the periapical area, bone is destroyed. Calcified bone is removed during the walling-off process by the inflammation. A definite area of bone loss appears on the X ray as a radiolucency which means the area is darker because the X rays have less bone to travel through than where the bone is complete from outer to inner surface of the alveolar process (fig. 27.18).

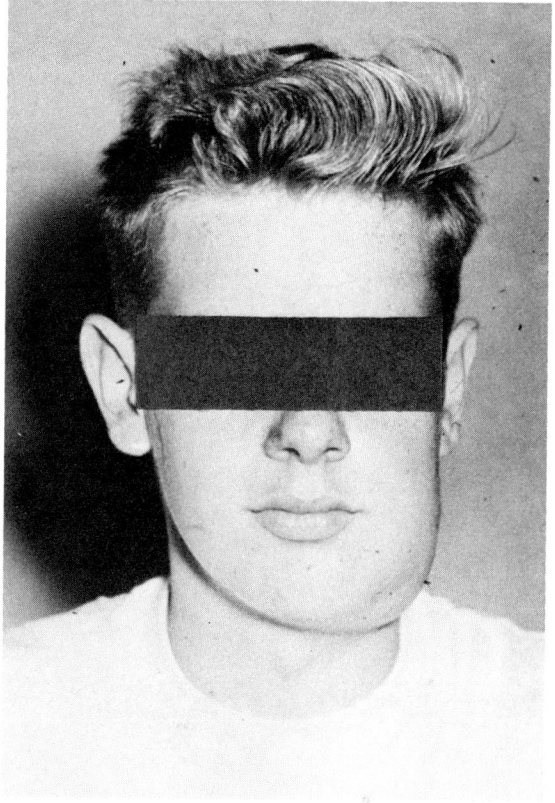

Fig. 27.24. Periapical infection with acute swelling

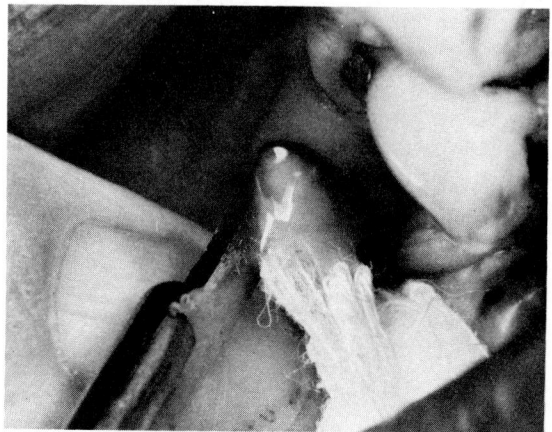

Fig. 27.25. Lancing acute abscess

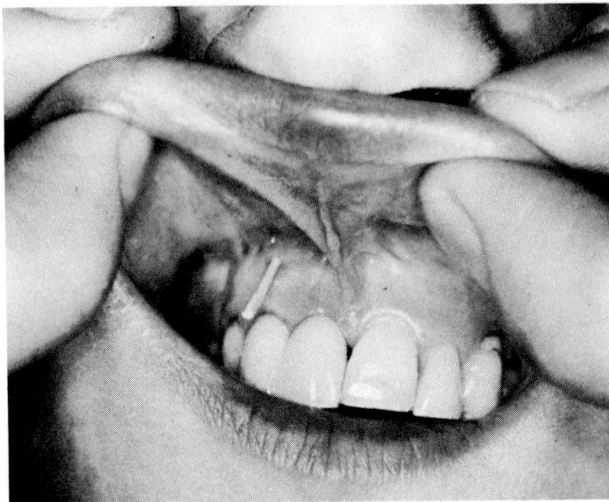

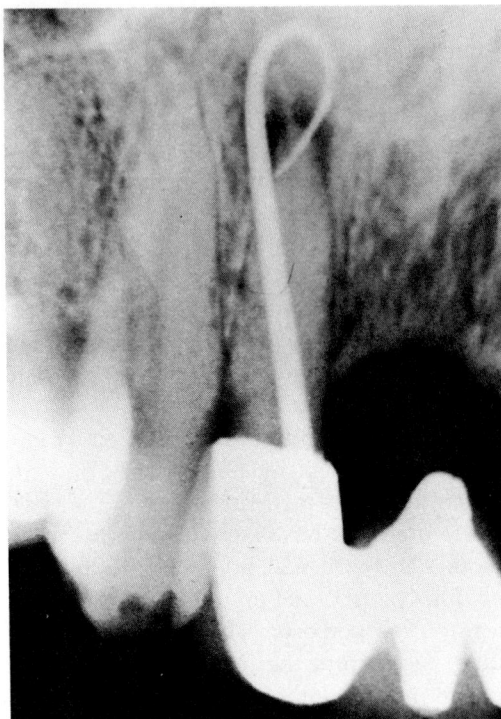

Fig. 27.26. (above) Gutta-percha marker in fistulous tract; (right) X ray of marker in place.

If the body's defenses are fairly evenly balanced with the invading infection, the severe inflammatory reaction does not occur, and an abscess may form without too much concern by the patient. Sometimes a fistula forms, providing drainage of the pus to the outside. While the fistula keeps the tooth comfortable, it does not eliminate the infection. Patients recognize the outer opening of the fistula as a "gum boil" (fig. 27.10).

At times it is necessary to trace the course of the fistulous tract to its source in order to determine which tooth is causing the problem. The dentist inserts a gutta-percha point or wire probe into the tract, and X-rays it in position (fig. 27.26).

Granuloma

The walling off of the periapical infection is usually accomplished by granulation tissue, and consequently, such lesions are called *granulomas*. If the wall of the sac is lined with epithelium, the lesion is called a *cyst*. If a tooth bearing a cyst is extracted and the cyst remains in the jaw, it is called a *residual cyst*.

With few exceptions, the chronic periapical conditions discovered during routine radiographic examination are granulomas (fig. 27.28). The patient may give a history of toothache of short duration which he thought did not require dental attention; or the death of the pulp and its extension periapically may have been so gradual that the patient was unaware of any serious trouble.

Since most of the lesions which wall off root ends with infected pulp canals are granulomas, a more detailed description of their microscopic structure is important for the dental assistant to more fully understand the problem involved and the dentist's treatment of the problem.

Fish presented an excellent means of describing the periapical granuloma by dividing the area into four zones:[3]

1. infection,
2. contamination,
3. irritation, and
4. stimulation.

Figure 27.27 shows a diagram of a root canal which contains necrotic and probably infected tissue. The necrotic area may be infected with organisms which gained entrance to the canal through a carious lesion, a pulp exposure caused by trauma, or perhaps through a transient bacteremia which may have allowed bacteria to have access to an area of low resistance

3. E. W. Fish, "Bone Infection," *J.A.D.A.* 26 (May 1939): 691-712.

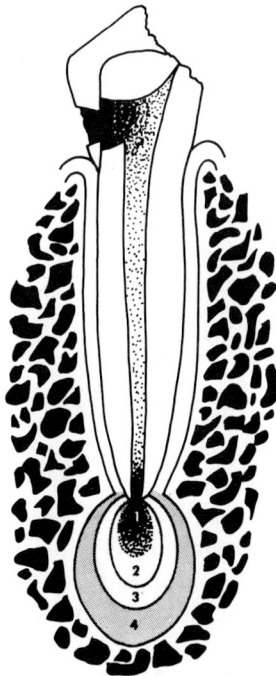

within the pulp tissue. On the other hand, the tooth may have been traumatized without fracture but with subsequent death of the pulp. In such cases, the pulp may not demonstrate microorganisms by routine culturing methods. Whether the toxins are produced by bacteria or break-down products of decomposed tissue, they have an irritating effect on periapical tissues.

1. The *zone of infection* is the area adjacent to the apical foramen. It represents an area in which the toxins exuding from the root canal are in their most concentrated state. Microorganisms may also be present. The microscopic picture is that of acute inflammation, with PMNs (a type of leukocyte) and macrophages dominat-

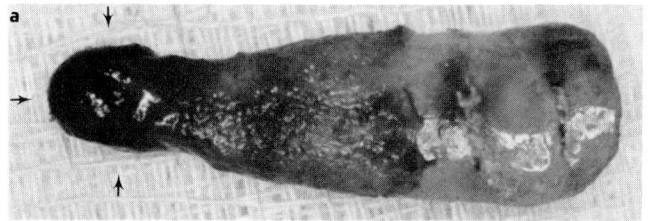

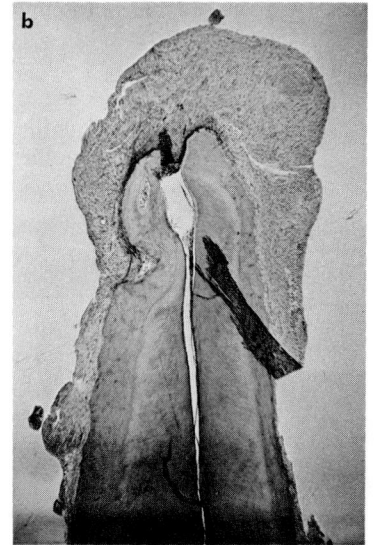

Fig. 27.27. Four zones of a periapical granuloma as described by Fish: (1) infection, (2) contamination, (3) irritation, (4) stimulation.

Fig. 27.28. Cross-specimen of tooth with sac on apex.

ing the scene. The function of the PMNs is to devour any bacteria present. The macrophages reinforce the PMNs in attacking bacteria and remove the debris from the area.

2. In the *zone of contamination,* the toxins are becoming diluted by the exudate from the blood. (*Exudate* means fluid oozing out.) Microscopically, this area presents a picture of chronic inflammation with lymphocytes and plasma cells predominating.

3. The *zone of irritation* is still farther from the source, and the toxins become more dilute. Their effectiveness may be reduced to that of a mild irritant. Osteoclasts may be found attacking the bone. (An osteoclast absorbs and removes bone.)

4. In the fourth zone, the *zone of stimulation,* the toxins are so dilute that they act as a stimulant to osteoblasts and fibroblasts, whose respective functions are to build new bone and tissue. Thus, there is present an active core of inflammation which gradually changes to an area of healing at the periphery as the toxins become diluted and lose their destructive effectiveness.

When a well-organized granuloma is present, an area of healing exists which would require only the removal of the source of irritation within the root canal to allow complete regeneration of periapical bone and periodontal membrane. The principle of intracanal therapy for periapically involved teeth is based on this premise.

The virulence of the toxins may be very close to the threshold of defensibility of the inflammatory process and held in check by only a small margin. The histologic picture may show a thin peripheral sac of granulation tissue filled with purulent material. Although proper intracanal therapy should remove the irritant inaccessible to the inflammatory process and allow periapical regeneration, this purulent mass may be self-sustaining and require intervention. Such residual infections have been observed following intracanal therapy, or following extraction of teeth where such periapical areas have not been properly curetted at the same time as tooth removal. Unfortunately, it is impossible to diagnose the histologic condition without viewing prepared sections of the tissue under a microscope.

If toxins exuding from the root canal are highly virulent (extremely poisonous) and maintain or increase their strength, the area will become larger. However, if the virulence is reduced, the condition will become static, and granulation tissue will make up the bulk of the lesion.

An acute apical abscess is entirely made up of the zone of infection, while the disease is actively spreading. When the inflammatory process becomes effective in counteracting the infection, the zones of irritation and stimulation become established.

Periodontitis

Periodontitis is an advanced stage of gingivitis, affecting the tissue supporting the teeth. As the disease progresses, the periodontal membrane is destroyed and alveolar bone is resorbed forming a *pocket.* If not treated with success, the teeth or tooth involved will lose so much support that a periodontal abscess may form or removal of the tooth may eventually become necessary. This disease is commonly referred to as "pyorrhea." It is preventable if attention is given to the first signs of poor oral health. It is treatable provided sufficient tissue remains to support the tooth—if the causative factors are corrected first.

Periodontosis, or diffuse alveolar atrophy, is a degenerative disease the end result of which is similar to that of periodontitis. Simplifying their differences to some extent, we might say that periodontosis is similar to periodontitis except for the lack of inflammatory reactions.

Control of Dental Caries

In any disease, many people are inclined to look for assistance or cure in a "tube" of this, a "bottle" of that, or a "shot" of some wonder drug to banish the difficulty. This is true in respect to dental caries as well.

Dental caries can only be corrected by the use of dental restorations. Teeth which have been damaged by dental caries cannot repair themselves. Caries *activity*, however, can be strongly influenced by personal habits. A correction of dietary habits combined with an improvement in oral hygiene can and does work wonders with the majority of individuals. This does not have particularly wide appeal because it does not consist of a "tube," a "bottle," or a "shot"—just the application of time and effort. This application often falls victim to the lethargy of which we are all guilty to some degree.

Fluoride in community drinking water has proved its usefulness in reducing the incidence of dental caries. The direct application of stannous fluoride to teeth has also proved dramatically effective. These methods are only helpful, however, if we exercise control of other areas of strong influence such as oral hygiene and diet control at the same time. "The most successful method today of keeping our own natural teeth is simply good oral hygiene."[4]

With a better understanding of the significance of the attachment of dental plaque in relatively thick, large masses, and the rapidity with which these organisms with their enzymes can produce acid within the plaque, oral hygiene can be made more effective than before. *First, the plaque must be removed at least daily.* This involves proper toothbrush technique and the proper use of dental floss. The use of both must be carefully taught the patient. *Secondly, food must be removed from the mouth as soon as possible after eating,* remembering the time element in the production of acid within the plaque. This removal of food can be accomplished by eating coarser foods last, rather than finishing with a dessert. Thorough rinsing and the use of toothbrush and dental floss are also helpful. The chewing of a small piece of paraffin wax or sugar-free gum immediately after eating is a good detergent, aiding in cleansing the teeth and in stimulating flow of saliva which dilutes and washes away food residue from tooth surfaces. (See chap. 29.)

Diet for Control of Caries

Some individuals have an unusually high degree of susceptibility to dental decay. These people should adhere rigidly to a special diet for the reduction of decay. If the problem is less serious, they may follow the diet less strictly, remembering that its extreme form is intended for individuals with a very high rate of decay.

Food habits in general warrant a careful scrutiny to improve general nutrition as well as to limit or eliminate foods which are high in refined starches and sugars. Sumter S. Arnim, D.D.S., Ph.D., of the University of Texas, Dental Branch, has suggested a dietary regime for caries control, which is given here. The patient's physician should be consulted before the dietary change is made in case any item should be restricted or omitted. In the list of foods to be included each day, the amount indicated is a minimum; the patient may use as much as he wants. The value of raw fruits and vegetables, such as celery, carrot, or apple, taken at the end of the meal should be stressed.

---

4. Hussein A. Zaki et al., *Clean Teeth Brighten Your Smile*, p. 1.

INCLUDE DAILY:

One pint of milk—whole, skim, or buttermilk.
One egg.
Vegetables, especially leafy greens and yellow.
  A raw one daily.
Potato—cooked in the skin is best.
Butter or substitutes, enriched margarine.
Cream, cheese, other fats.
Lean meats, poultry, fish, liver.
Fresh fruits, or unsweetened fruit juice, canned
  or fresh.
Citrus fruits.

LIMIT:

Bread to 1 or 2 slices a meal. At least half
  should be whole wheat.
Biscuits to one a day.
Cereals to one serving a day—cooked are best.
Hot breads to one piece, if made without sugar.

PREFERABLY OMIT OR GREATLY RESTRICT:

Sugar, syrups, molasses, jams, jellies, preserves,
  honey, candy, soft drinks, sundaes, ice
  cream, sherbet, milk shakes, sodas, cookies,
  crackers, cakes, pastries.
Fruits canned or prepared with sugar.
Salad dressings (purchased) with sugar or
  starch.
Sweet pickles, ketchup, chili sauce.

GENERAL SUGGESTIONS:

1. Use no sugar-sweetened chewing gum. It
   contains one-half teaspoonful sugar to the
   stick. Sugar-free gums following meals may
   be helpful.
2. Finish your meal with a piece of raw fruit
   or a raw vegetable, such as celery, carrot,
   apple, or orange.
3. Substitute oranges, apples, and other fresh
   fruits or vegetables for that in-between-
   meal snack that so often consists of candy,
   sweet carbonated beverage, cake, peanut
   butter and jelly sandwich. Natural cheeses
   contain minerals and vitamins as well as
   the needed calories that tend to develop

strong, healthy individuals. It should be
noted that many "process" cheeses contain
sugar.

The most successful method of stopping
carious lesions is the use of restorations. Restorations have served for many, many years as
effective agents for controlling the ravages of
this disease. When the diseased portion of the
tooth is surgically removed by the dentist and
the remaining tooth substance correctly prepared to receive a restoration, and that restoration is placed, one may safely assume that
the carious process has been stopped. Unfortunately, that portion of the tooth which has
not been protected with a restoration is still
susceptible to dental caries.

Careful mouth examinations, with X rays,
at regular intervals are necessary for early
diagnosis. It is especially important that we
instruct our patients (and follow our own advice) to have all carious lesions treated as soon
as we detect them. It is the dentist's responsibility to prevent the ravages of this universal
disease by using all means at his disposal:

> *Early Diagnosis,*
> *Preventive Measures,* and
> *Restorations Properly Made.*

Summary

Oral pathology is a study of the diseases of
the mouth.

Inflammation is the body's defense against
injury and disease. The cardinal symptoms of
inflammation are redness, swelling, heat, pain,
and impairment of function.

Diagnosis of oral pathology is not simple.
There are clinical and differential diagnoses.
A number of conditions which are pathological are commonly observed in the dental office. Learn them from your text.

Dental caries is decay. The four stages of
progress of dental caries are (1) formation of

a small cavity in the enamel of the tooth, (2) enlarged cavity beginning to make inroads in the dentin, (3) penetration of the caries process into the pulp chamber, resulting in infection of the pulp, and (4) formation of a periapical lesion with the death of the pulp.

The pulp responds to irritation of caries and if neglected can result in periapical abscess and granuloma.

Periapical granuloma is described by dividing the area into four zones: (1) infection, (2) contamination, (3) irritation, and (4) stimulation.

Periodontitis is an advanced stage of gingivitis.

Dental caries can be controlled by daily removal of plaque, removal of food from the mouth as soon as possible after eating, eating proper foods, and having careful examinations at regular intervals, followed by adequate care of any diseased areas.

The dentist's responsibility is to prevent the ravages of caries by means of early diagnosis, preventive measures, and restorations properly made.

Study Questions

1. Describe inflammation.
2. Familiarize yourself with the definition of oral pathologic conditions described in this chapter.
3. Describe caries and explain how and why it occurs.
4. Describe pulp reaction to dental caries.
5. Describe a periapical granuloma, dividing the area into Fish's four zones. Clarify each zone.
6. What is periodontitis?
7. What is the best method of keeping your natural teeth?
8. What is the most successful method of stopping carious lesions?
9. What means for preventing caries does the dentist use?

Bibliography

JENSEN, JAMES R., and SERENE, THOMAS P. *Fundamentals of Clinical Endodontics.* Dubuque, Ia.: K/H Publishing Co., 1972.

MASSLER, MAURY, and SCHOUR, ISAAC. *Atlas of the Mouth.* 2nd ed. Chicago: American Dental Association, 1958.

ZAKI, HUSSEIN A.; BANDT, CARL I.; and FOLKE, LARS E. A. *Clean Teeth Brighten Your Smile.* Minneapolis, Minn.: University of Minnesota Press, 1971.

28 Drugs, First Aid, and Emergency Care in the Dental Office

Drugs in the Dental Office

A *drug* is any substance which is used as a medicine.

While many people tend to associate all manner of evils with the word *drug*—usually thinking of drug addicts and drug addiction—in its true meaning it is used to indicate those substances which are used to help mankind fight disease.

It is true, however, that many drugs are helpful when used in prescribed quantity but act as poisons if used in an excessive quantity. It is also true that many drugs are helpful when used for one purpose and become very dangerous if used for another purpose.

Learn to exercise care in all procedures in which you use or dispense drugs upon the order or instruction of your dentist.

Your dentist has received training in pharmacology—the science which deals with the nature, properties, and use of drugs—which is required by law. He is, therefore, the one person in the dental office who is qualified and licensed to prescribe drugs for use by your patients. It is your obligation to follow his instructions exactly and carefully.

Should you discover that you cannot remember how much premedication you are to give a patient, *do not guess.* If you find that you do not know for certain what is used to refill the topical anesthetic bottle in the instrument cabinet, *do not guess.* Ask your dentist. *Be certain.*

If you wish to broaden your knowledge of pharmacology as it applies to the practice of dentistry, one of the books most commonly available in any dental office is *Accepted Dental Therapeutics,* which is published annually by the American Dental Association. It lists commercial products which are currently accepted by the Council on Dental Therapeutics and describes nearly all the official and non-official therapeutic items which are of demonstrated usefulness in dental practice. It well deserves your study because of its specific and thorough application to dental practice.

Throughout this book you will find comments regarding drugs and medications used in various situations in the dental office. "Sterilization," "Anesthesia," and "First Aid and Emergency Care" make use of many of the more common drugs in dental practice. Medications dispensed directly to the patient for use prior to an appointment, or for use at the conclusion of an appointment, make up a number of contacts with drugs requiring the greatest care.

If you are instructed to give a patient a preoperative medication to be taken at home before the next appointment, place that medication in a small "drug" envelope with *instructions clearly written* on the envelope regarding the time at which the medication is to be taken. When handing this envelope to the patient, repeat the instructions. If the medication is in capsule form, mention that the capsule is to be taken with water. Occasionally you will find individuals whose experience with medications is so limited that they will not be quite sure whether the capsule is to be taken apart to make the powder available or whether the capsule itself is safe to swallow. Be sure the patient understands completely.

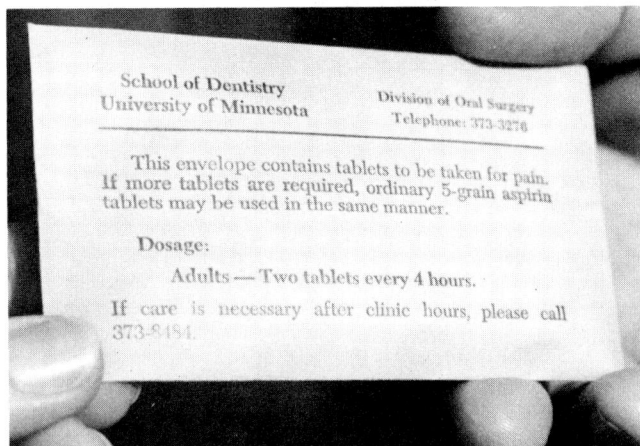

Fig. 28.1. Envelope with instructions handed to patient.

This medication should be noted on the patient's record.

If you are instructed to give a patient a medication in the dental office, for example an APC tablet, place that medication in a disposable paper cup. In a second disposable cup bring water for the patient's use in swallowing the tablet, holding the cup near its bottom rather than at the upper edge where the patient's lips will be placed in drinking. You say to the patient, "I am going to give you a pill. Will you hold out your hand, please?"

You then pour the tablet from the paper cup into the palm of the patient's hand, and at the same time extend your hand with the cup of water so that the patient may take the cup easily with his free hand.

Stand by the patient to be sure that the medication is taken as requested. Occasionally the patient will question the purpose or kind of medication given. Refer the question to the dentist.

Remember that drugs or medications can be dangerous. Never be careless in handling or working with them. *Keep labels in good condition at all times. Do not guess.*

Most drugs used in dentistry are prescribed by the dentist as a written order or prescription to the pharmacist who supplies the medication for the patient. There are, however, many preparations used in the office during the treatment of the patient, such as anesthetics, disinfectants, surgical dressings, medicated cements, irrigating solutions, desensitizing pastes and solutions, cauterizing agents, and many topical and systemic drugs, which must be carefully handled and monitored. Some solutions may be caustic if carelessly placed or may stain skin and clothing if spilled. Learn to respect these drugs for what they can offer in the treatment of patients as well as for the problems they can create if misused. For further information of the specific use of drugs in the practice of dentistry, consult *Accepted Dental Therapeutics,* published by the American Dental Association. It is an excellent compendium[1] of acceptable brands of drugs used in dentistry.

First Aid and Emergency Care

The dental assistant's association with a health profession makes it desirable for her to have formal training in first aid. The American Red Cross courses are most commonly available.

Certain types of emergencies are more common in a dental office. Recognition of these emergencies should be developed. For example, if a patient begins to faint, your dentist might have his back turned at the moment, and your quick attention may prevent the patient from losing consciousness.

What you are permitted to do for emergency care will depend on your dentist. For example, it is nice to know that a pressure pack

1. A compendium is a summary of knowledge of a specific field. It gathers together and presents in concise or in outline form all the essential facts and details of a subject.

in a tooth socket will help clotting and reduce hemorrhaging, but legally only the dentist or the patient himself can place that pack in the socket. The more likely emergencies which may be encountered in the dental office are syncopé (fainting), several forms of shock, procaine allergies, hypertension, hemorrhage, convulsions, and respiratory failure.

Dental procedures are the source of considerable tension and strain to some patients. If the patient is in good health, as are the majority of patients who come to the dental office, these stresses and strains may not bring on any unusual symptoms. However, every dental office will, at times, have a patient who suffers a reaction, from one cause or another, which requires that the patient be handled properly and quickly to prevent serious consequences. It is most important that the type of disturbance and its cause be recognized as early as possible. This is necessary in order that difficulties which are not serious may be recognized as such, and difficulties which *are* serious may be handled with due regard for the responsibilities involved.

In any emergency a primary attempt should be made to call the attention of the dentist to the problem. If the dentist is not available, procure medical assistance as rapidly as possible *after* taking the necessary preliminary precautions required by the condition of the patient.

Syncopé (*Fainting*)

The term *syncopé* refers to a sudden lack of circulation of blood to the brain. The most common conditions which are likely to cause syncopé (fainting) are fear, emotional disturbance, and pain. The lack of circulation is the result of a temporary lowering of the pulse pressure, which creates a shortage of blood supplied to the brain. A feeling of uneasiness and lightheadedness usually precedes the actual syncopé, or faint.

The picture of syncopé is quite startling. The skin is pale, cool, and clammy. The pupils are dilated and do not become smaller when in a strong light. Pulse pressure is weak, and respiration is slow, feeble, and irregular.

Usually the patient will indicate when he feels faint. Where the patient is will determine your action. If he is already in the dental chair, lower the backrest to a horizontal position so that the head is level with, or lower than, the body, as in the Trendelenburg position. A cold towel should be placed on his forehead. This may keep the patient from losing consciousness or allow him to regain consciousness if he has already fainted.

If the patient is in the beginning stages of syncopé and still conscious, his head may be placed between his knees, with his arms hanging loose. Place your hand on the back of his head and instruct the patient to apply upward pressure against your hand with his head, as though attempting to sit up. The patient's exertion will bring blood to the brain quickly and help avoid syncopé. Aromatic spirits of ammonia are furnished in small, cloth-packaged vials. A vial may be broken and briefly held under the patient's nose because the spirits act as a reflex stimulant. Be sure to use it sparingly, as the ammonia is quite strong and will be offensive to the patient.

If the patient happens to be standing and is likely to fall before he can be seated, do not

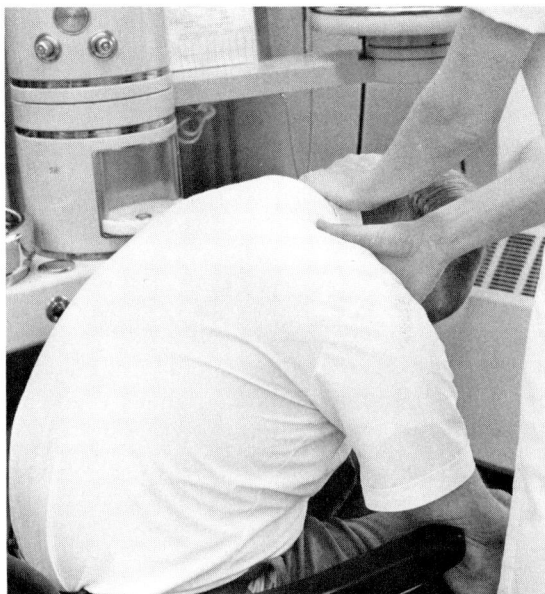

Fig. 28.3. Patient applying upward pressure against dental assistant's hand.

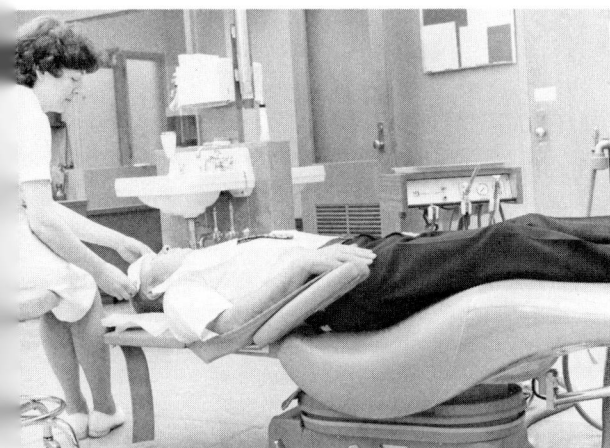

Fig. 28.2. Patient in horizontal position

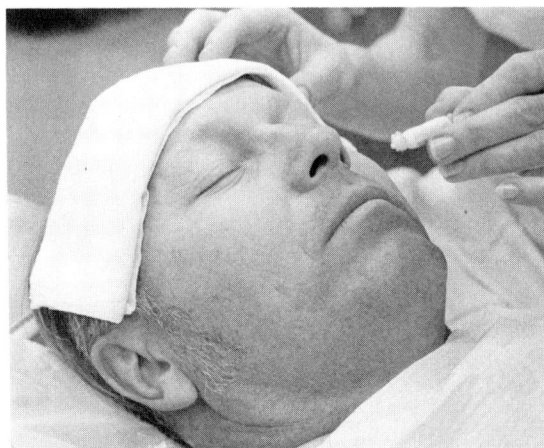

Fig. 28.4. Ammonia being administered

hesitate to have him lie down quickly on the floor.

Tight clothing should be loosened in all cases of syncopé. A short period of oxygen inhalation will be very helpful.

After such recommended treatment for syncopé, the patient may appear to recover quite rapidly but should not be placed in an upright position too quickly, nor should an effort be made to continue dental procedures immediately unless it is necessary. Give the patient sufficient time to readjust to the situation before proceeding. Better overall progress will frequently result.

Circulatory Reactions

Syncopé may be involved in a mild circulatory reaction or in a severe circulatory reaction or collapse. If the reaction is mild, the total effect is usually self-limiting.

Severe circulatory reactions or collapse, however, is extremely serious and requires immediate attention. It may occur with no warning. Circulatory collapse involves cardiac arrest, or stoppage of the heart, and every effort must be made to reinstitute cardiac rhythm rather than to desert the patient and seek medical help.

Learn to feel for a carotid pulse, rather than the usual radial pulse. The radial pulse, if a pulse is present at all, will be too faint to be identifiable; the carotid pulse would be more easily felt. The carotid pulse is best felt just ahead of the sternocleidomastoid muscle in the neck area by depressing the tissues firmly with three fingers held together. If no pulse is detected, promptly feel the chest and, with the ear pressed to the rib cage, listen for a heartbeat. The pupils will not respond to light stimulus, as is also true in milder syncopé.

The dentist will generally have taken charge of the patient, leaving the assistant free to secure medical assistance if the dentist so instructs her. If the dentist is not available,

the assistant must not desert the patient but, rather, must be able to apply the necessary emergency measures. *Circulation must be reestablished within three minutes to avoid irreversible CNS damage.*

Oxygen inhalation or mouth-to-mouth resuscitation should be started at once. Closed chest resuscitation methods can be applied by the dentist while the assistant cares for the breathing.

If cardiac arrest is suspected, the chair should be adjusted so that the unconscious patient is lying horizontal, with the chest supported by the backrest. Begin external cardiac massage by placing the palm of the right hand over the sternum and the left hand on top of the right. The sternum is then depressed one

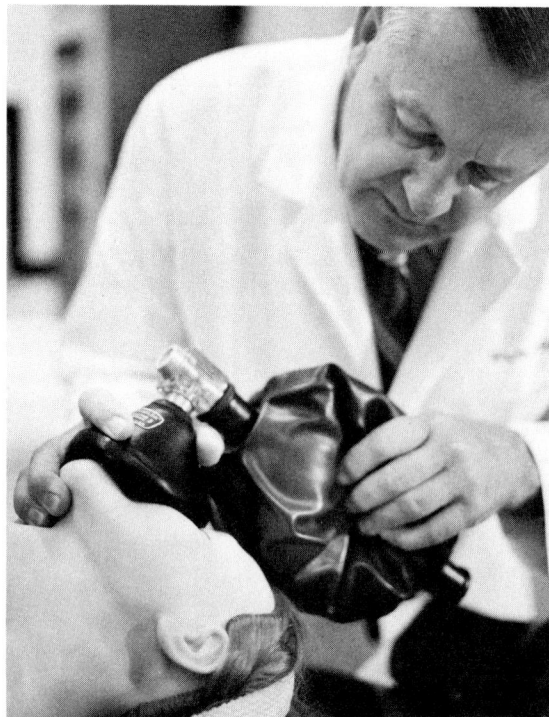

Fig. 28.5. Artificial respiration with a portable respirator demonstrated on model. Chin is pulled upward and forward to pull the tongue forward and maintain an open airway.

and one-half to two inches every second. If the patient is also suffering from pulmonary arrest, necessitating mouth-to-mouth resuscitation, and if you are alone with the patient,

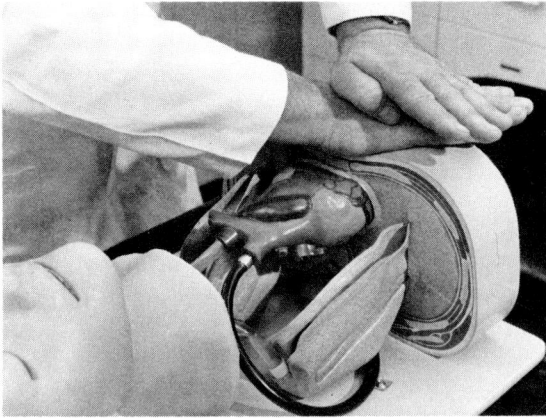

Fig. 28.6. External cardiac massage demonstrated on model to show hand positions and effect of compression on heart. The sternum should be depressed 1 1/2″ to 2″, 45 to 60 times per minute.

compress the sternum fifteen times and give two quick inflations of the lungs through mouth-to-mouth contact. If there are two people available for first aid, the lungs should be inflated after each fifth compression of the sternum. This process should be continued until spontaneous pulse returns.

Mouth-to-Mouth Resuscitation

When a patient suffers pulmonary arrest, the head should be tilted back and the mouth and throat explored with the fingers to remove any mechanical obstructions, such as loose dentures. The aspirator may be used to remove any accumulated fluids which may be obstructing the airway. *If the patient is breathing,* administer oxygen. Inhalation of aromatic ammonia may be used to support the oxygen administration. *If the patient is not breathing,* close the nose with the thumb and forefinger of one hand. With the other hand take a firm grip on the mandible and hold the mouth open.

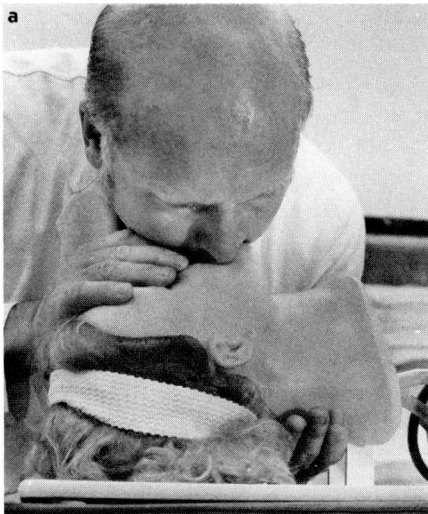

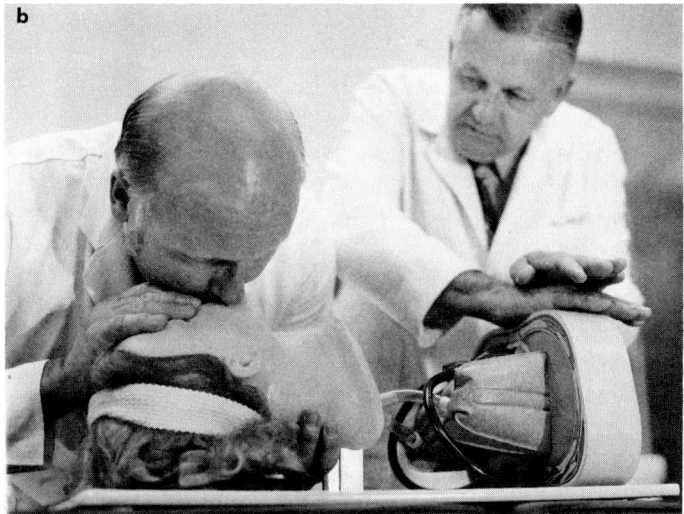

Fig. 28.7. (a) Nasal openings closed by thumb and forefinger of right hand; head tilted up and back with left hand to open air passage; mouth occluded and air forced into lungs by resuscitation. Repeat 12 times per minute for adults, 20 times per minute for children. (b) Combined mouth-to-mouth resuscitation and external cardiac massage demonstrated on model.

The patient's head should be tilted back with the neck fully extended. Lift the lower jaw forcefully upward or lift the neck to accomplish the same purpose. Then cover the patient's mouth completely with your mouth, so that it is airtight, and blow air into the lungs until you visibly see the chest rise. Remove your mouth, let the patient exhale, and repeat the procedure approximately twelve times a minute (twenty for children). When the patient has established his own breathing pattern, oxygen may be administered. Any administration of drugs for cardiac or pulmonary arrest should be done by either the dentist or the physician.

A discussion of procedures and a rehearsal are a desirable part of the training of the entire office staff. If plans are practiced for the various types of emergencies, competent action by the office staff is far more certain.

Convulsions (Adult and Infantile)

Convulsions are irregular, intermittent, and variable muscular contractions involving large areas of the body. Generalized convulsions are usually accompanied by a loss of consciousness. Such seizures are much less common in adults than in children and generally are much more serious in nature. Oxygen should be given for such seizures.

Convulsions may occur in a person who is subject to epileptic seizures. A history of taking Dilantin-sodium or a steady intake of barbiturates is indicative of susceptibility to such seizures. If Dilantin has been taken steadily over a period of time, the soft tissues of the mouth will show a marked hypertrophy (overgrowth), which should arouse suspicion of an epileptic history.

It is possible for some people to have a convulsion without being subject to epileptic seizures. Fever, indigestion, and nutritional deficiency can be causative factors.

A person experiencing such a seizure will frequently gnash his teeth violently and seriously lacerate the tongue and cheeks. A bite block, towel, or other soft object may be held between the jaws to prevent such damage. *Never* put your fingers or hands in the mouth of a person experiencing a seizure. The force of the jaw clenching is great enough to break bones.

The patient should be held in the chair to protect him from flailing his arms, falling, or bumping his head against the dental unit or cabinets, or otherwise harming himself.

A child or an adult known to be subject to epileptic seizure should be premedicated as an aid in prevention.

Regardless of the type of convulsion, keep the patient warm and prevent him from harming himself. No doubt your dentist will contact the patient's physician for whatever instructions the physician deems essential.

Shock

Shock covers a broad range of difficulty. It becomes a matter of degree. A very mild state of shock may produce nothing noticeable in the patient's physical appearance. Severe shock may leave the patient unconscious. Shock can result in symptoms of varying degrees of severity between these two extremes.

It is unusual to see more severe forms of shock than syncopé in the dental office. The rules for treating serious shock are similar to those for care of the person with syncopé. Keep the patient warm and loosen tight items of clothing, such as belts and collars, and call the patient's physician.

Insulin Shock

Diabetic patients can experience a condition known as insulin shock. It is imperative that you immediately call the physician of a patient who is experiencing insulin shock. Records of a diabetic patient should be marked with some arresting color to indicate that this patient is diabetic. The physician's telephone number should be written in bold digits where it can be easily seen in order to facilitate the telephone call which could be necessary to save a life. If a diabetic patient appears to be going into, or is already in, a state of shock, *rush* to phone his physician.

Allergies

Patients should be questioned regarding their possible allergic problems as part of the history when they register in the office. The most positive means of avoiding difficulties is to omit the use of drugs to which the patient reports a previously unfavorable reaction. If they are not sure of their response to proposed drugs, their physician should be consulted. Although allergists do not consider skin sensitivity an absolute indication of hypersensitivity, if the tests *are* positive, some other agent should be used. For example, sensitivity to a local anesthetic is occasionally encountered. With the variety of solutions available today, an alternate choice is no problem.

Chest Pain

If the patient experiences chest pain which persists, adjust the chair so that he is sitting upright, administer oxygen, and call his physician.

Hypertension

The term *hypertension* is used three ways:

1. It means a disease called "essential hypertension."
2. It means a symptom associated with heart-blood vessel-kidney disease.
3. It means a symptom of arteriosclerosis (hardening of the arteries).

Hypertension is an increased blood pressure and is usually uncommon before thirty years of age. A systolic pressure of over 150 mm. of

mercury is suggestive of hypertension, and in severe cases, systolic pressures of over 250 mm. of mercury are not unusual.

The treatment of essential hypertension is aimed more at relief of the symptoms than at curing the disease. Attempts are made to lower the blood pressure to a degree which will minimize the symptoms.

Anything which results in an elevation of blood pressure or causes nervousness should be avoided in hypertensive patients. Premedication will materially reduce nervousness but should be given only if your dentist has given the instructions to do so or has consulted with the physician acquainted with the patient's medical history. The physicians of all hypertensive patients are usually consulted by the dentist before proceeding with extractions or extensive oral surgery.

The usual local anesthetic is not used on these patients because no vasoconstrictive agent should be used. Most local anesthetic solutions are available without a vasoconstrictor and should be kept in stock in the office for use on such patients.

Hemorrhage (Bleeding)

The control of hemorrhage during and following dental surgery may be a problem. Extraction sockets or other surgical sites in the mouth may continue hemorrhaging due to

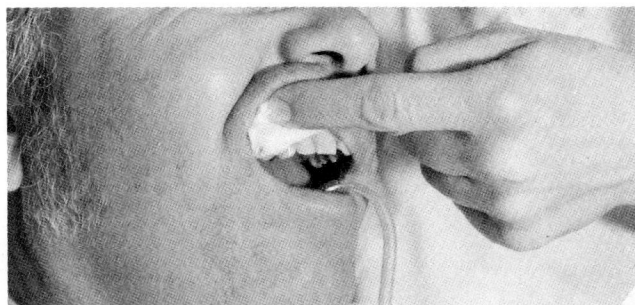

Fig. 28.8. Pressure packing to control hemorrhage

improper clotting or partially severed vessels, either in the bone or soft tissue. Pressure packing by holding gauze over the wound for three to five minutes is the most reliable method of stopping hemorrhage in a patient with normal clotting time. Occasionally it is necessary for the dentist to place additional sutures where indicated at the wound site to tie off the bleeding vessels.

Several hemostatic agents are being used to assist in the clot formation when it is necessary. Oxidized cellulose, a specially treated material which is capable of being gradually dissolved in relatively undamaged or normal tissue, may be placed in the wound and sutured in position. Therefore, when surgery is contemplated, it is very important to have materials for suturing available, as well as the hemostatic agents.

Epistaxis (nosebleed), should it occur to a patient, may be stopped with a large piece of cotton moistened with cold water and packed as high as possible in the nostril. Cold packs on the nose and lifting the head until the nose assumes a horizontal position (not low in relation to the rest of the body) are also helpful. An epinephrine pack might be used for a young person, but definitely not for an older patient, particularly one with any history of a cardiac disturbance.

Summary

Drugs are exceedingly important but potentially dangerous. Learn to exercise care in all procedures in which you use or dispense drugs. Be certain about the use of each drug. Do not guess. Follow the accepted procedures for dispensing drugs and be certain that your patient takes the drugs you are directed to give him.

It is wise for a dental assistant to have formal first aid training. Certain emergencies which can arise in the dental office need accurate and prompt care. You should know what to do for syncopé, circulatory reaction, respiratory reaction, convulsion, shock, procaine allergy, hypertension, and hemorrhage,

Study Questions

1. Discuss the values and dangers of drugs.
2. Why must you keep labels in good condition so that you know what is in containers?
3. Describe the following emergencies and explain the dental assistant's role in meeting them:

syncopé	circulatory restriction
cardiac arrest	chest pain
convulsions	hemorrhage
shock	epistaxis
allergies	

4. What is hypertension?

Bibliography

Accepted Dental Therapeutics. 34th ed. Chicago: American Dental Association, 1972.

BEESON, P. B., and McDERMOTT, W., eds. *Cecil-Loeb Textbook of Medicine.* 11th ed. Philadelphia: W. B. Saunders Co., 1963.

BERLONE, I. J. *Dental and Medical Emergencies and Complications.* 1st ed. Chicago: Yearbook Publishers, 1959.

BURKETT, L. W. *Oral Medicine.* Philadelphia: J. B. Lippincott Co., 1961.

JACKSON, C., and JACKSON, C. L. *Diseases of Nose, Throat, and Ear.* 2nd ed. Philadelphia: W. B. Saunders Co., 1959.

LITWIN, R. I., and SNEDDON, E. H. "A Simplified Approach to Cardiac Arrest." *Oral Surg.* 14 (November 1961): 1283.

PANUSKA, HAROLD J. "Dental Office and Hospital Emergencies." *Northwest Dentistry* 41, no. 3 (May-June 1962): 157-159.

29 | *Personal Oral Hygiene*

Oral Hygiene

For decades the dental profession attempted to care for oral health needs with a treatment-oriented philosophy and practice.

We have seen that treatment alone cannot save teeth. Dental decay and periodontal disease destroy the teeth and their supporting structures faster than the nation's dentists can treat them.

Dental researchers have proved that sound preventive practices coupled with good restorative treatment is the only way adequate health care can be achieved. Proper oral hygiene and toothbrush technique form the foundation for those sound preventive practices.

The dental health team must accept the responsibility for patient education in *Personal Oral Hygiene* in addition to the long-recognized responsibilities for

1. *restoration* of all carious, defective, or missing teeth,
2. *preservation* of the soft tissues and supporting structures, and
3. *maintenance* of the dental arches in a healthy state of function and aesthetics.

Frequently, too little attention has been given to POH education: teaching the patient how to give his mouth the correct daily care which is so important in maintaining good oral health.

It is also necessary to motivate him to continue his home care treatment.

Teaching the dental patient proper home care is a responsibility which should be and is delegated to the dental assistant. In order to teach the patient, the methods of home care must be learned and practiced by the dental assistant. Some of the basic information will be discussed here, but it must be emphasized that there are many ways to accomplish the same objective. Each dentist may have a somewhat different method he will wish to teach. The methods of brushing the teeth and the types of brush to use are subject to variation.

Plaque

The salivary glands (the parotids, the submaxillary, and the sublingual glands) produce a clear, alkaline, and usually viscid (to a greater or lesser degree) fluid called saliva. The saliva enters the mouth in three general areas: one in each cheek approximately opposite the buccal surface of the upper first or second molars and another in the floor of the mouth nearest the lower anterior teeth. Mucous glands, which are present wherever there is a mucous membrane—the lining of the mouth—add their mucous secretion. Saliva contains the enzyme called ptyalin which begins the conversion of starches in food to maltose (a sugar). Saliva also contains serum-albumin, globulin, and cell debris.

A yellow-white sticky substance, *mucin,* is a precipitate of saliva which combines with bacteria, food, and cell debris in the mouth to form a gelatinlike layer on those surfaces of the teeth which are somewhat sheltered. The surfaces which are constantly rubbed by the tongue, lips, or cheeks, or are scoured in the process of chewing food, do not accumulate this gelatinous layer which is called a *bacterial plaque.*

Plaque is the principal cause of dental caries and periodontal disease. If you can teach your patients to eliminate this slippery mass of microorganisms from the surfaces of the teeth through meticulous brushing and flossing techniques, their dental diseases will be all but eliminated. The maintenance of a healthy dentition is dependent on a plaque-free mouth.

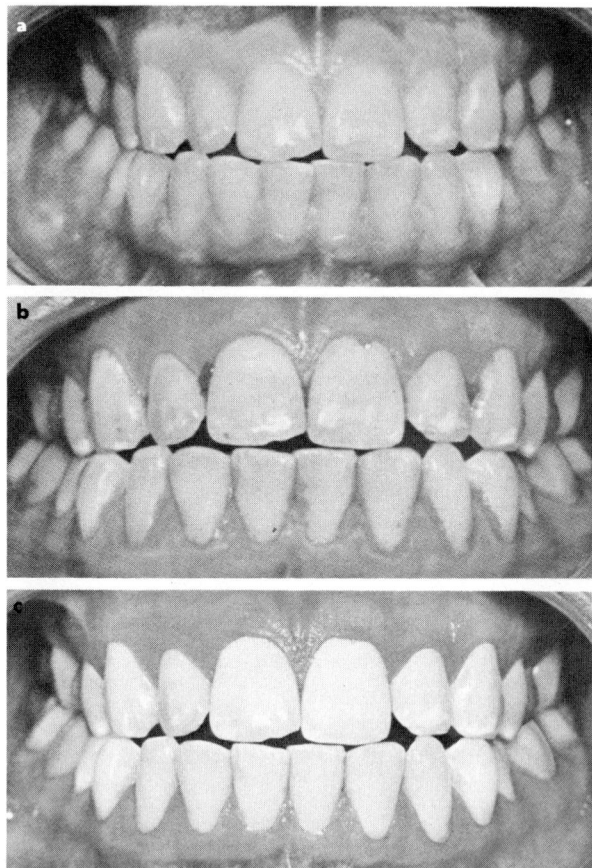

Fig. 29.1. Plaque staining: (a) Patient has brushed teeth, apparently clean. The patient is now instructed to chew and dissolve a disclosing tablet thoroughly, swish the liquid throughout the mouth for sixty seconds, spit it out, then rinse with a mouthful of water; (b) Results of the staining; (c) Mouth after the second brushing. Reprinted from Hussein A. Zaki, **Clean Teeth Brighten Your Smile** (University of Minnesota, 1971).

Calculus

Various salts, such as the salts of calcium and phosphorus, are also precipitated from saliva. The gelatinous matrix of the bacterial plaque provides a base for the accumulation of these salts, and eventually a hard, cement-like substance evolves which is impossible to remove with a toothbrush. The substance is calculus. This particular type of calculus is *salivary calculus.* When calculus forms on the teeth, it must be removed with scaling instruments as the first stage of the dental prophylaxis. If allowed to accumulate, it collects progressively into the subgingival area as well and compounds the periodontal problems. Loss of supporting bone occurs, and pockets of infection are created.

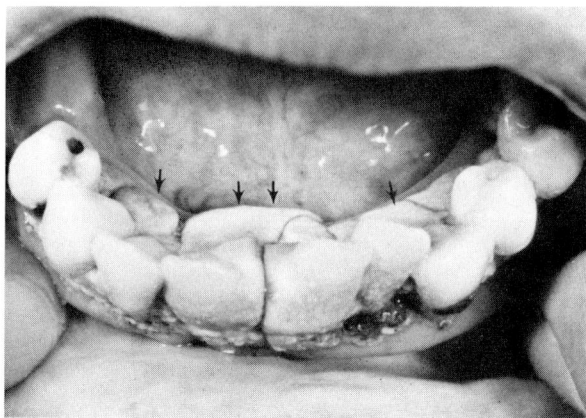

Fig. 29.2 Calculus

Stains

The most commonly seen stains are those caused by smoking. The brown or blackish stains are tobacco tars precipitated on the tooth surface and are extremely difficult to remove. Once the teeth are thoroughly cleaned, the patient can often retain a nice appearance, in spite of smoking, by doing a very thorough brushing job, and especially if he is encouraged to smoke cigarettes not more than half-way through. (But why smoke at all?)

Green stain on the gingival third of the tooth is sometimes seen in children. Less commonly, a red or red-brown stain is seen. These stains are caused by chromogenic bacteria attached to the remains of *Nasmyth's membrane,* a covering present over the unerupted enamel crown of the tooth. The stains are extremely disfiguring but can usually be removed by the dentist.

Dental Prophylaxis (Prevention Through Cleaning)

Dental prophylaxis is an operation for which scaling instruments and polishing pastes are used to remove the hard and soft accretions and stains from the tooth surfaces and the gingival crevices.

Scalers are necessary to plane the surfaces of the teeth and free them from all calculus deposits. The prophylaxis paste is used to remove all soft accretions and leave a smooth, polished surface.

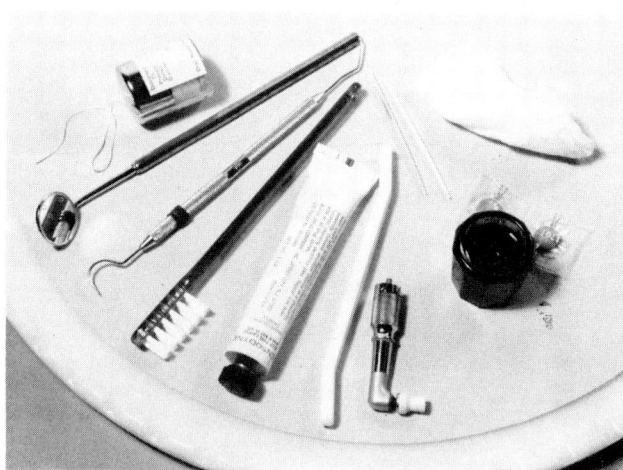

Fig. 29.3. Armamentarium for POH

Flour of pumice, a powdered grit made from lava rock, was formerly the powder of choice for prophylaxis. Today, however, less harsh cleaning agents containing zieconium not only clean the tooth surfaces well, but leave them highly polished and less susceptible to plaque formation. These commercially prepared powders also contain fluoride for its topical effect against caries.

The paste is used with brushes, rubber cups, and dental floss to eliminate all plaque and debris from pits, fissures, and interproximal surfaces.

The prophylaxis contra-angle is one made specifically for use with rubber cups. A regular contra-angle is used to hold the prophylaxis brushes. The grit in the cleaning pastes can gain access to the interior gears of the contra-angles, and consequently these instruments must be meticulously cleaned after each use to keep the gears functioning properly and to effect sterilization between patients. Care on your part will greatly increase the service your office can expect from these contra-angles (or right angles).

Stains and calculus can also be removed with the ultrasonic instrument that gently

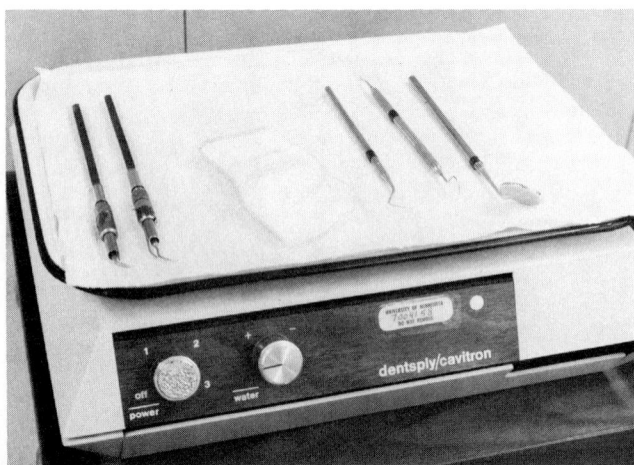

Fig. 29.4. Cavitron prophylaxis instrument

and quickly removes attached debris with an instrument tip which vibrates or oscillates twenty-five thousand cycles per second (fig. 29.4).

Dentifrice

The patient should be told that the choice of toothpaste or powder is entirely a question of using the one he prefers. *It is not what the adult patient puts on the bristles—it is what he puts on the handle that is important.*

The formation of calculus begins with the accumulation of food deposits and the retention of bacterial plaques for a period of time. If plaque is removed as thoroughly as possible on a daily basis, the dentist or hygienist can easily complete the cleansing of those areas which the patient cannot readily reach or which he misses. The daily removal of as much as possible of these soft accumulations reduces the irritation and inflammation and provides exercise for the gums.

The Council on Dental Therapeutics of the American Dental Association has supported the use of stannous fluoride dentifrices as aids in reducing the incidence of dental decay, along with the usual programs of dental care.[1]

Toothbrushes and Toothbrush Technique[2]

A variety of toothbrushes are available for patients to buy. The patients should be instructed to purchase a soft-bristled brush, bristles which will not injure the delicate gingival tissues and yet will be stiff enough to adequately reach and clean the gingival areas

1. Council on Dental Therapeutics, "Reclassification of Crest Toothpaste," *J.A.D.A.* 69, no. 2 (August 1964): 195-196; idem, "Evaluation of Cue Toothpaste," ibid., pp. 197-198.
2. Courtesy Lactona Products Division, Morris Plains, N. J., with adaptation by the authors.

and interproximal spaces as well as the easier-to-brush occlusal surfaces.

The method of brushing you teach your patients is the decision of your dentist. The objective is to deplaque all surfaces of the teeth. Although method is important, there are many ways to brush teeth and successfully accomplish the objective. Whatever the method, it should be specific and should be mastered by your patients under your instruction. One method, a modified Charters-Stillman method, is illustrated in figures 29.5 through 29.12.

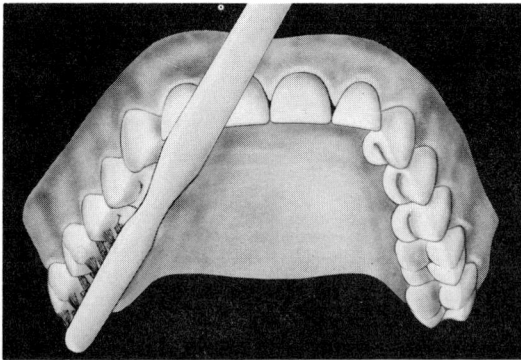

Fig. 29.5. Start on the **right** side and brush the occlusal surfaces of the upper teeth; next, the lower teeth. The ends of the bristles reach into the fissures and pits of the teeth to dislodge food debris. Use short, horizontal strokes with reasonable pressure. Memorize and then follow a definite toothbrushing routine as instructed by your dentist. Allow time for each successive brushing step and do not neglect a single tooth surface.

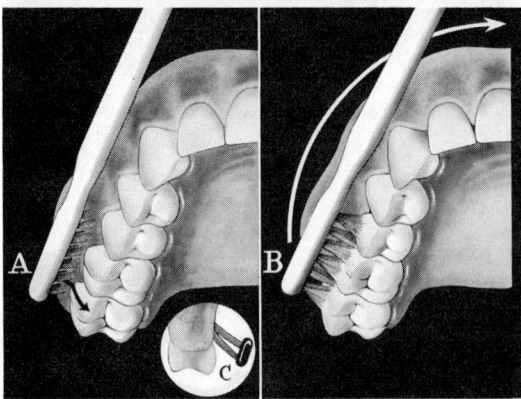

Fig. 29.6. With handle horizontal, place brush on gums above the buccal surfaces on three posterior teeth upper **right** side (fig. A). The bristles are directed toward roots of teeth with their sides touching the gums. With sweeping stroke, move brush downward to the occlusal surfaces. As the bristles enter the spaces between the teeth (fig. B), with a gentle vibratory motion cleanse these areas and stimulate the soft tissue. Fig. C shows sides of bristles with downward sweeping stroke over the gums. After brushing the three posterior upper teeth, move on around the arch, using the same strokes.

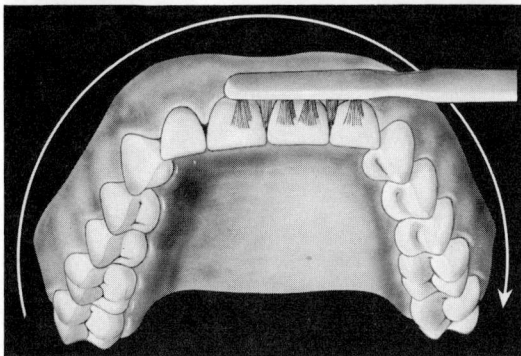

Fig. 29.7. This picture shows the brush moved on around to the **upper** anterior teeth. Use the same downward sweeping stroke as shown in figure 29.6. Care is taken so that the ends of the bristles do not pierce or otherwise injure the gums.

Continue around to the **upper** teeth on the left-hand side, using the same method as shown in 29.5 and 29.6 until all the facial surfaces of the upper teeth have been brushed.

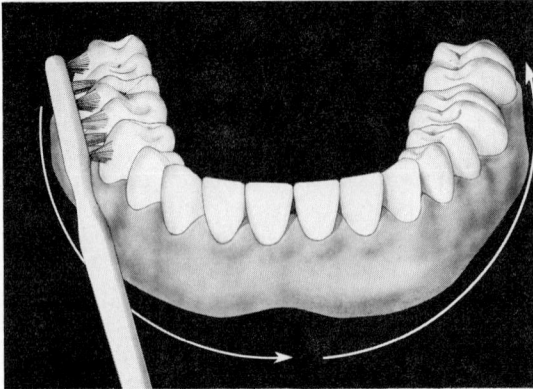

Fig. 29.8. Next, brush the facial surfaces of the **lower** teeth beginning with the posterior teeth on the right side and on around the arch to the left until every **lower** facial surface has been brushed. The same strokes and method as described in illustrations 29.6 and 29.7 for the upper teeth are used. Note that on the **lower** teeth the sweeping stroke is **upward.**

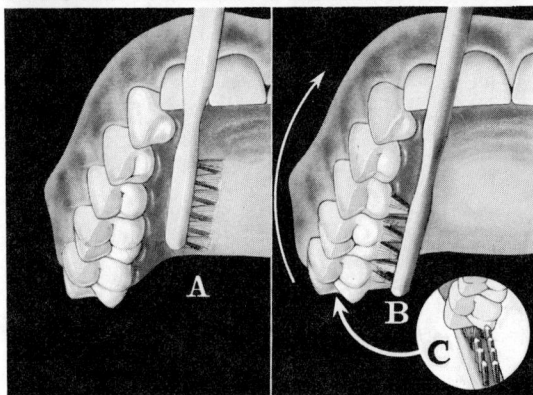

Fig. 29.9. Now brush the **lingual** surfaces of the three posterior upper teeth on the **right.** Place the sides of the bristles (fig. A) towards the center of the palate; use a sweeping stroke and move the brush to the lingual surfaces of the teeth until it is in position B. Use a gentle rotary motion; the ends of the bristles work into the spaces between the teeth.

Figure C shows how the distal surfaces of the last molar teeth, both upper and lower, are cleaned with a few short strokes. The toe or end of the brush is used.

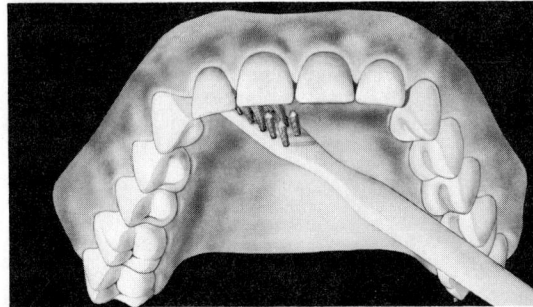

Fig. 29.10. Now clean the **lingual** surfaces of upper anterior teeth. The brush handle is in a more vertical position. The stroke is downward toward the occlusal surfaces with a gentle vibratory motion. When the lingual of upper teeth are brushed, use the same method for inside surface of lower anterior teeth.

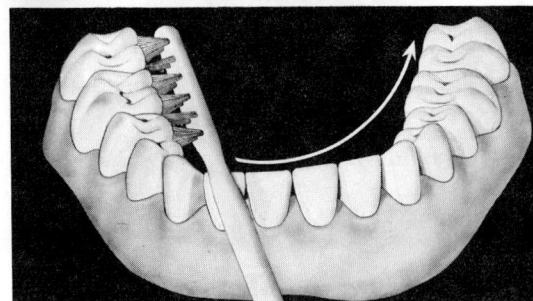

Fig. 29.11. To clean **lingual** surfaces of lower posterior teeth, the toe or end of the brushhead is used with controlled rotary motion. The tufts work into the spaces between the teeth. The brush is moved around the arch until no **lingual** tooth surface is neglected.

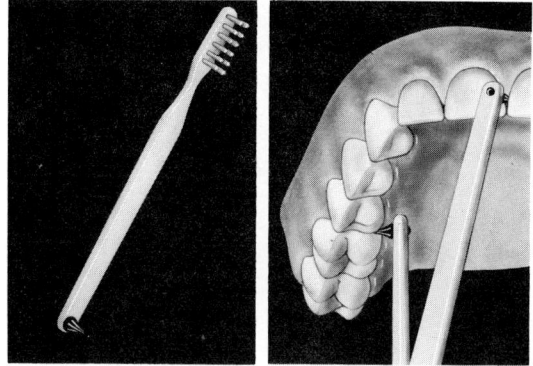

Fig. 29.12. Proper instruction at a dental office is the basis for effective stimulation of gum tissue and cleaning of spaces between the teeth with the rubber stimulator tip. Reasonable pressure with the tip is exerted against gum tissue. Intermittent action forces stagnant blood from the capillaries and it is replaced with a fresh supply. This is not adequate, however, to clean the interproximal areas. These hard-to-get-at areas are cleaned by flossing.

Another widely accepted and popular brushing technique, the Bass technique, utilizing short back-and-forth strokes of the bristles pointed into the gingival and interproximal areas, is well presented in the publication *Clean Teeth Brighten Your Smile.*[3]

Electric Toothbrushes[4]

Many brands of electrically powered toothbrushes have been introduced in recent years. They have varied widely in their construction, cost, and operating methods. The Council on Dental Therapeutics included powered toothbrushes in its evaluation program in order to provide authoritative information to dentists and the public, as well as to encourage manufacturers to establish adequate testing of their products.

Regardless of the manner of movement of the head of the particular electric toothbrush, it is possible to alter to a considerable degree the direction of the brush movement on the

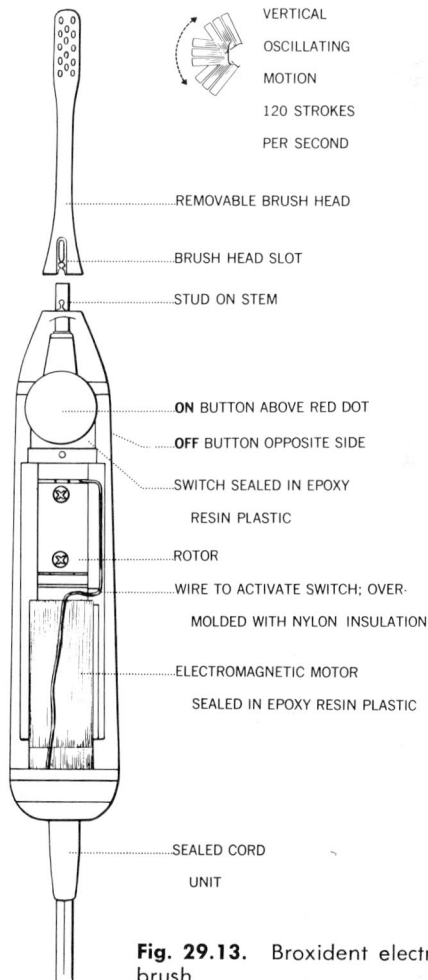

VERTICAL
OSCILLATING
MOTION
120 STROKES
PER SECOND

REMOVABLE BRUSH HEAD
BRUSH HEAD SLOT
STUD ON STEM

ON BUTTON ABOVE RED DOT
OFF BUTTON OPPOSITE SIDE
SWITCH SEALED IN EPOXY
RESIN PLASTIC
ROTOR
WIRE TO ACTIVATE SWITCH; OVER-
MOLDED WITH NYLON INSULATION
ELECTROMAGNETIC MOTOR
SEALED IN EPOXY RESIN PLASTIC

SEALED CORD
UNIT

Courtesy E. R. Squibb & Sons, N. Y.

Fig. 29.13. Broxident electric toothbrush.

3. Hussein A. Zaki et al., *Clean Teeth Brighten Your Smile.*
4. Council on Dental Therapeutics, "Current Status of Electric Toothbrushes," *J.A.D.A.* 69, no. 3 (September 1964): 404-6; idem, "General Electric Automatic Toothbrush Classified in Group A," ibid., pp. 407-8; idem, "Broxodent Classified in Group B," ibid., pp. 408-9.

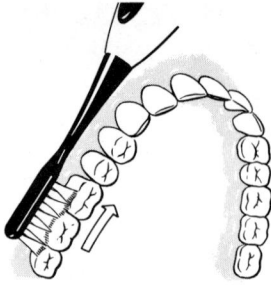

Fig. 29.14. Brushing the upper buccal surfaces.

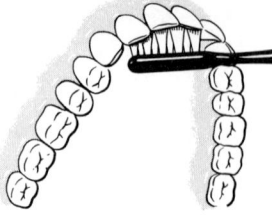

Fig. 29.15. Brushing the upper anterior lingual area.

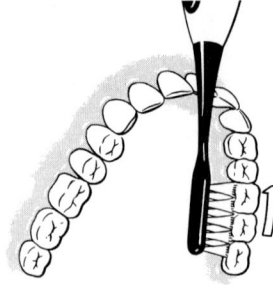

Fig. 29.16. Brushing the upper posterior lingual area.

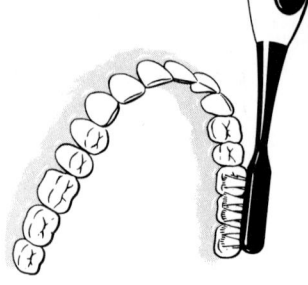

Fig. 29.17. Brushing the upper chewing surfaces.

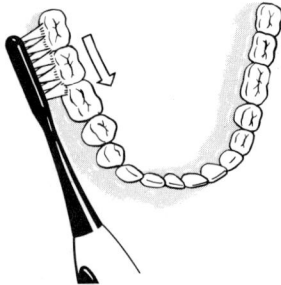

Fig. 29.18. Brushing the lower buccal surfaces.

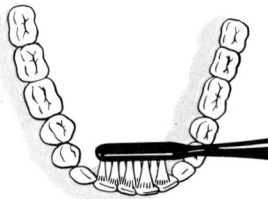

Fig. 29.19. Brushing the lower anterior lingual area.

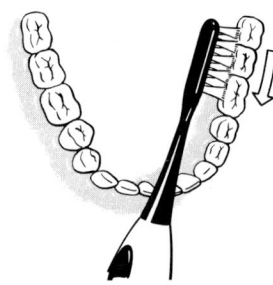

Fig. 29.20. Brushing the lower posterior lingual area.

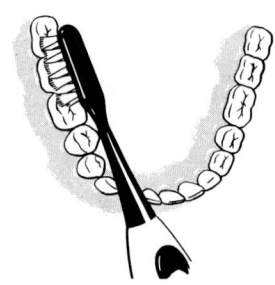

Fig. 29.21. Brushing the lower chewing surfaces.

teeth and gums by holding the brush handle in various positions. The series of drawings above illustrate a method of using one of the electric toothbrushes classified at this time by the Council on Dental Therapeutics.

The electric toothbrush can be an invaluable aid for persons with limited function of the hands and arms, such as persons with arthritis and patients in hospitals and nursing homes.

Flossing

Flossing is a process of cleaning the areas between the teeth with pieces of dental floss. Flossing may be accomplished by holding the dental floss firmly between the fingers and inserting it gently between the contact areas of the teeth. Care must be taken not to "snap" the floss through the contact and damage the interdental papilla. The proper procedure is to pass the floss through the contact at a forty-five-degree angle to the occlusal plane, moving it slightly back and forth (fig. 29.22).

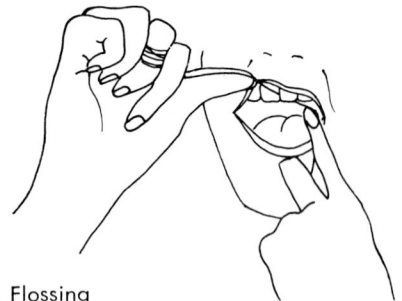

Fig. 29.22. Flossing

Cleaning with the floss is accomplished with an up-and-down motion, drawing the floss subgingivally as comfort permits. Floss in an unorganized pattern, making sure to polish the interproximal surfaces of all contacting teeth.

Water Jets

Another device marketed as an aid for oral hygiene delivers a stream of water to flush debris from hard-to-reach areas. One popular device is the water pik (fig. 29.23). This instrument projects a jet of water at adjustable pressures to wash out debris. Although this instrument cannot accomplish complete cleansing and plaque removal, it can remove debris from under fixed bridgework and around orthodontic appliances. It can also be used following brushing and flossing to rinse interproximal spaces where gingival recession exists. Care must be taken not to use too forceful a jet stream, which may harm the gingival attachment.

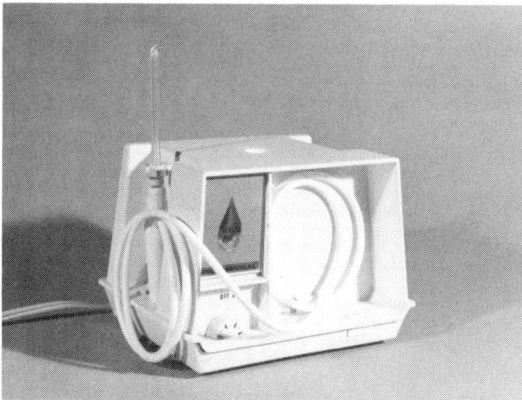

Fig. 29.23. Water pik

Summary

Oral hygiene is the most important area of preventive dental care, yet few patients are properly instructed or are willing to exert the effort it takes to administer proper oral hygiene.

Bacterial plaque forms on the teeth and must be removed quickly and thoroughly or calculus will form. Calculus is impossible to remove with a toothbrush. Stains are caused by smoking, drinking tea, or eating certain foods which stain.

Dental prophylaxis removes the accumulation which the patient has not removed by expending enough energy on the handle of his toothbrush. With proper care it is possible to keep one's natural dentition a lifetime. Without such care, artificial dentures become a likely possibility.

Study Questions

1. What forms the foundation for sound preventive practices for adequate health care?
2. What does POH mean?
3. Describe plaque and explain its effect on teeth.
4. Describe dental prophylaxis.
5. Explain the statement "what he puts on the handle of the toothbrush is important for the adult patient."
6. Describe a good method of toothbrushing.
7. Describe flossing.
8. Of what value is a water jet?

Bibliography

"Oral Hygiene Devices and Aids in Oral Health." In *Guide to Dental Materials and Devices*, pp. 148-157. Chicago: American Dental Association, 1972-73.

OSHIRO, R. S.; STOOKEY, G. K.; and MUHLER, J. C. "Laboratory and Clinical Studies Concerning Development and Evaluation of a New Mechanical Toothbrush." *J. Periodontology* 41 (January 1970): 23-29.

"Toothbrushes." In *Accepted Dental Therapeutics*, pp. 239-240. Chicago: American Dental Association, 1972.

ZAKI, HUSSEIN A.; BANDT, CARL I.; and FOLKE, LARS, E. A. *Clean Teeth Brighten Your Smile.* Minneapolis, Minn.: University of Minnesota Press, 1971.

30 | *Dental Specialties*

A dental assistant for a specialist will have some duties which are peculiar to the practice of the specialty. In this chapter the brief descriptions give a general idea of the particular work of each specialty discussed.

Two of the specialties, *oral pathology* and *dental public health,* have been omitted since they do not commonly require assistants. The other specialties are discussed in alphabetical order.

Endodontics

Endodontics (*end-* "within" + *dont,* "tooth") is that specialty of dentistry which deals with the diagnosis and treatment of irritated or infected pulps of teeth and their periapical tissues. Its purpose is to retain such teeth as healthy functioning organs. To thoroughly understand the problems involved in the treatment of pulpal and periapical disorders, the dentist must have a sound knowledge of the origin and effect of the various irritants which may attack the tooth, the ability to utilize diagnostic aids to their best advantage, and the faculty to correlate subjective and objective symptoms to arrive at a correct diagnosis. The correct treatment is the goal. Correct diagnosis is the means to that goal.

As a dental assistant, you will record much of the patient's history and symptoms and assist in performing such tests as vitality testing to help the dentist arrive at his diagnosis. Patients frequently come to the dental office with pain, and this pain is most often of pulpal origin. Such patients not only need immediate attention, but also a bit more understanding and gentle care.

Figure 30.1 illustrates diagrammatically the treatments performed by the endodontist. Although any of these may be performed by the general practitioner of dentistry, some dentists prefer to refer selected cases to the endodontic specialist.

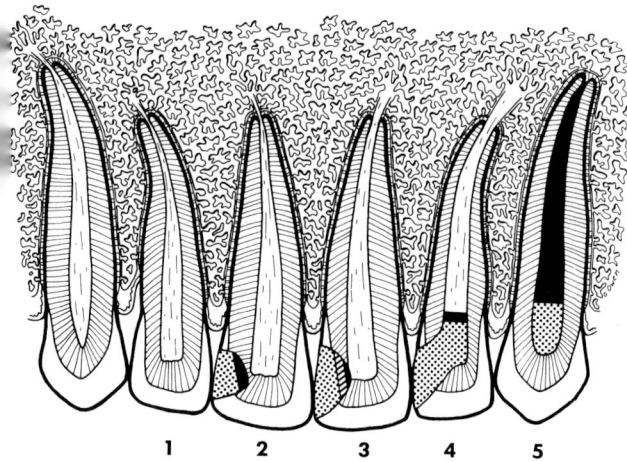

Fig. 30.1. Conservative endodontic treatments

The chart in figure 30.1 diagrams the scope of endodontic therapy. It can be seen that the treatment of pulpal and periapical conditions may be divided according to various objectives.

1. *Desensitization of dentin* is the treatment of dentin exposed through normal gingival recession, periodontal disease, or surgical intervention on adjacent tissues.
2. *Pulp protection* refers to the placement of an insulating, protective, and perhaps anal-

gesic cement or paste on the pulpal or axial wall of dentin when fractures of the tooth or the removal of deep caries approximates but does not expose vital pulp tissues.
3. *Pulp capping* is a superficial treatment of vital dental pulps exposed through trauma or during caries removal. This is an attempt to stimulate a hard tissue healing over the exposed area and to insure continued vitality of the remaining pulp tissue.
4. *Pulpotomy,* or partial pulpectomy, is the removal of part of the vital pulp tissue and the treatment of the remaining pulp stump or stumps in an attempt to stimulate hard tissue healing over the exposed wound(s) and maintain the vitality of the remaining pulp tissue. In principle, this latter operation is identical with pulp capping; however, the site of capping is selected at a more favorable position in this procedure.
5. *Root canal therapy,* or complete pulpectomy, is the removal of all pulpal tissue, followed by sterilization and filling of the root canal(s).
6. *Apical curettage* is the surgical removal of pathologic periapical tissues which may be done following root canal therapy or simultaneously with it.
7. *Apicoectomy* is the removal of a portion of the root apex performed concurrently with apical curettage where indicated.

The problem in pulpal therapy is to determine through correct diagnosis which treatment is indicated for any given case. This can be accomplished by properly correlating the probable etiology with the subjective and objective findings and intelligently evaluating all available information individually and collectively.

Occasionally roots must be sacrificed through root amputation or *hemisection,* retaining the remaining tooth structures for restoration (figs. 30.2 and 30.3).

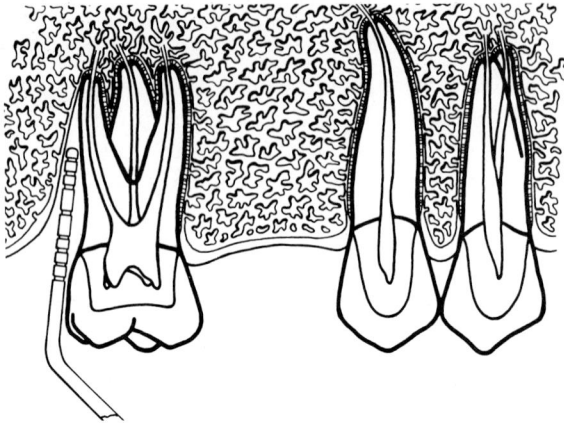

Fig. 30.2. Root amputation

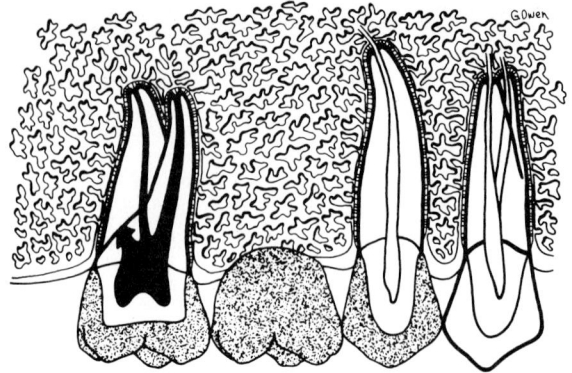

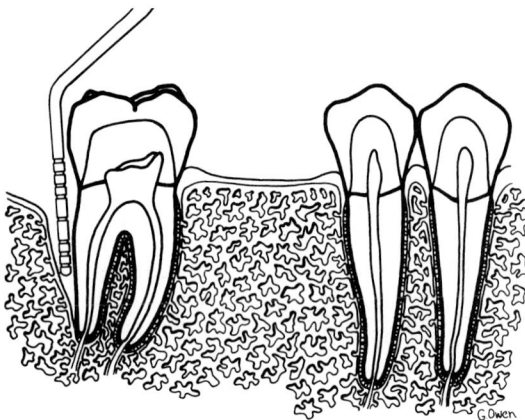

Fig. 30.3. Hemisection

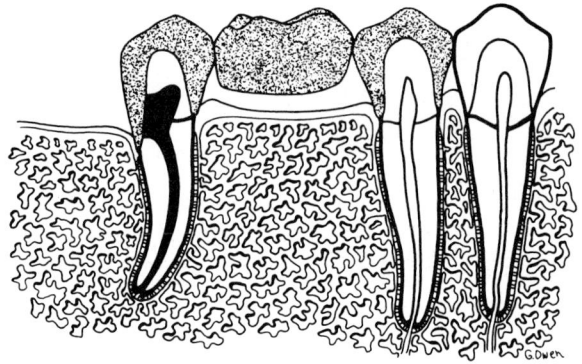

A thorough knowledge of microbiology and sterilization methods is paramount to the practice of endodontics. The assistant will be called upon frequently to work with the endodontist on surgical cases as well as the routine procedures performed under rubber-dam isolation.

Oral Surgery

Oral surgery is a specialty concerned with the removal of teeth and the treatment of frac-tures of the jaws and other abnormalities within the dental area.

Preoperative care and postoperative care are important parts of good oral surgery. Sterilization and anesthesia are necessary areas of understanding and use in the oral surgeon's office.

Patient reassurance is also of utmost importance. Most patients are apprehensive and need to feel confidence in their oral surgeon and his staff.

Fig. 30.4. X-rays (a) before and (b) after impaction removal.

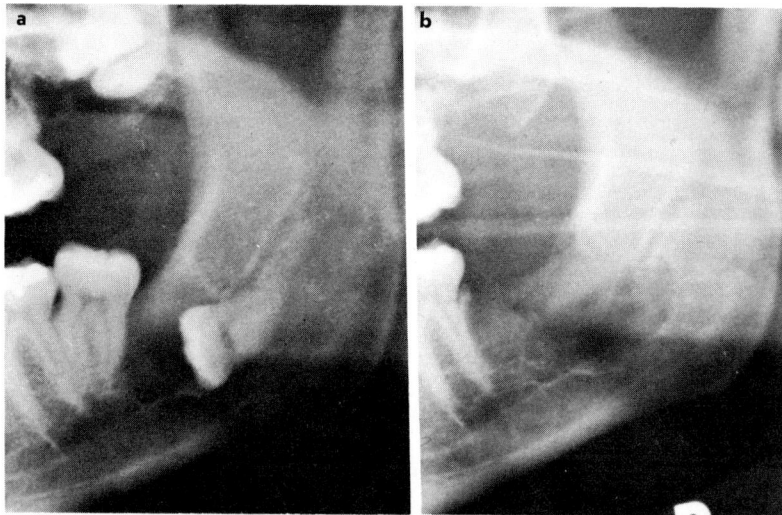

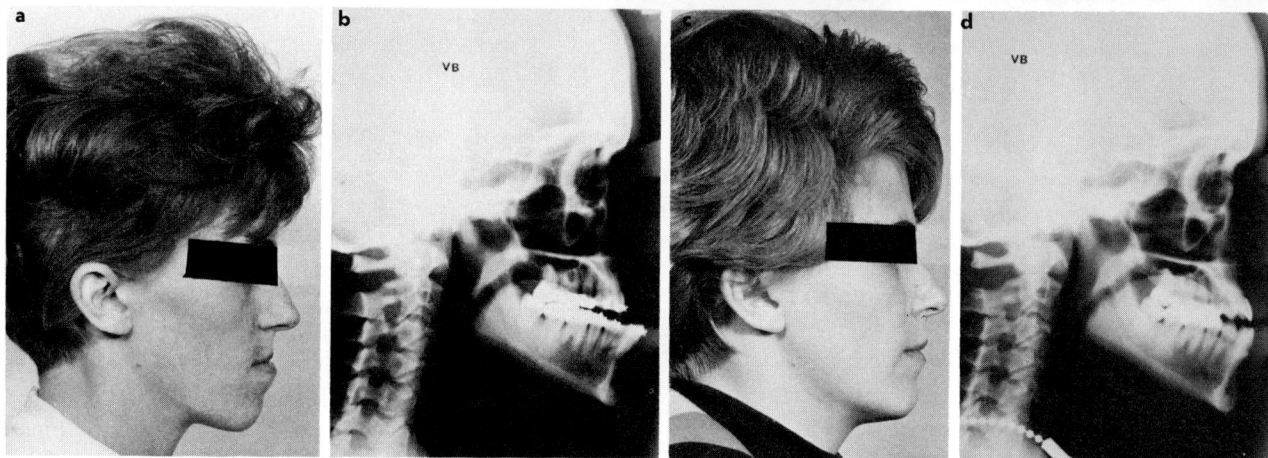

Fig. 30.5. Before (a, b) and after (c, d) prognathism

The assistant to the oral surgeon must assume responsibility which may affect a patient's comfort and, on occasion, may affect his ability to live. It is extremely important, therefore, that she learn her duties explicitly and perform them with accuracy.

Maintenance and Use of Accurate Records

1. Patient registration must be complete and accurate.

2. If surgery is to be performed for a minor, the parent's consent form must be attached to the minor's chart, dated and signed by the parent or guardian.

3. A brief, accurate medical background (history) must be written about the patient or by the patient at the direction of the oral surgeon. It includes systemic diseases, use of anticoagulants or insulin, bleeding tendencies, and inquiry into his history of an-

esthesia. Type of drugs used and the degree of results are important.

4. History of anesthesia—past history and notation of allergic reactions, if any—and the required preoperative preparations should be noted. It is the duty of the assistant to verify that the patient actually took the preoperative medication as requested. The assistant is in attendance during induction of anesthesia and through the recovery period.

5. The assistant should verify that the necessary X rays, both intraoral and extraoral, are in the operatory.

6. If the patient is to have general anesthesia, the assistant should suggest that the patient be escorted to and from the office. If the patient is to be hospitalized, the procedure should be explained to the patient.

Asepsis

1. Sterilization of instruments and materials by use of autoclave, dry heat, and cold sterilization is the responsibility of the assistant.

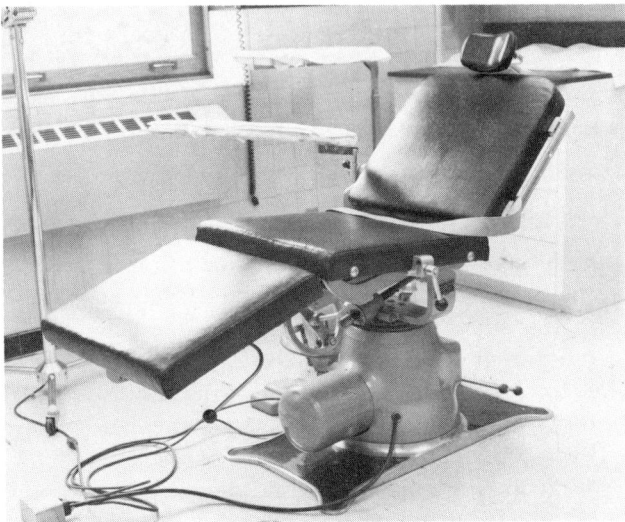

Fig. 30.6. Operating table-chair

2. The assistant should know when to use each type of sterilization.

3. She must be certain that she has sterilized when sterilization is necessary.

Surgical Assistance

1. Selection of proper instruments.

2. Knowledge of procedure to be carried out and the surgical steps involved to hasten the surgical movements.

3. Aspiration of operative site and oral pharynx of fluids, hemorrhage, and foreign bodies.

4. Give proper support to the jaw during procedures and correctly use retractors to aid and maintain good, clear operative field.

5. Know the intent of dressings and the use of them in oral surgery.
   a. Keep the surgical field free from infection.
   b. Support the incision and protect it. Absorb drainage extraorally.

Postoperative Duties

1. Accompany patient to recovery area.

2. Check full airway; note color, type of breathing, and pulse. Report abnormal findings to oral surgeon.

3. Have drugs available for all emergencies.

4. Know all the principles of first aid and understand mouth-to-mouth resuscitation and procedure for external cardiac massage.

Postoperative Responsibilities

1. Care of wounds.

2. Medications used locally.

3. Technique to remove sutures.

4. Proper dismissal of patients.

The assistant in oral surgery receives her instructions from her dentist, but she must have the ability and knowledge to carry them out skillfully.

Orthodontics

Orthodontics[1] (*ortho*, "straight" + *dont*, "tooth") is that science which has for its objective the prevention and correction of malocclusion of the teeth.

Have you worn "braces" on your teeth?

This assorted group of wires and bands applied to a young person's teeth is correctly termed an *orthodontic appliance*. Its most obvious purposes are to realign that person's teeth into a more pleasing appearance and to establish normal function.

The effect produced by a successful orthodontic treatment, however, extends much further than that simple statement. "More pleasing appearance" is made up of many more factors than alignment of the visible front teeth. Very commonly it includes a complete

1. Lawrence McIver. Personal communication covering section on orthodontics.

alteration of the relationship of *all* the teeth, for example:

1. An orthodontic treatment may involve changing within the same dental arch the original relationship of the teeth to each other.
2. An orthodontic treatment may involve changing the original relationship of the lower arch to the upper arch.
3. An orthodontic treatment may involve changing the original relationship of the anterior sections of both arches to the rest of the facial structures, such as lips, or to the upper lip and nose (seen in profile).

Orthodontic treatment is a complex specialty. Besides achieving the improvement in appearance which is the chief interest of both the patient and the parents, the orthodontist must also restore normal function (ability to chew)

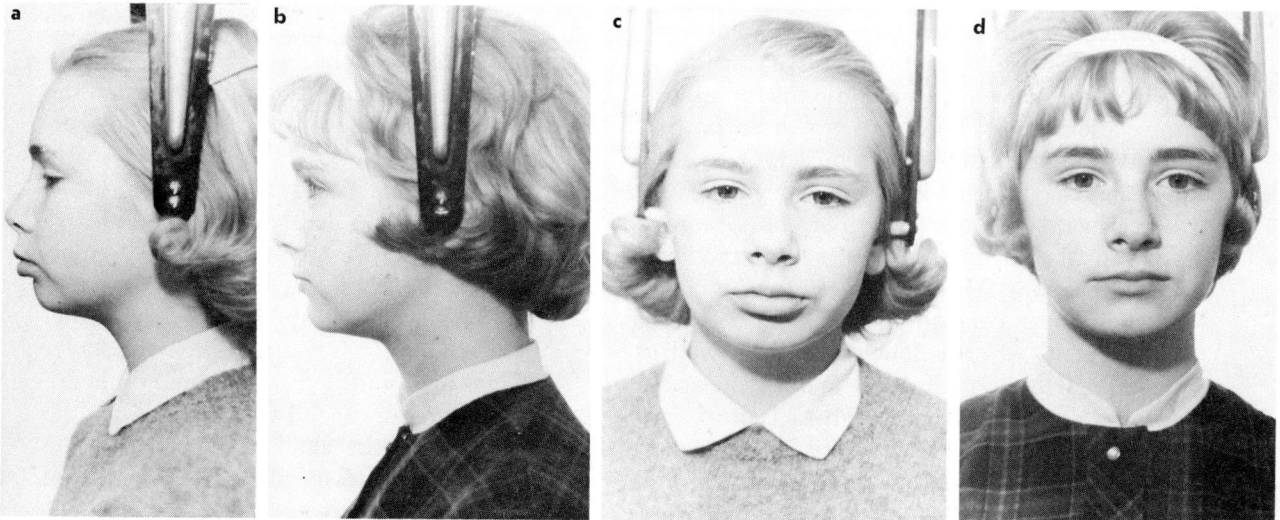

Courtesy Dr. L. W. McIver, Minneapolis

Fig. 30.7. An orthodontic patient before and after treatment: a and c are side and front views before treatment; b and d are side and front views after treatment.

Set I

Set II

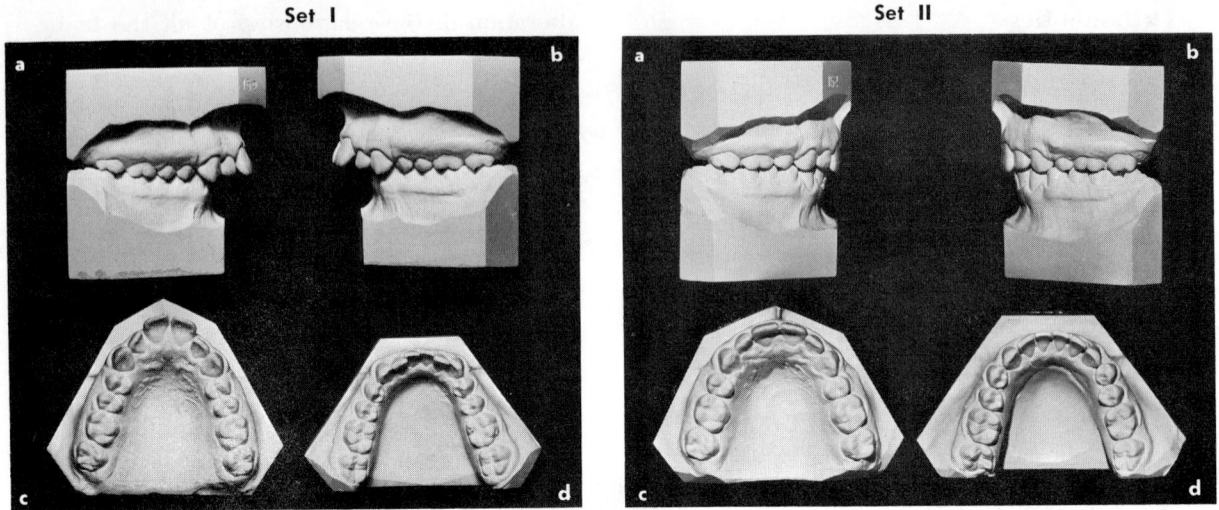

Fig. 30.8. Casts of an orthodontic case before and after treatment. Set I is before treatment. Set II is the same mouth after treatment. Notice the alignment of the teeth in the arch: (a) right profile, (b) left profile, (c) upper arch, (d) lower arch.

to the complete mouth in order to achieve a correction which is stable and healthy for the individual.

Malocclusions which occur have many variations, causing difficulty in classifying them. In order to achieve a common basis for analyzing various cases, however, it is essential that some form of classification be used. One of the most commonly used is the form developed by Dr. Edward H. Angle, who became a pioneer specialist in this field in 1892 while practicing in Minneapolis, Minnesota. Dr. Angle's classification dates back to 1899. The assistant in the specialty of orthodontia would do well to memorize the classification and at the same time to match each class with a typical case from the collection of her dentist's orthodontic models made from cases before treatment.

Angle's Classification

Class I. All cases of malocclusion in which the lower dental arch and body of the mandible are in normal mesiodistal relationship to the anatomy of the skull.

Class II. Division 1. Cases in which the lower dental arch and body of the mandible are in bilateral, distal relationship to the anatomy of the skull and in which the upper incisor teeth show labial axial perversion.

Subdivision. Cases in which the lower dental arch and body of the mandible are in unilateral, distal relationship to the anatomy of the skull and in which the upper incisors manifest labial axial perversion.

Division 2. Cases in which the lower dental arch and body of the mandible are in unilateral, distal relationship to the anatomy of the skull and in which the upper central incisors are in lingual axial perversion.

Subdivision. Cases in which the lower dental arch and body of the mandible are in unilateral, distal relationship to the anatomy of the skull and in which the upper central incisors are in lingual axial perversion.

Class III. Cases in which the lower dental arch and body of the mandible are in bilateral mesial relationship to the anatomy of the skull.

Subdivision. Cases in which the lower dental arch and body of the mandible are in unilateral, mesial relationship to the anatomy of the skull.

Parts of the Orthodontic Appliance

The orthodontic appliance is made up of several parts. That part which is fitted to an individual tooth and cemented to that tooth after it has been fitted is called a *band.* Many bands may be used as part of an individual orthodontic appliance.

Another part of the orthodontic appliance appears to be a wire, usually following the shape of the dental arch around the outside (buccal and labial surfaces) of the teeth but at times placed on the inside (lingual) surfaces of the teeth. The wire is correctly called an *arch wire.*

The arch wire is used to apply gentle, steady pressures to the teeth which the orthodontist wishes to move. The arch applies pressure to the band which is cemented solidly to the tooth. At times *rubber elastics* will be used between arches to produce an intermaxillary pressure, or force.

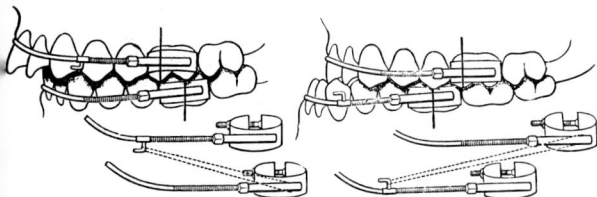

Courtesy Dr. L. W. McIver, Minneapolis

Fig. 30.10. Patient wearing a cervical anchorage

A commonly used device is a "head band," called a *cervical anchorage.* A wire arch is inserted in the bands on the farthest back teeth in the upper arch. This wire exerts even pressure on all the teeth of the upper arch. To the front of this wire arch are soldered two wire head-band anchors which extend across the face and along the cheeks on the outside of the head. The ends are curved like a cup hook. An elastic band with wire eyes at each end is attached to the hooks of the mouth arc "feelers" and fits around the neck. Thus, by means of anchoring the arch wire around the neck, steady pressure is maintained on all the upper-arch teeth for whatever length of time the orthodontist prescribes. Usually youngsters are to wear them twelve hours out of each twenty-four. They put them on after school or after dinner and wear them all night.

When the elastics or cervical anchorage devices are to be worn, the young patient (as

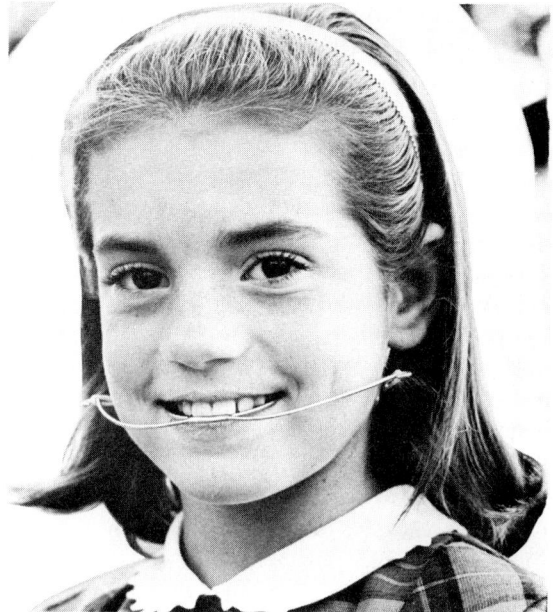

Courtesy S. S. White Co., Philadelphia

Fig. 30.9. Intermaxillary rubber elastics

well as the parent) often needs reminding to see that the elastics are worn *constantly,* or the head band is used nightly if the orthodontist so instructs. Often you are in a better position than the orthodontist to encourage the patient.

Study models are widely used in orthodontics as records of progress in treatment. Alginate materials are perhaps most commonly used as an impression material for these models. A detailed and specific method of trimming the models is used, for which the steps and method are outlined in chapter 36, "Models and Dies."

The construction of orthodontic appliances involves the use of banding material, attachments of many kinds (attached to the bands or arches), arches of various types, and soldering or electric spot-welding equipment. Instruments include contouring and bending pliers, crown shears, band drivers, cementing instruments, mirrors, and explorers. If arch wires are placed lingually to the teeth, the appliance is called a *lingual appliance.* If the arch wires are placed labially to the teeth, the appliance is called a *labial appliance.*

Methods of radiographic cephalometry are used in many orthodontic offices. Lateral head plates in specific positions at specific distances are made as an additional source of information in the treatment of the individual. These large plates involve processing of extraoral film cassettes, often used with intensifying screens to shorten the exposure required. (See "Radiography," chap. 40.)

Your orthodontist may use either or both intraoral and extraoral photography. He may use black-and-white or color film. Photography is used as a means of recording case progress and results. These procedures, when used, are so organized that their use is routine, with positioning of both camera and patient controlled for purposes of accurately repeating various views. Lighting also is standardized so that exposures are always the same.

The active movement of teeth and their placement in the dental arch may continue over quite a long period of time. Many orthodontic cases are completed within two years, but some cases may exceed two years.

At the conclusion of active treatment, a *retainer* or *retention appliance* is constructed for each case. A retainer is a device which holds the teeth in correct position until they stabilize. Most of the retainer appliances are removable by the patient. You may have occasion to use your influence to encourage the patient to wear the retainer as he has been instructed. Retainers are not as complex as the original appliances but do require occasional inspection and adjustment. They are frequently a combination of plastic and metal.

Duties of an Orthodontic Assistant

The duties of the orthodontic assistant may be grouped into three main divisions.

Laboratory Work

1. Soldering bands or spot-welding bands.
2. Making the plastic part of retainer appliances.
3. Making plaster casts of impressions taken by the orthodontist for records.
4. Trimming plaster casts on a model trimmer, as precisely required for records.
5. Developing cephalometric X rays.

Chair Assisting

1. Seat the patient for impression taking, band forming, or appliance adjustment.
2. Prepare cement for placing bands when ready.
3. Remove excess cement from bands and teeth after the orthodontist has cemented the bands.
4. Take photographs, when required, for records.
5. Maintain supply of ligature wires cut to correct length.

6. Keep small envelopes, as required, filled with various sizes of rubber elastics.
7. Make up headgear kits as required.

Secretarial Work

1. Making appointments. The time required for various types of appointments is important. New patient examination, securing history of new patients, consultation with parents, construction of appliances, adjustment of appliances, construction of retainers and removal of appliances, retainer adjustments, and final records—each may require a different block of time.
2. Letter writing. There are likely to be more letters written in the orthodontic practice than in general practice. An important letter in any orthodontic practice should be that which is sent to the referring dentist, thanking him for the referral and often including a note on the case involved.
3. Bookkeeping.
4. Ordering supplies.
5. Maintaining an accurate recall file for patients under observation.
6. Maintaining an accurate active treatment file.
7. Maintaining an accurate retention file.

Pediatric Dentistry

As a specialty, pediatric dentistry—children's dentistry—is similar in many respects to the general practice of dentistry for adults. The assistant's duties are very similar.

However, the differences which *do* exist are very important. Your knowledge of working with children is necessarily increased.

The care in what you do—what actions are seen by children—is accentuated. Duties must be performed with speed and accuracy. The smaller child's attention span is limited. It is necessary to work quickly and efficiently before he tires. However, your physical move-

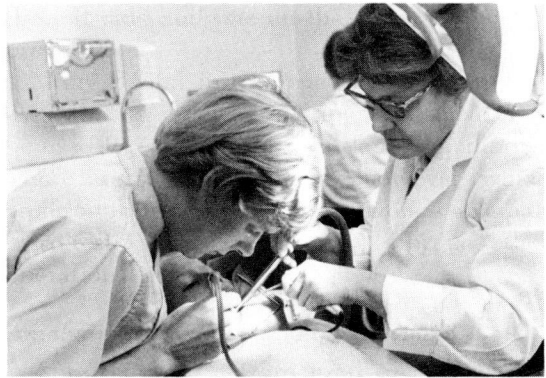

Fig. 30.11. Pediatric dentistry

ments near him must be slow and deliberate, your manner easy-going and relaxed. Quite a combination! Mix the amalgam quickly and accurately—but be leisurely and relaxed in attitude. Insert the saliva ejector gently and slowly—but quickly have ready whatever instrument your dentist needs.

Your speech should be calm and reassuring. It is a good idea to refresh your memory about the psychology of the particular age group of the child you have as a patient at that moment. If you have memorized the age-group characteristics given in chapter two, you can pause a moment and review the characteristics before you greet the child patient. After a few weeks of this approach, the psychology will become such a routine part of your mental equipment for your job that you won't have to think of it.

Children are a challenge. They can be the best patients and the most fun if properly approached by the dental health team.

Periodontics

A periodontist is a specialist who works with diseases "around the tooth." *Peri is* a Greek prefix meaning "around" and *odont* (as you already know) means "tooth."

The tissues around the tooth which the periodontist usually treats are these:

Gingivae (or gums);

Periodontal ligaments which attach the teeth to the bone socket of the mandible and maxilla; and

Cementus, the surface covering the roots of the teeth.

The periodontist is interested in the following symptoms:

Bleeding of gums during toothbrushing.

Unpleasant breath which persists.

Loose, soft gums, red instead of pale pink in color.

Separation of teeth from gums.

Drifting teeth, or teeth which are changing position.

Teeth which feel loose, or mobile.

Many people have periodontal diseases. It is the most common cause of loss of teeth. The first stage of periodontal disease is *gingivitis* (inflamed gums). If this disease is not treated and corrected, the second stage—or more advanced condition—is called *periodontitis*. (The layman is accustomed to calling it pyorrhea.)

Gingivitis is sometimes neglected because the bleeding and swollen gums (which are its first symptoms) cause very little discomfort, and people are inclined to think that this condition is perfectly normal.

If gingivitis is not treated, the more advanced condition, periodontitis, is the result. The inflammation spreads around the roots of the teeth, the gums become separated from the teeth, and pockets appear which are collectors of food particles, calculus, bacteria, and even pus. As the disease progresses, bone is lost around the root of the tooth. Eventually the tooth itself is lost because there is nothing to hold it in position.

Periodontal diseases are caused by the following conditions:

1. Plaque.
2. Calculus (tartar) which irritates the tissue surrounding the teeth.
3. Malocclusions: improper hitting of the occlusal surfaces of the teeth which produces uneven pressures on some teeth.
4. Missing teeth not replaced by a bridge or partial.
5. Bruxism: clenching and grinding of the teeth, especially during sleep—and sometimes during the day.
6. Inadequate nutrition.
7. Worn-out restorations, whether crowns, partials, or bridges.

The periodontist diagnoses the problem for the patient by examination, case history, X rays, and case study. He *treats* the conditions, educates the patient in proper care of his

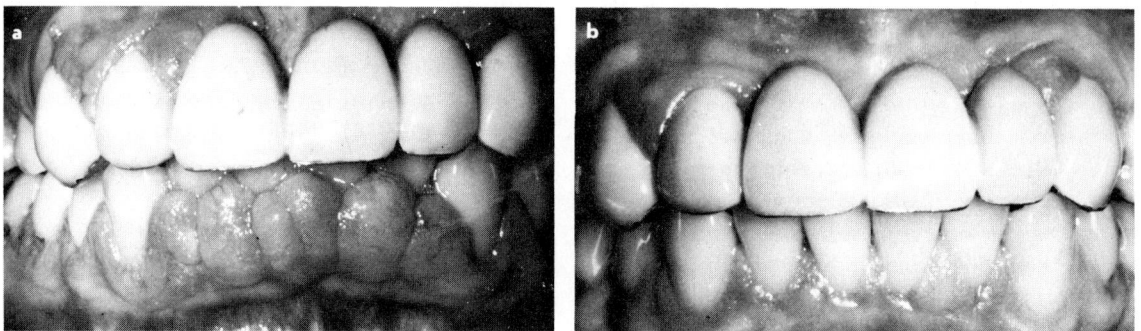

Fig. 30.12. Pre- and post-operative periodontic treatment: (a) Dilantin hyperplasia, preoperative condition; (b) condition following periodontal treatment.

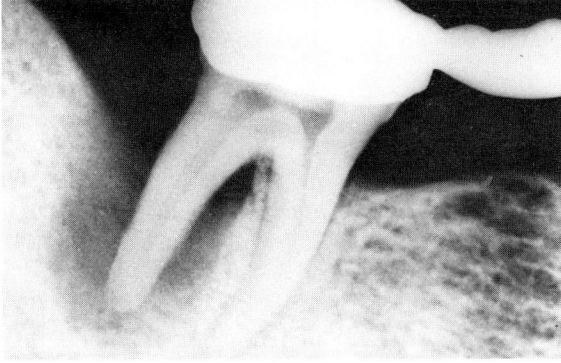

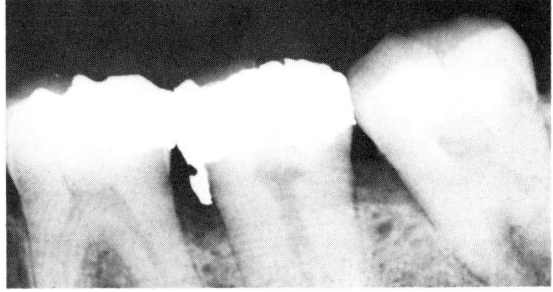

(left) **Fig. 30.13.** X ray of bone loss
(above) **Fig. 30.14.** X ray of overhang

mouth, and has the patient return at regular intervals for examination. He makes certain that the patient is providing the proper home care and uses X rays as necessary to determine the continued health of the part of the mouth which is not directly visible.

In treating the condition he may do one or many of several things. Basically, he removes the causes of the periodontal disease. This means he starts with the removal of calculus, then removes diseased gum tissue if any, corrects malocclusions, has missing teeth replaced, and constructs splints or other appliances to control the movement of loose teeth or correct harmful mouth habits. Finally, most importantly, he *educates* the patient to the necessity of proper care of the mouth.

Prosthodontics

Prosthetics (*Prosthesis*, "a putting to" + *Odont*, "tooth") refers to the artificial replacement of a missing natural part. Thus, an "artificial leg" is a *prothesis*, a prosthetic device to replace a missing leg. If a person has lost a tooth, he may have a *bridge* made—a fixed prosth*odont*ic appliance to replace the missing tooth. If he has lost many, but not all, teeth in one arch, he may have a *partial denture*. If he has no teeth left in one arch, he must use a *full denture. All* of the replacements are really

prosthetic appliances or, in the dental sense, prosthodontic appliances.

If a person needs full dentures, he may have emotional problems in adjusting to the idea of losing his remaining natural teeth. To most people dentures mean old age. Modern den-

Fig. 30.15. A three-tooth bridge.

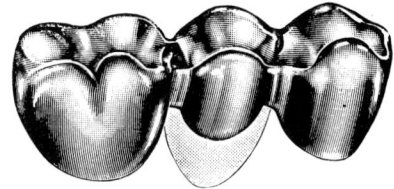

Courtesy J. M. Ney Co.

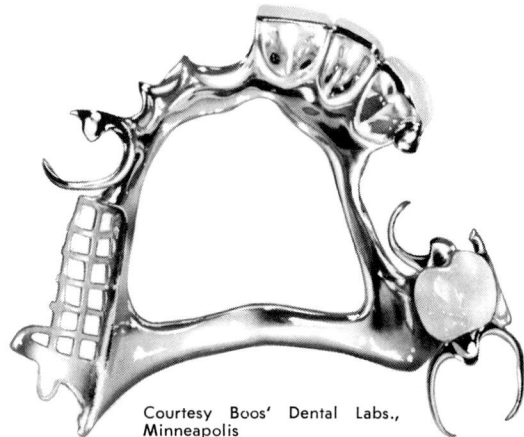

Courtesy Boos' Dental Labs., Minneapolis

Fig. 30.16. Upper cast partial denture frame with a "tube" tooth and three Steel's facings in place.

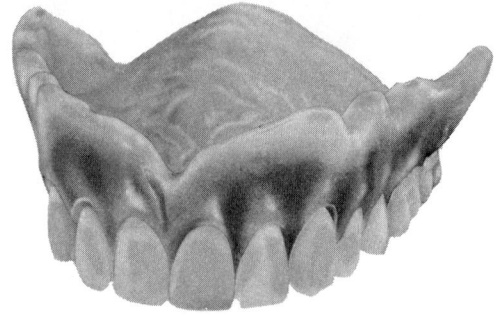

Courtesy Boos' Dental Labs., Minneapolis

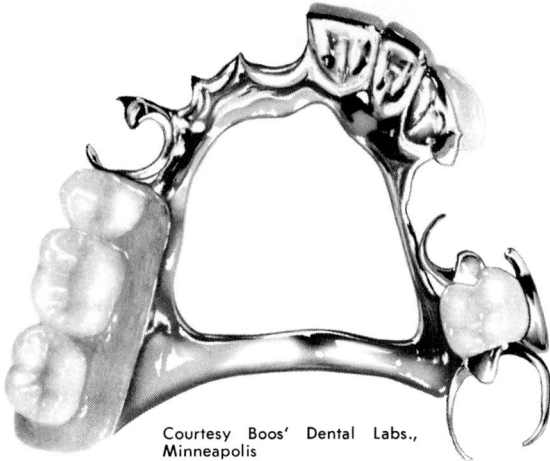

Courtesy Boos' Dental Labs., Minneapolis

(left) **Fig. 30.17.** Acrylic saddle portion completed on same partial which appears in figure 30.16.

(above) **Fig. 30.18.** A full upper denture

tistry can create dentures which are amazingly natural replicas.

Summary

The duties of the assistant to the specialist will vary from those of the assistant to the general practitioner.

Endodontics is concerned with correct therapy for the conservation of natural dentition for a lifetime. There are seven treatments which are performed in an endodontic practice. The assistant must be well educated in microbiology and sterilization.

The oral surgeon removes teeth and treats fractures of the jaw and abnormalities within the oral cavity. The oral surgeon's assistant must maintain and use accurate records, be certain asepsis is maintained where necessary, assist with surgery, perform postoperative duties, and be prepared for emergencies.

The orthodontist prevents and corrects malocclusions and reestablishes normal function and pleasing appearance. The assistant has three areas of work: laboratory, chair assisting, and secretarial work.

Pediatrics dentistry is dentistry for children, and assistants to the pediatric dentist must not only be prepared to assist at the chair, but must be acquainted with the necessary psychology and techniques of working with children of all ages.

Periodontists treat diseases around the tooth. The assistant must be able to educate patients in home care as well as assist at chairside and maintain asepsis where necessary.

The prosthodontist prepares artificial replacements. In addition to impressions and chairside assisting, the dental assistant must be aware of techniques of meeting patients' emotional problems over artificial replacements.

Study Questions

1. Describe each of the following specialties and explain the areas of work for the assistant:

endodontics	pediatric dentistry
oral surgery	periodontics
orthodontics	prosthodontics.

2. What are Angle's classifications?

Bibliography

JENSEN, JAMES R., and SERENE, THOMAS P. *Fundamentals of Clinical Endodontics.* Dubuque, Ia.: K/H Publishing Co., 1972.

THE DENTAL OFFICE ...
ITS ARMAMENTARIUM

PART SIX

AND MAINTENANCE

A lawyer can practice law and a teacher can teach almost anywhere there are people gathered together willing to listen. A dentist is unable to perform dentistry (except for minimum services) unless he has a well-equipped and well-maintained office. This office should be attractive as well.

A dentist's education is the most costly of all the professions, and the practice of dentistry generally requires a more expensive installation and higher overhead than does the practice of a physician, an attorney, or any other professional man.

The investment in office and equipment in starting a practice is relatively high. Replacement must be considered constantly in view of improved equipment, instruments, and techniques. In order to preserve the equipment and instruments over their useful lives, it is necessary to give considerable thought to their proper treatment and care.

The purpose of this part of your text is to acquaint you with the physical plant with which you and your dentist work—office, equipment, and instruments—and to instruct you in the care of these valuable tools of dentistry.

31

The Dental Office...
Its Atmosphere,
Housekeeping,
and Maintenance

Atmosphere

Office atmosphere is one of the very important factors in patient relations. People enjoy being in colorful, attractive, clean, well-organized surroundings. Many offices today have background music which helps patients relax and adjust to office routines.

While it is not the responsibility of the dental assistant to provide the colorful, attractive surroundings, it *is* her responsibility to see that they remain attractive and clean. If music is used, it is also her responsibility to see that the volume is at the proper level.

Components of the Dental Office

Dental offices may have several rooms. The dental assistant should know the names and purposes of these rooms. The *reception room* is normally the room a patient enters, a place for him to relax before his appointment. Usually there is a coat rack or closet, comfortable furniture, and reading material. Most dentists provide a small-scale table and chairs for their child patients. These require more careful watching because children are inclined

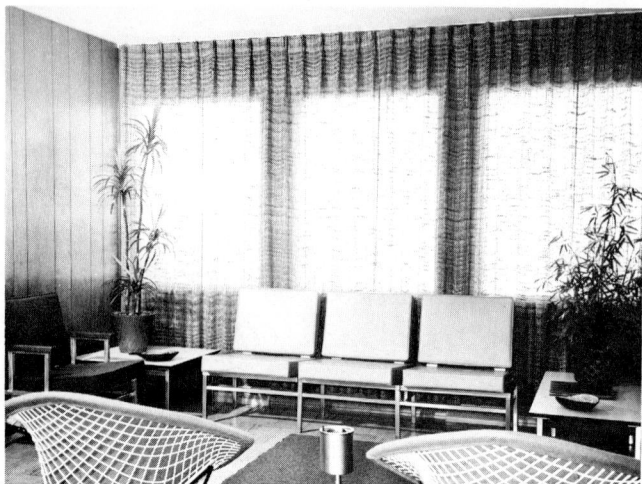

Fig. 31.1. A dental reception room

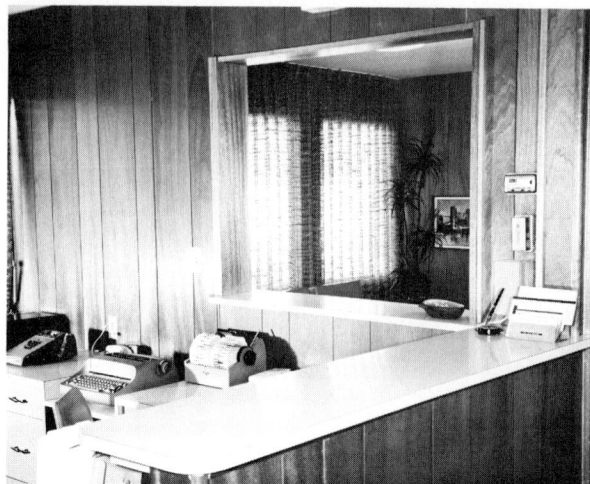

Fig. 31.2. The business office

to leave the magazine or book where they finish using it.

The *business office* most frequently adjoins the reception room in order that the business secretary may acknowledge entrants to the reception room. Usually there is a counter or window in the reception room which opens into the business area so that the secretary may continue to do her work between arrivals.

Some dentists have a *private inner office* where they present cases, conduct their professional business, and keep their library of dental journals and textbooks.

The *laboratory* is a room in which all the laboratory preparations to be done in the office are performed. The *darkroom* is used for X-ray developing, washing, and drying.

The *operatory* is the room which is furnished with the necessary equipment to perform all dental operations. There may be several operatories. In an office where there is more than one operatory, each room may be designed for special operations—or they may be exact duplicates.

The dental office today ought to be beautiful, and the colors should be restful and relaxing. We hope that your dentist provides this atmosphere for his patients; but regardless

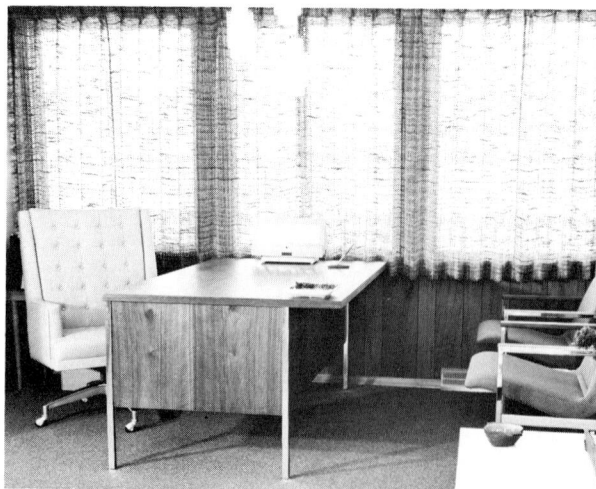

Fig. 31.3. A private office where the dentist may present cases.

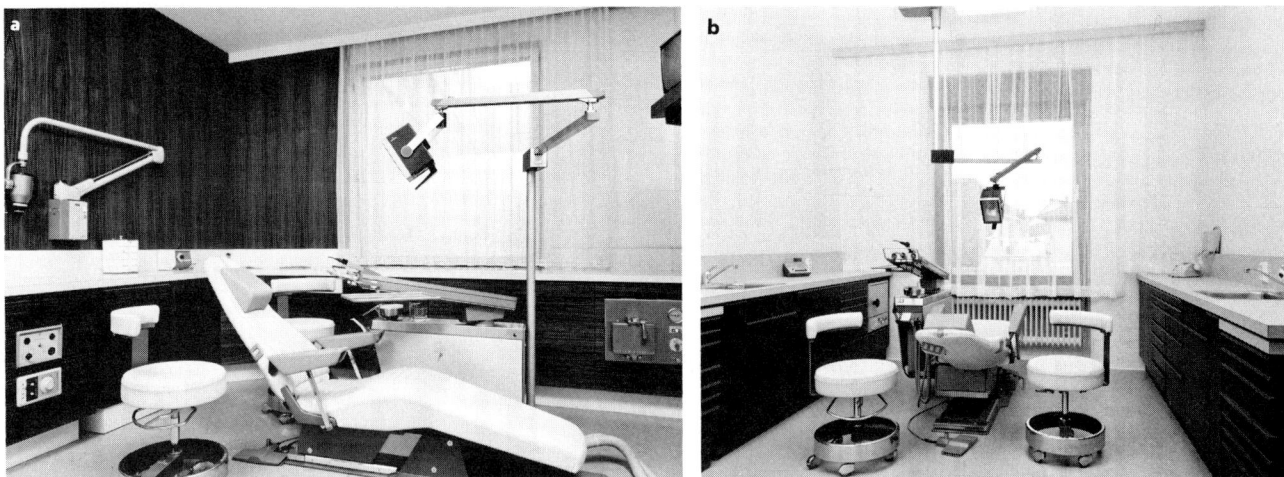

Fig. 31.4.   (a) A contemporary operatory including Siemens T2-S chair 2000E unit, operating light, stools for dentist and chair assistant, sink in corner, and wall-mounted X ray. (b) A modern operatory installed in an older office building. Note the stools, chair, unit, light placement, and two sinks (one for dentist, one for chair assistant). Built-ins permit storage at site of work.

of what kind of atmosphere he provides, the dental office must be immaculately clean, neat, and attractive. The equipment must be in excellent working condition as well as sparkling with good grooming.

This chapter is devoted to helping the assistant maintain the kind of office the most fastidious person will enjoy entering. Please don't be reluctant about doing some tasks which may seem to be the most menial labor. Sometimes it is necessary to do actual housecleaning. Accidents do happen; occasionally there is need for the assistant to perform janitorial work.

A clean, attractive office, perhaps with musical background of a relaxing nature, provides an atmosphere of congeniality for the dentist, the dental assistant, and the patient.

Housekeeping and Maintenance

The following daily routines are reminder lists of jobs to be done on a regular basis each day. Referral to these lists will help reassure you that the office is at its best at all times.

Daily Routines

Opening the Office

Open the office one-half hour before appointment time of the first patient, or at the regular time for office hours to begin, whichever is earlier.

Open enough windows and open all the doors to give the office a thorough airing.

Turn on all necessary switches. Prepare all equipment needed.

See that all instruments are sterilized and placed in their proper drawers or on the proper trays. Instruments left in cold disinfectant overnight should be dried and returned to their proper places, ready for use. Rubber bulbs, hoses, or other plastic or rubber parts can be wiped either with gauze moistened with a disinfectant or with a disposable disinfectant pad.

Dust *everything* in all rooms carefully; wipe all surfaces of equipment. Extend the arm of the X ray and wipe all crevices with care. Scrub footrests with soap and water or other designated cleaners.

See that everything is neatly and properly arranged, from magazines to equipment.

Illumination in all rooms should be correct for the existing conditions.

When you have finished, walk through all the rooms again as if you had never seen them before. Look around, from the patient's actual position in the reception room and operatory.

Place patients' records for the day in the proper operating rooms.

During the day, keep the office looking as neat as possible. Check it occasionally.

Closing the Office

Clean the instruments and remove debris of the last patient's appointment. Cutting instruments may be left in cold disinfectant solution overnight, if necessary. Other instruments may be prepared for sterilizing upon arrival the next workday, unless needed for the first patient; but they should be washed with soap and brush and rinsed whether they are to be sterilized immediately or left until morning.

Whenever possible, setups for the first patient of the next workday should be prepared.

Turn off all equipment.

Elevate chairs completely for easier access to the floor by the cleaning crew.

Check all windows. Be sure that heating or air conditioning is properly set for the night.

Leave no office records out. Appointment book, receipt book, records prepared for the next workday, etc., should be placed together in a closed drawer, cabinet, or filing case.

Cover all office equipment, such as typewriters, adding machines, and copiers.

Any patients for the next workday who have not been contacted by telephone should be called at this time for appointment reminder.

Double-check to see that all sterilizers, units, lights, water valves, and air compressors are turned off and no radiographs are left in the washing tank.

Take all outgoing mail with you and mail it. Be certain that the office door is locked.

Care of the Laboratory

The laboratory is the workshop of the dental office for those procedures which require preparation for completion outside the patient's mouth. Since these procedures are directly related to the welfare of the patient, the laboratory should be kept as scrupulously clean as any other part of the dental office. It is frequently as visible to the patient as the operating room. By its cleanliness and general good order, it forms a part of the total impression the patient receives of the dental office.

Making the Office a Place of Beauty

An office can be charming and attractive without losing its efficiency. No matter what furnishings and decor your dentist desires in his office, the addition of natural or artificial plants and flowers add a touch of beauty appreciated by most patients.

Whether the dentist selects the plants or leaves it up to the assistant, she is responsible for the care of these plants. When the assistant is not familiar with a particular plant, she should consult a florist or the library to learn how to care for it. There are many pamphlets which are helpful in determining the care of plants.

Routines Which Keep the Office Beautifully Clean

Equipment in a dental office will vary a great deal in age, type, and condition of maintenance. Breakdown of equipment may be reduced and smoother operation assured by proper maintenance of each piece. A carefully planned schedule for this work takes a minimum of time to execute once the schedule is set up in written form. The list of jobs may seem long, but each item requires only a few seconds or minutes to perform. A Come-up file assures your proper care of all items of equipment as they require care.

Each item of equipment listed in this chapter is followed by a series of suggestions for proper maintenance. These suggestions are general. They apply to the equipment produced by most manufacturers. For answers to questions about the care of a particular piece of equipment in your office read the instruction booklet from the manufacturer.

Finishes

Several pieces of equipment in the dental office have similar finishes. The care of each finish is the same regardless of where it is found.

CHROME AND STAINLESS STEEL Wipe with a clean, damp cheesecloth pad daily. Polish with a dry cloth. If stains or finger marks remain, use a nonscratching cleanser and then polish. Stainless steel will respond well to good soapsuds, a rinse, and a dry polishing.

ENAMEL Wipe with a clean, damp cheesecloth pad daily and dry with a soft cloth.

Wax lightly every two months.

Every six months use a cleaner before waxing the surface.

If chipping occurs, touch up the spots with enamel finish which can be purchased at your dental supply house.

WOOD Furniture generally remains more beautiful when kept waxed. One nationally known teacher of home economics recommends that furniture be thoroughly cleaned, then waxed daily with a carnauba-base wax until one hundred coats of wax are built up. Weekly waxing will protect the piece.

Daily dusting is essential to maintain a clean dental office.

Scratches may be hidden with one of the many commercial stains available for that purpose.

LEATHER SURFACES[1] For normal use apply a cloth dampened with lukewarm water to a mild soap, such as castile, and rub briskly over the surface of the leather. Next, remove soapy film with another damp cloth, since even the film of the mildest soap may cause discoloration if left on the leather. Finally, rub briskly with a dry cloth to bring back the original gloss.

Never use oils, varnishes, or furniture polishes on upholstery leather since most of these compounds contain solvents which attack the finish of the leather.

Occasionally, abnormal conditions of wear, such as the increased acidity in the atmosphere of large cities, necessitate the use of a more effective material for cleaning and preserving the finish of upholstery leather than is possible with the use of soap and water. We recommend an upholstery leather cleaner and dressing.

PLASTIC SURFACES Wash with a mild soap or detergent, rinse well, and dry. If this procedure is not suitable for a special plastic, the manufacturer's label will so indicate.

DRAPERIES—CURTAINS—RUGS—UPHOLSTERY—SLIP COVERS Watch for signs of soil. The varying conditions of each practice determine the length of time between cleanings. A practice located in the heart of an industrial center may find draperies or curtains soiled in less than a month. A residential, air-conditioned office may find yearly cleaning sufficient.

Commercial cleaning of rugs or draperies is usually preferred. Check to find a reputable cleaner. Be sure that both you and the dry

---

1. Information supplied by the Lackawana Leather Company, Hackettstown, New Jersey, to the S. S. White Dental Manufacturing Company for the care of colored leather upholstery.

cleaner know the size of the rugs and draperies before they are cleaned. A reminder to him to be certain that they are returned the same size as they were before cleaning assures you of well-fitting draperies and rugs on their return.

Curtains may be commercially-laundered or home-laundered as your dentist desires.

Spots on upholstered furniture should be removed promptly with one of the many detergents available for this purpose. Seasonal dry cleaning may be necessary, depending on the particular type of practice.

Slip covers may be home-laundered or dry-cleaned as your dentist chooses. They should be cleaned as soon as soiled since they look better and wear longer if they receive proper care.

POTTERY AND GLASS Wash with soapy water, rinse, and polish dry.

LINOLEUM—RUBBER TILE—ASPHALT TILE—CORK—PLASTIC TILE In most offices janitor or cleaning services care for floors, but there are counter tops occasionally made of these materials.

There are cleaners on the market today which clean these finishes without the use of water. Most of them contain a wax which helps maintain a beautiful finish. The cleaners are labeled for the surfaces on which they may be safely used. A cleaner-wax suitable for one may harm another.

A soapy cloth, followed with a clear-water rinse, is suitable. Be sure to wipe the surface dry when it has been rinsed. The trick is to avoid any excessive quantity of water in cleaning these glued-on surfaces.

Summary

Office atmosphere is a very important factor in patient relations. Keeping the office clean and attractive is essential to the successful practice of dentistry.

The dental office may be divided into a reception room, business office, private office, laboratory, darkroom, and operatory—or several operatories.

Planning and executing routines for the numerous jobs which must be done to create a clean, attractive office is an important part of the dental assistant's work.

Study Questions
1. Why is it essential to maintain a clean and attractive office?
2. What components are there in a dental office?
3. How can a dental assistant maintain a clean and attractive dental office?
4. Describe the routines for opening the office.
5. Describe the routines for closing the office.

32 Dental Equipment and Maintenance

Dental Equipment—Old and New

The design of dental equipment has undergone more rapid change since the mid-fifties than at any other period in the previous one hundred years. Although many dental offices are still served by the hydraulic-pump-type chair, illustrated in figure 32.1, and a floor-mounted dental unit similar to that illustrated in figure 32.2, the contour motor chair coupled with a mobile chair-mounted or cabinet-mounted unit (fig. 32.3) is more characteristic of the modern dental office or clinic.

The belt-driven handpiece, the workhorse of restorative dentistry two decades ago, has been almost completely replaced by air-powered handpieces.

Dental cabinets may be wall-hung or mobile. Usually the dental assistant's cabinet is mobile, allowing her to place it in a position most convenient for her as she assists at the chair (fig. 32.3). The mounted cabinets will often have an additional sink, one for the dentist and one for the assistant.

Whatever the style of the dental unit, it usually has the following components:

High-speed contra-angle handpiece,

Low-speed high-torque handpiece with contra-angle,

Three-way syringe (air, air-water, and water from the same jet),

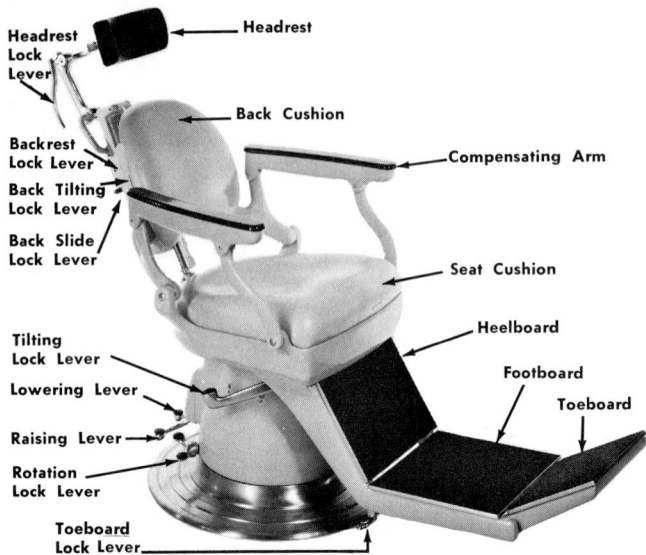

Headrest Lock Lever

Headrest

Back Cushion

Backrest Lock Lever

Back Tilting Lock Lever

Back Slide Lock Lever

Compensating Arm

Seat Cushion

Tilting Lock Lever

Lowering Lever

Raising Lever

Rotation Lock Lever

Heelboard

Footboard

Toeboard

Toeboard Lock Lever

Courtesy Weber Dental Mfg. Co.

(above) **Fig. 32.1.** Older type dental chair
(right) **Fig. 32.2.** Older type dental unit
(below) **Fig. 32.3.** Lounge-type dental chair and unit.

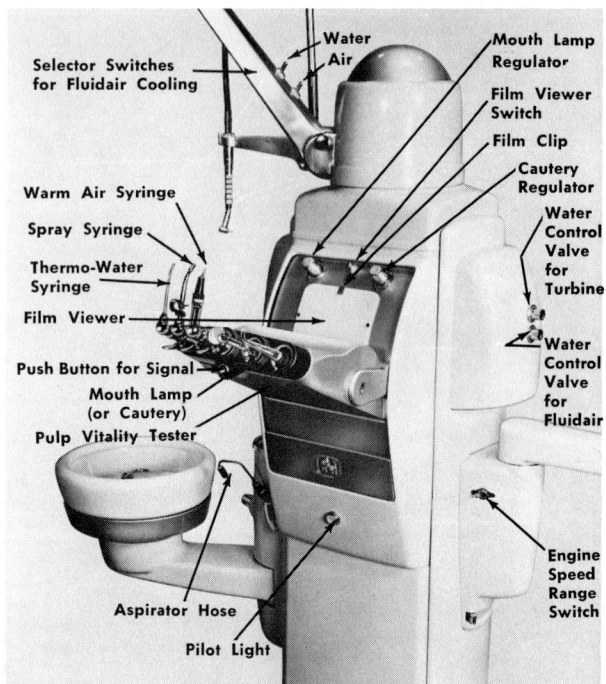

Selector Switches for Fluidair Cooling

Water
Air

Mouth Lamp Regulator

Film Viewer Switch

Film Clip

Cautery Regulator

Warm Air Syringe

Spray Syringe

Thermo-Water Syringe

Film Viewer

Push Button for Signal

Mouth Lamp (or Cautery)

Pulp Vitality Tester

Water Control Valve for Turbine

Water Control Valve for Fluidair

Engine Speed Range Switch

Aspirator Hose

Pilot Light

Courtesy Ritter Dental Mfg. Co.

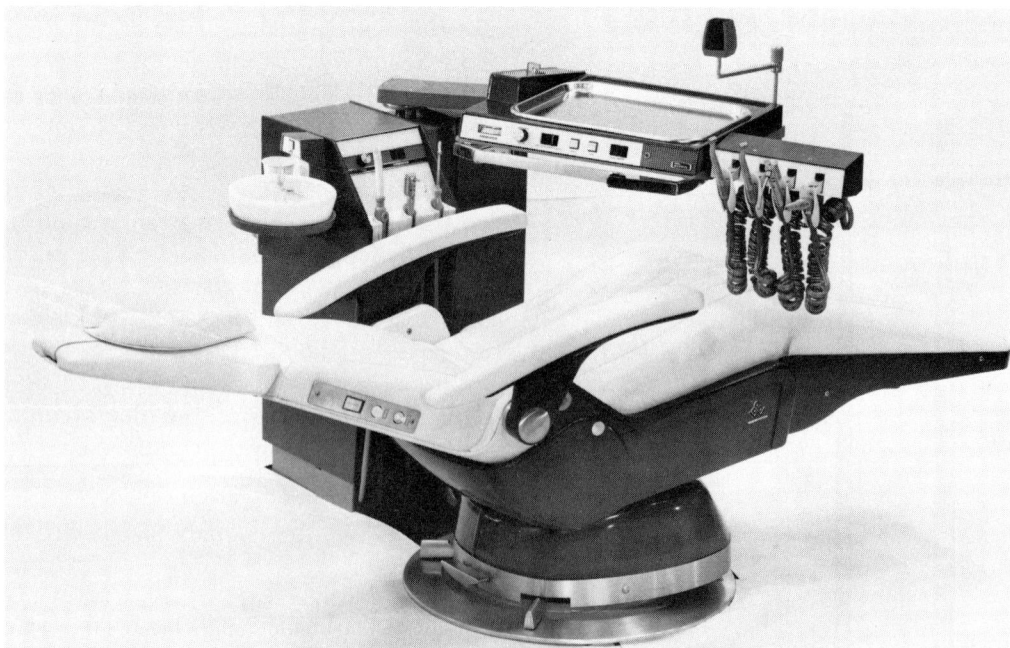

Courtesy S. S. White Co.

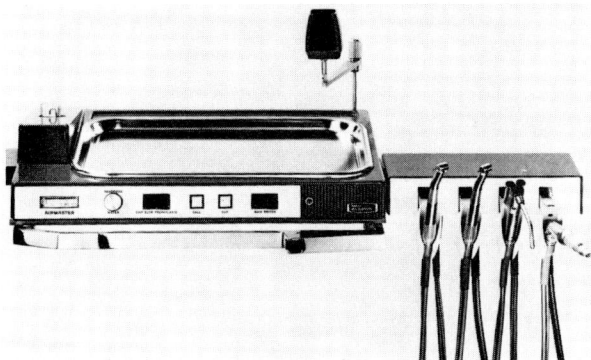

Courtesy S. S. White Co.

Fig. 32.4 An instrument panel of a modern dental unit, with contra-angle, handpiece, and syringe.

Saliva ejector,

High-volume evacuation,

Cuspidor or evacuation cup.

Although they are still available, units with a motor-powered belt-driven handpiece have all but disappeared from the market.

An oral evacuator is used to remove water, saliva, scraps of material, or any other foreign matter, from the patient's mouth. It provides a clear field (good visibility) for the dentist as he works.

Separation tanks are arranged to trap solid debris, permitting the liquids to be collected in a separate tank or to be automatically directed into a waste line when the motor of the evacuator unit is turned off. *The solid materials must be removed by the assistant at regular intervals to insure proper functioning of the evacuator.*

When the cuspidor is eliminated, usually a second suction line or hose will provide a cup which can be used by the patient to empty his mouth when necessary to supplement the evacuator. These occasions will be rare if the low-pressure evacuator is operated in a skillful manner by the dental assistant. The evacuator tip must be used both to remove water

and debris from the patient's mouth and at the same time to keep soft tissues retracted (out of the way). In some areas of the mouth this will seem an impossible problem in dexterity, but it can be developed with practice. The most rapid way to acquire this skill is to observe the manner in which a skilled person manipulates the tip of the evacuator while working with the dentist, then try to repeat the positions yourself.

Regardless of age, all equipment requires expert care. The general instructions given in this chapter for the care of equipment must be supplemented with the specific instructions supplied in manual form with each piece of equipment when it is purchased. Your dentist may have this material available and on file. If not, such information may often be obtained by sending the name of the equipment, the model and serial number, and any other identifying information, to the manufacturer, with a request for the instruction or operating manual.

Care of Dental Equipment

The type of finish used on dental equipment will indicate the care required to keep the piece looking new. Refer to the previous chapter on "Housekeeping" for directions regarding the proper care of various finishes, such as enamel, chrome, leather, etc.

The Dental Unit

Some offices may use a conventional *engine arm and handpiece* for slow-speed operation as an adjunct to high-speed equipment in at least one operatory. This mechanism is one of the common dust-catchers—it requires constant attention to maintain an undeniably clean appearance around every pulley, joint, and crevice. It should be carefully wiped at least daily to remove accumulated dust and fuzz. Turn the parts of the arm to the left and right, up and down, and check the undersides of all parts as well as the portion you see most easily. Remember to take "the patient's point of view" in all cleaning procedures.

The *motor* which operates the handpiece through the pulleys and arms requires occasional lubrication. Your maintenance manual will give the necessary lubricating instructions.

The dental engine is made to run by the use of a *rheostat,* an electric control which is placed on the floor behind the dental chair, convenient to the foot of the dentist. It resembles a small hatbox with two little paddles sticking out on opposite sides. It is also known as a *foot controller.*

Dental units which have a *bracket table* or instrument table attached to an arm may have a gas burner or electric heater coil which is partially enclosed in a metal cup to catch any materials which might drip when heated. Wax drippings may accumulate in this cup when the burner is used; the assistant should remove the drippings and polish the cup with a piece of cotton saturated with chloroform.

Another dust trap on a conventional-type dental unit is the *cuspidor bowl* or evacuator cup. This should be cleaned as thoroughly as possible between patients, in addition to very thorough cleaning at least daily. A mild soap or cleanser should be used. Always look at this item from the "patient's point of view," because it can be left with unclean areas which are not visible to a person standing beside it but are visible to a person seated in the dental chair.

Cuspidors are also designed to trap or catch material which might tend to clog the drain. The device used for this purpose is called a *metal trap,* usually consisting of a removable strainer and cup in the center of the cuspidor. It is essential that this be removed and cleaned whenever a patient has emptied solid materials from his mouth, such as pieces of impression material. In such cases the cleaning opera-

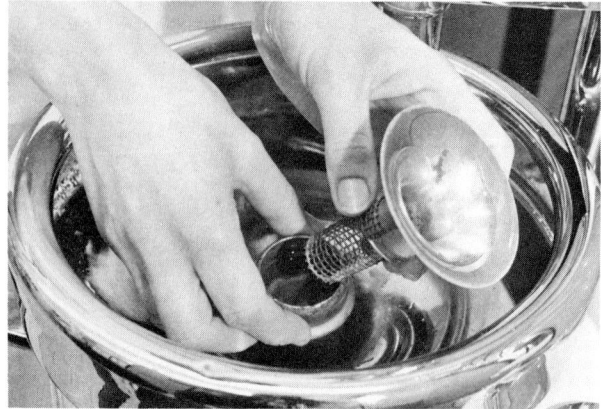

Fig. 32.5. Cleaning the cuspidor screen

tion is best done between patients. Very small scraps of amalgam, however, do not necessitate cleaning the trap until the end of the day.

Another part of the conventional dental unit which requires daily care is the *saliva-ejector screen.* The saliva ejector is composed of a flexible tube, about four feet long, attached to the unit at one end, with a short rubber collar at the free end into which a saliva ejector is placed (a piece of plastic or metal shaped

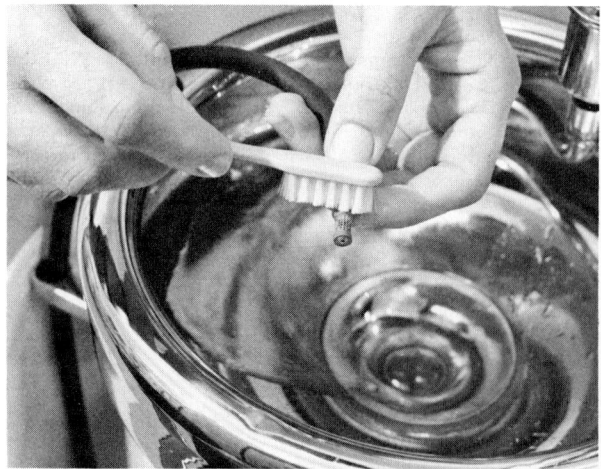

Fig. 32.6. Cleaning the saliva ejector screen

somewhat like a question mark). Its purpose is to remove saliva from the patient's mouth, when it is required, in order to keep the work area as dry as possible. Most offices will use a disposable type of saliva ejector made of plastic. These are discarded after use; metal types must be most carefully flushed after use and sterilized by the method of choice in the office. At the end of the day, flush very warm water through the hose of the saliva ejector; detergent may be added to the water.

The water supply to the cuspidor, as well as to the water syringe on a conventional dental unit, is caused to flow through a screen or strainer. This water-supply screen is usually positioned so that you can remove and clean it regularly without much difficulty. This should be done every three months, unless this time interval allows a considerable amount of material to collect in the screen. If this is true, increase the frequency of cleaning until only a small amount of debris needs to be removed each time. Much accumulation tends to cut down the flow of water to the necessary devices on the unit and also reduces the amount of suction available for the saliva ejector. To clean the water supply screen:

Turn off the main water valve.

Place a container under the plug containing the water-supply screen.

Remove the plug, catching any water which may drain from the pipes.

Clean the strainer and replace.

Turn on the main water valve.

Open the saliva ejector and cuspidor flush valves for a moment to expel any air which may be in the pipes.

Remove and clean the *cuspidor trap* of amalgam scrap every day. Place the trap contents on a piece of paper to dry, then into the scrap-amalgam jar.

Every morning wash the *glassware* with soap and water. If it is necessary, use a nonscratching cleanser.

Summary of Care for the Dental Unit— Conventional Type

DAILY

Clean finish as needed.

Wipe engine arm.

Clean gas-burner or electric-coil cup of wax drippings.

Clean cuspidor bowl thoroughly and repeat as needed during the day.

Wash glassware.

Remove and clean saliva-ejector screen. Flush with warm water through hose.

Remove and clean the cuspidor trap.

LESS FREQUENT JOBS

Every two weeks oil the dental engine.

Every three months clean the water-supply screen.

Every six months care for the foot controller as directed.

Care of the Dental Chair

Care for the various finishes of the chair parts as directed in the section on finishes in chapter thirty-one.

The footrest of the dental chair becomes dirty every day. It should be scrubbed daily, upon opening the office.

When the chair back is movable, it slides up and down to adjust to the height of the individual patient. It moves on sliding channels in the back assembly, and these channels need to be wiped with a lightly oiled cloth each week.

At least once a week depress the chair to its lowest limits and then elevate it to its highest position. This lubricates the guideways of the hydraulic mechanism.

The seat and headrest should be treated as directed in the section on care of finishes. Headrest covers should be changed between patients.

If seat covers are used, determine the type of material and clean accordingly.

The elevation of the motor chair is changed by operating levers. Every three months these levers should be oiled. Some chairs have a metal shell which must be removed for access to the oilholes.

Under the seat of the chair you will find a tilting lock. Every three months it should be wiped well and then oiled.

The headrest lock assembly (with which the position of the headrest may be altered and set again) should be oiled lightly every six months.

The motor of the chair has an oil reservoir. At six-month intervals this reservoir should be checked and brought to the proper level.

Check the instructions which the manufacturer of the chair in your office gives for the type of oil to use for lubrication.

The Dental X ray

Care of the X ray is relatively simple. The finishes should be cared for as directed in chapter thirty-one.

Every two months oil the supports on either side of the X-ray head. They are called *trunions*.

Every six months put one drop of oil on the head retainer.

Use only the oil recommended by the manufacturer.

The Dental Cabinet

Dental cabinets should be cleaned at the beginning of each day and checked throughout the day for dust and debris which may have collected on the top or drawer surfaces as a result of the treatment activity. Occasionally, medications, cements, or other materials may be spilled inadvertently. Adhering sticky ce-

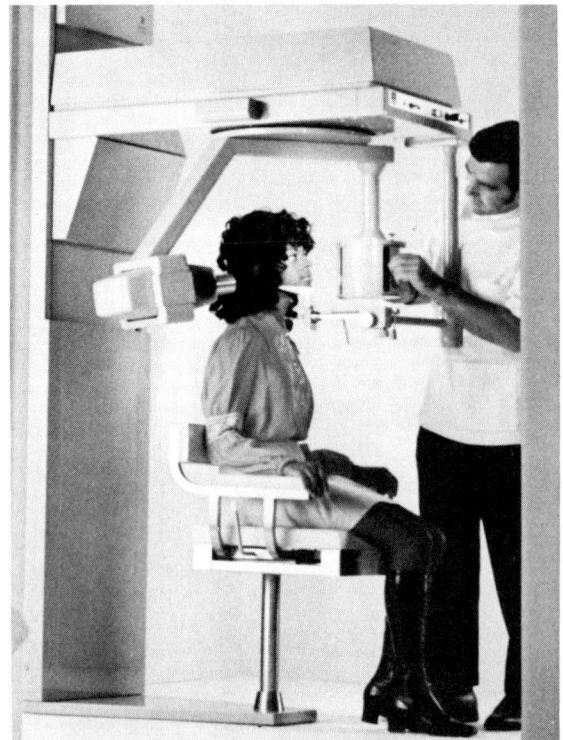

Courtesy General Electric Co.

Fig. 32.7. G.E.-100 remote control X-ray unit, with compact control and wall support for tubehead.

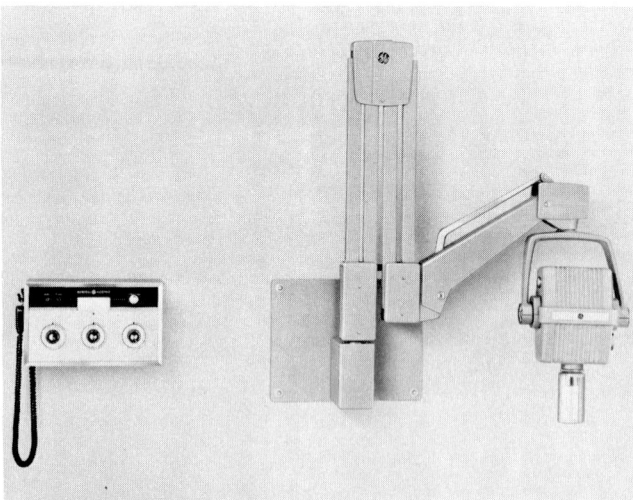

Courtesy General Electric Co.

Fig. 32.8. The panoramic X ray

ments may be cleaned by cotton dampened with xylol. Along with the cuspidor, unit, and chair, the cabinets should be checked for cleanliness before seating the next patient.

The Surgical Cabinet

The surgical cabinet contains *sterile* instruments for extraction and other surgery. They must be sterile at the time of their use.

As the instruments are sterilized, they are placed on autoclaved towels which completely cover all shelves.

Care must be taken in handling these towels so that they remain sterile.

When required, the surgical cabinet is cleaned, freshly autoclaved towels are placed on the shelves, and all instruments are resterilized and replaced.

To place autoclaved towels or sterile instruments in the surgical cabinet, use sterile tongs.

The Water Sanitizer

If boiling water is used for disinfecting instruments, check the water level several times daily, being sure that the instrument tray is fully covered when it is in the lowered position.

Remove the water completely and scour the inside of the boiler and tray once a week. Use cleanser and a cloth. If the water in your community is exceptionally hard, heavy deposits will accumulate. It may be necessary to clean the inside of the boiler daily.

Sterilizer tablets may be purchased which, when put into the water sanitizer, prevent corrosion, rust, and staining of steel instruments.

If scale should begin to accumulate which cannot be removed with normal cleaning, fill the boiler with a 10 percent solution of hydrochloric acid and boil about fifteen minutes. Then scour with cleanser and a cloth or brush.

Maintain the outside of the water sanitizer as suggested under "Chrome and Stainless-Steel Finishes," chapter thirty-one.

The Oil Sanitizer

The oil sanitizer usually holds a pint of oil. When it is necessary to fill it, use a pint measure. If none is available, fill the reservoir until the tray, in the down position, is covered completely.

Oil does not evaporate; it becomes dirty. When it shows discoloration or is obviously dirty, warm it slightly and pour directly down the sink drain. If your aim is good, you will not have a messy cleaning job in the sink.

When the sanitizer is empty, scour inside with a cleanser and a cloth. Wipe dry and clean.

Refill with one pint of clean oil.

The outside is cleaned according to the directions for chrome and stainless-steel finishes. Hard caking of carbon may occur. If it does, this will have to be removed with a flat blade, exercising due care to prevent scratching the metal of the sanitizer.

The Ultrasonic Cleaner

An excellent device for cleaning instruments prior to sterilizing is an ultrasonic cleaner. See figure 32.9.

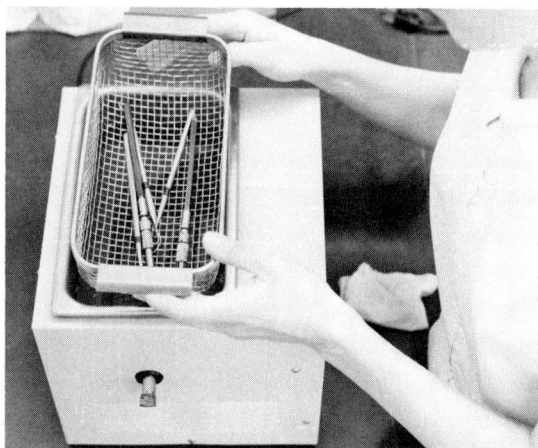

Fig. 32.9. A basket of instruments is being placed into the ultrasonic cleaner for cleaning.

The Autoclave

Only distilled water is used in the auto-clave. It may need to be replenished during the day. Be sure that you check the water level before each use. Be certain that you fill it or refill it only with distilled water.

Once each month drain all the water from the reservoir. Scrub the inside of the reservoir and the chamber with soap and lukewarm water. Rinse thoroughly and rub dry. Refill with distilled water.

Every six months the autoclave is to be thoroughly cleansed. Prepare a commercial auto-clave cleanser and use as directed.

The outside of the autoclave is to be cleaned according to the directions given for chrome and stainless-steel finishes.

All moving parts are to be oiled or greased regularly. Use light oil or silicone grease on door hinge and center hub of locking attachment on the door.

Discharge valve screens should be removed and cleaned. Directions come with your particular autoclave.

Check rubber gasket on the inside of the door, if present. If the gasket is worn so that steam escapes, replace it.

Summary

Dental equipment design has changed drastically in the last twenty years. Since the equipment used is expensive and replaced only infrequently, the office in which you work may have a variety of types of equipment.

Familiarity with the operation and care of equipment in your office is important. Routines to help you maintain it are given in this chapter and in chapter thirty-one.

Study Questions
1. Describe the modern dental office equipment.
2. What components are usually found on the dental unit?
3. How do you care for the dental unit? dental chair? dental X ray? dental cabinet? surgical cabinet? water sanitizer? oil sanitizer? ultrasonic cleaner? autoclave?

33

Instruments... Their Use, Care, and Identification

NOTE: This chapter is divided into two parts: Part one is a discussion of instruments and armamentarium utilized in dentistry and the care which the dental assistant must give them. Part two is composed of illustrations which will permit the dental assistant to recognize the instruments found in the office in which she works.

Part One: Use and Care of Instruments

Dental instruments—so many tiny heads—each for a specific purpose! Each type of instrument may have a variety of similar—but slightly different—forms. This area of dental assisting can be quite confusing.

This chapter contains descriptions of the use and care of dental instruments. Some are larger instruments, such as handpieces. Others are hand instruments—the innumerable objects the dentist uses in the patient's mouth. They are hard to recognize at first because many look so similar.

Instruments are grouped according to purpose and should be studied in connection with their use in the office. There are pictures to help familiarize you with these tiny-headed objects which are so important. Although an excavator and a gingival margin trimmer look very much alike, they are used for different purposes. One has a curved-spoon edge, the other a beveled, knifelike edge. If you confuse them, it could be frustrating to your dentist to be handed the wrong instrument.

Clean, sterilized instruments are placed either on tray setups or in the cabinet drawers according to a plan which satisfies your dentist. Ordinarily, instruments used together are grouped together regardless of whether your dentist prefers to use the left-hand third drawer for amalgam instruments or any other specific drawer.

Cement bottles should be in the same drawer as the slabs and spatulas used for cement.

Mirrors, cotton pliers, and explorers—all are usually kept in the same drawer to facilitate setups.

Cutting instruments used in tooth preparations should be grouped in neighboring drawers.

If tray setups are used in your office, a group of stainless-steel or fiber-glass trays are kept in a special section of the work area. Each tray has a complete set of instruments on it for a specific dental operation. When a patient is scheduled for a recall, you have only to pull one of the trays which have been set up for recalls and place it in the proper work area. This procedure means faster change-over between patients and allows the dental assistant to replenish the trays in moments which are not pressured.

Instruments are expensive. They are carefully formed, delicate, and not to be subjected to misuse. Flaming, which can ruin the temper of the metal, should be avoided. (Without temper the instrument dulls very easily. Temper is sometimes called "the ability to hold an edge.")

Another misuse of the instrument is to drop it. Dropping can deform the working end. Since the instrument is valuable only so long as it is exactly shaped to perform an explicit task, the slightest malformation ruins it. Please take care of your instruments.

A good assistant is careful to keep all instruments in their proper places. She replaces them promptly after sterilization. She is positive that they are clean.

The sterilization of most of these instruments is considered postoperative sterilization—to sterilize the instrument after use. (See chap. 26.)

The Dental Unit and Its Accessories

The dental unit is considered to contain an evacuator, a three-way syringe, a dental light, and two handpieces—one for high-speed and one for low-speed operation. The unit may be floor-mounted or mobile; the light may be ceiling-mounted or part of the unit. For purposes of identification we will consider these items to be included in the dental unit:

Dental Light—Evacuator— Three-way Syringe

The *dental light* should be cleaned frequently; the handles should be routinely disinfected between patients.

The *evacuator* has removable tips which should be autoclaved after each use. It is used to keep the site free from debris and water. It affords the dentist better visibility of the area he is treating. The dental assistant operates the evacuator.

The *three-way syringe* delivers water, air, or both, as required by the operation.

The Handpieces (Figs. 33.1-33.3)

On the dental unit, the instruments which require the most care are the two handpieces and their accessories.

A handpiece, one of the basic instruments of dentistry, is used to prepare teeth for restorations and to clean the surfaces of teeth.

A handpiece is held by the dentist in his hand and is used with a variety of burs, stones, wheels, cups, and diamond instruments which the dentist selects and attaches to the end. He then turns on a speed control, usually with his foot, causing the bur or tip to revolve at a speed which the dentist can vary.

The figures on page 409 illustrate several types of handpieces: a low-speed, motor-driven straight handpiece with contra-angle which is inserted in the straight handpiece when needed; the electrotorque, a medium-speed, motor-driven handpiece, capable of being carried on house calls; an air-driven ultraspeed handpiece used for all high-speed preparations—air-driven in contrast to motor-driven.

The sleeve-type, friction-bearing handpiece, used for many years, operated at speeds up to 10,000 rpm. If it was used at higher speeds, its friction-type bearings became hot, making the handpiece uncomfortable for the dentist to hold and dangerous for the patient. The handpiece became hot enough to burn the patient's lips or cheeks.

These handpieces are still used for prophylaxis and removal of deep caries. They are also used with finishing discs and stones. These operations require high torque and slow speed without generating unnecessary heat.

When the sleeve-type friction bearings were replaced by ball bearings, it was discovered that the handpiece would operate at speeds up to 25,000 rpm without undue heat and wear. Consequently, the ball-bearing handpieces have replaced the friction-bearing types as a clinical instrument, whether air- or belt-motor-powered.

The *utraspeed handpieces* are usually air-turbine types and operate generally at 100,000-600,000 rpm. Their construction is very different from the conventional types. Instead of an electric motor to drive them, they use compressed air supplied to the handpiece through a very flexible rubber tubing, which is also the means of supplying water spray to the cutting instrument and the area being prepared. This handpiece is necessary in bulk tooth reduction in cavity and crown preparation where slow-speed operation not only is more time-consuming and traumatic to the tooth, but does not offer the ease of operation and control of the cutting tip for the dentist.

The handpiece is also described by its shape. There are contra-angles, right angles, and straight handpieces. Their uses vary, but the principle of their operation is the same.

There are several types of handpieces. *The dental assistant should learn the uses and care of those found in her office.* Each handpiece comes with the manufacturer's directions for maintenance. Follow the instructions scrupulously.

Care of Standard-Speed Contra-Angles and Right Angles

After each use run the contra-angle or right angle in the cleaner recommended by the manufacturer, then in the lubricant solution, for the specified time. Wipe with a gauze moistened with seventy percent alcohol.

When replacing the contra-angles and right angles in the tray used for their storage, it is preferable to place the recently prepared instruments behind those already in the tray. When removing one for use, always remove the front instrument. This helps rotate the use of instruments to equalize the amount of wear.

Care of Ultraspeed Handpieces

Follow the manufacturer's instructions accurately when caring for ultraspeed handpieces. Usually they may be wiped with ethyl or isopropyl alcohol; some may be autoclaved. Check with care. They are expensive, delicate instruments.

Care of Standard Handpieces (Low-Speed)

A ball-bearing handpiece is a delicate precision instrument and requires meticulous care to remain optimally functional. The sheath should be removed from the handpiece assembly daily, and any excess oil should be wiped off. If oilholes are present at the bearing sites, place a drop of oil in each hole. The manufacturer's directions will be specific in this detail. Follow the directions for care.

The handpiece may be sterilized or disinfected for each patient in one of two ways. The outer shell of the handpiece is called the *sheath*. This is removable. If extra sheaths are available in the office, after use each is sterilized in the autoclave or sanitized in the water sanitizer or cold disinfectant solution. A clean one is placed on the handpiece for the next patient. If extra sheaths are not supplied, the sheath should be wiped thoroughly with a gauze moistened with seventy percent alcohol before the next patient is seated.

The underside of the handpiece pulley, the side facing the sheath of the handpiece, is often missed in wiping. Be sure that it is kept clean.

The entire handpiece assembly, including the *wrist joint*, should be removed once each week under average conditions and run through the oil sanitizer, if one is available in the office. Some types of handpieces may be disassembled for this process. Ask the dental supply salesman about the handpiece used in your office. It should be sanitized twenty minutes from a cold start in the oil sanitizer.

If an oil sanitizer is used for the handpiece, remove the handpiece, while still hot, after the required sanitizing time and drain thoroughly and immediately on a paper bib. When cooled sufficiently, wipe off any remaining excess of oil, reassemble, and replace on engine arm. Wipe the sheath with a gauze wet with seventy percent alcohol and place on handpiece assembly. Holding a disposable tissue over the wrist-joint assembly, run the engine wide open for fifteen seconds, holding the engine arm extended. The disposable tissue will catch oil which spatters from the wrist-joint pulleys.

In the next few pages we will consider the cutting instruments used in handpieces: burs, diamond instruments, prophylaxis brushes and cups, small mounted abrasive stones, and unmounted abrasive stones used with mandrels.

The flexible wire scratch brush is used for removing debris lodged in the rough surfaces of the bur (fig. 33.4).

Accessories for the Handpieces

Dental Burs (Figs. 33.5, 33.6)

The "drill" with which the dentist prepares a tooth for a restoration is correctly called a *bur*. Dental burs are supplied in two types of material: one is the regular steel bur; the other is a carbide bur. Regular steel burs are used at operating speeds of up to 10,000 rpm. Carbide burs are used at speeds up to 600,000 rpm.

Carbide burs are more expensive than regular steel burs, but they last much longer. They must not be immersed in cold disinfecting solution unless the manufacturer specifically indicates that this is permissible.

Manufacturers place a distinguishing feature on their carbide burs: the shank may be colored brown or gold, it may have grooves conspicuously placed around it, it may have other types of markings; or the shape of the bur at the "neck" may differ markedly. Learn to identify all the brands of carbide burs used in your office so that you will not confuse them with regular steel burs. They are usually stored for use in a bur block different from the block in which regular steel burs are stored.

All burs may be cleaned by brushing well with a "scratch brush" (see fig. 33.4). They must be cleaned thoroughly. Regular steel burs may be sterilized in the dry-heat oven, in oil sanitizers, or in an autoclave. Carbide burs should be sterilized according to the manufacturer's recommendations only.

Burs for contra-angles are supplied with either friction-grip or latch-type shanks. The straight handpiece is designed to hold only the long-shanked burs. The standard latch-type contra-angle will hold standard angle and short-shank burs. A miniature-head latch-type contra-angle is required for miniature burs. Some manufacturers also make a long-shanked bur for contra-angle use. Gear-type contra-angles for slow speed are also available with friction grip. High-speed handpieces, such as air turbines, use burs which have a more slender shank, referred to as a *friction grip* or *FG type*. These burs are all carbide.

Domestic burs (burs manufactured in this country) are numbered according to a specific numbering system which most dentists use. Imported burs may be numbered differently.

Friction-grip and latch-type burs are kept in separate bur blocks, properly labeled. The diagram of burs in figure 33.6 will show you the *shapes* of burs; the size numbers give you some understanding of the gradations in size of each shape of bur.

Diamond Instruments (Fig. 33.7)

Diamond instruments cut harder structures more quickly than burs and are used particularly to "open" a tooth, i.e., to get through the enamel, or to do major shaping as for a full-crown preparation. They are used in a handpiece—usually in those handpieces capable of very high speeds.

Diamond instruments used under a constant stream of water or a water-air spray are very easy to keep clean. If they are used without a stream of water or water-air spray, the job is more difficult and heat is generated which will damage the pulp. The surface of the disc or wheel tends to become clogged with the fine debris of the grinding operation. The longer this debris remains on the surface of the dia-

mond instrument the more difficult it is to remove and the more heat is generated.

Diamond instruments should be cleaned in the ultrasonic cleaner immediately after use. If an ultrasonic cleaner is not available, immerse instruments for five minutes in a solution of soapy water.

Using a stiff-bristled toothbrush, brush the surface of the instrument until completely free of debris, rinse, and then dry by blowing with the air syringe.

If the debris will not come free, mount instrument in the slow handpiece, run engine as slowly as possible, and gently hold a rubber ink eraser against the cutting surface of the instrument, moving eraser back and forth across the surface until clean. Be careful of your fingers! Rinse with clear water and dry as before.

If, through some circumstance, diamond instruments should become coated with dried blood and mucus which will not brush off, they may be cleaned by soaking in an ordinary paintbrush cleaner.

Diamond instruments which are filled with amalgam may be cleaned most safely by soaking overnight in mercury, then running slowly against an ink eraser.

Keep all diamond instruments in holders for that purpose, clean and ready for use.

Dental Prophylaxis Right-Angle Brushes and Cups (Fig. 33.8)

A patient recall appointment includes a prophylaxis—which to the patient means cleaning his teeth. A special right angle may be used on the handpiece with cups and brushes which clean and polish the surfaces of the teeth.

It is possible for the prophylaxis brushes and cups to be mounted in the regular handpiece, but the abrasive material used to clean the teeth can work its way into the handpiece and wear it out sooner than necessary. A prophylaxis right angle is designed to prevent this wear from occurring. You may find either used in your dentist's office.

If a hygienist is caring for the patient, she may use brushes, rubber cups, and porte-polishers for the recall visit.

Mandrel (Fig. 33.9)

A mandrel is used to attach small grinding stones or sandpaper discs. It is a rod of metal —a shank which is inserted into the handpiece. A mandrel with no cutting instrument attached to it is equipped wth a pin or tiny screw in the end. The dentist attaches a paper disc or an unmounted stone with this pin or screw to the mandrel and then inserts the mandrel into the handpiece. Some stones are mounted stones and are attached permanently to a mandrel. These are simply inserted into the handpiece. There will be some mandrels available if your office uses polishing discs and unmounted stones. Mandrels are available for straight (conventional) handpieces and for (conventional) contra-angles. The latter are shorter than the former.

Stones (Fig. 33.10)

The handpiece can be used with mounted or unmounted stones to do many grinding operations—on surfaces in the mouth, on artificial teeth, on casts, and on any material which needs to be finished.

There are several types of stones used for different purposes as well as overlapping purposes. If the stones are green, they are carborundum; if they are red, they are aluminum oxide; and if they are gray, they are heatless stones, i.e., they produce little heat when being used.

Stones which are permanently attached to a mandrel are referred to as mounted stones; those which must be mounted on a mandrel before they can be used in the handpiece are unmounted stones.

Basic Setups

No matter what dental operation is to be performed, certain instruments are utilized. We refer to them as a *basic setup*. They are placed on the tray for every patient who is seated in the dental chair. They include dental mirrors, explorers, and cotton pliers.

Dental Mirrors (Figs. 33.11-33.13)

Dental mirrors are supplied with short stems fixed to a circular mirror. There are two types of stems: plain or simple for use with a plain handle, and cone-socket for use with a cone-socket handle. Dental offices usually use one type or the other. The mirror itself is available in two types, plane and magnifying. The plane type gives the same image as a hand mirror, whereas the magnifying type gives an enlarged image. Mirror sizes vary. They are listed either by inches in diameter or by a size number (1-5).

Explorers (Fig. 33.14)

Explorers are used most commonly to examine the teeth. Most of them are double-ended, that is, they have a point on each end. They will be different points. A number on the handle identifies the design of the explorer. When the points become bent or dull, the instrument must be replaced.

Cotton Pliers (Fig. 33.15)

Cotton pliers are long tweezers with bent, pointed ends. They are used to take materials to and from the mouth.

Miscellaneous Armamentarium

Certain materials are used commonly in dentistry but are not necessary for every operation. The following materials and instruments are such.

Rubber Dam (Fig. 33.16-33.20)

Most dental operations are performed with better visibility and better results when the "field of operation" is isolated and completely dry. Cotton rolls and cotton-roll holders of various kinds are commonly used for this purpose, in addition to low-pressure evacuators or saliva ejectors.

The ideal method of achieving this, however, is by applying a rubber dam to the teeth under operation. Rubber dam is supplied either as precut 5″ x 5″ or 6″ x 6″ squares or in a roll five or six inches wide, in light or dark color. The dam also comes in various thicknesses. It is usually coated lightly with talc to prevent sticking.

A piece of rubber dam approximately seven inches in length is cut off the roll. The rubber-dam punch is used to make a series of small holes in this piece. Holes are usually made for a few teeth to the mesial of the one under operation and at least one to the distal, if one is present. The position of the holes corresponds to a spot in the center of the occlusal or incisal surface of the teeth involved, and in that same relative position to each other hole. That is, if holes were to be punched for a complete set of sixteen teeth in one arch, they would be placed in exactly the same curve as the arch itself. A rubber-dam template may be used as a guide to positioning the holes until sufficient experience is gained.

The rubber dam is lubricated lightly with Vaseline around each punched hole, as an aid in slipping the rubber dam over each tooth. The rubber dam is then placed in the mouth, with the punched holes over the corresponding teeth, and the dam is slipped down over each tooth for which holes have been punched, slipping the edge of the rubber dam through the contact first. At the cervical area of each tooth, the rubber dam is tucked downward under the "free gum margin" into the gingival crevice for a good seal against moisture. Saliva, as well as any interference from the tongue or cheeks, is well controlled. A *rubber-dam retainer* is usually placed on the most distal tooth to hold the rubber down in position. A *rubber-dam retainer forceps* is used in placing the clamp. Dental floss is sometimes used in addition to a rubber-dam retainer, or alone, as a ligature around the cervical portion of some or all of the teeth exposed through the rubber dam.

A rubber-dam frame or holder is then positioned to secure the sheet of rubber dam. The elastic band of the holder goes around the back of the patient's head and is adjusted to hold snugly. When a saliva ejector has been inserted (sometimes under the rubber dam and sometimes through another hole punched in the dam for that purpose), the field is clear and ready for the operative procedures.

Weights are sometimes clipped to the lower edge of the rubber dam as an aid in holding this edge down, out of the dentist's way.

Gauze napkins, called rubber-dam napkins, are available for use under rubber-dam applications. This gauze is shaped like the piece of rubber dam except for a large opening cut out of the gauze for the mouth, since the gauze is designed to lie between the rubber dam and the skin of the face. The use of a rubber-dam napkin makes a rubber dam much more comfortable for the patient. Moisture which may seep between the skin of the face and the rubber dam is otherwise extremely uncomfortable.

The application of rubber dam is more easily performed with the help of the dental assistant to hold the rubber in position before the retainer is placed, as well as in using a piece of dental floss to help force the rubber dam down between teeth when the contacts are so tight as to make it difficult.

Observation of the problems involved will show the dental assistant many ways to assist in this procedure.

Anesthetic Syringes (Figs. 33.21-33.22)

The instrument with which the dentist injects a local anesthetic is called a *syringe*. The most commonly used type in dental offices consists of a barrel with open sides. A plunger mechanism is inserted into one end of the barrel and has a barb on the end to engage the rubber plug in the local anesthetic *cartridge*. The other end of the plunger mechanism has a crossbar or round disc for the dentist's thumb. The end of the barrel containing the plunger mechanism opens in some manner to permit the insertion of the cartridge. This may be a spring device or a screw device. Examine the type used in your office. Learn how it operates.

The other end of the barrel contains the mounting mechanism for the needle. A portion at the end of the barrel is threaded, with an opening in the center through which part of the injection needle extends inside the barrel. This end of the needle perforates the "fixed" plug or cap of the anesthetic cartridge and communicates with the solution inside. As the plunger is depressed, the solution is discharged.

Needles for Anesthetic Syringes
(Figs. 33.23-33.24)

Needles are manufactured in various gauges which are indications of the outside diameter of the needle. The gauges used in dental offices are 25, 26, 27, 28, 29, and 30. Twenty-five-gauge would be the heaviest needle with the greatest diameter; and thirty-gauge would be the finest needle with the smallest diameter.

To insure a sterile and sharp needle every time, presterilized disposable needles are used. Each needle is individually sterile, protected within a two-piece plastic case. It is generally necessary to remove that section which covers the short end, attach the needle to the syringe by holding the remaining plastic sheath, then remove the remaining portion of the plastic

sheath when ready for the injection. The ampule is inserted into the syringe barrel prior to attaching the needle.

When reusable needles are received from the supply house, they will have a *stylet* (a tiny wire) inserted in the *lumen* (the hollow passage which extends the length of the needle). *The stylet must be removed prior to use.*

The length of the needle is also variable. The longest one commonly used is one and seven-eighths inches long, and the shortest is just one inch.

Local anesthetic solutions are most commonly supplied to the dental office in cans of fifty glass tubes, called *ampules* or *cartridges*. The glass tube, or ampule, is closed at one end by a rubber plug which rests completely inside the tube. This is the "movable" plug which faces the plunger when inserted in the syringe. The other end of the ampule is also closed, either with a rubber stopper, which has a shoulder extending over the glass wall, or a metal cap with a small rubber center. This is the "fixed" plug, which faces the needle when inserted in the syringe. The fixed plug should be wiped with a solution of seventy percent ethyl alcohol before insertion in the syringe.

Proper preparation before and proper care after use of anesthetic syringes are most important. Improper care can result in infection of a patient. The ideal method of providing care for anesthetic syringes is to autoclave them.

Always prepare the syringe as if it were to be used on yourself!

Preparation of Syringes for Use—
Autoclaved

If presterilized needles are used in your office, the syringe body alone needs sterile handling and storage.

If presterilized needles are *not* used, proceed as follows:

1. After autoclaving, store the syringes with a sterile cotton roll protecting the needle or place them in seventy percent alcohol in a syringe storage jar.
2. If stored with a sterile cotton roll over the needle, leave the roll in place, open the syringe and insert the anesthetic ampule with the fixed plug toward the needle. Test for delivery as before. Replace the cotton roll.
3. Place the syringe on the tray or working top, preferably covering it with a disposable tissue.

Care of Syringes After Use— Autoclaved

If presterilized needles are used, the used carpule is removed from the syringe. Replace the original sheath over the working end of the needle and remove the needle from the syringe. With a pliers, bend and crush the portion of the needle not covered in order to prevent its reuse. Do not stick yourself. The needle is no longer sterile.

If presterilized needles are not used, proceed as follows:

1. Remove the old cartridge.
2. Examine the tip of the needle. Before sterilizing syringes, form the habit of always checking the needle for sharpness. Draw the needle backward over a piece of gauze. If it snags on the threads of the gauze, the needle should be replaced with a new one before sterilizing the syringe. This procedure is more reliable than examining the needle visually.
3. Autoclave the syringe and needle. Syringes must be autoclaved for fifteen minutes at fifteen pounds of pressure and are placed above other instruments in the autoclave load. Place a single cotton roll alongside each syringe, to be slipped over the needle when the load is removed from the autoclave. Be careful not to touch the needle with your fingers.

Storage of Sterile Syringes

A *syringe jar* is sometimes used for storage of sterilized syringes. This is a tall jar which has a round glass plate mounted inside near the top. This plate has four holes in it, each large enough to permit the passage of a syringe barrel. This plate supports the syringes in position (with their needles attached if reusable needles are used). Alcohol in the jar will completely cover the hub end of each syringe. A glass cover is provided for the jar.

When a syringe is to be used, carefully remove it from the syringe jar, being sure not to touch any surface or any foreign object with the hub.

Attach the sterile disposable needle, leaving the plastic cover on, if used.

Open the syringe, insert the cartridge of local anesthetic with fixed plug down, close the syringe, remove the plastic needle cover, and test for delivery. If the solution does not squirt out through the needle, rotate the cartridge in the syringe by using a thumb and forefinger on the open sides of the barrel. If the solution does not come out through the needle, open the syringe and remove and replace the ampule with a slight twisting motion.

If the syringe is to be placed in the operatory some time before use, replace the plastic protective cover on the needle. Place the syringe on the cabinet top, preferably covering it with a disposable tissue so that the patient will not see it.

Transfer Forceps (Fig. 33.25)

A transfer forceps is an instrument commonly used in the dental office. It is different from surgical forceps and is used to transfer sterile instruments from the autoclave to the sterile cabinet or storage. The transfer forceps is stored in a sterile container designed for the purpose.

Cement Slabs and Spatulas (Fig. 33.26)

Cement slabs and spatulas are stored in one of the cabinet drawers. Whenever a cement is required under a restoration, a slab and spatula must be used. These require special clean-up care. If the slab is glass, it must be cleaned for the next use.

Cement is best removed from glass slabs and spatulas immediately after the dentist has used the amount he desires. Take slab and spatula to the sink. Lay the slab in the sink and run warm water on it. Hold the spatula in the stream of water, rubbing it with thumb and forefinger to remove all traces from both sides and edges. Then pick up the glass slab and rub it also with your fingers, under running water, until all traces of cement are removed. Wash both slab and spatula with soap, then rinse completely with water and dry. Return to storage.

If not cleaned immediately, place both slab and spatula under a light stream of cold water and let stand. The cement will set up and, when hard, will flake off quite easily. If slabs and spatulas are not free from scratches, it may be necessary to keep a solution of bicarbonate of soda in which to soak both before rubbing with fingers to clean. Thoroughly rinse off soda solution.

The bicarbonate of soda solution may also be applied to the dry cement with a cotton pellet, if preferred.

Never use one spatula to cut the cement off another spatula. Never use metal to remove cement from the slab. Slabs and spatulas will remain free from scratches and much easier to keep clean if these two rules are followed.

Benzene or fingernail polish remover will remove the rubber-base impression materials from soiled spatulas. Use a gauze to apply and wipe.

Another form of slab is a pad of parchment or heavy paper sheets. These parchment mixing pads are made of individual sheets sealed together at the edges. One small area is left unsealed. It is at this point that a clean cement spatula may be inserted and the used sheet of parchment or paper removed by drawing the spatula around the gummed edge in the same manner as you use a letter opener.

Still another form of slab is a pad of clear plastic sheets.[1] These are also sealed on the edges; each sheet is disposable. This particular type is most useful for temporary cements which, as a rule, are very difficult to clean from glass or will soak through the parchment types of pads.

Twelve Small, But Important, Items

Bib or Napkin Holder (Fig. 33.27)

A napkin or bib holder is used to hold a towel or paper napkin across the chest of a patient in order that any debris or splashing from the mouth will not soil his clothes. At each end of the holder is an alligator clip or clasp. Attach the holder to one side of the napkin, lay the napkin across the patient's chest, under his chin, slip the chain around his neck, and fasten the holder to the other side of the napkin. Be careful that the cold chain does not rest on bare skin. It is an uncomfortable sensation.

Carbon Paper (Fig. 33.28)

Whenever a restoration is completed, it is necessary to check the articulation to be certain that the teeth are in proper occlusion. Carbon paper is used for this purpose. It has carbon on both sides, and when the patient taps his teeth together or bites on this paper, at the direction of the dentist, marks are left which enable the dentist to see whether the

1. Caulk Resinslab.

restoration needs further carving for correct function.

Cotton Holder (Fig. 33.29)

This metal receptacle is kept filled with clean cotton for the dentist to use according to need during dental operations.

Dappen Dish (Fig. 33.30)

This dish has a cup in each end—one is smaller than the other. Small amounts of medicament or prophylactic paste are placed in this dish for the dentist's use.

Dental Floss and Dental Tape Dispenser (Fig. 33.31)

Dental floss and dental tape are used in oral hygiene as well as in general dental work. The dispenser provides convenience in the use of both materials.

Medicament Bottles

Medicament bottles are usually kept in a drawer easily accessible to the dentist.

Bottles should be clearly labeled. Type on white paper the name of the medicament. Trim close to the typing. Put all labels on bottles in a uniform position. They may be taped on with a strip of cellophane tape, such as Scotch-brand mending tape, which covers the label completely. Be sure that the label is straight. Replace all labels every six months, or sooner if defaced.

If a label printer is available, effective labels can be made more easily. The tape used is already gummed for application to any surface.

Bottles should be kept clean at all times. It is much easier to keep them clean if no more than one-fourth inch of medicament is placed in any bottle. In the event of spillage, only a small quantity is out of control.

There are exceptions to this rule for quantity of medicaments:

1. Keep a greater quantity in each bottle of solutions which evaporate very quickly, such as alcohol, chloroform, or similar clear solutions.
2. Keep a lesser quantity in each bottle of caustic solutions, such as phenol. These potentially dangerous solutions are used more safely if a cotton pad is kept saturated in the bottom of the bottle so that there is no free liquid to spill and perhaps burn you.

Check medicament bottles daily to see that there is a usable supply in each.

Saliva Ejectors (Fig. 33.32)

A small tube placed in the patient's mouth to remove the saliva which collects during dental operations is called a saliva ejector. The hook-shaped tube is connected to a suction hose. (This is the saliva-ejector hose on the conventional dental unit.) The open end of the ejector is hung over the teeth and lips. This end of the ejector rests on the floor of the mouth where it draws up all the saliva within reach.

The most commonly used saliva ejectors are disposable plastic tubes. A new one is used for each patient and then thrown away after use. If metal saliva ejectors are used, they must be *sterilized* between patients.

Self-Retaining Cotton-Roll Holders (Fig. 33.33)

A device which holds a cotton roll on each side of the lower arch in order to keep the tooth dry is called a self-retaining cotton-roll holder. Each holder uses two cotton rolls. The holder clamps into position by means of a flat brace which slips under the patient's chin and can be locked against the outside of his jaw.

The upper arch is kept dry by inserting the cotton roll between the cheek and arch. None is required on the lingual side of the upper arch.

Towels—Clean

It is the dental assistant's responsibility to see that a clean towel is available at each lavatory where the dentist and the dental assistant wash many times every day. The towels are supposed to be *clean*. Replace them frequently enough to be certain that they look clean to the patients.

Pulp Tester (Fig. 33.34)

If there is a question regarding the health of a specific tooth, the dentist may check it with a pulp tester to see whether the tooth is still alive.

Waste Receptacle (Fig. 33.35)

A waste receptacle should be available for the dentist to deposit any debris or used cotton pellets, etc., he may wish to throw away during dental operations.

Quick-Filling Water Syringes (Fig. 33.36)

Rarely will you see this type of syringe in the modern dental office, but for many years this instrument was the only means of flushing an area of the mouth. The syringe is filled with water or mouthwash solution by squeezing the bulb to exhaust the air and allow it to refill with the desired liquid. The point of the syringe is then aimed at the area to be flushed, and the water is squeezed out.

Instrument Sharpening Devices

Instrument sharpening is an important activity in the dental office. Sharp instruments are essential in certain operations.

Arkansas Stone and Motor-Driven Sharpeners (Figs. 33.37-33.39)

Arkansas stone is a sharpening stone used to sharpen instruments. Arkansas stones are available in several shapes in order that many types of instruments can be sharpened.

The Arkansas sharpening stone is commonly found in dental offices as a flat stone; others used are grooved and cylindrical stones of various sizes. These are not motorized but depend on handwork by the operator to produce the desired edge.

Most dentists who sharpen their instruments prefer to do so themselves. If an individual dentist wishes his dental assistant to sharpen instruments, he will quite likely teach her the necessary skills. The angle at which the instrument is held against the stone determines the bevel of the blade; therefore the dentist must teach his assistant what he wishes done with each instrument he asks her to sharpen.

Care of Sharpening Stone

The Arkansas sharpening stone is of extremely high quality and fine grade and requires good care. Before it is used, oil is applied to produce a finer edge and keep from clogging the stone with debris.

After it has been used, wipe the stone clean with a lintless cloth, apply a few drops of oil, and put the stone away.

Motor-driven instrument sharpeners should be cleaned only according to the manufacturer's instructions. Most of these sharpeners use a synthetic abrasive stone rather than an Arkansas stone.

Hand Instruments

Hand instruments are difficult to recognize quickly until you become familiar with them.

The hand instruments are held in the dentist's hand, so they have a handle. They also have a shank and a working head. The handle varies in size and weight depending on the use of the instrument. The shank is straight or bent at an angle—not always the same angle. The angle is designed so that a specific area in the mouth can be reached with that particular instrument.

You will learn the instrumentation sequence more easily if you recognize that the type of operation determines the basic instrument set-up, but that within the basic instrument set-up the location of the operation (that is, upper or lower teeth, mesial or distal surfaces, left or right) also introduces some variations in the specific instrument your dentist requires. Therefore it is necessary that you not only know what type of operation is being performed, but that you also know *where* it is being performed in order to effectively *serve instruments to your dentist as he requires them. They must be placed in his hand in the position in which he will use them.*

Instrument Numbering

Instruments must be identified, especially for reordering; thus a numbering system has been devised. The numbers indicate important information about the instrument.

The first number toward the operative end, reading from left to right, indicates the width of the blade in tenths of a millimeter; the second number indicates the length of the blade from the center of the angle to the end in millimeters; the third number indicates the angle of the blade with the shaft in hundredths of a circle or centigrades.

However, some cutting instruments have four formula numbers, and this occurs when the cutting edge of the instrument is at an angle, in which case the second number of the formula indicates the angle of the cutting edge; the third number indicates the length of the blade; and the fourth number indicates the angle of the blade with the shaft.

If *R* or *L* appears in the number of an instrument, this indicates that the instrument is for use on the right or left side of the cavity. The instruments are identical except that their shapes are reversed so that one is usable on the left side and one on the right side *of the preparation.*

Many dental instruments have overlapping uses; that is, a certain cutting instrument may be used for several different dental operations. There are some instruments, however, which are used for specific purposes, such as an amalgam restoration, and are used for no other operation.

Amalgam Instruments (Figs. 33.40-33.43)

Amalgam carriers are used to carry amalgam from the squeeze cloth to the preparation, where the dental assistant releases the amalgam and the dentist condenses it into the preparation with amalgam pluggers or condensers.

When the preparation is completely filled with amalgam, the dentist carves or shapes the still-soft amalgam with a carver. (Carvers are also used to carve tooth anatomy in wax when making crowns. This use will be discussed in chap. 37.)

Cutting Instruments (Figs. 33.44-33.46)

A group of instruments which may be used in any dental restoration are all cutting instruments of various types. We speak of them as cutting instruments because they are used to cut either soft tissue or hard tissue in the mouth. Strictly speaking, burs and discs are also cutting instruments; but these are rotary cutting instruments and can be considered with the handpiece with which they are used. This section defines "hand" cutting instruments—those held in the dentist's hand.

Several of the cutting instruments are *chisels* in various forms: hatchets, hoes, enamel hatchets, and gingival margin trimmers. Notice the tiny variations in the working end of each of these instruments and learn to know those which your dentist uses.

Spoon excavators are cutting instruments used to scoop out decay. They have a small curve to their head like a spoon. The edge is sharp and can cut the decay which is then held in the curve of the spoon.

Trimming knives are very thin-bladed knives used to trim soft tissues. Ideally they should be resharpened after each use.

Scalers are used for prophylaxis and in periodontics. In the general practitioner's office, the greatest use will be for prophylaxis. These instruments are used to remove deposits of calculus (tartar) from around the teeth. There are many shapes of scalers.

The periodontist has some instruments which are used exclusively for periodontia. In addition to scalers used by all dentists for some operations, the periodontist uses curettes, files, and polishing instruments.

Matrix and Matrix Holders (Fig. 33.47)

When an amalgam restoration includes a proximal surface, a matrix band is necessary to hold the amalgam in place until it has been carved and is ready to set. If the location and complexity of the preparation require it, the dentist may make his own matrix band from matrix material. He will usually use a continuous matrix holder, such as the Tofflemire. Most matrix operations, however, can be accomplished with the matrix holder and matrix bands which are purchased ready to use.

Gold-foil Instruments (Figs. 33.48-33.53)

Gold-foil restorations require special instruments. There are gold pluggers, files, holding instruments, annealing instruments, and pellet placers—all for use with gold-foil preparations. There are burnishers which are used for polishing any metal—but especially gold.

Plastic Filling Instruments (Figs. 33.54-33.56)

Another group of instruments are called plastic filling instruments. These titles have the true use of plastic. Plastic means *moldable*; hence, these instruments are used to *shape*

plastic material. Amalgam is plastic before it sets; cements are also plastic before setting occurs. The dentist is not asking for a polyethelene bag or a Tupperware cup when he asks for a plastic instrument—he means an instrument used for shaping a restoration material which can still be moved.

Sable Brush (Fig. 33.57)

A sable brush is used to "paint in" an unfilled plastic material such as a methyl methacrylate restoration.

Contouring Pliers (Fig. 33.58)

Temporary covers, children's steel crowns, and orthodontic appliances usually need to be shaped. Contouring pliers are used for this purpose. Notice there are several different shapes for the heads of these pliers.

Orthodontic Band Driver (Fig. 33.59)

An orthodontist needs a band driver for use on orthodontic appliances.

Instrumentation for Five Specialties

Endodontic Armamentarium (Figs. 33.60-33.64)

In endodontics a special chairside sterilizer is needed. This glass bead sterilizer maintains a temperature of approximately 440° Fahrenheit. It will disinfect an instrument in ten seconds and will sterilize in four minutes. It is used at the chair to disinfect the blades of reamers and files during endodontic treatment.

The specialist in endodontics also uses reamers, files, broaches, pluggers, and separators. These instruments are used exclusively for endodontic treatment. Reamers, files, and broaches are similar in use and shape. They are used to clean and shape the root canal. The broaches have needlelike projections on their surfaces. The pluggers and separators are similar to each other in service. They are used to pack gutta-percha points into the canal which has been prepared by use of one or all of the first three instruments.

Crown and Bridge Instruments (Figs. 33.65-33.70)

Generally speaking, the instruments and materials illustrated in figures 33.65-33.70 are used for fixed prostheses.

Crown and bridge scissors are used to cut copper bands and other metals.

Crown forms are used to make an acrylic cover for a tooth which is prepared and requires protection until the crown has been finished, ready for cementation.

Periodontic Armamentarium (Figs. 33.71-33.72)

The periodontist, the dentist who treats the area surrounding the teeth, uses probes, scalers, curettes, elevators, sharpening stones, gauze sponges, knives, needle holders, suture scissors, and suturing materials, in addition to the basic setups for operative dentistry. He also uses a number of instruments used in general dentistry.

Surgical Instruments (Figs. 33.73-33.93)

Surgical instruments are used by an oral surgeon or by a dentist with a general practice who performs any oral surgery. The surgical instrument most commonly known to the layman is a forceps.

Surgical forceps are used to remove teeth. There are many shapes, each designed to be used in a particular location in the mouth.

Other instruments are used in oral surgery, some of which are also called forceps. Examples are tissue forceps, hemostatic forceps, and splinter forceps. In addition to forceps, the surgical armamentarium may include the following instruments, and others, depending on the choice of the oral surgeon: needle holder, gauze packer, tissue retractor, chisels, rongeurs, curettes, scalpels, and elevators.

Care of Forceps

Forceps which are autoclaved for sterilization can be treated with an oil emulsion before processing.

Forceps may gradually become stiff in the joint, making them difficult or impossible to use. Three suggestions for correction of this condition follow. Start with the first. If that method does not succeed, proceed to the second, and finally, as a last resort, to the third.

1. Apply a few drops of dental engine oil to the joint and work it briskly for a minute.
2. Hold the forceps under very cold water and continue to open and close the forceps.
3. Soak the forceps overnight in penetrating oil. This can be obtained at most hardware stores. The forceps should be immersed in the penetrating oil, with the beaks of the forceps opened as wide as possible. Upon removal from the oil, wipe the forceps with a disposable tissue, briskly open and close several times, then wipe with a gauze moistened with seventy percent alcohol. Now sterilize as usual.

Care of Sterile Surgical Instruments

All surgical instruments are usually stored in some area where they are protected from contamination. They are transferred from the autoclave to the storage area by means of transfer forceps. Following are the two most frequently used methods of storage:

1. Autoclaved, covered-tray setups: one tray for each surgical operation.
2. Autoclaved surgical packs: each pack a complete set of instruments for one single operation. The packs are stored in the surgical cabinet.

If the volume of surgery does not warrant the duplication of instruments necessary for multiple tray or pack setups, the selection of surgical instruments, including forceps, is stored in the surgical cabinet in drawers lined with autoclaved towels.

Prostheses

Impressions, articulators, and facebows are important adjuncts to the preparation of a prosthetic device.

Impression Trays (Figs. 33.94-33.97)

Following surgery there is usually a need for a prosthetic replacement—whether it is a bridge, partial, or full denture. In order to make a prosthesis, the dentist must use impression trays to reproduce the dental arch or quadrant. With this impression the dental assistant can make a cast which will permit the dentist to create the reproduction outside the mouth. The trays used must have special care to keep them looking nice for the patient. They are usually aluminum or plastic. If they are not treated properly, they soon become scratched and marred. A patient may feel uncomfortable if a tray inserted in his mouth looks as if it had been given rough treatment. He may wonder where the tray has been. Treat trays gently—according to the following directions.

Impression trays, when returned by the laboratory after use, are usually not thoroughly cleansed. They should first be cleaned of all foreign material. Scrape plaster off when necessary, being careful not to raise rough spots on the surface of the tray.

If compound is sticking on the tray, pass the tray through a gas flame until the compound is softened, then wipe off with disposable tissue or cloth.

Give the tray a very light daubing with Vaseline, flame the tray lightly to melt the Vaseline, wipe with a disposable tissue to remove excess Vaseline. Now sterilize the tray.

To brighten trays periodically, boil in a pan of water containing one tablespoon of detergent to each pint of water.

There *are* some special trays made of a very soft, low-fusing metal which, like plastic, cannot be held in a flame.[2] Check with your dentist to see whether he does or does not have some trays of this type.

Articulators (Fig. 33.98)

Articulators are the mechanisms used in the construction of dentures which resemble in various degrees the movement of upper and lower jaws. Many different kinds with varying degrees of complexity are used. One rule applies to all articulators: keep them clean. Dust-proof storage is important. One good method is to place each articulator in a clear plastic (polyethylene) bag. The more complex, the more important it is that it be kept clean and free from dust.

After completion of a denture case, be sure to remove completely all traces of plaster, wax, and other debris. Parts that slide against one another or parts that are hinged should be oiled lightly with a good grade of light oil. When rings or bars are used to mount casts in the articulator, keep them clean by giving them a very light coating of Vaseline prior to use. Check with your dentist on the care he desires you to give these instruments.

Do not handle any articulator roughly. They should be handled much as you would your most expensive china at home.

The Facebow (Fig. 33.99)

The purpose of using a *facebow* is to discover the proper relationship of the patient's upper jaw to the patient's center of rotation of the temporomandibular joints and to transfer this relationship to the articulator. The articulator, a mechanical means of duplicating the

2. Page's lower edentulous trays.

movements of the mandible in relation to the maxilla, will then more closely duplicate the actual relationship of the jaws as they exist in the patient. The success of the entire process, of course, rests upon how accurately the original location of centers of rotation is made and how accurately the transfer is made.

A facebow consists of a U-shaped rod or bar. At the ends of the U are adjustable rods or pointers which slide at right angles from the bar and may be locked at various degrees of extension.

Along that part of the facebow which lies between the two straight end sections are one, two, or three clamps constructed to hold other rods when tightened. One clamp is used to hold a rod which has on its end a forklike smaller U about the size of an average dental arch, called a bite fork. A second clamp, if present, may be used to hold a pointer to control the vertical positioning of the facebow by always being placed in contact with a specific landmark on the face, such as the infraorbital notch or rim. A third clamp, when present, is used as an aid in holding the facebow in proper relationship to the articulator when the actual transfer of the record is to be accomplished.

The dentist first establishes the center of rotation of the temporomandibular joints of a patient by one of two methods. (1) He may use a type of hinge axis locator which consists of a rod placed in the external auditory meatus (the external opening of the ear). The rod has a short arm to which a clamp is attached to hold a pencil in such a position that as the rod is rotated in a short arc, the pencil inscribes an arc thirteen millimeters in front of the external auditory meatus. With a ruler, another line is then drawn from the upper border of the external auditory meatus to the outer canthus of the eye, intersecting the arc previously drawn. This point of intersection is considered an approximate indication of the center of ro-

tation of the temporomandibular joint. This is marked on both sides of the face.

(2) The dentist may use another device, called a *kinematic* facebow, to more exactly locate the centers of rotation of the temporomandibular joints. This device consists of a mechanism called a clutch which is attached to the lower arch of the dental patient. From this mechanism a pointer arrangement is extended to the area in front of the external auditory meatus. The pointer has some means by which its position in the vicinity of the ear may be adjusted. The dentist will teach the patient the manner in which he wishes the patient to open and close his jaws with a steady, rhythmic, short arc. As the motion proceeds, the dentist adjusts the pointer until it points to only one spot throughout the movement. This spot will be the exact center of rotation of the temporomandibular joint.

The bite fork is now either embedded in the upper trial denture (if full dentures are being constructed) or covered with a layer of hard pink wax into which the patient makes indentations of his natural teeth (if the natural dentition is to be balanced). This is thoroughly chilled in cold water and is reinserted in the patient's mouth. The transfer bow is now slipped onto the bar of the bite fork—loosely, to allow for positioning the sliding rods or pointers at the ends of the U over the marks indicating the center of rotation of each temporomandibular joint. The distance each sliding rod or pointer is extended from the U bar must be as nearly as possible equal on both sides of the facebow. The U bar is then locked tightly to the rod of the bite fork. The second clamp, if present, is tightened when the pointer has been placed on the selected landmark. The entire assembly is removed from the face of the patient. It is now ready for attachment to the articulator and the mounting of the casts.

There may be various other details involved, depending upon the procedure used in a particular dental office, as well as the type of equipment used. These variations may include *bite registrations* which may be made in several ways, and perhaps at different stages in the procedures for occlusal equilibration (balancing a natural dentition) or for full-denture construction. A bite registration is a record of the way the teeth of the upper and lower jaws fit together, necessary in occlusal equilibration and denture construction. It is important to verify the occlusion as work progresses, and the bite registration permits the dentist to make this verification. Make notes of the particular requirements of your office until you have thoroughly learned the procedures and are able to have the proper materials and equipment ready for use at the proper time.

Summary

If, as you read through this summary, you find that there are comments which do not seem clear, perhaps it will be helpful to review that section of the chapter before you try to answer the questions in the Workbook or go on to the next chapter.

Dental instruments vary in size and shape. Minute differences are important. Learn to recognize the fine points and their uses so that you are a help to your dentist—so that you can anticipate his need and have the correct instrument ready.

Cutting instruments have sharp blades. Some are designed for the right or left side of a preparation.

Instruments are expensive and delicate. Handle with care. Keep them sterilized or clean, depending on their use. Keep them as you would like to have them kept for use in your own mouth.

A basic setup is a mirror, an explorer, and cotton pliers.

Handpieces are conventional, high-speed, and ultraspeed. Learn to care for them according to the instructions given for each type.

Dental burs are classified for the type of handpiece in which they are used and also by their shape. Learn to recognize them by both classifications.

Diamond instruments cut harder structures more quickly than burs and are used to open a tooth or do major shaping as for a full-crown preparation.

Prophylaxis handpieces, cups, and brushes are used for cleaning teeth.

Mandrels are metal shanks which fit into a handpiece and on which a disc or unmounted stone can be mounted.

Stones, either mounted or unmounted, do grinding and finishing operations.

The stones used for sharpening instruments are different from the mounted stones put on the handpiece to grind and finish dental prostheses. Learn to care for the sharpening stones used in your office.

Hand instruments have a handle, a shank, and a working head. They are fine, minute heads, and the differences are very important and sometimes hard to recognize. Instruments are numbered in a fashion which identifies them for reordering and also gives important information about the instrument—width, length, and angle of the blade.

Amalgam carriers, pluggers, condensers, and carvers are used only for amalgam restorations.

Cutting instruments are those which are used to cut either soft or hard tissue in the mouth. There are chisels, hatchets, enamel hatchets, hoes, gingival margin trimmers, and trimming knives. Spoon excavators are used to scoop out decay; scalers are used for prophylaxis and in periodontics.

Matrix tools are used to make a band fit around a prepared tooth when a temporary wall is needed until the amalgam is packed and carved in the shape of the original tooth.

Special instruments are needed for gold-foil work: pluggers, files, annealing instruments, pellet placers, burnishers, and holding instruments.

Plastic filling instruments are used to shape and trim plastic material before it is set.

Contouring pliers are used to shape temporary covers and crowns.

A pulp tester is used to determine the vitality of a tooth.

Rubber dam is used when the field of operation needs to be kept dry.

Anesthetic syringes need special care, for they must be sterile when used for a patient.

Surgical instruments include several types of forceps as well as other instruments used exclusively for surgery, including elevators.

When surgery has been performed, a prosthesis is usually required, and impression trays are necessary to take an impression in order that the prosthetic device may be prepared.

Finally, articulators and facebows are useful in creating prosthetic devices which may be constructed for the patient who has had surgery and requires rehabilitation. It does not matter whether it is one tooth, several teeth, or full dentures.

Learn the care and use of all these instruments.

Part Two: Visual Identification of Instruments

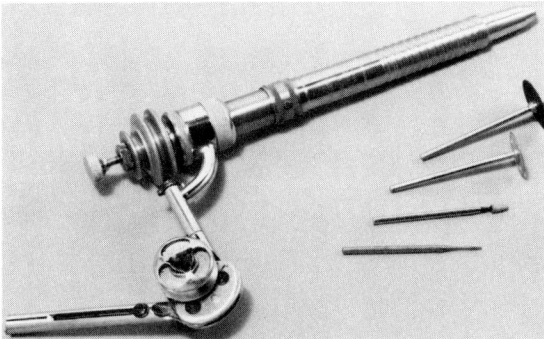

Fig. 33.1. Ball-bearing handpiece

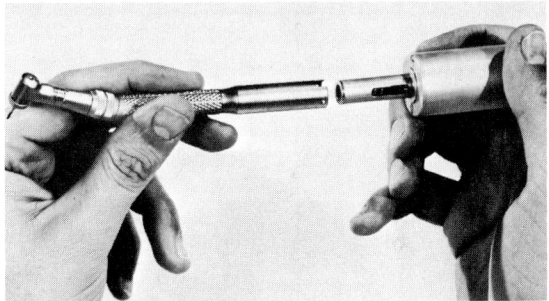

Courtesy Kerr Mfg. Co.

Fig. 33.3. Kerr electrotorque motor and handpiece

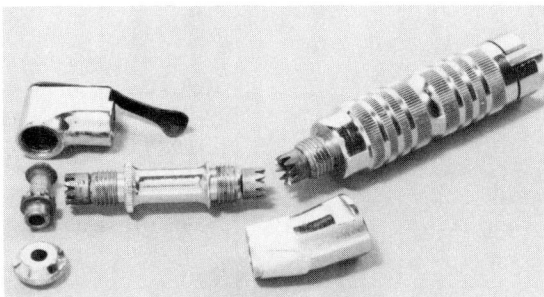

Fig. 33.2. Latch-type contra-angle disassembled

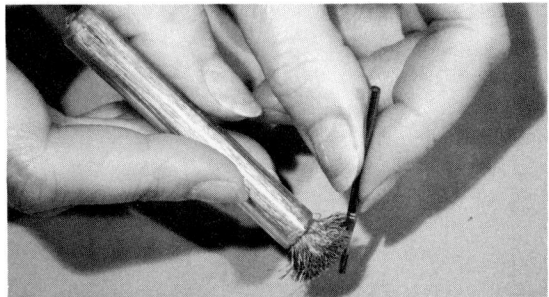

Fig. 33.4. Cleaning bur with scratch brush

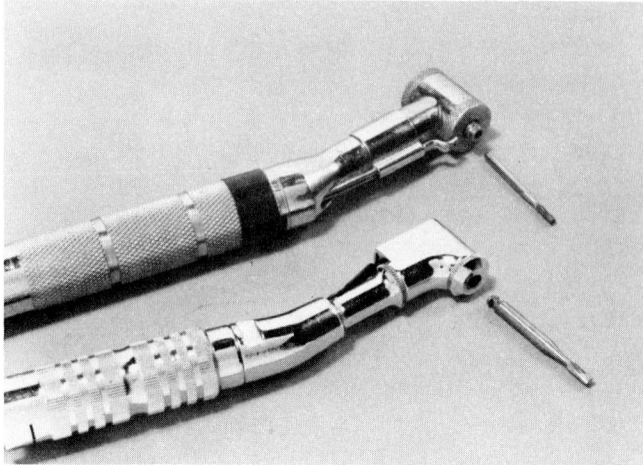

Fig. 33.5. Friction-grip and latch-type burs

(below) **Fig. 33.6.** Kerr Tungsten-Carbide burs classified by shape and size.

	Round	Inverted Cone	Plain Fissure	Straight Crosscut Fissure	Plain Tapered Fissure	Tapered Crosscut Fissure	Round-Nose Fissure
Friction Grip	¼ ½ 1	33½ 34 35*	55 56	555 556	169 169L 170	699 700 699L*	1057
	2* 4 6	37 37L	57* 57L	557 558*	170L 171 171L	701 701L	1557
Right Angle and Straight Handpiece	1 2 3 4	33½ 34 35 36	57 58	557 558	170	700 701	
	5 6 7 8	37 38 39	59	559 560	171	702 703	

*Available in short shank

Courtesy Kerr Mfg. Co.

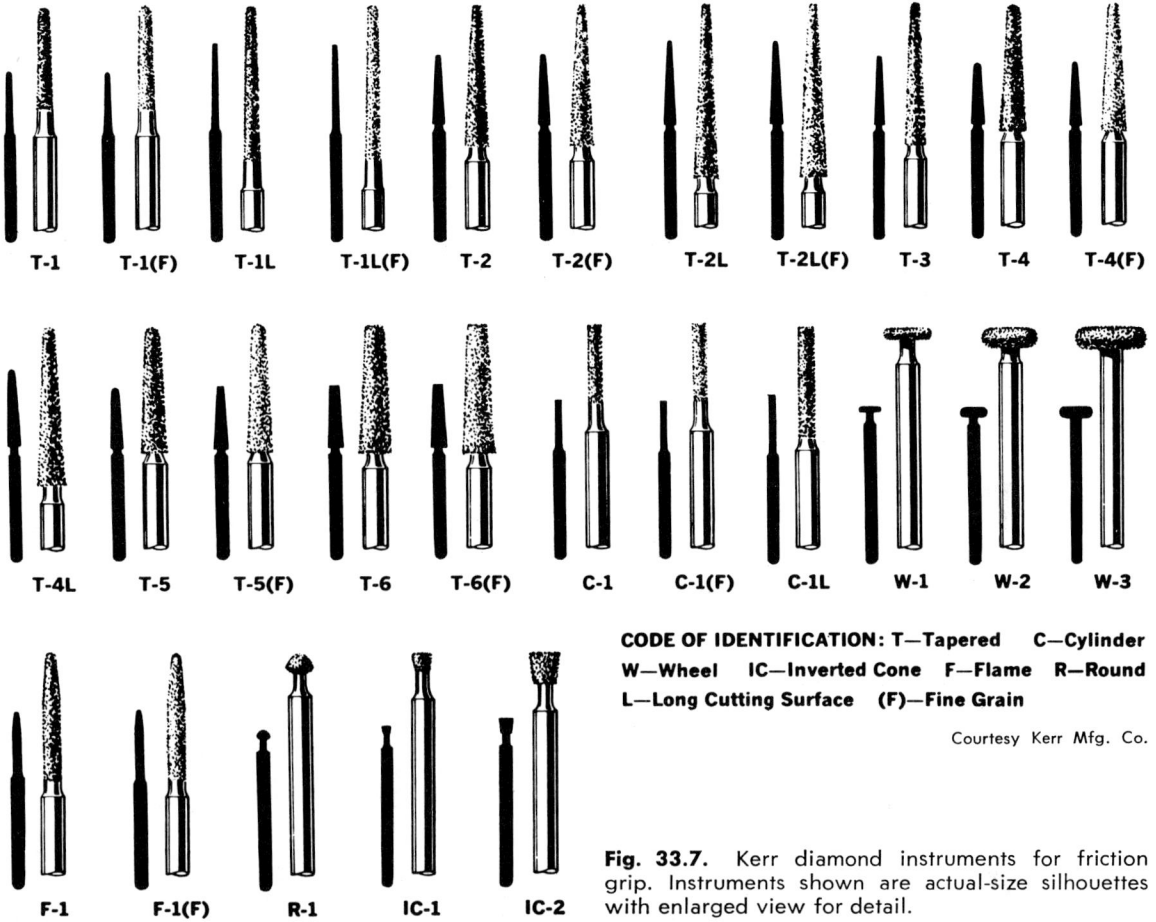

CODE OF IDENTIFICATION: T—Tapered C—Cylinder W—Wheel IC—Inverted Cone F—Flame R—Round L—Long Cutting Surface (F)—Fine Grain

Courtesy Kerr Mfg. Co.

Fig. 33.7. Kerr diamond instruments for friction grip. Instruments shown are actual-size silhouettes with enlarged view for detail.

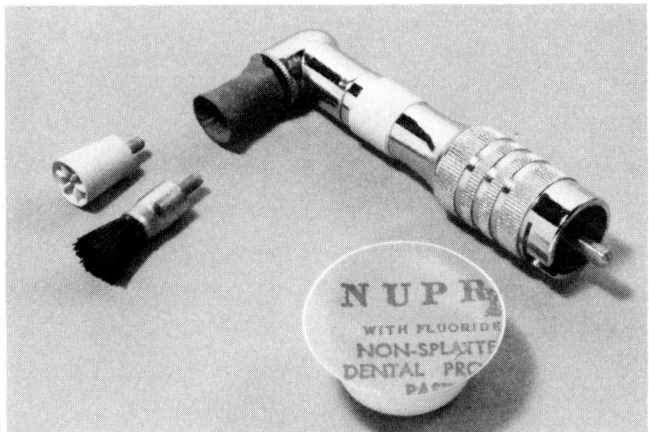

Fig. 33.8. Prophylaxis right angle and cups

Fig. 33.9. Mandrels

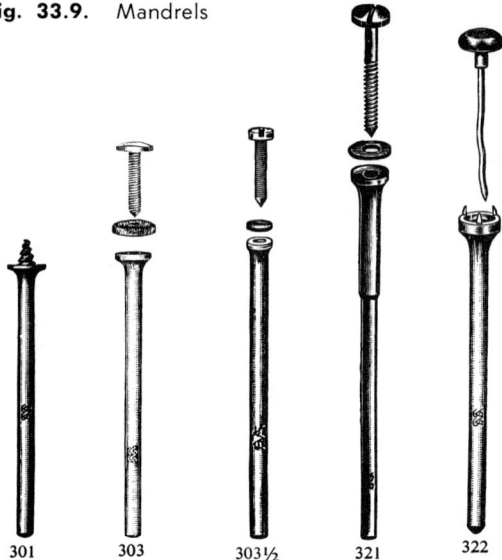

301	303	303½	321	322
Screw with Shoulder	**Dr. Huey Screw Head**	**Screw Head for Small Disks**	**Disk and Wheel**	**Morgan-Maxfield Improved For Disks**

Courtesy S. S. White Co.

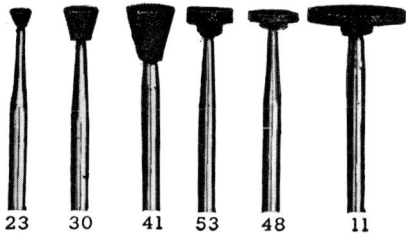

23 30 41 53 48 11

Courtesy S. S. White Co.

Fig. 33.10. Mounted stones

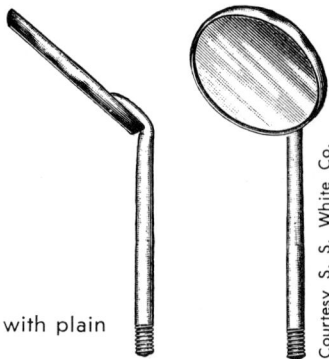

Fig. 33.11. Mirrors with plain or simple stem.

Courtesy S. S. White Co.

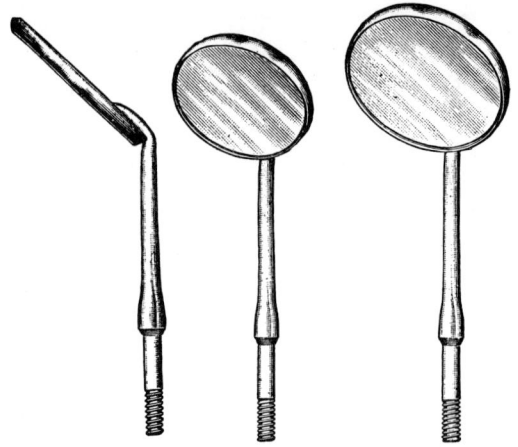

Courtesy S. S. White Co.

Fig. 33.12. Mirrors with cone-socket stem

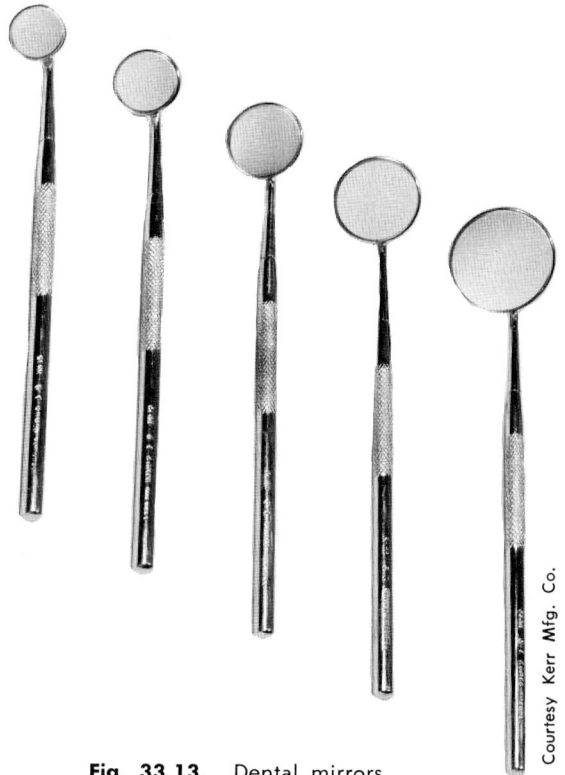

Courtesy Kerr Mfg. Co.

Fig. 33.13. Dental mirrors

2   3   5   6   7   9   10   11   12   13   14   17   18   20   21   22   23

EXP 1
EXP 2
EXP 3
EXP 5
EXP 6

Courtesy S. S. White Co.

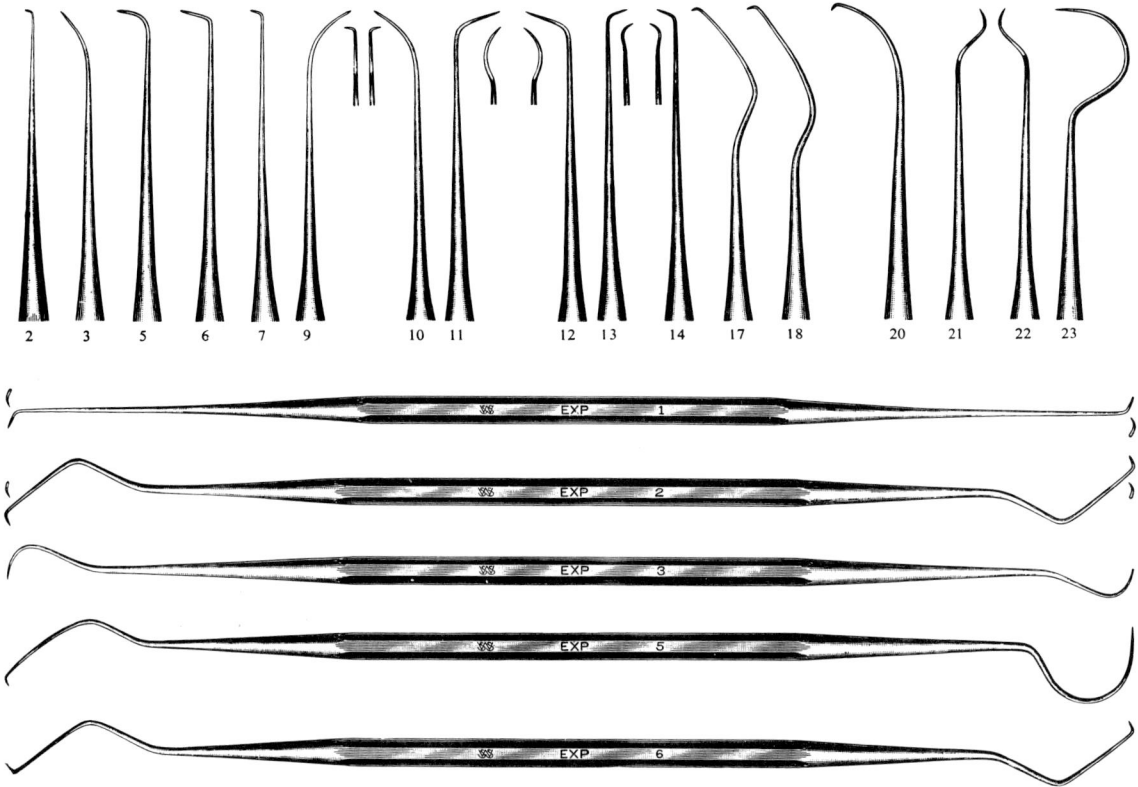

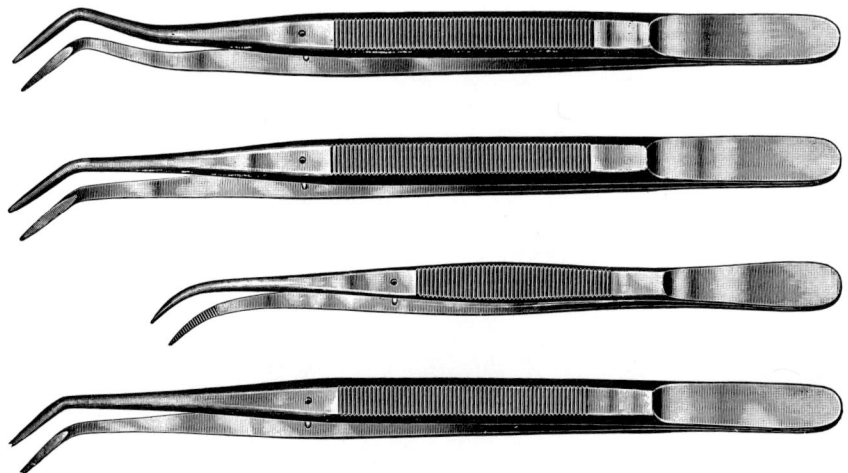

Fig. 33.14. Explorers, single- and double-ended

Courtesy S. S. White Co.

Fig. 33.15. Cotton and dressing pliers.

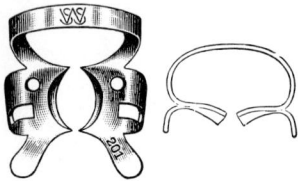

201. Upper Molar.

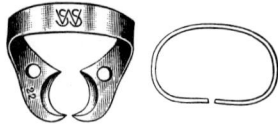

22. For upper and lower bicuspids. Flat jaws. For same clamp with dam-engaging projections.

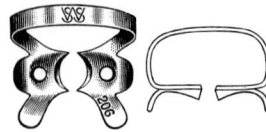

206. For upper and lower bicuspids

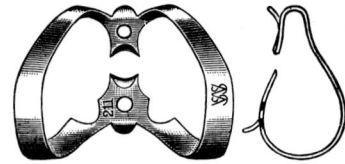

211. Universal for labial cavities on the twenty anterior teeth

Courtesy S. S. White Co.

Fig. 33.16. Assortment of rubber-dam clamps: molar, bicuspid, and anterior

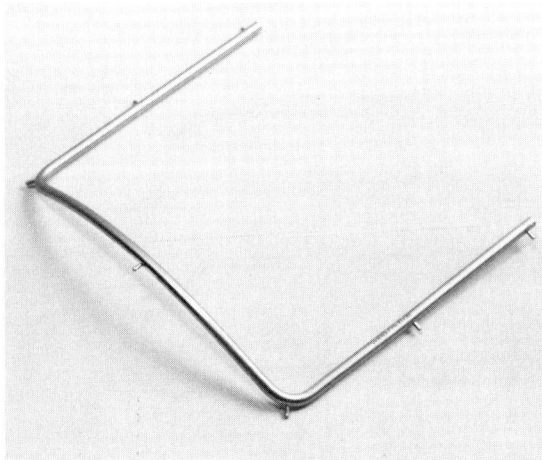

Fig. 33.17. Young's rubber-dam frame

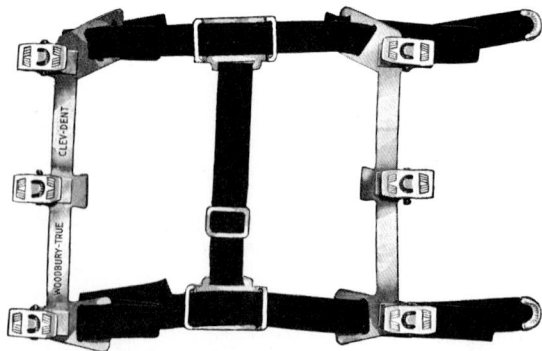

Courtesy S. S. White Co.

Fig. 33.18. Woodbury-True rubber-dam holder

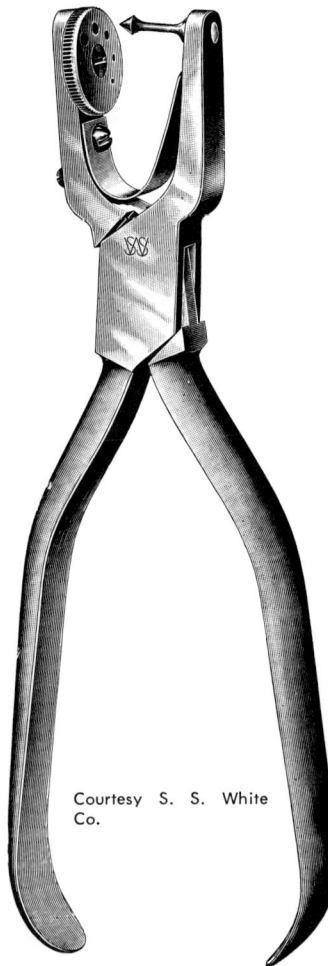

Courtesy S. S. White Co.

Fig. 33.19. Perfected rubber-dam punch.

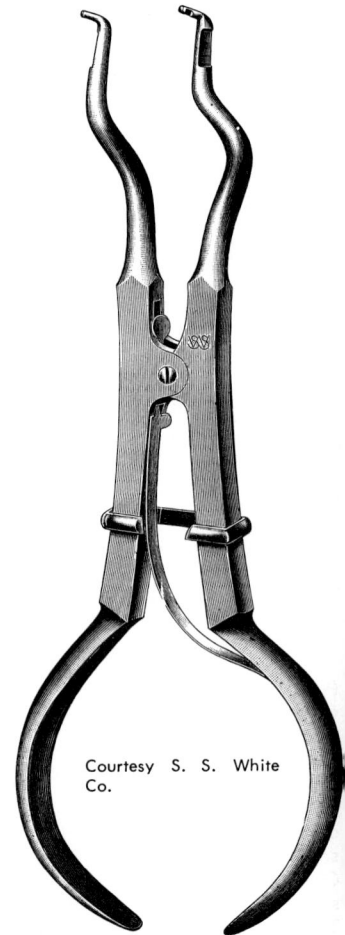

Courtesy S. S. White Co.

Fig. 33.20. Brewer universal rubber-dam clamp forceps.

Courtesy Astra Pharmaceutical Products, Inc.

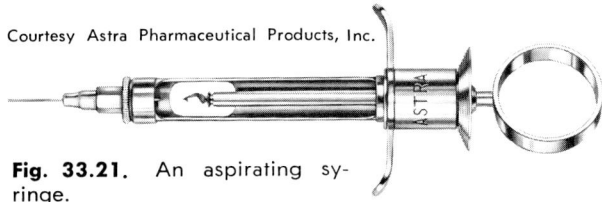

Fig. 33.21. An aspirating syringe.

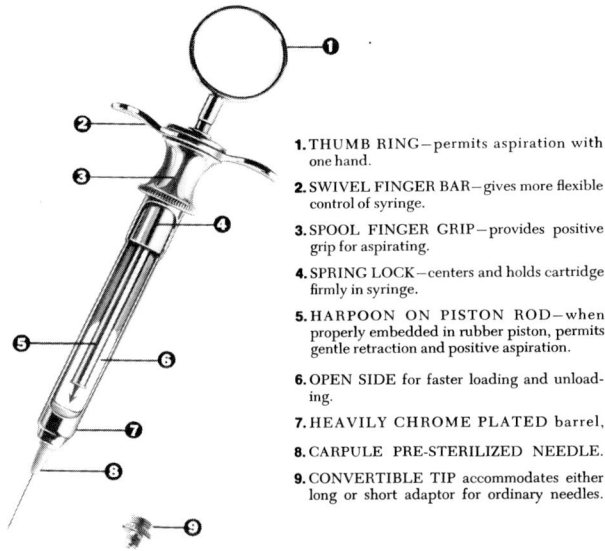

1. THUMB RING—permits aspiration with one hand.
2. SWIVEL FINGER BAR—gives more flexible control of syringe.
3. SPOOL FINGER GRIP—provides positive grip for aspirating.
4. SPRING LOCK—centers and holds cartridge firmly in syringe.
5. HARPOON ON PISTON ROD—when properly embedded in rubber piston, permits gentle retraction and positive aspiration.
6. OPEN SIDE for faster loading and unloading.
7. HEAVILY CHROME PLATED barrel,
8. CARPULE PRE-STERILIZED NEEDLE.
9. CONVERTIBLE TIP accommodates either long or short adaptor for ordinary needles.

TO LOAD

Drop Carpule Pre-Sterilized Needle in syringe and remove needle cap (Fig. 1). If ordinary needles are used, screw convertible tip into end of syringe barrel, insert needle into adaptor and attach to convertible tip.

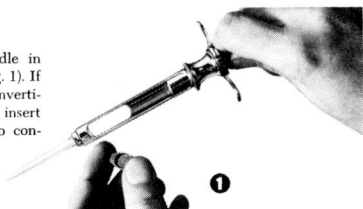

Fig. 33.22. A series of illustrations giving the directions for the use of an aspirating syringe. Aspiration is held mandatory by leading anesthesiologists today, particularly in using modern, highly potent, fast-acting local anesthetic solutions. It is the only sure way to avoid injecting into a blood vessel. Thus, aspiration will increase patient comfort and tolerance and make local anesthesia, the safest known, still safer by minimizing systemic reactions. Good anesthesia can be obtained more consistently as the solution will not be rapidly dissipated by the bloodstream. The Carpule "Aspirator" enables you to aspirate routinely before every injection—positively, safely, easily—while using the cartridge system of injection with its many conveniences and advantages.

Retract spring lock with piston rod as far as possible holding syringe with open side facing up (Fig. 2). After disinfecting the cartridge diaphragm, place cartridge into syringe barrel *piston end first.*

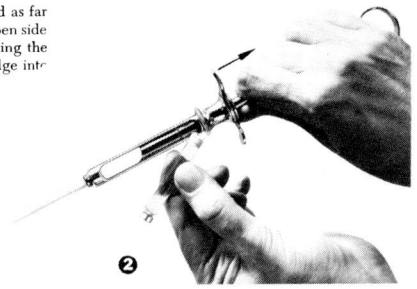

TO ENGAGE HARPOON

Release the piston rod—the spring lock will automatically seat cartridge onto needle. Impel the harpoon into the rubber piston with quick jab of thumb ring.

With practice it will be found possible to engage harpoon in rubber piston before cartridge is seated on needle by holding cartridge against syringe barrel with thumb and finger (Fig. 3). The cartridge will be seated on needle as harpoon becomes engaged.

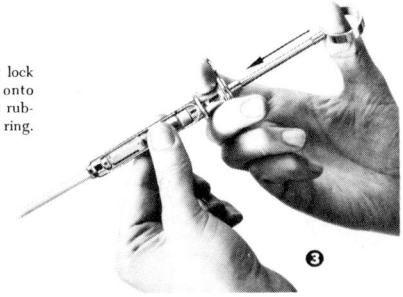

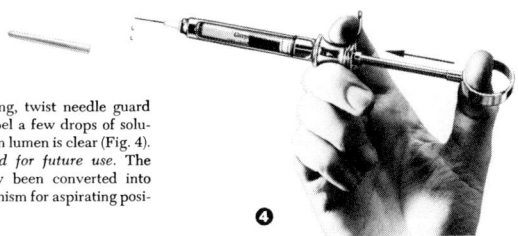

Just before injecting, twist needle guard to remove and expel a few drops of solution to make certain lumen is clear (Fig. 4). *Save needle guard for future use.* The cartridge has now been converted into an effective mechanism for aspirating positively.

TO ASPIRATE

The aspiration by means of the syringe will be performed by the dentist.

Inject solution slowly drop by drop ahead of point as it is advanced through the tissues until site of main deposit is reached. Then apply negative pressure to rubber piston by retracting thumb in thumb ring.

Attempting to retract rubber piston creates negative pressure in the cartridge. If the point of the needle is in a blood vessel, blood will be drawn into the distal end of the cartridge. In this case, withdraw needle slightly and change direction of insertion. Aspirate again.

If needle is *not* in a blood vessel, piston should not be expected to move back *and should not be forced.* Complete injection, *injecting slowly.*

POSTOPERATIVE PROCEDURE

Retract spring lock with piston rod as far as possible using one hand. This will disengage the harpoon from the rubber piston *without* pulling it out of the cartridge. Turn syringe over to allow the assembly to drop out (Fig. 5).

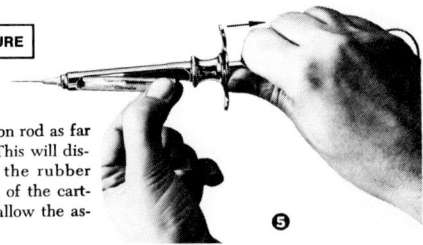

Fig. 33.22 (Continued)

DO NOT HOLD CARTRIDGE WITH OTHER HAND WHILE DISENGAGING THE HARPOON. To do so will pull the rubber piston out of the cartridge.

If the procedure requires the use of more than one cartridge, retract the spring lock with the piston rod, turn syringe over, as to remove assembly, and then instead bend cartridge out of the plastic hub. Insert second cartridge and proceed as before.

CAUTION: It is recommended that each needle be broken before discarding to prevent unauthorized use. This is best accomplished by *replacing the needle guard* and bending the cannula back and forth inside until it breaks.

SYRINGE MAINTENANCE

To disassemble the syringe, unscrew spool finger grip from barrel. After unscrewing the thumb ring from the piston rod, the spool grip, spring and harpoon housing (lock) may be slipped off the piston rod.

Rubber pistons are impregnated with paraffin wax to facilitate smooth mechanical action. Hence, when the harpoon of the "ASPIRATOR"

is embedded in, and then removed from, the cartridge piston, it is likely to accumulate particles of paraffin.

It is recommended that these particles be removed by brushing periodically with the brush used for scrubbing other instruments. A clean harpoon will engage the rubber piston to best advantage.

HARPOON REPLACEMENT

Although the harpoon is extremely durable and engineered for long service, use over an extended period of time could result in diminished sharpness. If a new harpoon is

needed for this or any other reason, a replacement is readily available and the change-over as indicated in the section "Syringe Maintenance" is simplicity itself.

About the Needles You Employ With This Instrument

The Carpule Aspirator is a precision instrument designed to increase the safety of all injections and protect your patients from intravascular injections. Positive protection against such injections will be enhanced if you will heed the advice of leading authorities on aspiration and *use no needle finer than 25 gauge* since the viscosity of blood is such that it may not flow freely through lumens of finer gauge.

All Cook-Waite needles—Carpule Pre-Sterilized, "Laminex" or Rustless Steel, possess the exclusive Huber Dental Point—a scalpel-sharp point located where a point should be located: on the mid-axis of the needle. Because of this point, *no needle, however fine the gauge,* can offer your patients a more pain-free injection. We hope this fact is reassuring to you as you begin to use your new Carpule "Aspirator".

Courtesy Cook-Waite Labs., Inc.

Fig. 33.22 (Continued)

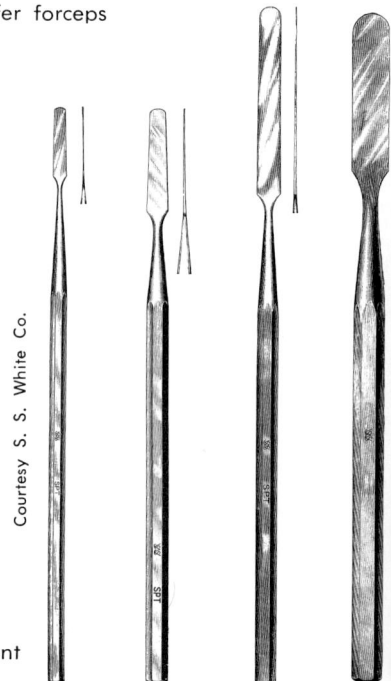

Courtesy Bard-Parker Co.

Fig. 33.25. Transfer forceps

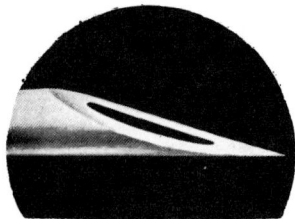

Fig. 33.23. The bevel of a standard hypodermic needle, enlarged to show its construction as a hollow tube. Magnified 19 times.

Courtesy Cook-Waite Labs., Inc.

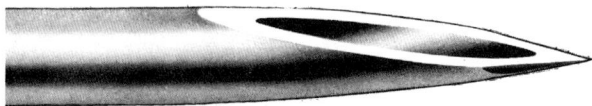

Courtesy Cook-Waite Labs., Inc.

Fig. 33.24. The bevel of the Huber dental needle, showing its construction which places the point at the center line of the long axis of the needle.

Courtesy S. S. White Co.

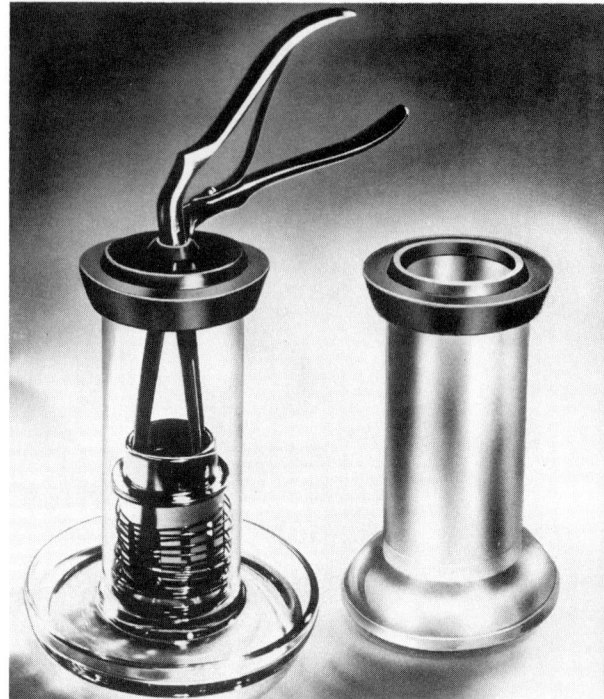

Fig. 33.26. Cement spatulas.

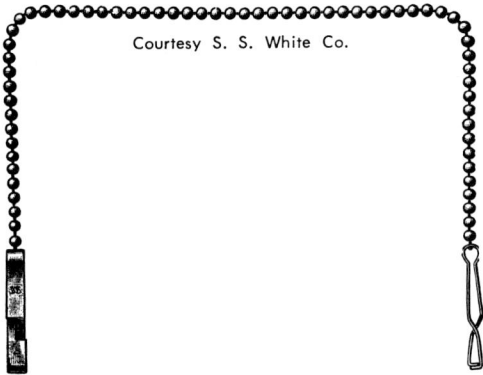

Courtesy S. S. White Co.

Fig. 33.27. Napkin holder

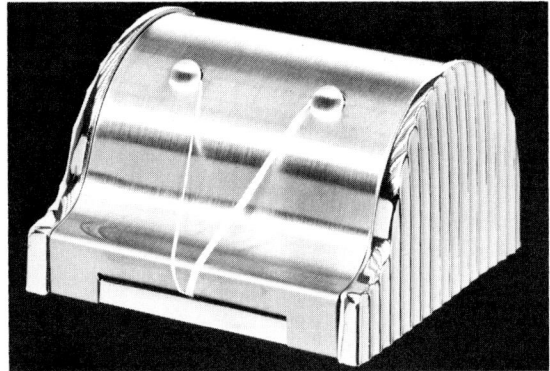

Courtesy Johnson & Johnson

Fig. 33.31. A dispenser for dental floss and dental tape.

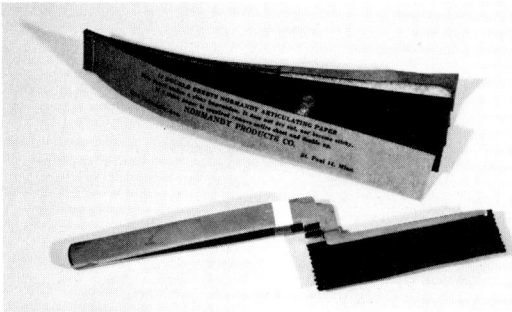

Fig. 33.28. Articulating paper with holder

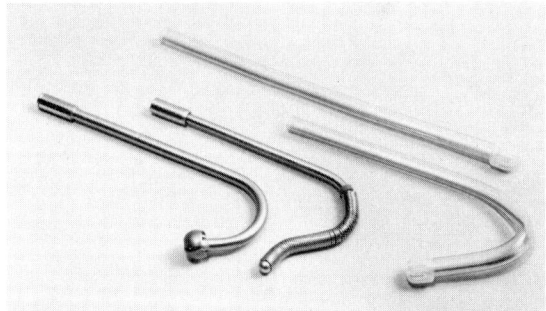

Fig. 33.32. Saliva ejector

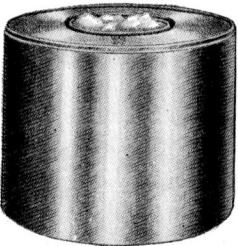

Fig. 33.29. Cotton holder.

Courtesy S. S. White Co.

Courtesy S. S. White Co.

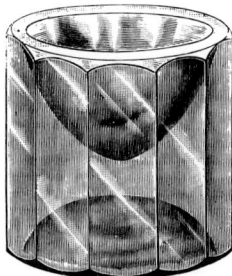

Fig. 33.30. Dappen dish

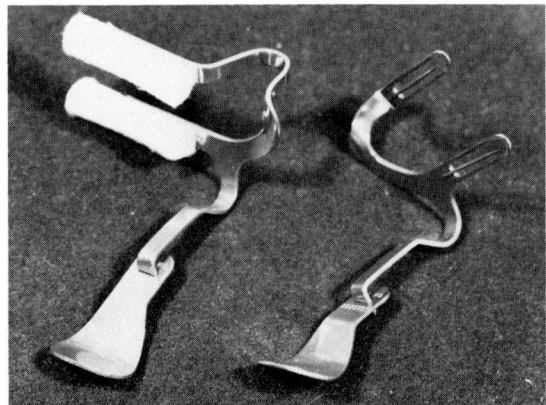

Courtesy Garmers Mfg. Co.

Fig. 33.33. Cotton-roll holders

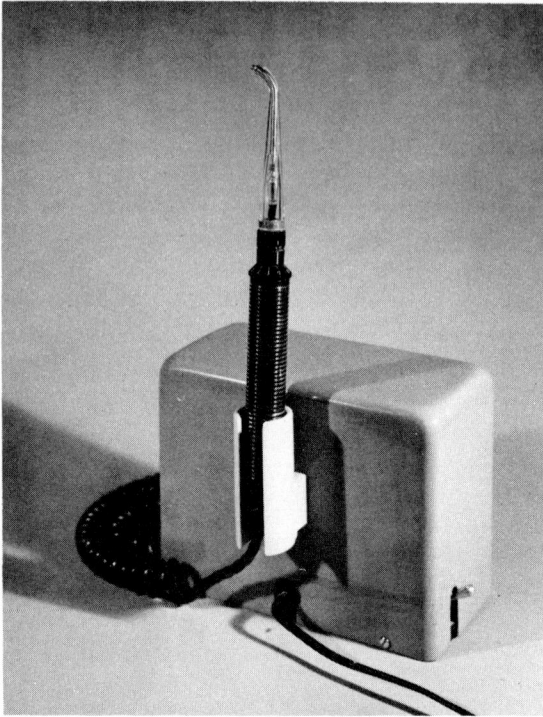

Courtesy Ritter Dental Mfg. Co.

Fig. 33.34. A pulp tester

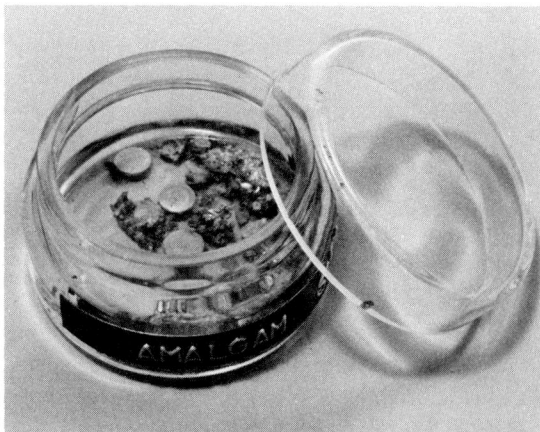

Fig. 33.36. Quick-filling water syringe.

Courtesy Clev-Dent

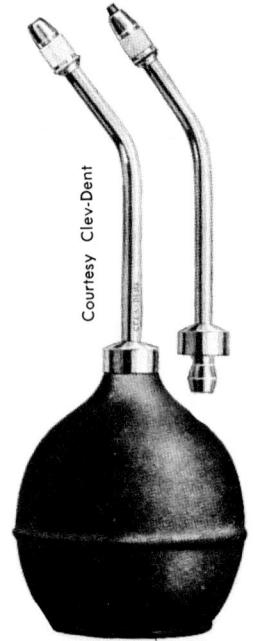

Courtesy Clev-Dent

Fig. 33.37. Bates Arkansas sharpening stone No. 5. It is made for the purpose of sharpening all types of instruments, such as chisels, gouges, lancets, knives, excavators, and elevators. It has four grooves—1 mm., 2 mm., 3 mm., and 4 mm. The reverse side is flat to take care of all kinds of knives and chisels.

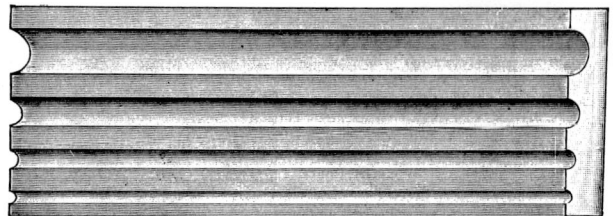

HU-FRIEDY MFG CO

Courtesy Clev-Dent

Fig. 33.38. Gracey Arkansas files. Designed for all types of scalers with a curette type of blade. No. 1 is 3/16" x 4", No. 2 is 1/4" x 4", and No. 3 is 3/8" x 4".

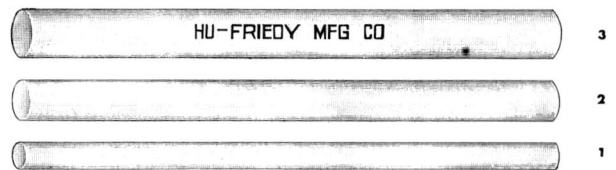

Fig. 33.35. Waste receptacle

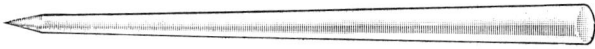

Courtesy Clev-Dent

Fig. 33.39. Gracey Arkansas cone No. 299. An individual stone for scalers and pyorrhea curettes.

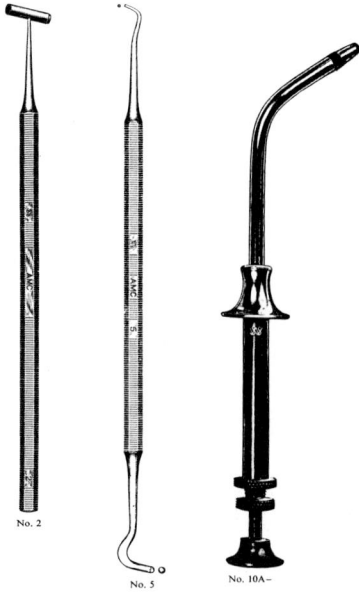

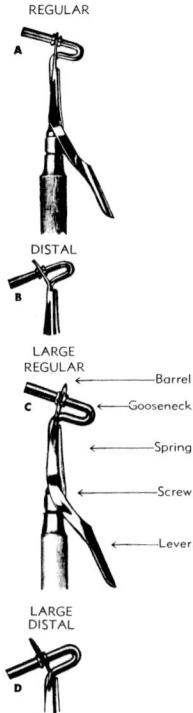

No. 2

No. 5

No. 10A–

REGULAR

A

DISTAL

B

LARGE
REGULAR

C

— Barrel

— Gooseneck

— Spring

— Screw

— Lever

LARGE
DISTAL

D

Place your finger under the lever when filling carrier. Press the lever to expel the amalgam. Maintain pressure on the lever to attach first amalgam in the cavity. To clean use a little heat on the barrel (over an alcohol lamp or Bunsen burner) and press the lever several times. *Do not heat the spring.*

Fig. 33.40. Amalgam carriers

Courtesy J. W. Ivory, Inc.

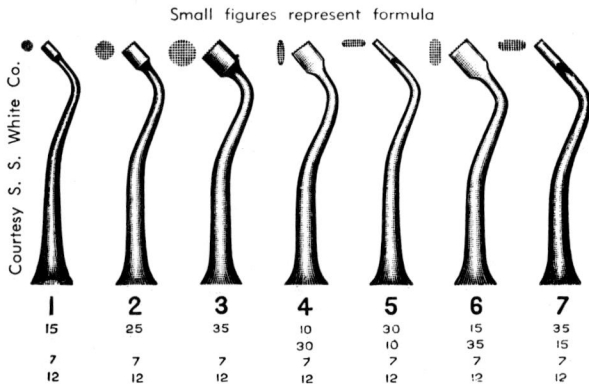

Courtesy S. S. White Co.

Fig. 33.42. Hollenback's amalgam condensers

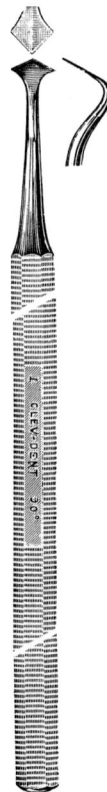

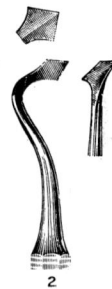

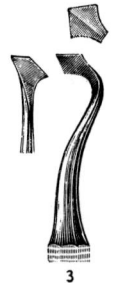

Courtesy S. S. White Co.

Small figures represent formula

1	2	3	4	5	6	7
15	25	35	10	30	15	35
			30	10	35	15
7	7	7	7	7	7	7
12	12	12	12	12	12	12

Fig. 33.41. Black's amalgam pluggers

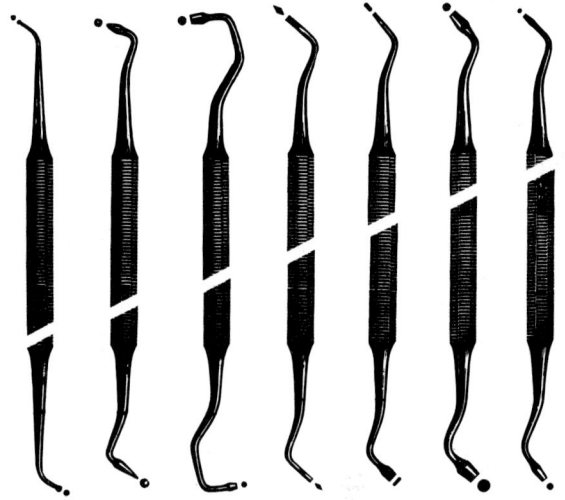

Courtesy Clev-Dent

2

3

Fig. 33.43. Frahm's carvers

Ordinaries—Hatchets

2	3	4	5	6	7	8	9	10	11	12	20	22	23	24
12	10	8	6	4	14	12	10	8	6	4	12	9	5	4
5	4	3	2	2	6	5	4	3	2	1	5	3	2	1
6	6	6	6	6	12	12	12	12	12	12	23	23	23	23

Ordinaries—Hoes

25	26	27	28	29	30	32	34	35	42	44	45	46
14	12	10	8	6	4	12	8	6	4	12	10	8
6	5	4	3	2	1	5	3	2	1	5	4	3
6	6	6	6	6	6	12	12	12	18	23	23	23

Hoes

47	48
6	4
2	1
23	23

Enamel Hatchets

49	50	51	52	53	54
20	20	15	15	10	10
9	9	8	8	6	6
12	12	12	12	12	12
L	R	L	R	L	R

Gingival Margin Trimmer

77	78	79	80
15	15	15	15
95	95	80	80
8	8	8	8
12	12	12	12
L	R	L	R

Gingival Margin Trimmers

73	74	75	76
20	20	20	20
95	95	80	80
9	9	9	9
12	12	12	12
L	L	R	R

Spoons

61	62	63	64	65	66	71	72
20	20	15	15	10	10	10	10
9	9	8	8	6	6	6	6
12	12	12	12	12	12	23	23
L	R	L	R	L	R	L	R

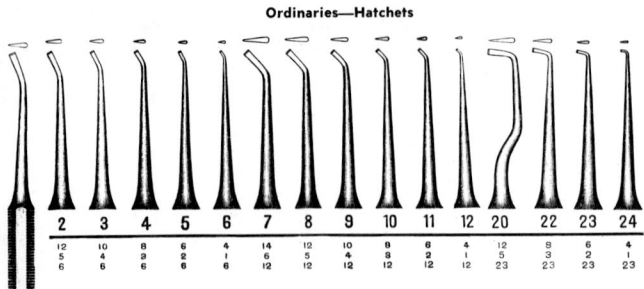

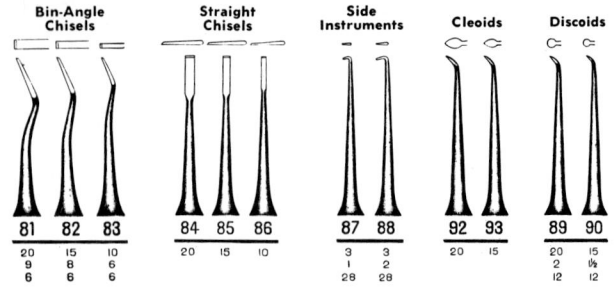

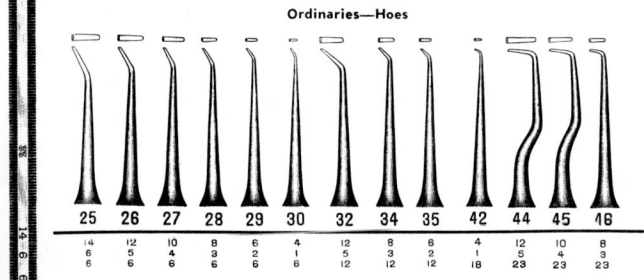

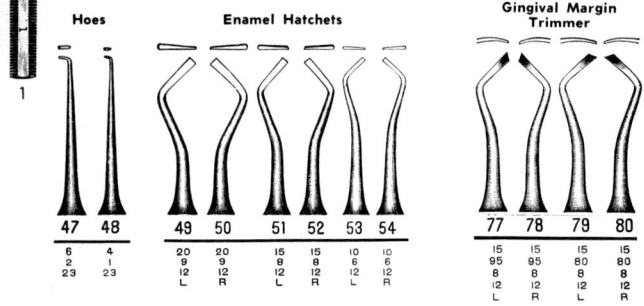

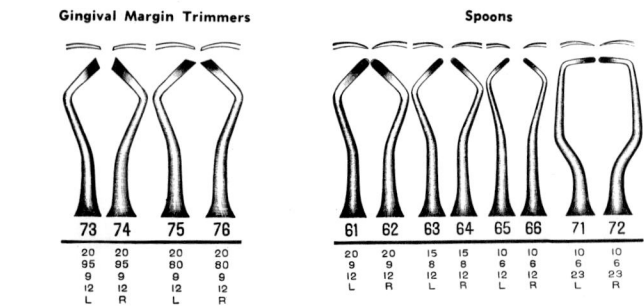

Fig. 33.44. Black's cutting instruments

Bin-Angle Chisels

81	82	83
20	15	10
9	8	6
6	6	6

Straight Chisels

84	85	86
20	15	10

Side Instruments

87	88
3	3
1	2
28	28

Cleoids

92	93
20	15

Discoids

89	90
20	15
2	¼
12	12

Long Handle—Nos. 1 to 12, 20, 22 to 30, 32, 34, 35, 42, 44 to 54, 61 to 66, 71 to 90, 92, 93—Carbon Steel

Long Handle—Nos. 2, 4, 5, 8, 10, 11, 20, 22, 23, 26, 28, 29, 32, 34, 35, 44, 46, 47, 49 to 54, 61 to 66, 73 to 89, 92, "TARNO"

Double-end—Nos. 49-50, 51-52, 53-54—Carbon Steel

Double-end—Nos. 61-62, 63-64, 65-66—"TAR-NO"

Courtesy S. S. White Co.

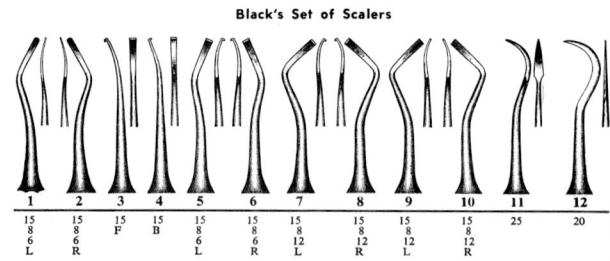

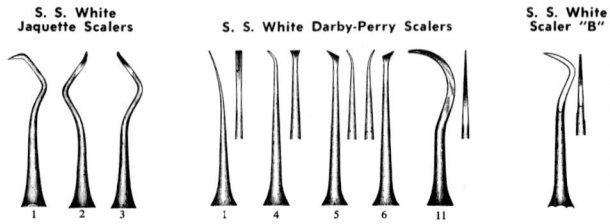

Fig. 33.44 (Continued)

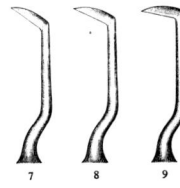

7	8	9

Fig. 33.45. G. V. Black's trimming knives and files.

Courtesy S. S. White Co.

Black's Set of Scalers

1	2	3	4	5	6	7	8	9	10	11	12
15	15	15	15	15	15	15	15	15	15	25	20
8	8	8	8	8	8	8	8	8	8		
6	6	F	B	6	6	12	12	12	12		
L	R			L	R	L	R	L	R		

S. S. White Jaquette Scalers

1	2	3

S. S. White Darby-Perry Scalers

1	4	5	6	11

S. S. White Scaler "B"

Fig. 33.46. A selection of scalers

Dr. W. A. Jaquette's Scalers

Baylor Scalers

2   3

University of Southern California Scaler No. 128

CLEV-DENT 1 JAQUETTE SCALER

CLEV-DENT 1 BAYLOR

CLEV-DENT 2 BAYLOR

Courtesy S. S. White Co. and Clev-Dent

1   2

Fig. 33.46 (Continued)

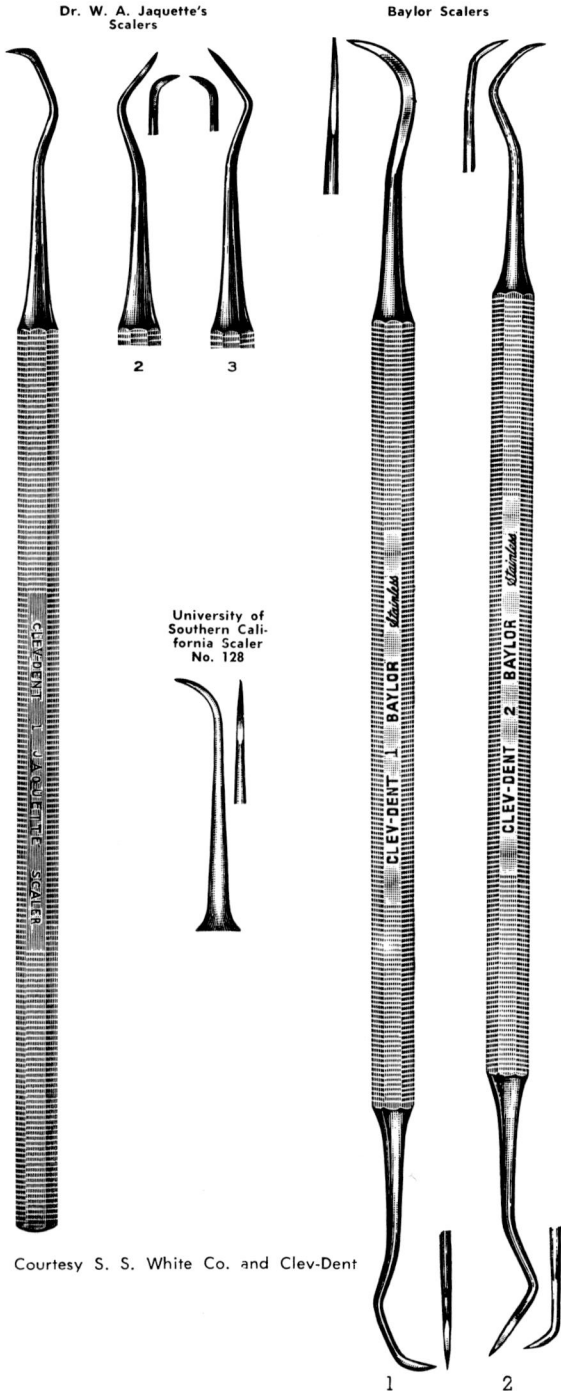

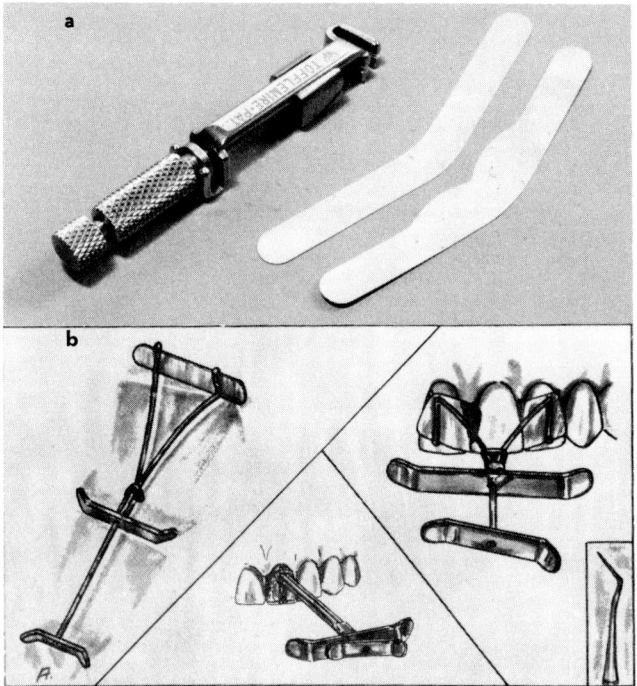

Fig. 33.47. Matrix retainers: (a) Tofflemire matrix retainer; (b) Garmers anterior matrix retainer.

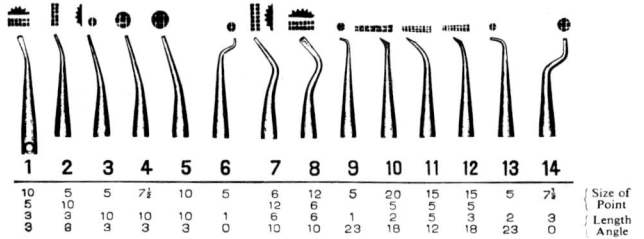

1	2	3	4	5	6	7	8	9	10	11	12	13	14	
10	5	5	7½	10	5		6	12	5	20	15	5	7½	Size of Point
5	10					12	6		5	5	5			
3	3	10	10	10	1	6	6	1	2	5	3	2	3	Length
3	8	3	3	3	0	10	10	23	18	12	18	23	0	Angle

Nos. 1, 2—for Automatic Mallet and Cone-socket Handle
Nos. 7, 8—for Automatic Mallet and Cone-socket Handle

Courtesy S. S. White Co. and Clev-Dent

Fig. 33.48. G. V. Black's gold pluggers

1   2   3   4   5   6

Courtesy Clev-Dent

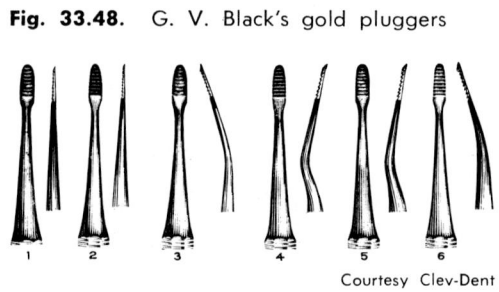

Fig. 33.49. G. V. Black's files

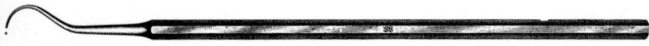

Courtesy S. S. White Co.

Fig. 33.50. G. V. Black's holding instrument

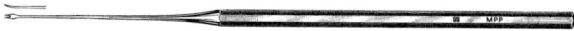

Courtesy S. S. White Co.

Fig. 33.51. Pellet placer

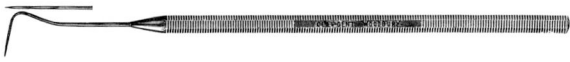

Courtesy Clev-Dent

Fig. 33.52. Woodbury's annealing instrument

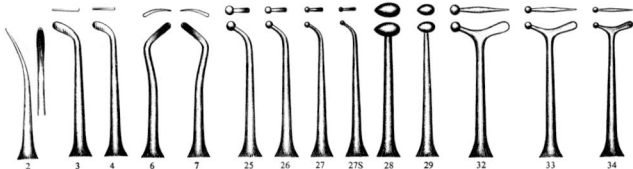

Courtesy S. S. White Co.

Fig. 33.53. A selection of burnishers

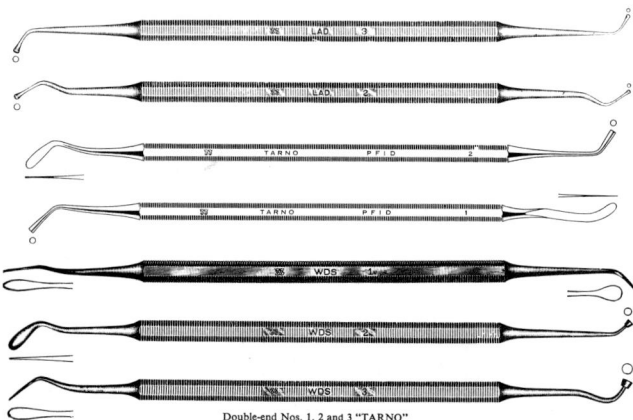

Double-end Nos. 1, 2 and 3 "TARNO"

Courtesy S. S. White Co.

Fig. 33.54. Plastic double-end filling instruments

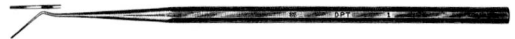

Courtesy Clev-Dent

Fig. 33.55. Darby plastic trimmers

Courtesy S. S. White Co.

Fig. 33.56. Texton trimmer No. 1, double-ended

For use with Nealon Brush Technique for quick-curing resins

Courtesy Clev-Dent

Fig. 33.57. Red sable brush No. 00.

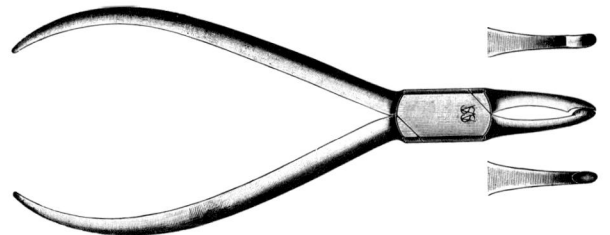

Courtesy S. S. White Co. and Rocky Mountain Dental Products Co.

Fig. 33.58. Contouring pliers

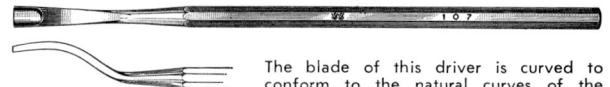

The blade of this driver is curved to conform to the natural curves of the surface of the tooth, thereby bringing the entire working end in contact with the edge of the band. The offset reduces slipping, also aids in seating "hard to get at" bands.

Courtesy S. S. White Co.

Fig. 33.59. Band driver No. 107 for orthodontic use

Fig. 33.60. Chairside sterilizer for endodontic use.

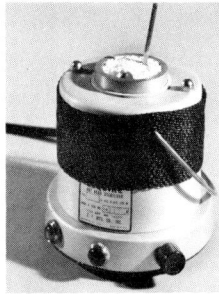

STYLE B—Short Handle

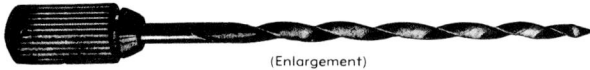

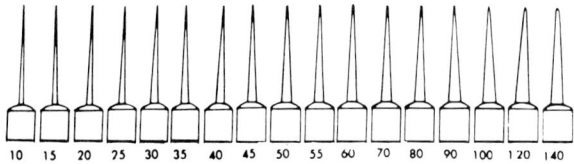

(Enlargement)

10 15 20 25 30 35 40 45 50 55 60 70 80 90 100 120 140

Size—Numbers above also indicate (in hundredths of a millimeter) the D¹ dimension of the instruments.
Length of Blade—21 mm, 25 mm, 30 mm.
Packed—6 reamers to box, 6 assorted 10 to 35, or 40 to 70, or 80 to 140.

Courtesy Star Dental Mfg. Co.

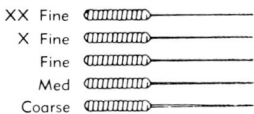

Fig. 33.61. Reamers used for endodontics

FILE, Long Handle Style D

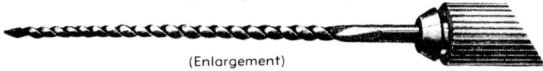

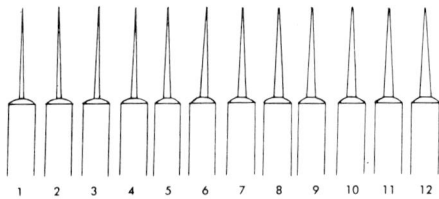

(Enlargement)

Length of Blade

26 mm, sizes
1 to 12
30 mm, sizes
1 to 12

1 2 3 4 5 6 7 8 9 10 11 12

K TYPE following existing size progressions and tolerance

Courtesy Star Dental Mfg. Co.

Fig. 33.62. Files used for endodontics

BROACH Barbed, Short Handle

(Enlargement)

Courtesy Star Dental Mfg. Co.

XX Fine
X Fine
Fine
Med
Coarse

Fig. 33.63. Broaches used for endodontics.

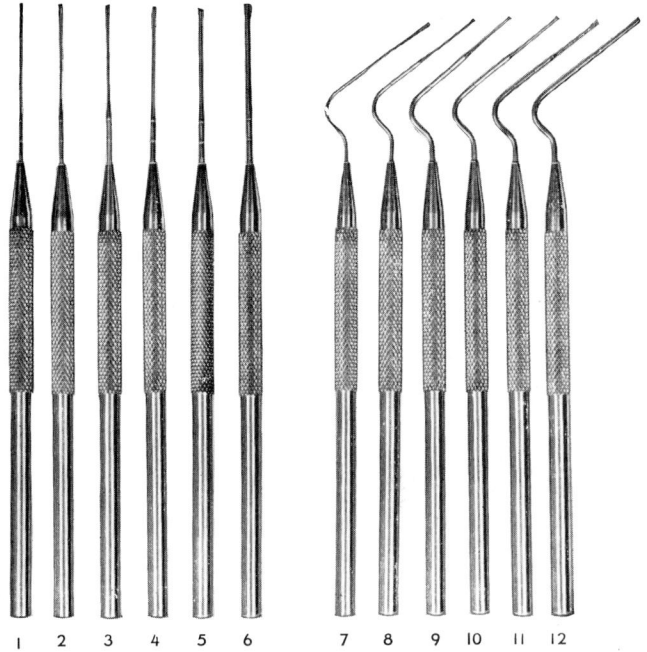

1 2 3 4 5 6   7 8 9 10 11 12

Courtesy Kerr Mfg. Co.

Fig. 33.64. Root canal pluggers used for endodontics

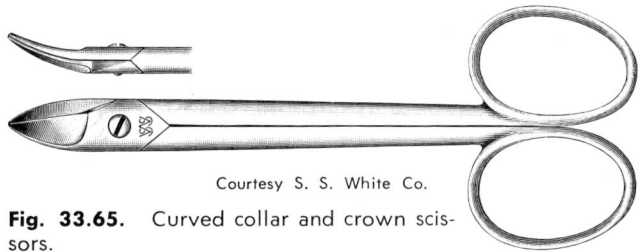

Courtesy S. S. White Co.

Fig. 33.65. Curved collar and crown scissors.

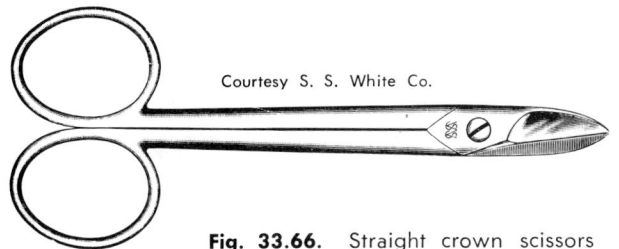

Courtesy S. S. White Co.

Fig. 33.66. Straight crown scissors

Crandall Copper Bands are made in fourteen sizes, 30 and 36 gauge, one-half, five-sixteenths and one inch long, annealed and unannealed.

5/16" and 1/2" long, 30 and 36 gauge—
In bulk, 100 of one number

5/16" and 1/2" long, 30 and 36 gauge—
Box of 12 of one number
Box of 25 of one number
Box of 100 assorted

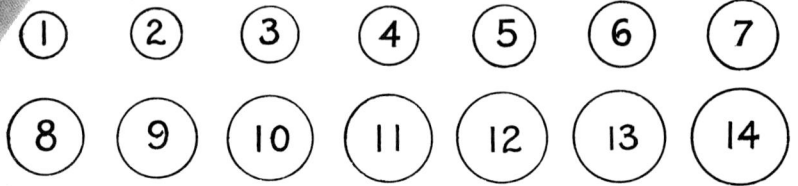

1" long, 36 gauge—
Box of 12 of one number
Box of 25 of one number
Box of 100 assorted

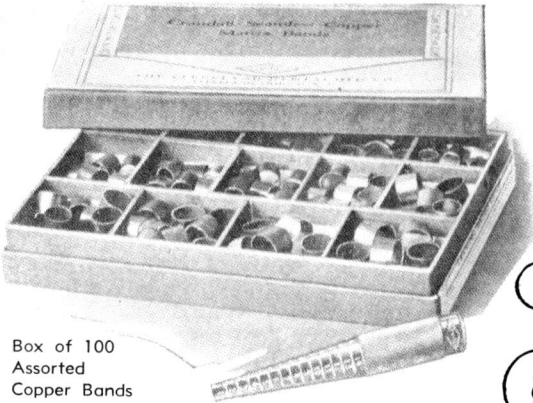

Box of 100
Assorted
Copper Bands

Courtesy Clev-Dent

Fig. 33.67. Crandall copper bands with circles to indicate size of bands

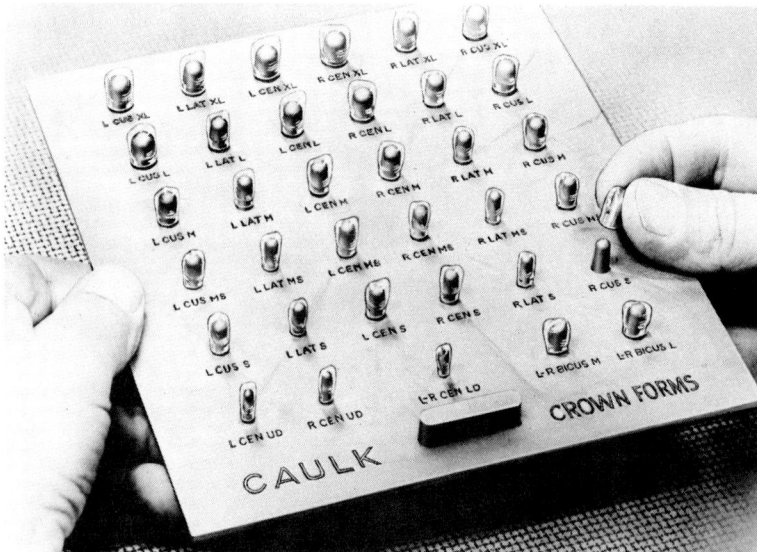

Courtesy L. D. Caulk Co.

Fig. 33.68. Crown forms on selection board

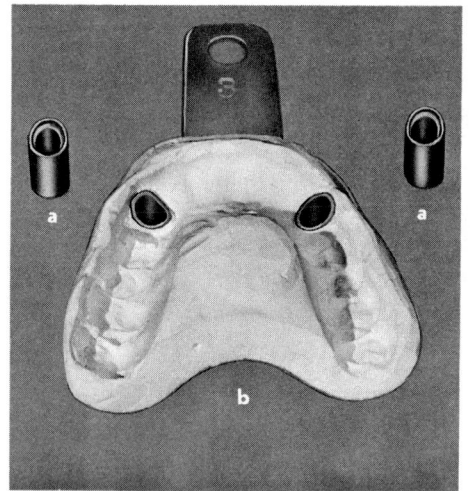

Courtesy Kramer Dental Studio

Fig. 33.69. Two "thimble" impressions (or copper bands) of synthetic jacket crown preparations and an impression removed in superimposed plaster tray.

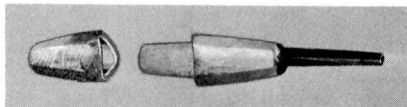

Courtesy Kramer Dental Studio

Fig. 33.70. Amalgam die made from a thimble impression with a "coping" made to fit the amalgam die.

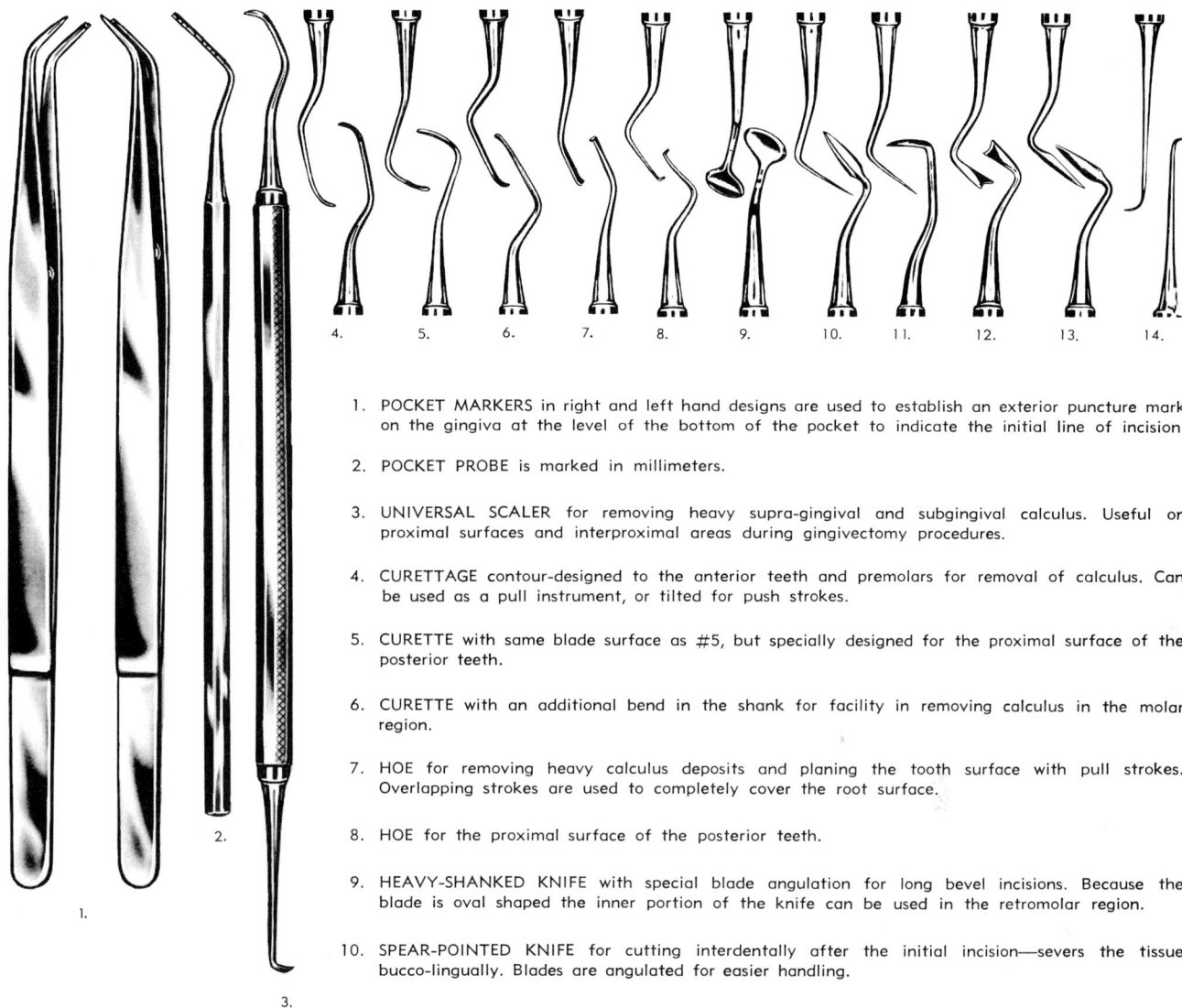

1. POCKET MARKERS in right and left hand designs are used to establish an exterior puncture mark on the gingiva at the level of the bottom of the pocket to indicate the initial line of incision.

2. POCKET PROBE is marked in millimeters.

3. UNIVERSAL SCALER for removing heavy supra-gingival and subgingival calculus. Useful on proximal surfaces and interproximal areas during gingivectomy procedures.

4. CURETTAGE contour-designed to the anterior teeth and premolars for removal of calculus. Can be used as a pull instrument, or tilted for push strokes.

5. CURETTE with same blade surface as #5, but specially designed for the proximal surface of the posterior teeth.

6. CURETTE with an additional bend in the shank for facility in removing calculus in the molar region.

7. HOE for removing heavy calculus deposits and planing the tooth surface with pull strokes. Overlapping strokes are used to completely cover the root surface.

8. HOE for the proximal surface of the posterior teeth.

9. HEAVY-SHANKED KNIFE with special blade angulation for long bevel incisions. Because the blade is oval shaped the inner portion of the knife can be used in the retromolar region.

10. SPEAR-POINTED KNIFE for cutting interdentally after the initial incision—severs the tissue bucco-lingually. Blades are angulated for easier handling.

11. DOUBLE-ENDED INSTRUMENT has spear-pointed blade on one end for use in the mandibular anterior region from the posterior direction; modified sickle scaler on the other end is elongated to use in the interdental area for debridement.

12. TRIANGULAR TISSUE RETRACTOR designed to lift off the gingival tissue after interproximal cutting. Concave blade edge fits against the cervical portion of the tooth.

13. SPEAR-POINTED KNIFE similar to #10 except the blades are offset for use in the posterior regions.

14. DOUBLE-ENDED INSTRUMENT has sharp spoon curette on one end for debridement in curettage procedure; other end has small scaler curette and can be used with either a circumferential or vertical stroke.

Courtesy Hu-Friedy Mfg. Co.

Fig. 33.71. Some instruments used by periodontists.

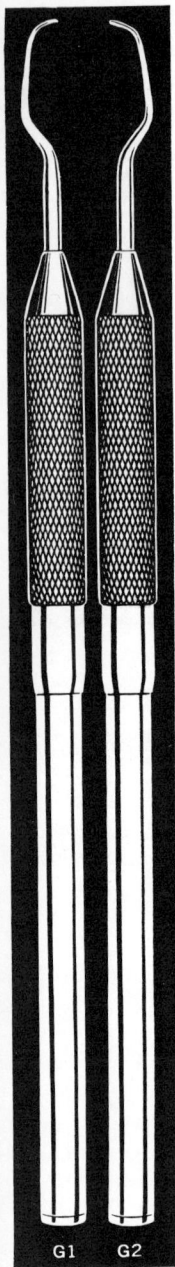

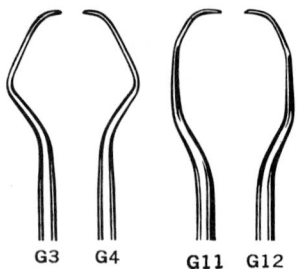

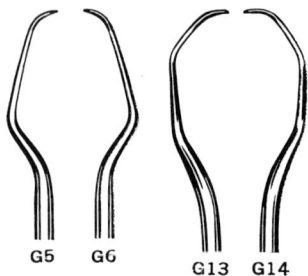

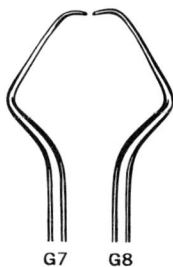

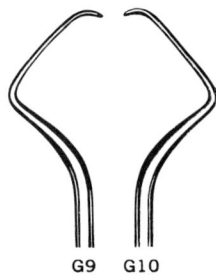

"Universal" as used in the description of forceps means that the forceps are equally efficient for extraction of teeth on right or left side and for upper and lower jaws as indicated.

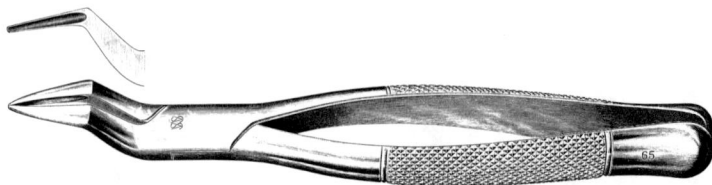

Fig. 33.73. Forceps, incisor and root, upper, No. 65

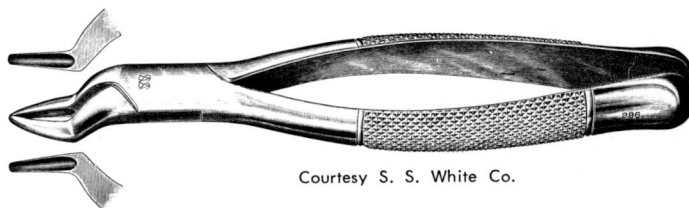

Courtesy S. S. White Co.

Fig. 33.74. Forceps, bicuspid, incisor, and root, upper, No. 286.

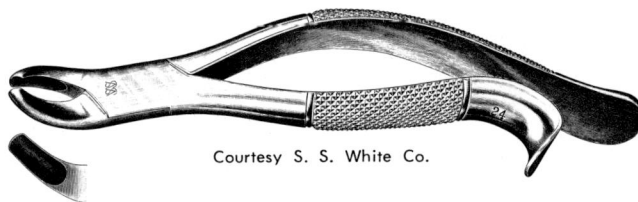

Courtesy S. S. White Co.

Fig. 33.75. Forceps, molar, upper, universal, No. 24

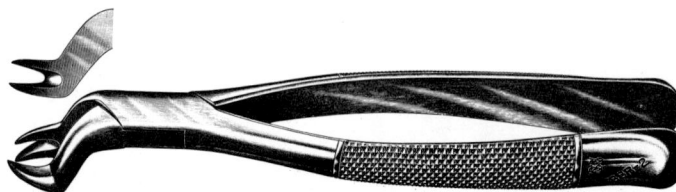

Courtesy S. S. White Co.

Fig. 33.76. Forceps, first and second molar, upper right, No. 88R-2.

G1 G2   G3 G4   G11 G12

G5 G6   G13 G14

G7 G8

G9 G10

Fig. 33.72. Gracey curettes, generally used in periodontics.

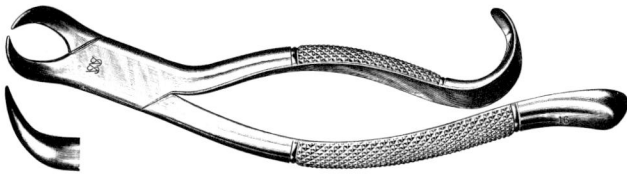

Courtesy S. S. White Co.

Fig. 33.77. Forceps, first and second molar, lower-universal-hornbeak, No. 16.

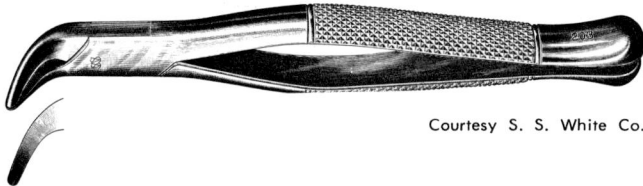

Courtesy S. S. White Co.

Fig. 33.78. Forceps, bicuspid, incisor, and root, lower-universal, No. 203.

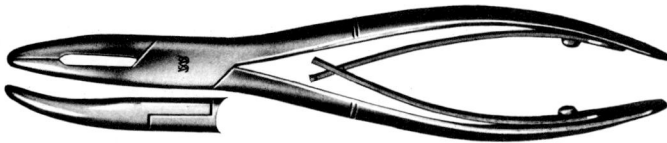

Courtesy S. S. White Co.

Fig. 33.79. Rongeurs, No. 1A, is a universal and may be used anywhere in the mouth for an alveolectomy and in many cases for removing small particles of roots; also in breaking down the process during extraction.

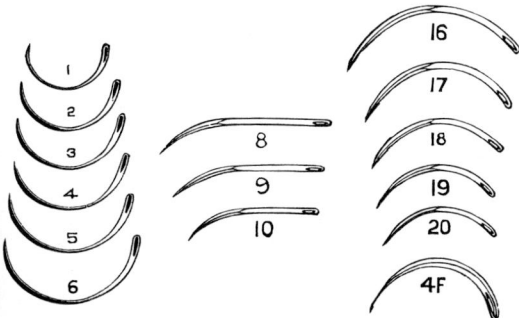

Courtesy Johnson and Johnson

Fig. 33.81. Exodontia sponge

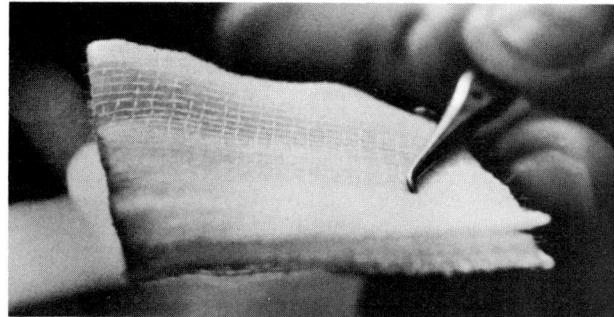

Courtesy Hu-Friedy Mfg. Co., Inc.

Fig. 33.82. Tissue forceps

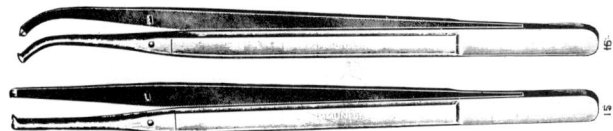

Nos. 1-2 — Provident, 6 in. over-all
Nos. 3-4 — The Mosquito, 5 in. over-all.

Courtesy Hu-Friedy Mfg. Co., Inc.

Fig. 33.83. Hemostatic forceps

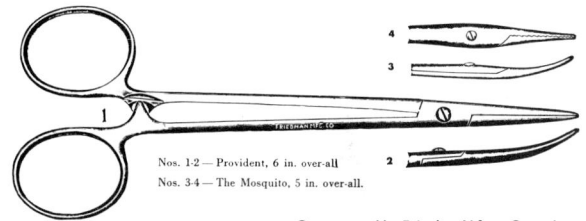

Courtesy Hu-Friedy Mfg. Co.

Fig. 33.80. Surgical needles

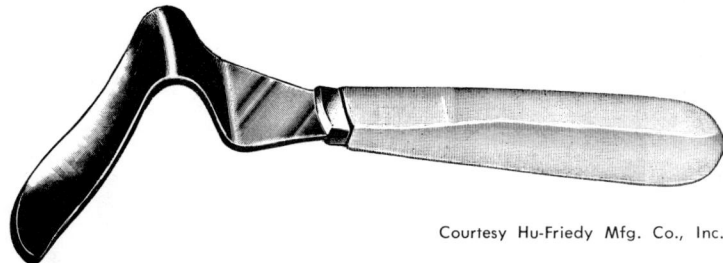

Courtesy Hu-Friedy Mfg. Co., Inc.

Fig. 33.84. Black cheek and third molar tissue retractor.

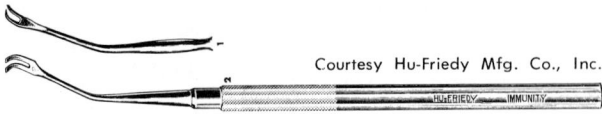

Courtesy Hu-Friedy Mfg. Co., Inc.

Fig. 33.85. Thoma tissue retractor

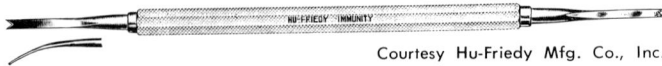

Courtesy Hu-Friedy Mfg. Co., Inc.

Fig. 33.86. Gauze packer

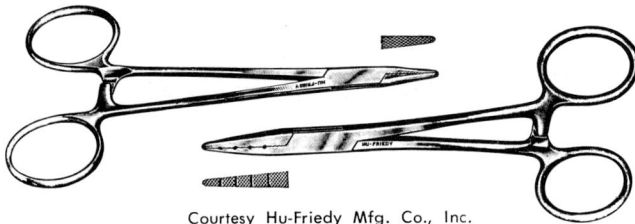

Courtesy Hu-Friedy Mfg. Co., Inc.

Fig. 33.87. Gardner and Abbey needle holders

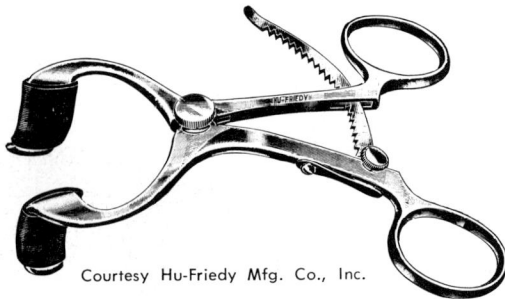

Courtesy Hu-Friedy Mfg. Co., Inc.

Fig. 33.88. Molt standard mouth gag

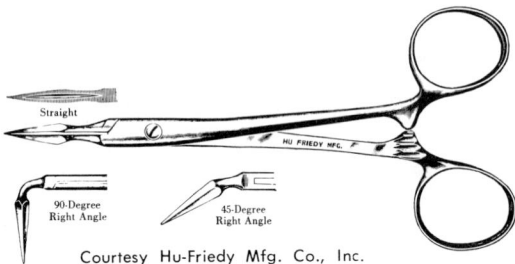

Courtesy Hu-Friedy Mfg. Co., Inc.

Fig. 33.89. Archer splinter forceps

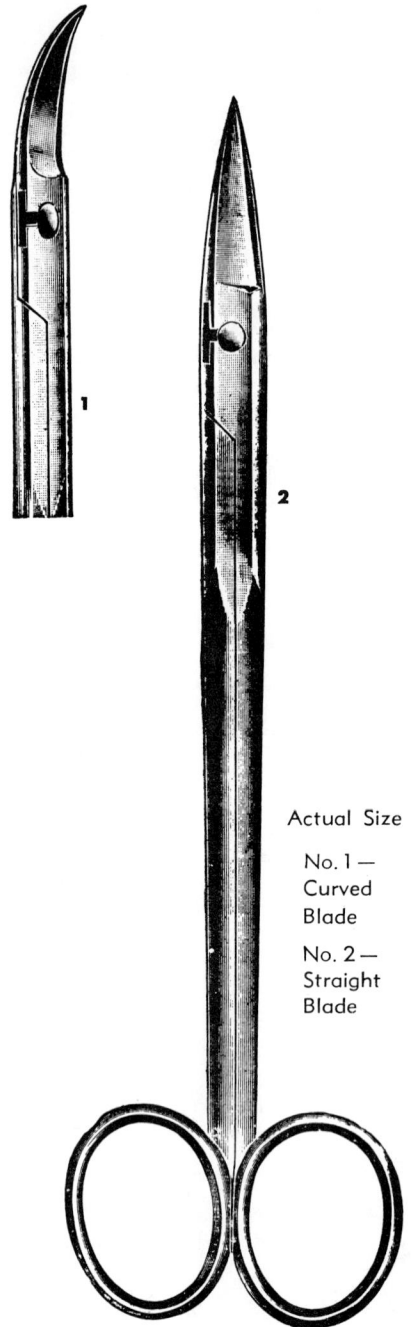

Actual Size

No. 1 —
Curved
Blade

No. 2 —
Straight
Blade

Courtesy Hu-Friedy Mfg. Co., Inc.

Fig. 33.90. Kelly surgical scissors

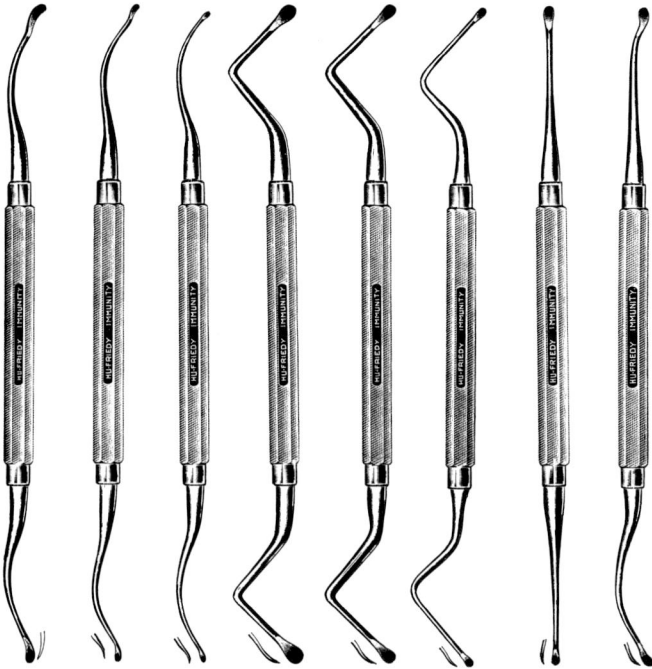

Courtesy Hu-Friedy Mfg. Co., Inc.

Fig. 33.91. Miller standard surgical curettes

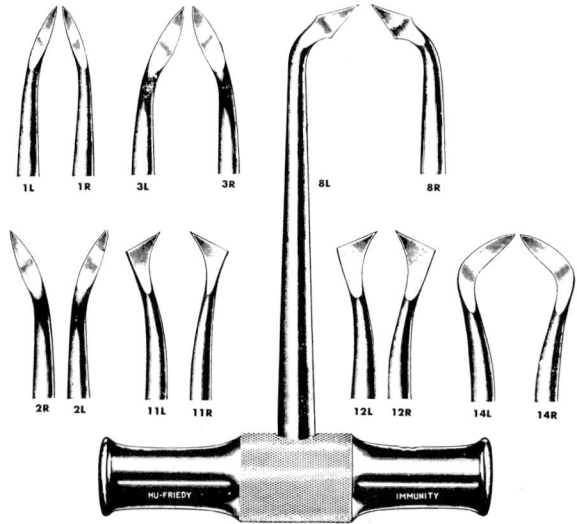

Courtesy Hu-Friedy Mfg. Co., Inc.

Fig. 33.93. Elevators

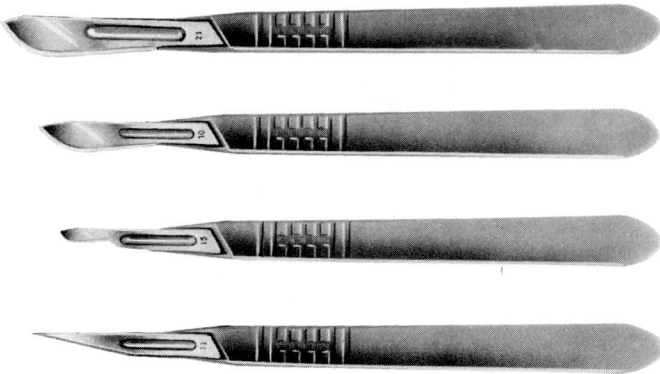

Fig. 33.92. Scalpels: (above) standard; (right) disposable

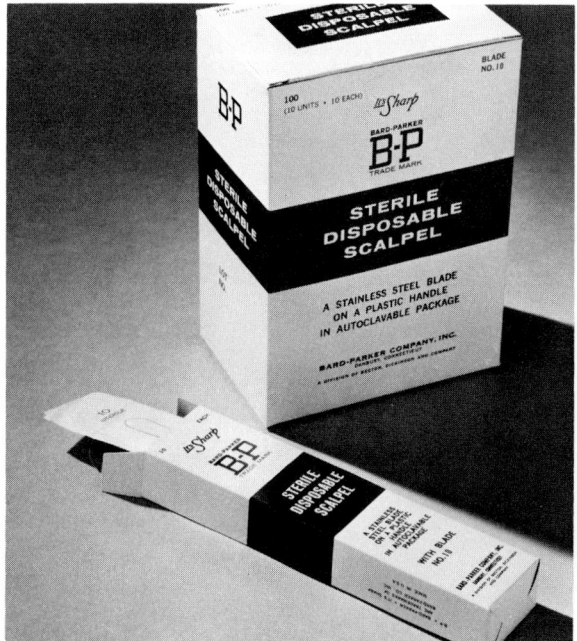

Courtesy Hu-Friedy Mfg. Co., Inc.

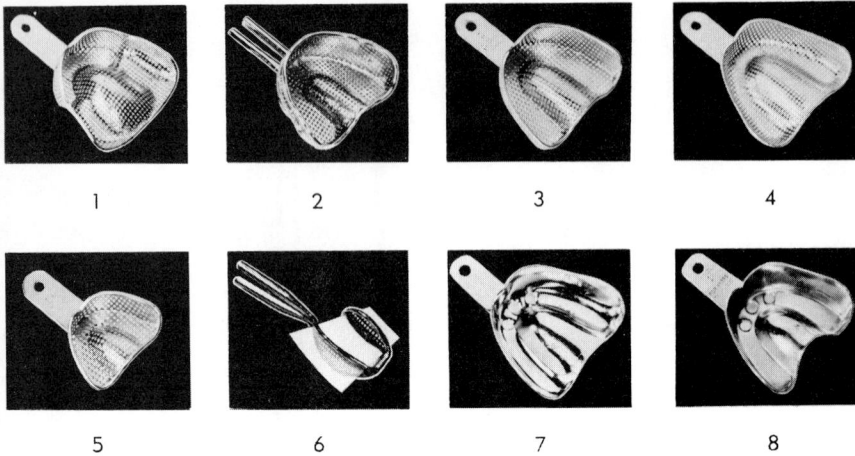

1. McGowan Immediate Denture Trays for use with alginate impression materials. Set of 8.
2. Frigidtrays for use with hydrocolloids: water-cooled. Sets of 6 and 8.
3. Coe Perforated Full Denture Trays for alginate impressions of the edentulous mouth. Set of 8.
4. Coe Perforated Trays for partials: inside peripheral lock. Regular or depressed anterior. Set of 6.
5. Cce Perforated Trays for orthodontics. Small size for childen. Set of 6.
6. Coe Check-Bite Trays for inlays, crowns and bridges.
7. Bunce-Kanouse Trays for edentulous mouths. Set of 8.
8. Coe Akers Trays for partials: for use with soluble plasters or other materials. Set of 9.

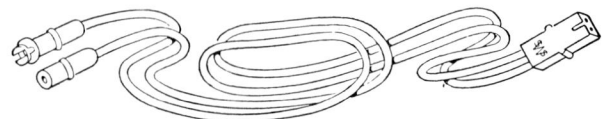

Courtesy Coe Labs., Inc.

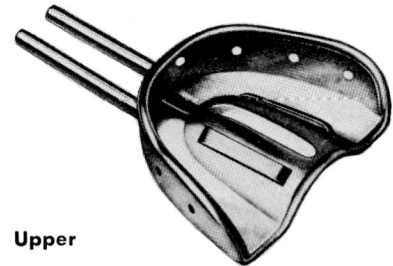

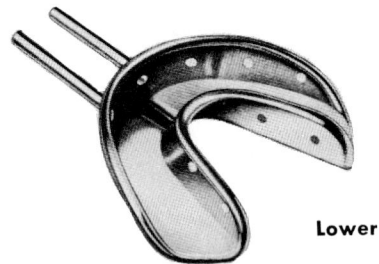

Fig. 33.94. Impression trays

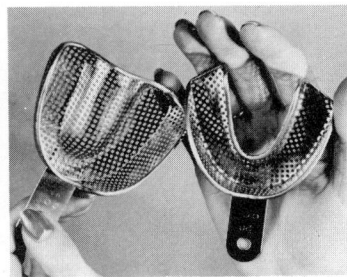

Fig. 33.95. Perforated trays, upper and lower, for dentulous mouths for use with alginate materials.

Courtesy Coe Labs., Inc.

Upper

Courtesy Coe Labs., Inc.

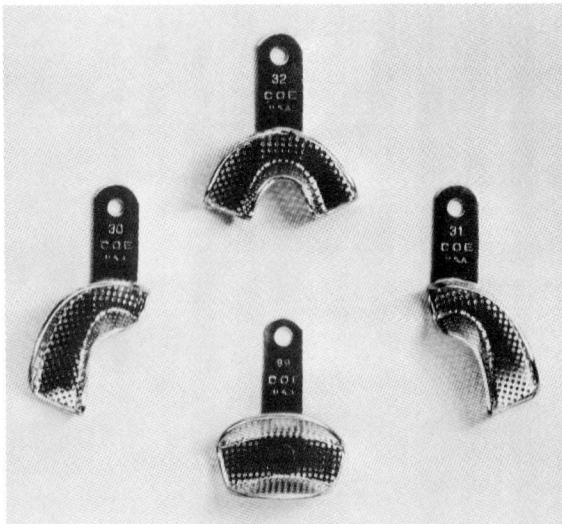

Fig. 33.96. Perforated trays, partial

Lower

Courtesy Coe Labs., Inc.

Fig. 33.97. Water-cooled trays and rubber tubing

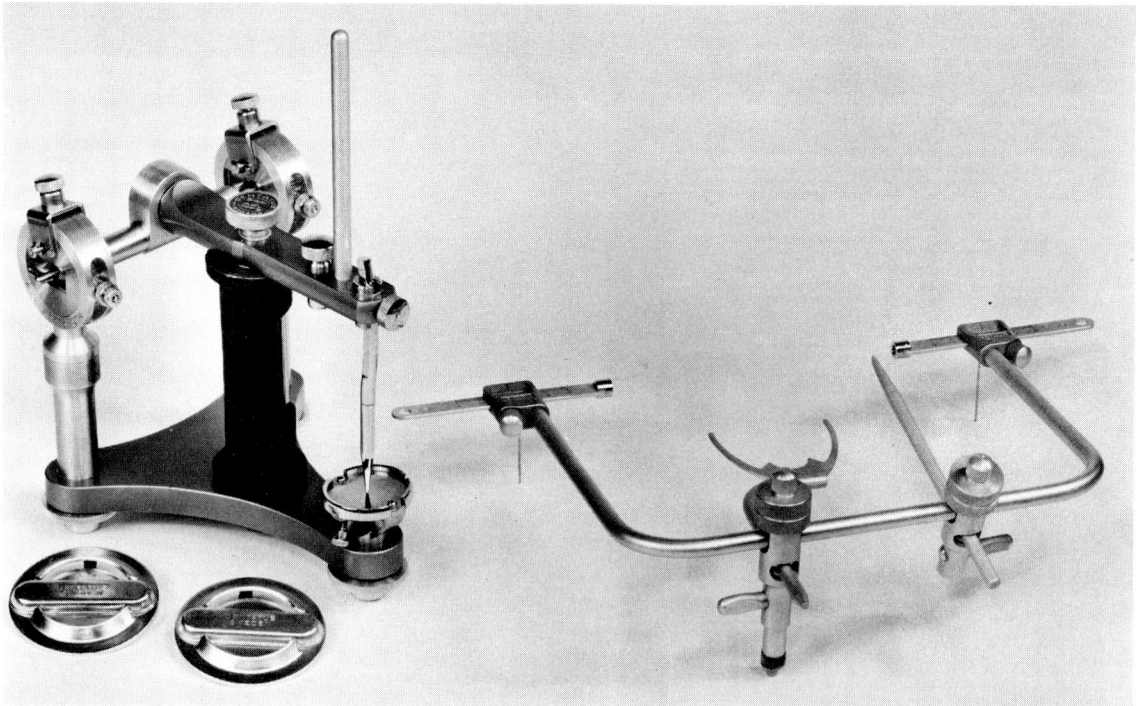

Courtesy Kerr Mfg. Co.

Fig. 33.98. Kerr Dentatus articulator and Kerr facebow

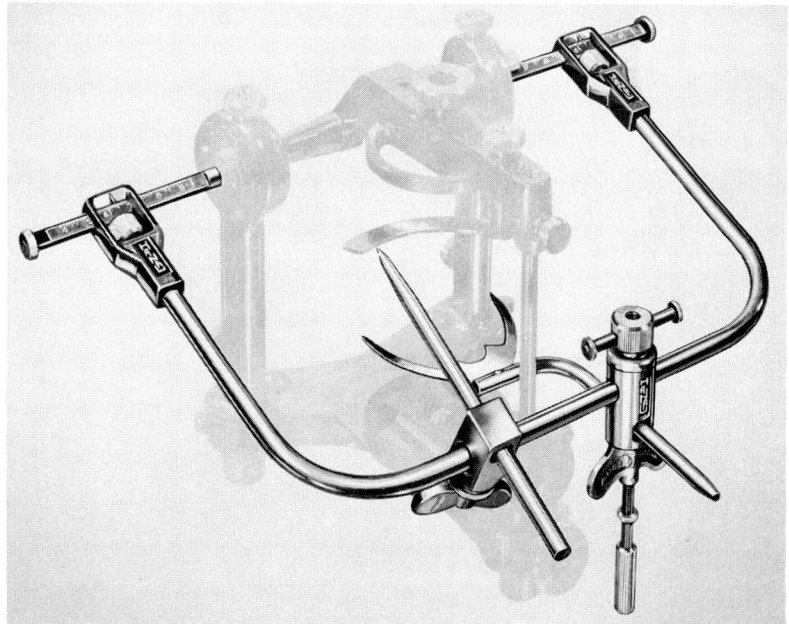

Courtesy Hanau Engr. Co.

Fig. 33.99. The facebow with bite fork and pointer, on a Hanau articulator.

PART SEVEN | # DENTAL MATERIALS AND LABORATORY PROCEDURES

Now that you have become acquainted with the armamentarium of the dental office, you can profit from understanding the materials which are used in dentistry—and the chairside and laboratory procedures which you will be performing.

The restorative materials of dentistry (used in the mouth), the materials which are used outside the patient's mouth, and the procedures you will use in preparing these materials are discussed in this section. In addition to being familiar with these materials and procedures, you must be capable of working with the materials and skilled in performing the procedures described. It really doesn't matter whether you work with them at the chair or in the dental laboratory.

Procedures which are associated with certain dental materials are discussed in the proper sequence following basic information concerning that material. However, these procedures, laboratory or chairside, require actual practice under supervision to attain the desired proficiency in their use. It is recommended that your instructor or dentist supervise your work until you have acquired the necessary skills.

34 | *Restorative Materials*

Biomaterials

One of the most fascinating studies with which the dental profession concerns itself involves the study of the many materials used in the performance of dentistry. No one area in dentistry interrelates with so many disciplines as do *biomaterials*. (*Bio* is from the Greek *bios* meaning "life." *Bio-* means "the relationship to or connection with life.") As the name suggests, these materials are directly associated with living tissues. They are usually used in the mouth and may be temporarily or permanently placed in contact with the teeth and/or surrounding oral tissues.

The environment of the oral cavity is considered restrictive for the following reasons:

1. The oral cavity is constantly moist;
2. The oral cavity is subjected to rather extreme changes of temperature (hot coffee and ice water);
3. The oral cavity is subjected to pH changes (acid-alkaline foods and beverages); and
4. The restorative materials may be placed under the stress and abrasion of masticatory (chewing) forces.

The foreign materials placed in the oral cavity must be unusually adaptable to survive in such an environment.

Consider that an important facet of dental care is the repair and restoration of oral structures damaged or destroyed by injury or dis-

TENET	ZINC OXIDE-EUGENOL	ZINC PHOSPHATE	SILICATE	UNFILLED PLASTIC	FILLED PLASTIC	COMPOSITE FILLING MATERIALS	AMALGAM	CAST GOLD	WELDED GOLD
Aesthetics	Does not detract; may enhance	Yes	Yes	Yes	Yes	Yes	No	No	No
Toxicity	Sedative	Needs liner or base for protection	Needs liner or base for protection	Needs liner or base for protection	Needs liner or base for protection	Needs liner or base for protection	No	No per se; cementing media may be	No
Solubility	Slightly soluble	Slightly soluble	Slightly soluble	Insoluble	Insoluble	Insoluble	Insoluble	Insoluble	Insoluble
Adaptation	For short period: Good	Good	Good	Fair	Fair	Good	Good	Fair	Good
Coefficient of Thermal Expansion	Not of practical importance	As a cementing media: Good	Good	Poor	Poor	Fair	Fair	Fair	Fair
Strength	Lacking	Adequate as a cementing media	Inadequate for masticating surfaces	Inadequate for masticating surfaces	Inadequate for masticating surfaces	Inadequate for masticating surfaces	Good	Good	Good
Anti-cariogenicity	No	No	Yes	No	No	No	No	No	No
Reparability	Not practical	Not a consideration	No	Yes	Yes	Yes	Yes	No	Yes
Manipulability	Good	Good	Good	Good	Good	Good	Good	Fair	Fair
Radiopacity	If opaquer is added	To a degree	No	No	No	Some have	Yes	Yes	Yes

Fig. 34.1. The ten tenets for restorative materials applied to each material

ease. Therefore, dental researchers are constantly challenged in their efforts to find the ideal restorative material. Unfortunately, the ideal restorative material has not been developed, and new products seem to appear more rapidly than researchers can properly evaluate. The practicing dentist finds it difficult to evaluate materials before incorporating them into his armamentarium because he lacks both time and the laboratory facilities for formal testing procedures.

The American Dental Association recognizes this problem and, in cooperation with the National Bureau of Standards, has established standards or requirements for materials which are to be certified for dentistry. Manufacturers must meet these standards if their products are to be listed by the American Dental Association as certified dental materials. The practicing dentist should restrict his selection of materials to the certified list.

As is true of most dental procedures discussed in this book, the discussion of dental materials will be limited to that which is fundamentally necessary for you to know and understand as a beginning dental assistant. If your curiosity is aroused by any individual material or by any particular phase of dentistry, further information is available in many forms to enlarge your knowledge and increase your value as a dental assistant. A text providing a more thorough background in dental materials will be found in the bibliography at the end of this chapter.

The non-dentally-oriented person is usually amazed at the restrictions the oral environment places on materials used to treat or correct oral deficiencies. Anything attached to, or in constant contact with, the oral tissues is subjected to a variety of physical and chemical changes which require properties of extremely fine dimension. These materials must also be biologically compatible with the oral tissue.

Ten Tenets for Restorative Materials

Ten tenets have been established for a filling material. Any currently available restorative material must be measured against these tenets:

1. *Aesthetics.* To most patients aesthetics is more important than biological or functional considerations, especially in anterior restorations. Aesthetics, therefore, must be a prime requisite of a filling material. To be aesthetically acceptable a material must not only match the variable colors within the crown of a single tooth from incisal to gingival, but it must also match the tooth's translucencies, opacities, and fluorescence. Furthermore, aesthetic appearance should not be lost as the restoration ages.

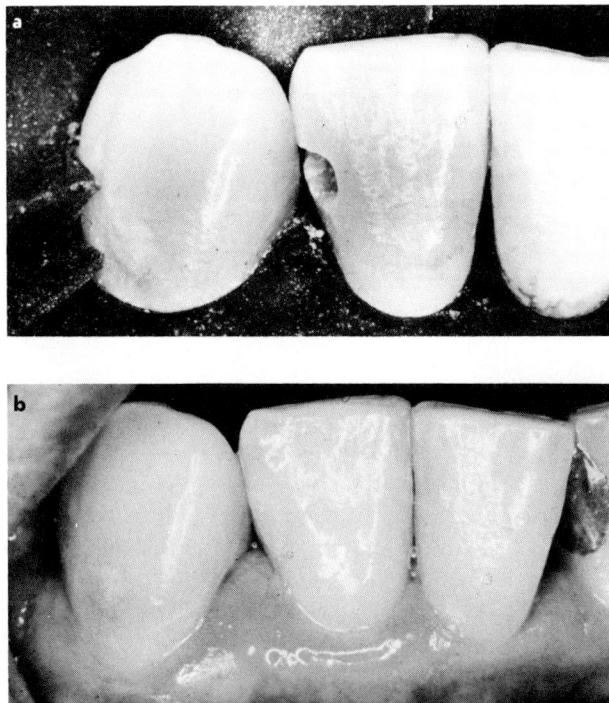

Fig. 34.2. (a) Pre- and (b) post-operative anterior restoration.

2. *Toxicity.* The most important biological consideration is toxicity. The material cannot be toxic to the adjacent gingival tissues or the pulp as it sets, polymerizes in the cavity, or after it is set. (Polymerization is the chemical reaction in which smaller molecules combine into larger molecules.) The material cannot contain toxic ingredients which may produce irreparable damage to any unprotected oral structures. Many manufacturers recommend a cavity liner, or furnish their own, to paint the inside of the cavity and thereby provide the necessary protection.

3. *Solubility.* A material which is soluble in saliva can only be considered temporary in nature. Such a material obviously cannot hold interproximal contact or maintain marginal integrity or contour.

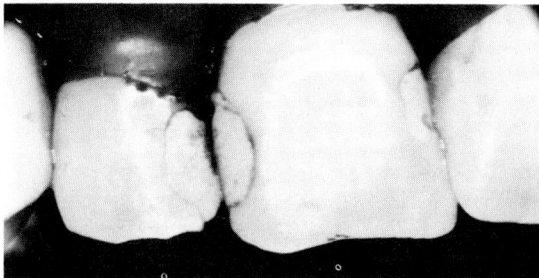

Fig. 34.3. Solubility-defective silicate

4. *Adaptation.* "Adaptation" and "adhesion" are terms sometimes wrongly but loosely used interchangeably. Adhesion is molecular binding; adaptation means modification to fit the conditions of the environment. An adaptable material in dentistry, then, is one which will adapt itself to the shape of the preparation in which it has been placed.

There is no material in dentistry today which will indefinitely adhere to vital tooth structure to insure marginal seal, although it would be desirable to have such a material.

Adhesion (the ability to chemically bond to tooth structure) and the maintenance of dimensional stability and contact with the tooth are important for the life of the restoration. The material must not only closely adapt to the enamel and dentinal walls of the cavity, but it must maintain this close contact or seal in a wet environment when subjected to wide temperature variables. A filling which does not accurately fit the cavity will fail quickly because caries can recur at the leaking margins.

5. *The coefficient of thermal expansion.* (An expression of the rate of expansion and contraction of a material as related to temperature change.) All things behave differently when subjected to temperature variations. In dentistry the coefficient of thermal expansion is extremely important when selecting materials for restorations. The material used should closely match the expansion and contraction properties of tooth structure. The patient may drink hot coffee or ice water. As these liquids pass over the tooth, the crown of the tooth and the filling material will expand and contract according to their own characteristics. If the filling material confined in the enamel of the crown or surrounding the tooth has a coefficient of thermal expansion much greater than the enamel, it will expand and contract much more than the enamel when exposed to these temperature extremes. The filling would then be smaller than the cavity prepared for it when the temperature decreases and larger when the temperature increases.

When the filling is smaller than the cavity (because ice water has passed over it), oral fluids, bacteria, and food debris can flow between the filling and the tooth. Discoloration by the debris can occur at this time, and caries-producing bacteria can enter all parts of the cavity. When the patient heats his mouth by drinking coffee, the filling then expands and the fluids are forced out. However, some residual bacteria and food debris *remain in the spaces between the tooth and filling.* The bubbling of fluids forced out at the margins of fillings subjected to temperature cyclings is called *percolation.*

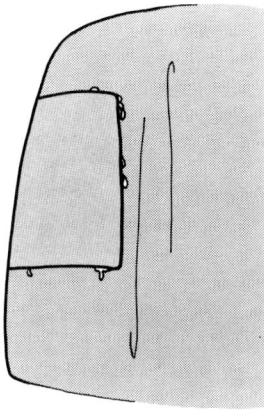

Fig. 34.4. Percolation

Now it is understandable that the coefficient of thermal expansion of the filling material should be similar to that of the tooth enamel because an extreme variation would eliminate from consideration an otherwise acceptable filling material.

6. *Strength.* The strength of a material, whether demonstrated by shear, tensile, or crushing tests, has not been adequately related to masticatory demands. However, a filling material used in areas subjected to stress must be able to withstand incisive or occlusal impact without flow and distortion. It should be as strong as enamel and match its ability to withstand the constant abrasive forces of wear.

7. *Anticariogenic activity.* (*Anti* means "opposite or against." *Cario* refers to caries or decay." *Genic* means "production thereof." Thus, a layman's definition of *anticariogenic* is "opposing the production of caries.") Anticariogenic activity of the material would be a desirable characteristic because it would help eliminate a recurrence and further invasion of caries at the margins of the restoration.

Although a material may release an anticariogenic substance such as fluoride when initially placed in contact with the tooth, to remain active it must continually release its anticariogenic substance. Once the material has set or solidified there can be no release of an anticariogenic component without a break-

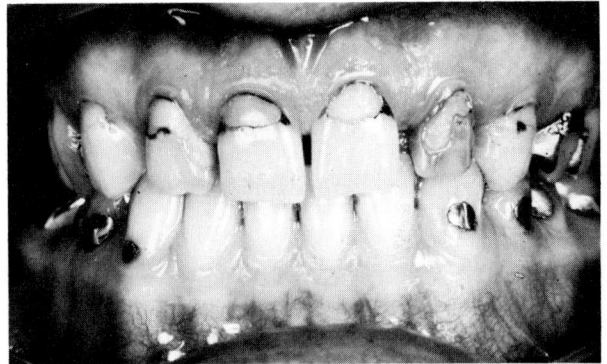

Fig. 34.6. Recurrent caries on margins

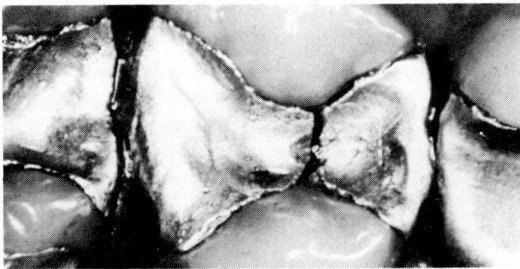

Fig. 34.5. Fractured amalgam

down or dissolution of the material. To do so means that the substance must go into solution in saliva. Any material which will continue to go into solution is soluble—and solubility leads to deterioration of the restoration. Thus, a material which has continual anticariogenic activity is also a material which does not make a permanent, strong, satisfactory restoration.

8. *Reparability.* Ideally, a material should be reparable. If a defect occurs in a restoration,

it should be possible to repair the defect without removing the entire restoration. It would be advantageous for a filling material to chemically bond to the previously polymerized restoration.

9. *Ease of manipulation.* A dentist wants a restorative material which can be manipulated easily. An acceptable material

(*a*) can be easily prepared and placed in the cavity,
(*b*) can be adapted to a cavity,
(*c*) can be properly contoured,
(*d*) will set in a clinically acceptable time, and
(*e*) can be polished satisfactorily.

If a material fails to meet these five qualifications, it will not be as readily accepted by the dentists as one that does meet the qualifications and is of comparable quality.

10. *Radiopacity.* (Not transparent to X ray.) *Radiopaque* materials look white on the X-ray film because X rays do not go through the materials. *Radiolucent* materials look dark because the X rays pass through them. If a restoration is radiopaque, the limitations of

the restoration are denoted by radiopacity. Although this quality is not vitally important, it is helpful because radiolucent recurrent caries can then be differentiated from the filling which is opaque on the X ray.

Figure 34.1 is a summarization of the application of these tenets to filling materials discussed in this chapter.

Dental Cements

The American Dental Association's *Guide to Dental Materials* classifies dental cements into the following categories:

zinc oxide-eugenol   silicate
zinc phosphate   zinc silicophosphate
copper phosphate   resin.

In addition to these categories, Phillips lists calcium hydroxide cements for pulp capping and carboxylate cements.[1] Silicate cement is the only one used as a restorative material. Although there are resin restorative materials, they are different from the cementing resin.

Zinc Oxide-Eugenol Cements

If a cavity is very close to the vital dental pulp, but does not actually expose it, a sedative or analgesic substance is placed on the dentin wall immediately over the near-exposure before placing the cement base. For decades the material of choice for this sub-base has been zinc oxide-eugenol. Many cements have been introduced under trade names for pulp capping, pulp protection, and root canal sealers. All of these cements are essentially zinc oxide and eugenol, but they contain other ingredients which enhance their physical properties. For example, if ethoxybenzoic acid

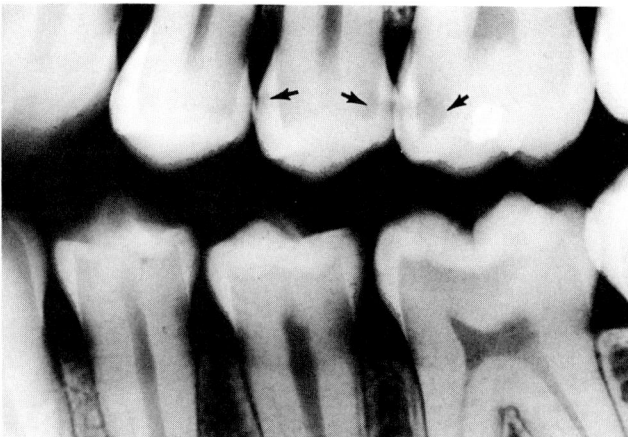

Fig. 34.7. Radiopacities and radiotranslucencies

1. Eugene W. Skinner and Ralph W. Phillips. *Science of Dental Materials* (Philadelphia: W. B. Saunders Co., 1967), pp. 460-486.

is added to the liquid, and fused quartz is added to the powder, the resulting cement provides strength for cementation, bases, and temporary fillings, while keeping the mild sedative effect of the eugenol, and serves as a luting (cementing) medium for cast-gold restorations as well as firm protective bases. Although such cements are known as EBA (for ethoxybenzoic acid cements), they are still considered zinc oxide-eugenol.

The Ten Tenets Applied to Zinc Oxide-Eugenol Cements

Although these cements are not exposed to view as a permanent material is, zinc oxide-eugenols do not detract from the aesthetics of a restoration and, when underlying thin sections of enamel and dentin, may actually enhance the aesthetics by masking undesirable effects of metallic restorations. Tissue adjacent to any material attached to the body and foreign to it must have an other-than-normal reaction. However, zinc oxide-eugenol cements are nonirritating to the point of being sedative. They do not have an exothermic reaction like the zinc phosphate cements and therefore will not irritate the pulp as a result of the setting process in the tooth. The oil base of these cements makes them less soluble in the mouth than zinc phosphate. They are still much too soluble and weak to be considered for restorations. Their adaptation is generally good for the short period they are exposed when used as temporary restorations. Their coefficient of thermal expansion and reparability are not of practical importance since solubility and strength negate their use for purposes other than bases, temporary fillings, and cementation. They are not considered anticariogenic. One of the major assets of these cements is their ease of manipulation. Most of these cements contain a trace of barium sulfate, making them radiopaque and distinguishable on an X ray.

Composition and Purpose of Ingredients

The labels of the commercial temporary cements usually denote the same basic common ingredients. The powders contain zinc oxide; the liquids contain an essential oil, usually eugenol.

Preparations vary in the types and amounts of additives incorporated in the powder or liquids to enhance the physical or antibacterial properties:

To increase the adhesiveness: rosin and olive oil or Canada balsam;

To accelerate the setting: zinc acetate or zinc stearate;

To increase the antibacterial effectiveness: phenol, thymol, thymol iodide, iodoform.

Zinc oxide and eugenol or any of the commercially prepared zinc oxide-eugenol-rosin cements may be used as an analgesic sub-base in unusually deep cavities. Other uses include bases under metal restorations, sedative treatments, capping exposed pulps, and temporarily cementing some form of protection over teeth prepared for crown or bridge placement.

Care of Equipment

A zinc oxide-eugenol-rosin cement should be mixed on a paper mixing pad. If a glass slab is used, it should be wiped clean immediately after mixing and washed with a rosin solvent such as xylol or chloroform. Washing with water will not remove the sticky rosin cement. Instruments used with zinc oxide-eugenol preparations must be wiped as soon as possible with a disposable tissue, then with a gauze moistened with chloroform. Wash with soap and water, rinse, and dry.

Mixing the Cement

The cement is supplied in two bottles, one containing powder and the other containing liquid. The consistency of the mix depends on the use for which it is intended. The liquid absorbs a considerable amount of powder; therefore, no more than two drops should be necessary for a sub-base. The cement can be mixed rapidly. It is to be as thick as possible for ease of handling.

Place two drops of solution near one end of the mixing tablet.

Place an amount of powder about five times the volume of liquid toward the other end.

First mix about half the powder with the liquid, spatulating rapidly and well into a smooth mix. Then add smaller portions, mixing thoroughly, until the mix is heavy.

Remove excess oil by blotting the mass on absorbent paper or cloth, leaving a soft, putty-like cement that is easily positioned and shaped in the cavity (fig. 34.8).

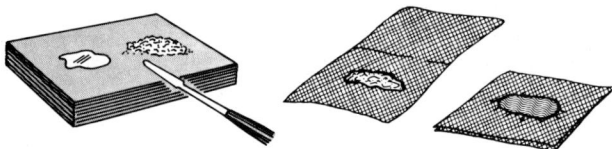

Fig. 34.8. Mixing zinc oxide-eugenol cement

Ample time can be used for mixing and handling since the material will not harden rapidly. It can therefore be prepared somewhat in advance of use, if desired.

The amount of cement needed should be closely approximated before being carried to the cavity. Too often the placing of the cement base becomes messy because too much cement is placed in the cavity, requiring tedious and delicate removal of the excess. Water acts as a catalyst for zinc oxide-eugenol cements; therefore, a pellet of wet cotton may be used to manipulate the cement in a cavity as well as to remove the excess cement.

Although individual preferences vary, cements mixed for retention of restorations in the cavity should be mixed to a toothpaste consistency in order to permit the proper seating of the restoration. Too thick a mix will prevent the restoration from reaching its prescribed position in the cavity and may necessitate redoing the entire operation.

Zinc Phosphate Cement

Zinc phosphate cement, a material at one time used for restorations, is now used only for thermally protective bases under metallic fillings and as a cement to retain gold restorations such as inlays, crowns, and bridges. This cement contains unreacted phosphoric acid which is irritating. However, the unreacted free acid is used up within a matter of hours and, consequently, is not a lasting irritant. Cavities receiving zinc phosphate cement bases, or restorations retained with zinc phosphate cement, should be painted with a protective liner, preferably containing calcium hydroxide, to prevent any chemical irritation to the dental pulp.

The Ten Tenets Applied to Zinc Phosphate Cement

Zinc phosphate cement is not used as a permanent restorative material per se. It is provided in many shades to offer an *aesthetic* background for cementation of fused porcelain restorations. Its *toxicity* is initially as severe as silicate cement, and a protective liner of cavity varnish or thin paste of zinc oxide-eugenol or calcium hydroxide is necessary for pulp protection. Although it *adapts* well to tooth structure, it has no *adhesion* when set. It is quite *soluble*, has a *coefficient of thermal expansion* within practical limits of tooth structure, is not considered *anticariogenic*, and has *strength* values commensurate with its uses. Although it is quite easy to *manipulate, reparability* is not a consideration with its clinical application. It is *radiopaque* to a degree and can be identified on X ray.

Composition and Purpose of Ingredients

Zinc phosphate cements are supplied as a powder and liquid. The powder is composed primarily of zinc oxide, with some magnesium oxide and traces of other metallic salts composing about ten percent of the total. The liquid, like that of silicate cement, is composed of phosphoric acid and water, buffered with salts of aluminum and zinc. These cements are all balanced by the manufacturer to provide the proper physical properties. *Bottles should be stoppered at all times when not in use to prevent the addition of water to the liquid on humid days or the evaporation of water on dry days.* The balance of acid and water in the liquid must be maintained as manufactured; otherwise the setting time and other properties of the cement will be severely affected.

When mixed, the cement sets as a hard, crystalline structure composed of a core of unreacted particles of powder in a matrix of zinc phosphate compounds. The consistency and setting time of the mix can be altered by varying the manner in which the cement is spatulated and varying the amount of powder incorporated into the mix. The necessary consistency and setting time will be determined by the purpose for which the mix is being prepared.

A Word of Caution

The reaction of the powder with the liquid generates heat and is called an *exothermic reaction.* If the cement is mixed too fast or on a warm slab and is placed in the tooth, the heat produced by this reaction could be enough to burn the dental pulp and cause the tooth to abscess. Consequently, the cement slab is always cooled in running water before it is used. It should not be cooled below the dew point, however, which is the point at which moisture from the air condenses on the glass. Should this happen, the cement will have excess water

in it and will set much too fast for use. If the cement liquid is placed on the slab long before it is to be mixed, water may evaporate from it, and the subsequent mix will set too slowly for practical use. Therefore, the cement should be spatulated on a cool slab, with small increments of powder added to the liquid at five- to ten-second intervals and the mixture thoroughly spatulated between additions. Total mixing time should be between one and one-half and two minutes. The amount of cement to be mixed as well as its consistency is directed by the use intended.

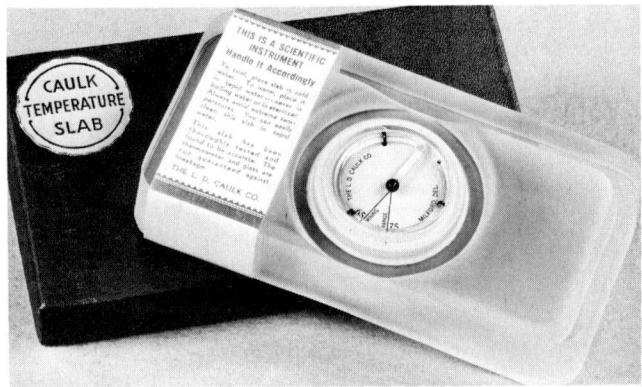

Fig. 34.9. Glass mixing slab with thermometer

Directions for Mixing the Cement

Cool and dry the glass mixing slab.

When your dentist indicates it is time to begin, place the required number of liquid drops on the slab. *Stopper the bottle.*

In another place on the slab place the necessary amount of powder. *Stopper the bottle.*

Form the powder into a thin, flat, rectangular shape with the spatula.

Divide the rectangle into halves, then into quarters, then into eighths.

Divide four of the eighths again to make sixteenths.

MIXING SCHEDULE OF ZINC PHOSPHATE CEMENT
total mixing time: 120 secs.

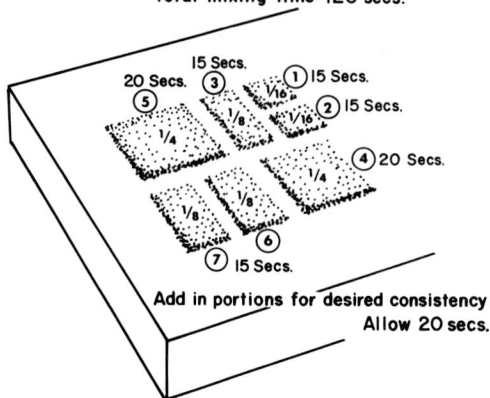

Fig. 34.10. Cement ready to mix

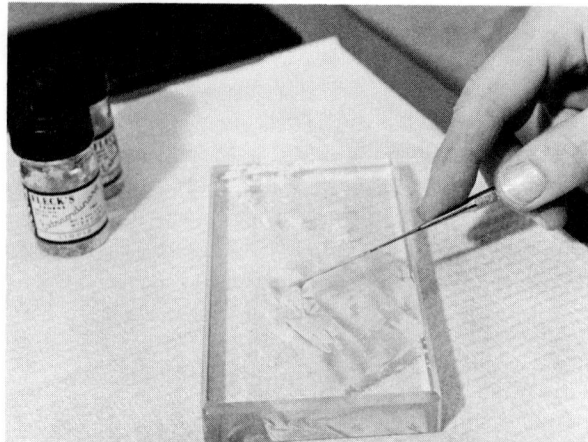

Fig. 34.11. Mixed zinc phosphate cement

Place your watch, with a sweep-second hand, near the slab where you can see it easily.

Draw the first sixteenth into the liquid and spatulate with the flat of the blade for thirty seconds.

Add the remaining sixteenths in turn and spatulate each for ten seconds.

Now add the eighth portions, spatulating each for ten seconds, except the last portion, which is spatulated for fifteen seconds.

There should be no unmixed particles of powder or liquid remaining around the edges when each portion is considered to be thoroughly incorporated into the mix.

Setting time may be delayed by first thoroughly spatulating a very small quantity of powder, about the size of a pinhead, into the liquid and permitting this to stand for two or three minutes before proceeding with further additions of powder. Rapid spatulation will hasten the setting time. If a heavy mix is desired, merely add more powder.

An excess amount of liquid is always provided in the bottle. The excess liquid should be discarded when the powder has been used up, and a new bottle of each should be opened when the next mix is required.

Powder which has been removed from the original bottle and placed on the slab but not used in the mix should *not* be returned to the original powder bottle.

Silicate Cement

Silicate cement is provided in a powder and liquid like zinc phosphate cement, *but it is a very different material.* Its setting reaction forms a gel matrix rather than crystals like zinc phosphate.

Deservedly or not, silicate cement has been the most commonly used anterior restorative material. A variety of shades are available, and this material closely resembles tooth structure in fluorescence and opacity. Its aesthetics, at least initially, is reasonably good. It cannot be applied in layered shades. Thus one shade must match tooth structure at the gingival as well as the incisal. If the destruction by caries has been extensive, the variance from yellow-orange gingival to gray incisal may more than challenge the ability of silicate cement to remain undetected.

*The Ten Tenets Applied
to Silicate Cement*

Set silicate cement is composed of unreacted powder particles (70 percent) held together by the gel matrix (30 percent). The matrix can be easily damaged irreparably on the surface of the restoration by dehydration. This damage is a common occurrence in mouth breathers. Silicate cement is also highly *soluble* in saliva which eventually causes deterioration of the surface comparable to dehydration. Loss of marginal integrity and contour of the resto-

cannot be placed in Class IV or Class VI cavities. Its *solubility* also dictates exclusion where proximal contact is involved. Such contact may be gradually lost, with the resultant loss of interproximal space.

The free unreacted phosphoric acid in the cement restoration has access to the subjacent dentin and thus to the dental pulp. It can seriously injure or even destroy this vital tissue. The irritating action can be arrested by a cavity liner, preferably containing calcium hydroxide. This acid *toxicity* may last for several

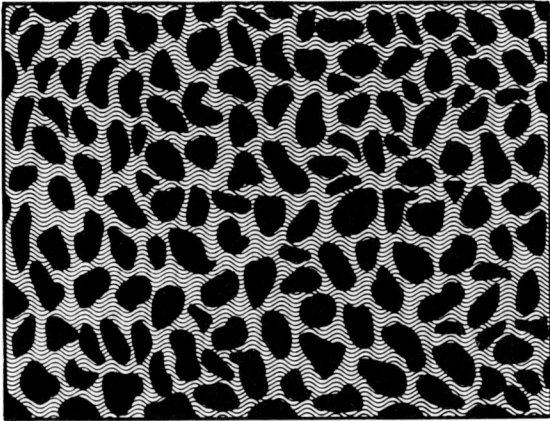

Fig. 34.12. Silicate matrix and particles

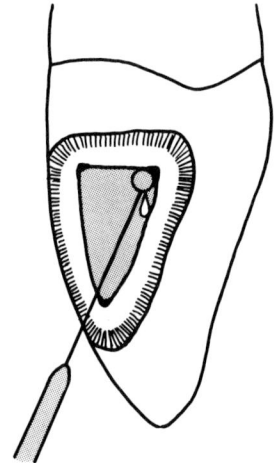

Fig. 34.13. Liner and base application.

ration is the result of this deterioration which sharply curtails its serviceability. Thus, the average life of a silicate cement restoration is considered to be approximately two years. This solubility has one advantage, however. It releases the fluoride component of the cement to create an *anticariogenic* atmosphere for the adjacent tooth structure. Silicate restorations are therefore desirable in caries-active mouths.

The vulnerability of the set silicate cement to incisal stresses makes this material of little value where such forces are active. Thus, it

weeks; therefore, lining is recommended for all cavities to receive silicate cement—even the innocent-looking shallow preparations which seem to have adequate dentin between cavity floor and pulp. Toxicity of the adjacent gingival tissues is not a problem. However, surface roughness created by dehydration or solubility is a problem. It attracts debris which in turn acts as a mechanical irritant and provides an excellent microbial breeding ground. Maximum service from a silicate cement restoration requires careful polishing to reduce the possibility of debris attraction.

The *ease of manipulation* and *adaptability* of silicate cement is satisfactory. Premeasured powder and liquid in capsules mixed mechanically eliminates most of the manipulative variables.

Placement of the cement in the cavity must be done in a dry field. Therefore, rubber-dam isolation is essential. The cement is confined to the cavity and surface-contoured with the matrix band. If the band is disturbed during the setting process, marginal integrity may be lost.

Silicate cement is *radiolucent* and, unfortunately, looks very much like caries on the radiograph. The diagnosis can usually be verified by clinical examination. The cement has some *anticariogenic* activity, and therefore it is unusual to have an active carious lesion under a silicate cement which is not detectable with an explorer tine. The *coefficient of thermal expansion* of the cement is very close to that of enamel, and consequently there is no percolation problem when extreme thermal variations occur in the mouth.

Silicate cement restorations are *not reparable*. They must be removed completely when a defect is detected. Dehydration would damage any remaining filling material during the isolation which is necessary for placement of the new material.

The Mixing of Silicate Cements

(If capsules containing premeasured powder and liquid are not used)

Silicate cement may seem to be much like the zinc phosphate cements, but it is a very different material. It is used to make a restoration in the labial, mesial, or distal surfaces, usually limited to anterior teeth. Silicate cement is *not mixed like the zinc phosphate cements. Do not consider them identical.*

The one and only function of spatulating silicate cement powder and liquid is to *wet* the entire surface of every particle of powder with the liquid. It is *not* the purpose of this spatulation to grind the particles into the finest dust possible so that the powder goes into complete solution with the liquid, nor is it desirable to crush the particles of powder in any way. The particles of silicate cement powder are accurately graded in size for maximum strength in the filling material.

As each powder particle is wetted by the liquid, the outside surface is dissolved, but the inside area remains intact in an undissolved state. These solid portions of the powder particles provide the necessary tough bulk for the filling material, just as the crushed stone of irregular shapes and sizes provides the aggregate in construction concrete. The spatulating of silicate cement powder and liquid actually involves (1) pushing or drawing as many powder particles as possible into the liquid and (2) under the strokes of the spatula, thoroughly *wetting* the entire surface of each particle as quickly as possible. Spatulation and mixing of the most commonly used types should be limited to one minute. If the material in your dental office requires different handling, instructions which accompany it will so specify. They should *always* be read thoroughly.

The manner of holding the spatula and manipulating it on the slab is not the prime factor in properly mixing silicate cement. The heavy consistency of the mix and the short time of spatulation are of much greater importance. *Mix it thick and mix it quickly* is a good general rule.

The slab should always be cooled (submerge in cool water in the sink for several minutes prior to use) to the ideal temperature range of 65° to 75° F. Then rub the slab dry with a clean towel. If the slab is chilled below the dew point and moisture condenses on the surface, rub the slab with a towel until the temperature of the slab is raised above this level. Dew point is defined as the variable temperature at which moisture vapor will condense. It varies, depending upon the amount of moisture in the air in relation to the temperature of the air and the temperature of the slab. (Remember to cool the spatula, too!) (See fig. 34.14.)

In routine office use, weighing the powder and liquid is impractical. If care is used in developing a proper procedure, it is unnecessary. Place sufficient powder on the slab to produce a mix of heavy consistency with a minimum of three drops of liquid; more drops if required (fig. 34.15).

The tendency to add small portions of powder to the mix to avoid an excess of powder invariably prolongs mixing beyond the recommended period of one minute or less and disrupts beginning matrix formations, producing a weaker restoration. The remedy is to draw four-fifths of the required powder into the three drops of liquid right at the start of the mix (fig. 34.16).

With light pressure, start wetting each powder particle, spatulating briefly and rapidly with a rotary motion within the smallest possible area (fig. 34.17).

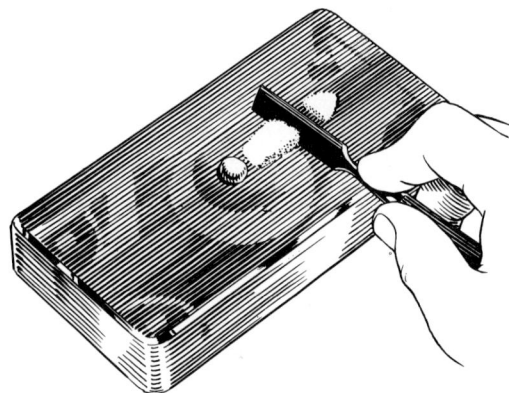

Fig. 34.14. Drying the cooled glass slab before mixing silicate cement.

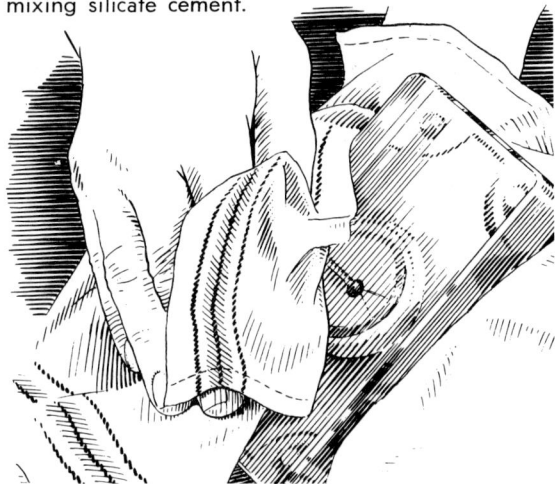

Fig. 34.16. Draw in most of the required powder immediately.

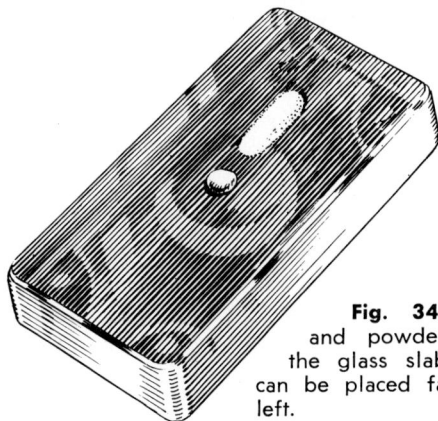

Fig. 34.15. Liquid and powder placed on the glass slab. The liquid can be placed farther to the left.

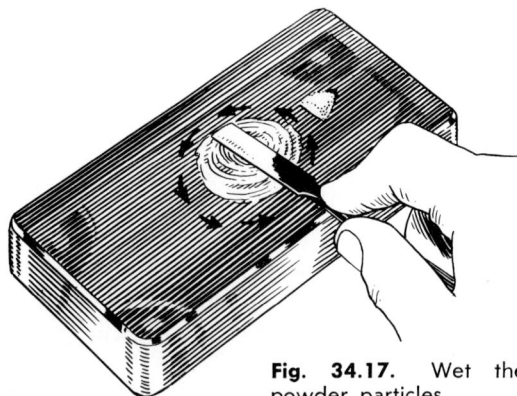

Fig. 34.17. Wet the powder particles.

Fig. 34.18. Adding final powder.

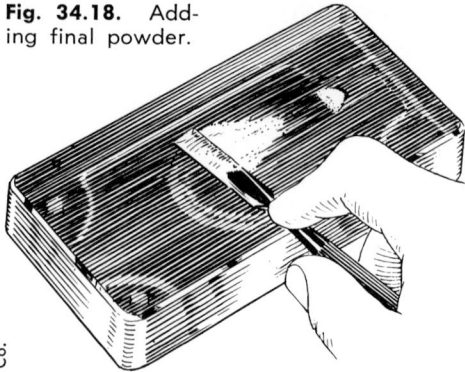

Fig. 34.20. Make sure the mix is not too thin.

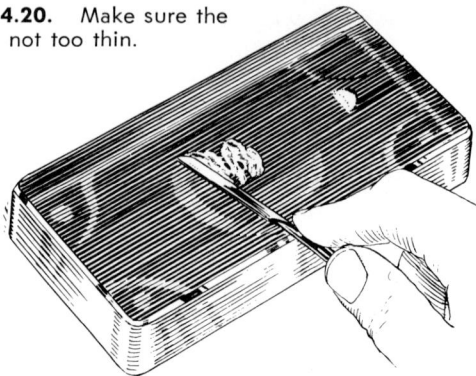

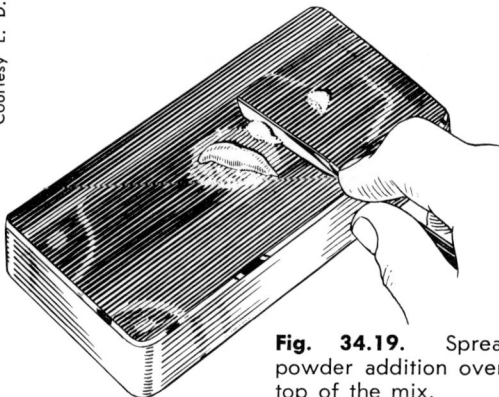

Fig. 34.19. Spreading powder addition over the top of the mix.

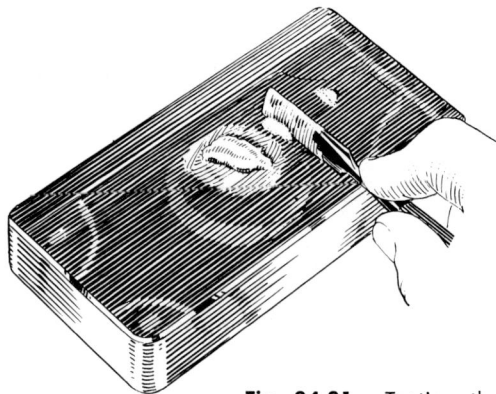

Fig. 34.21. Testing the mix.

If the surface has a high-gloss sheen, the mix is too thin and more powder is necessary (fig. 34.18).

Spread this powder over the mix and then combine it with a light, rotary spatulation (fig. 34.19).

If the surface still has a glossy sheen, draw more powder into the mix. Silicate mixes are generally too thin in consistency (fig. 34.20).

The mix is dull, having lost its lustrous sheen as the result of sufficient powder and correct spatulation. It now resembles bread dough of heavy texture. As the spatula is drawn over the mix, the surface breaks up into rough curls. These are the characteristics of the heavy consistency most essential for durability. Be sure

to complete the mix within one minute—preferably less (fig. 34.21).

Unfilled Plastic Filling Materials

Dissatisfaction with existing materials causes researchers to continue searching for a new material. Some of the research has developed three groups of materials: unfilled plastics, filled plastics, and composites—each with some advantageous properties and, as is to be expected, each with deficiencies.

Bonfil and Sevriton are examples of unfilled methyl methacrylate resins containing catalysts effective in causing polymerization (setting) of the material within the cavity in a clinically acceptable time, and yet not contributing to eventual discoloration of the restoration, as was true of similar products formerly available with a different catalyst system.

The Ten Tenets Applied to Unfilled Plastic Filling Materials

Methyl methacrylate was originally popular as *the* replacement for silicate cement. Then, through clinical experience, it was discovered that a built-in marginal failure existed: during polymerization or setting the filling shrinks two percent to seven percent, depending on the amount of liquid used in the mix. Other faults were also discovered; namely, color instability and a *coefficient of thermal expansion* approximately eight times that of enamel.

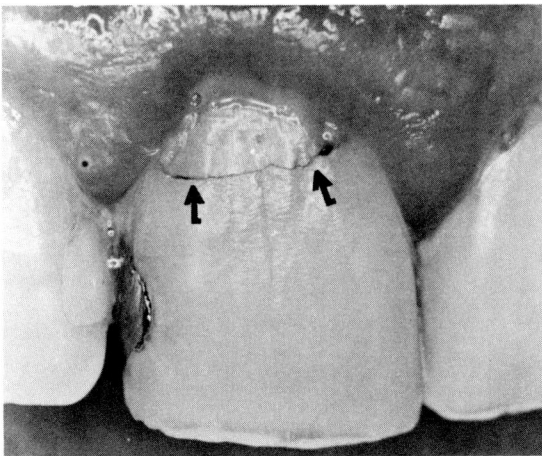

Courtesy L. D. Caulk Co.

Fig. 34.22. Defective plastic margins

Newer methyl methacrylates are now available. The discoloration problem is almost eliminated, but the excessive coefficient of thermal expansion remains. It can cause discoloration through marginal leakage.

The material is reasonably *adaptable* to cavity walls initially, but simple percolation with temperature cycling in the mouth causes lack of marginal seal which is easily demonstrated with tracer dyes and isotopes.

The paint-in technique of placement has minimized the problem of polymerization shrinkage, and it allows more than one shade of the material to be used in building the restoration from the gingival to the incisal, giving more latitude in achieving the desired aesthetics.

Fig. 34.23. Placing a bead of plastic in cavity.

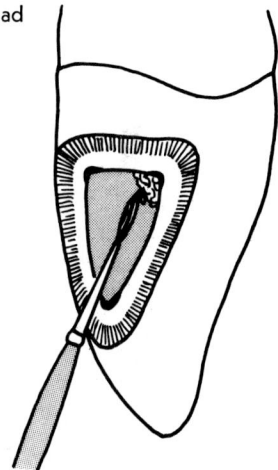

The irritation caused by the material can be all but eliminated by liners. Manufacturers either furnish or recommend such liners. Pulpal involvement resulting from the use of unfilled plastic materials is usually due to marginal failure rather than irritating ingredients.

Like silicate cement, these materials are *radiolucent.* Unlike silicate cement, they are not *anticariogenic.* Thus, recurrent caries can exist without being detectable by clinical or radiographic examination and may only be discovered when the pulp is irreversibly involved.

The plastics are particularly subject to flow and distortion under stress; and, therefore, they cannot be used where stress is involved and a permanent restoration is desired. They may be used with pin support (figs. 34.24, *a*, *b*, and *c*) temporarily, but must be examined carefully at regular intervals to detect possible marginal discrepancies which could lead to pulp damage. The filled plastics are better for this purpose since they have greater strength. Plastic materials are *insoluble* in saliva and can hold interproximal contact.

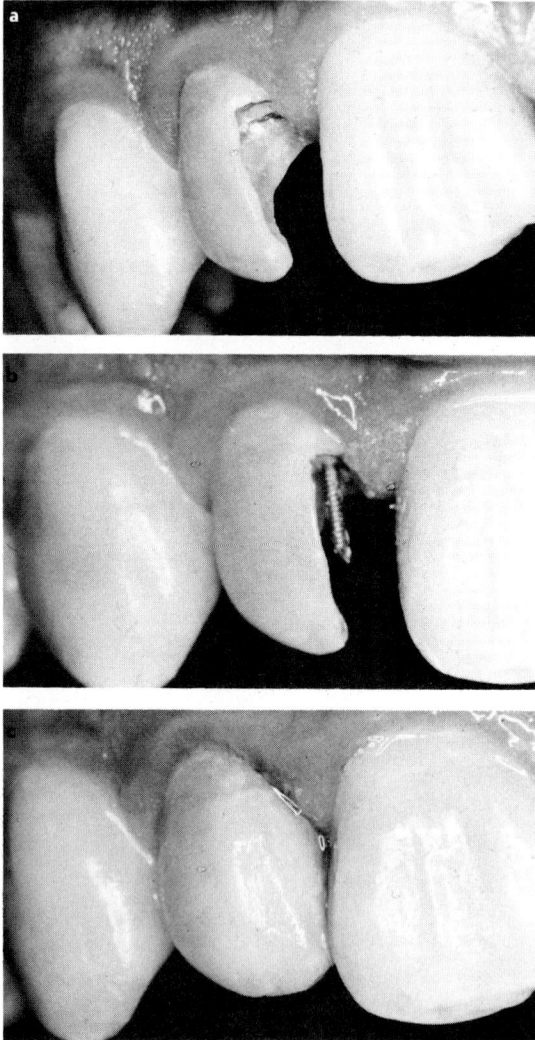

Fig. 34.24. Pre- and post-operative pin-supported plastic.

The placement of a methyl methacrylate restoration is not difficult, but it is exacting. The procedure varies with the type of material. Sloppiness in technique and inattention to detail will result in failure. These materials are easily contoured and finished. Where discrepancies exist, new material can be added which will polymerize to the old.

Filled Plastic Filling Materials

Some manufacturers have added fillers to methyl methacrylate, such as glass fibers or a combination of minute glass beads, powder, and fibers. Little, if any, improvement in the physical properties has resulted. These plastics are called *filled plastics*.

Composite Filling Material

New plastic matrices composed of a combination of methyl methacrylate and epoxy, called epoxoid, have been developed. These matrices can contain a large percentage (in excess of 70 percent) of glass filler in the form of beads, powder, and fibers (fig. 34.25), calcium hydroxyapatite or quartz—all silane-coated to molecularly bond to the matrix.

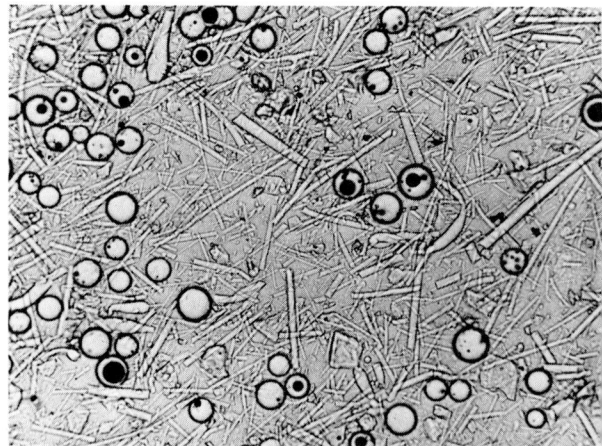

Fig. 34.25. Filled plastics—micrograph of beads and fibers.

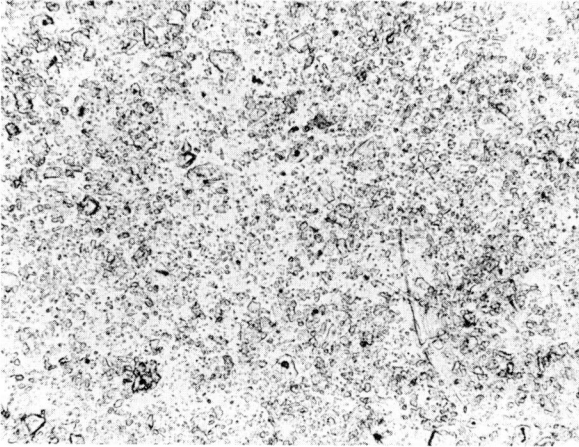

Fig. 34.26. Micrograph of hydroxyapatite

The Ten Tenets Applied to Composite Filling Materials

The fillers are designed to reduce the *coefficient of thermal expansion,* increase *strength* of the materials, and provide a refractory factor to the material, which makes it possible to draw color from the surrounding tooth structure. It is therefore possible to use one shade for all restorations. The color-matching properties of these materials are surprisingly good and stable but not completely consistent. (See fig. 34.2.) The materials containing quartz have more opacity and are more accurate in matching color in large restorations, especially those with no lingual enamel wall to mask the dark interior of the oral cavity.

Like other plastics, these materials are *radiolucent,* are not *anticariogenic,* and are subject to marginal leakage from a difference in *coefficient of thermal expansion* which is about four times that of enamel. Although more resistant to stress, they are not able to withstand the forces of mastication and will lose what marginal *adaptation* they have with the distortion caused by incisal or occlusal stresses. Since it is impossible to distinguish these plastic materials from caries on a radiograph, and since it is impossible to detect caries with the explorer tine when it recurs in the dentin by margin leakage, the use of any plastic, methyl methacrylate or epoxoid, filled or unfilled, is certainly a questionable procedure where stress is involved. With pin support they may be used temporarily (fig. 34.24).

The unpredictable setting properties of epoxoid base materials pose a serious problem. In general they have a flash set that is supposed to occur after allowing approximately one and one-half to two minutes' mixing-placing time. Most products allow an adequate, but hurried, mixing-insertion time. Exact techniques and efficiency of operation are essential.

Liners provided with or recommended by the manufacturers of filled plastics indicate that an irritating factor is present in the materials. When properly lined, this effect of the material on the pulp is no more severe than that of silicate cement over a calcium hydroxide liner. Materials containing glass beads and fibers as a filler have a rough surface when set. This surface is not appreciably improved by the available polishing methods. Polishing abrasives only dislodge the filler particles. The surface is then pocked, easily stained by food debris, and potentially irritating to the adjacent gingival tissues. Those with other fillers may be polished adequately. The filled plastics, methyl methacrylate or epoxoid, are *insoluble* in saliva and will maintain contact. They can be *repaired* by adding new material which will polymerize to the old restoration.

Silver Amalgam

"Silver filling" is a common term among lay people. You may have many examples of silver fillings in your mouth. However, the "silver filling" is not all silver. The American Dental Association's Specification Number One for

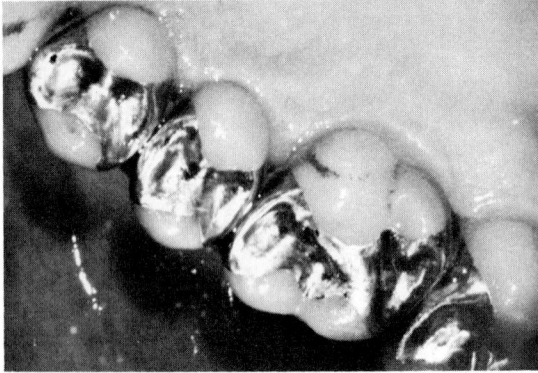

Fig. 34.27. Amalgam restoration in patient's teeth

Dental amalgam is the most widely used restorative material for posterior teeth. Although it has a high crushing strength, it has little tensile strength and is brittle and weak in thin sections. Therefore, it must be used in bulk. Amalgam is seldom used in anterior teeth. Because anterior teeth are translucent, amalgam shows as a dark mass if visible, or a shadow if the restoration is not visible.

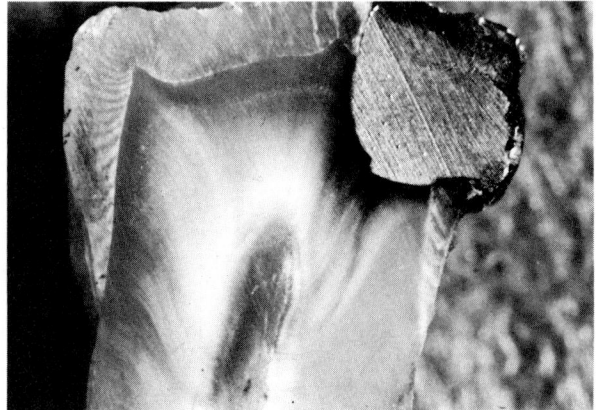

Fig. 34.28. Staining from amalgam

Dental Amalgam Alloys requires the composition to be within the following limits:

silver: 65 percent minimum
tin: 29 percent maximum
copper: 6 percent maximum
zinc: 2 percent maximum
mercury: 3 percent maximum.

Manufacturers who provide dental amalgam can design their alloy as they choose, provided it remains within the limits of these specifications. The range of materials in the alloy of these manufacturers varies according to their carefully guarded formulas.

When pure mercury and the alloy, composed of the above-mentioned metals, are mixed together, a chemical and physical reaction occurs between the alloy and the mercury. This process is called *amalgamation*. The product formed by this compound is generally referred to as *dental amalgam*. When it is inserted into prepared cavities in teeth, it is called an *amalgam restoration*. However, it is important to remember that this terminology refers to the dental use of the word. Actually, an amalgam is *any* metal combined with mercury. Dentists use the term to mean a *certain* alloy of metals when combined with mercury.

However, amalgam is the most satisfactory and popular restoration material for posterior teeth. Less time is consumed in completing an amalgam restoration than a restoration of other acceptable posterior materials; and at the same time, an amalgam restoration gives excellent service in the mouth.

Each of the metals in the alloy has a function to perform:

Silver (ag) is the main constituent of the alloy and contributes the properties of high expansion, strength, rapid setting, low flow, and silver color. Silver is not used alone with mercury because silver is difficult to amalgamate and has poor carving qualities.

Tin (sn) is added as a counterbalance to silver in the alloy. Tin reduces expansion, slows the setting reaction, and permits more rapid amalgamation and smoother carving. Tin must be added in proper amounts, however, because too much tin will cause an amalgam to be weak as well as to have excessive shrinkage, high flow, and too slow a setting reaction.

Copper (cu) imparts properties which are similar to those of silver. The amount used is never very large and is put into the alloy primarily to help harden it, to decrease flow, and to help stabilize the other metals. It also increases the expansion somewhat. Too much copper makes the alloy more susceptible to tarnish.

Zinc (Zn). When the specification for silver amalgam alloy was determined, practically every manufacturer of dental silver alloy was using zinc as a deoxidizing agent to help overcome melting and alloying problems. It is used in many industrial alloys as a scavenger to reduce oxides. Since zinc is not essential to dental alloys, there are dental alloys which contain no zinc; others may contain up to the maximum allowed by A.D.A. specifications. Zinc is known to react with moisture. Amalgam, therefore, should not be touched by the hand or come in contact with saliva at any time during manipulation. It should also be placed in the mouth under very dry conditions.

Mercury (Hg) in a small amount—up to three percent—is permitted to facilitate amalgamation.

After formulating the alloy, the metals are melted together and cast into bars, called *ingots.* The ingots are ground into small filings, and the filings are sifted to obtain controlled size (fig. 34.29). During the casting of the ingot and cutting of the filings, changes occur in the alloy. The alloy does not react consis-

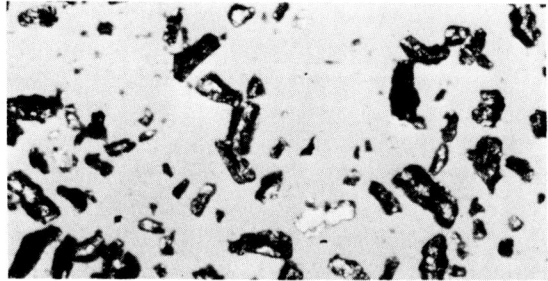

Fig. 34.29. Alloy filings

tently. It changes as it ages unless it is *annealed.* Annealing is a process which quickens the aging of the alloy, producing material of predictable physical properties. Thus, the important next step is the annealing of the alloy.

A carefully controlled annealing process stabilizes the alloy so that it does not change when stored. Annealing also makes it possible to have sufficient time in which to condense the amalgam in the cavity preparation and to carve it.

Alloy is also manufactured in the form of small spheres (fig. 34.30) which may be made either by atomizing molten alloy and permitting the tiny droplets to freeze in their spherical state, or by spreading alloy filings on trays and heating them to melting temperature. They will become spherical and congeal in that state if allowed to cool.

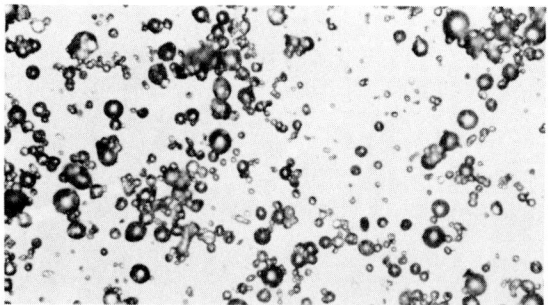

Fig. 34.30. Spherical particles

A third form of alloy is a combination of spheres and filings. Manufacturers claim the combination is easier to manipulate when placing it in the cavity.

Any of these alloys may be obtained as premeasured pellets. The pellets are desirable because the amount of alloy dispensed is more consistently accurate (fig. 34.31). Thus, alloys may be purchased as a loose aggregate of filings, spheres, a combination of the two, or as premeasured pellets.

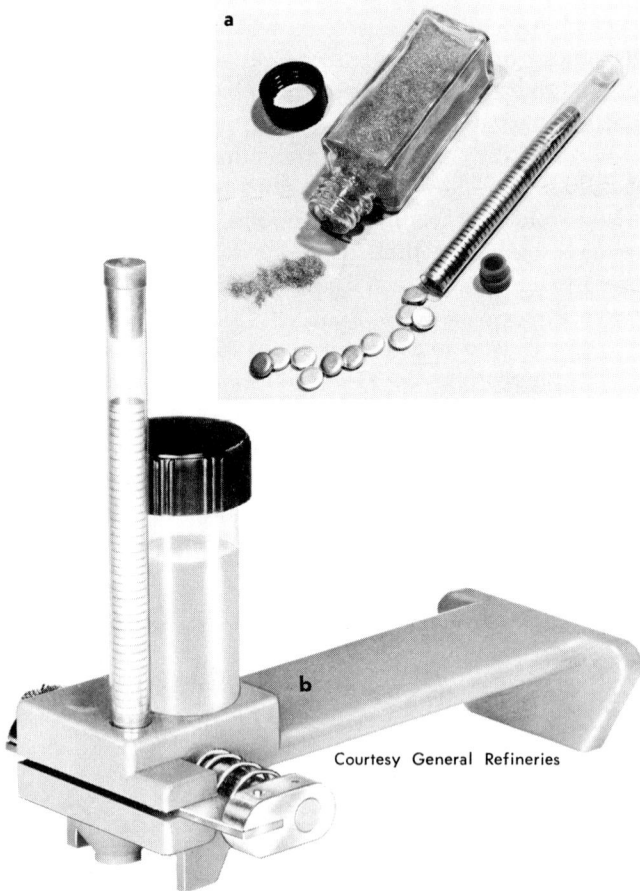

Courtesy General Refineries

Fig. 34.31. (a) Amalgam filings and pellets; (b) alloy pellet dispenser.

What Happens During Amalgamation?

When mercury is mixed with the alloy, it *coats the particle surface* and creates a complex series of reactions. The silver-mercury and tin-mercury compounds formed in this reaction harden the amalgam. The quality of the amalgam restoration is governed by the way these materials are handled. These new compounds formed on the surface of the alloy particles are not as hard nor as strong as the particles themselves and take up less volume than the original alloy particles in mercury, causing an initial contraction of the amalgam mass. However, there is still more free mercury in the mass whose molecules, during a period of time following condensation, diffuse through the mass, pushing apart the molecules of alloy and creating a setting expansion. Thus, the beneficial expansion required for a successful restoration is achieved. Toward the end of this reaction, the final small contraction which occurs is caused by the final reaction of this mercury upon alloy particles.

An expansion curve of amalgam which shows the initial contraction, expansion, and final contraction is illustrated in figure 34.32.

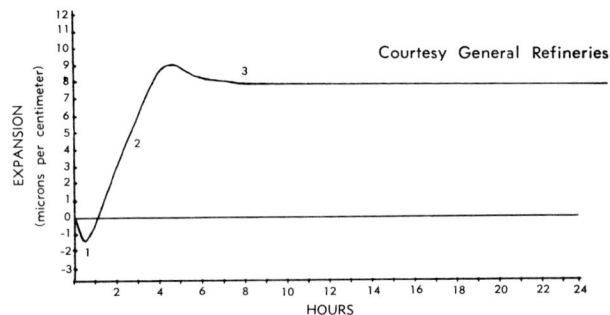

Courtesy General Refineries

Fig. 34.32. Curve showing initial contraction, expansion, and final contraction of setting amalgam. (1) Indicates the first joining of mercury and alloy forming gamma phases and initial contraction. (2) Diffusion phase or setting expansion. (3) Final combination of mercury and alloy forming additional gamma phases.

The amalgam in the restoration, then, is composed of particles of alloy surrounded and bound together by a new alloy formed by the interaction of mercury with the surface of the particles. The surfaces of filings and spheres need to be coated with mercury in order to react with it, forming the matrix which bonds the filling into one solid mass. The matrix formed is not as strong as the particles of alloy; therefore, the final restoration should have a minimum amount of matrix to hold the particles together. The more mercury added to the mix, the more mercury in the final restoration. It is impossible to squeeze out or condense out all the excess mercury. For these reasons, it is imperative that the mercury-alloy ratio be accurately measured. Such measurement insures adequate mercury to cover the

2. Remove as much free mercury as possible from the amalgam
   a. with the squeeze cloth, and
   b. during condensation in the preparation.

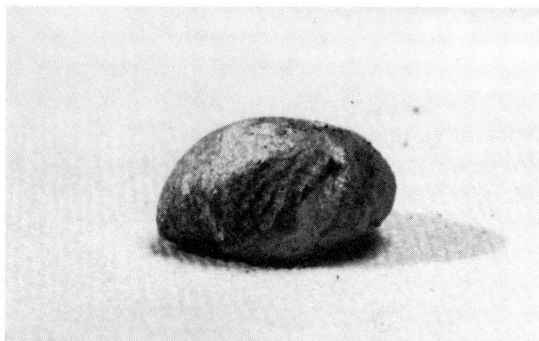

Fig. 34.34. Squeeze cloth with amalgam on it

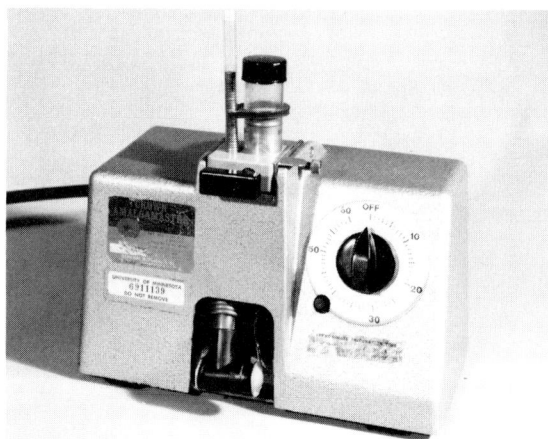

Fig. 34.33. Pellet mercury dispenser with amalgamator.

particles, but avoids the excess mercury which leads to a weaker filling. For the strongest restoration, keep the bonding matrix to a minimum. To do so follow these suggestions:

1. Control the original amount of mercury in the mix by accurate measurement.

One of the important variables in amalgam restorations which must be controlled is expansion. The manufacturer contributes to the control of this variable by the composition of the alloy, the method of heat treatment, and particle size. The factors of alloy-mercury ratio and method of *trituration* (mixing) are controlled by the dental assistant. The correct alloy-mercury ratio *must* be maintained since mixing time is based on this ratio. Measuring devices for filings are not too accurate and tend to become more erratic with repeated use; therefore, premeasured pellets (fig. 34.33) offer a more practical means of controlling alloy-mercury ratios. Amalgam restorations containing more than fifty-five percent mercury will have a shortened life due to excessive tarnish, corrosion, and weakness. Although some mercury can be squeezed out after trituration, and even additional mercury removed during condensation, all effort should be made to keep the initial mercury-alloy ratio under the fifty-five percent level.

To ensure complete surface coverage of each particle, the irregular shape of alloy filings requires more mercury in the mix than the regular shape of smooth, rounded particles. The diffusion of the liquid mercury over the surface area of spherical particles is more readily accomplished, and therefore less mercury is required initially when mixing spherical alloy. The need for less mercury is one of the major advantages in using the spherical form or the combination of spherical and filings over the use of filings alone. The amount of mercury necessary when mixing spherical alloy need not exceed fifty-two percent. It can be as low as forty-eight percent, thus assuring longer life for the restoration. Regardless of the form of alloy used, good amalgam restorations can be obtained by proper attention to mercury-alloy ratios and trituration by the dental assistant.

The Mixing of Amalgam

Before the invention of amalgamators, triturating was accomplished by using a mortar (a glass cup with a smooth, rounded bottom) and a pestle (a glass mixing rod rounded to fit the curve of the cup) (fig. 34.35). The dental assistant mixed the alloy and mercury by moving the glass rod (pestle) around the bottom of the mortar—much like blending with a spoon and bowl.

The same principle is now used with the amalgamator, which not only saves time but offers control of mixing through standardization of mixing time and method. (See fig. 34.33.) A tiny capsule serves as the mortar. A round ball which fits in the capsule serves as the pestle (fig. 34.36). The measured mercury and alloy are placed in the capsule (mortar) and the ball (pestle) is added. The capsule is closed and placed in the repository on the amalgamator. The timer is set according to the manufacturer's instructions. Timing is extremely important.

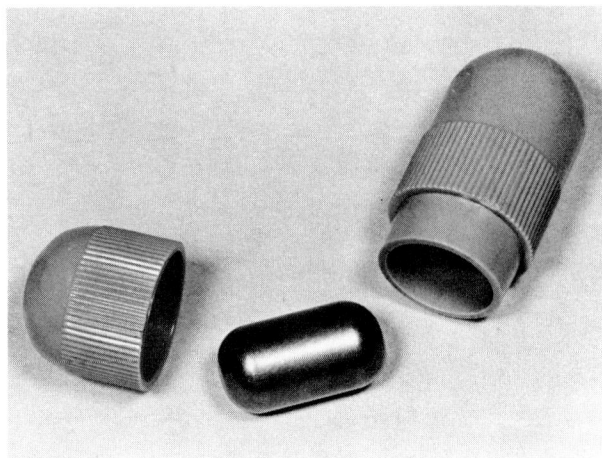

Fig. 34.36. Mortar and pestle for automatic trituration.

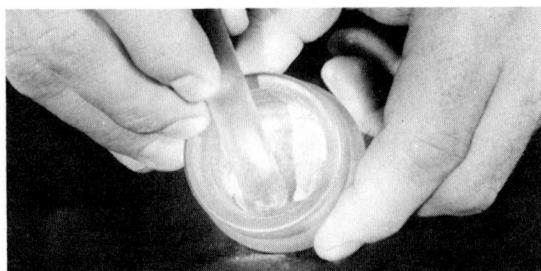

Fig. 34.35. Mortar and pestle being used to mix amalgam.

If the mass is undermixed, some of the particles will not be covered with mercury. This will result in an amalgam which is noncohesive and usually has excessive expansion, sometimes enough to cause the tooth to be painful. Overmixing, on the other hand, causes a breaking up or grinding up of the particles of alloy. This exposes so much alloy surface to the mercury that an excessive amount of bond material is formed, producing an amalgam which may have a reduced amount of expansion and possibly even a shrinkage. *Accurate timing prevents over- or undermixing.*

Following trituration, the mixed amalgam is placed on a squeeze cloth (fig. 34.34), and gross, excess mercury is removed by twisting finger pressure (fig. 34.37).

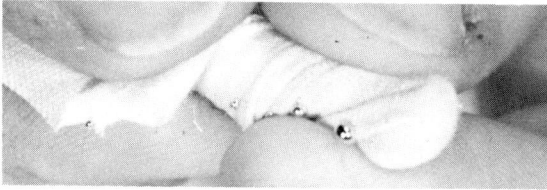

Fig. 34.37. Expressing excess mercury from mass of amalgam.

It is important that this excess mercury be deposited in a receptacle specifically for mercury. It must not be permitted to fall on the floor where a buildup of mercury contamination in the room would soon constitute a health hazard for everyone.

The alloy is now ready for placing in the cavity. To avoid contamination with moisture through hand contact, the alloy gun is loaded (fig. 34.38c) for placement of the alloy in the cavity (fig. 34.38d) by the assistant. The small increments of amalgam are deposited in the areas of the cavity at the direction of the dentist, who completes condensation following each addition. The amalgam restoration is then carved to proper anatomy contour, contact, and occlusion by the dentist.

A minimum of forty-eight hours must elapse before the restoration can be polished. Complete setting of the amalgam must occur. Polishing is necessary and important, not only for the appearance of the restoration, but primarily to prevent tarnish and corrosion. The life of the restoration would be seriously jeopardized by omitting the polishing procedure. The completed restoration is capable of withstanding the stresses of mastication and the corrosive

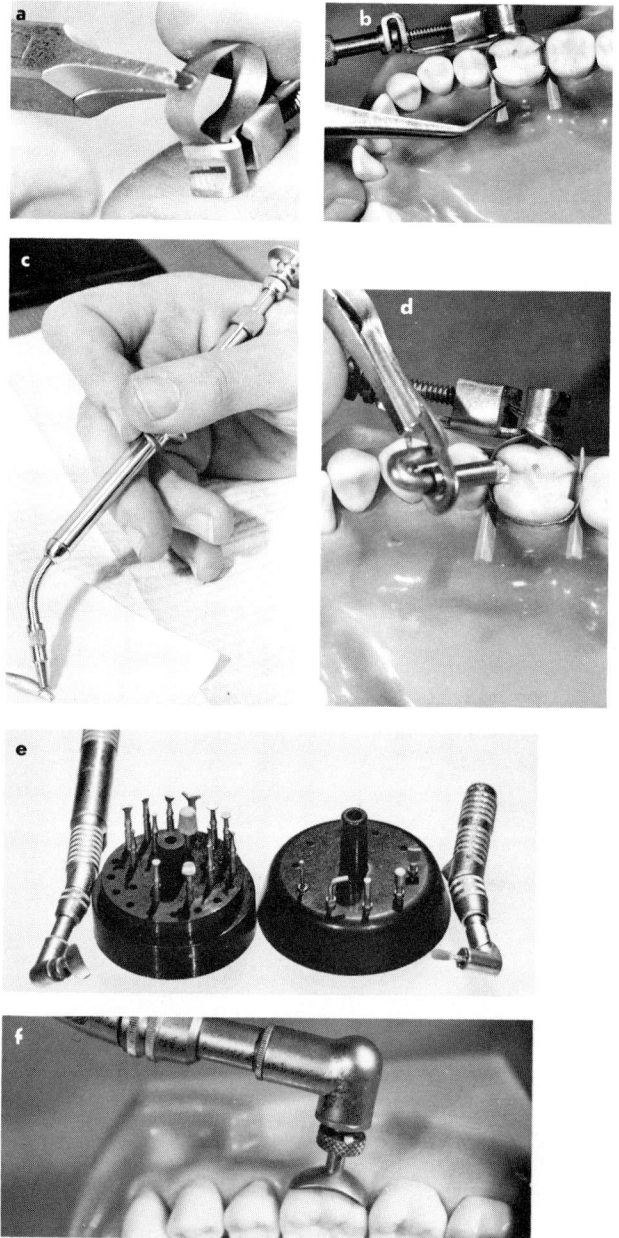

Fig. 34.38. The amalgam filling process: (a) contouring matrix band prior to placement; (b) placement of wedges to secure matrix band at gingival; (c) loading alloy gun; (d) placing alloy in cavity; (e) mechanical condensing instruments; (f) use of mechanical condenser.

environment of the mouth. Yet, fortunately, it has little or no effect on the adjacent tissues.

The *ten tenets as applied to amalgam* are shown on the summary found in figure 34.1.

Excess Amalgam

Usually there is some amalgam in excess of the amount necessary for the restoration. It has reclamation value. It should be kept in an amalgam scrap jar. (See fig. 34.39.) Scraps recovered from the cuspidor trap are also saved. The women's auxiliary or local dental societies often collect this scrap as a means of raising money for the Relief Fund for dentists in need.

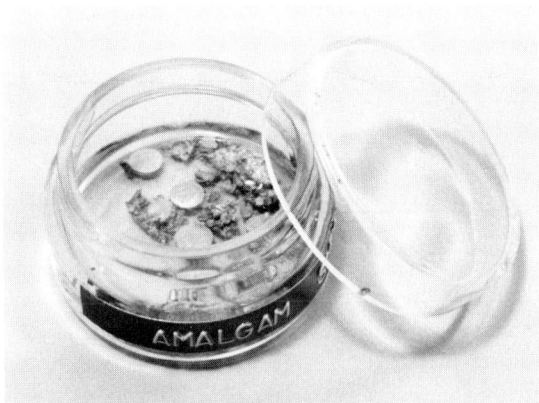

Fig. 34.39. Amalgam scrap jar for excess mercury and amalgam scrap.

Gold and Gold Alloys

Gold may be used in restorative dentistry in several forms. In the pure form it is provided as gold foil, crystalline or mat gold, or as a powder. Small amounts of powder are wrapped in pieces of gold foil for convenient handling. Pure gold is packed in the cavity preparation in a manner similar to amalgam. This restoration in gold may be completely contoured and polished at the same visit because no setting time is required.

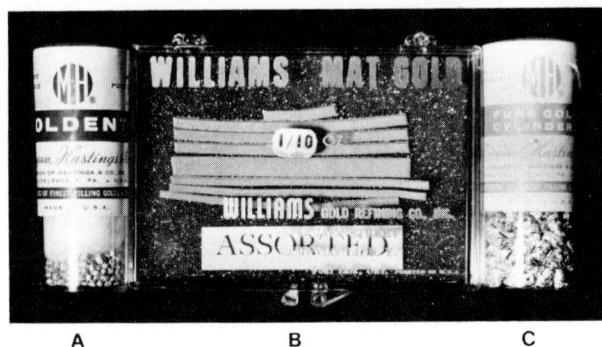

Fig. 34.40. (A) Powdered gold, (B) mat gold, and (C) foil.

Gold alloys are called casting golds. They are used to fabricate restorations outside the mouth which are later cemented to the tooth. Gold alloys are produced by combining gold with silver, copper, and small amounts of platinum, palladium, and zinc. By varying the amounts of the metals used in the manufacture of these alloys, casting golds of different hardness and strength for different dental uses are produced.

Welded Gold Restorations

Gold-foil restorations are made from cohesive or noncohesive gold. The pure gold, condensed into cavity preparations, molecularly bonds, forming a solid, *cohesive* restoration. If noncohesive gold is used, it is literally wedged into the cavity.

Decades ago gold foil was commonly used as a restorative material. Now amalgam or cast gold is used in the posterior of the mouth where ability to withstand masticatory stresses is essential. Silicate cement, composites, or fused porcelains are used in the anterior region because aesthetics is the primary concern of the patient. Thus, gold foil has been almost completely replaced; however, some dentists still create beautiful gold-foil restorations. It is therefore important that we understand the process of placing them.

Gold foil is basically in the same physical form as associated with the words *aluminum foil,* except that gold is capable of being made into the thinnest sheet of metal imaginable, about one-tenth the thickness of an average human hair. This foil is made by hand, "beating" the gold between layers of sheepskin until it has reached the desired thickness.

Gold foil is sold to the dental office as factory-prepared *cylinders* of various sizes, or in *books* of flat gold leaves. Both are sold by weight. In the case of a book, each contains one-tenth of an ounce of gold, and each sheet of foil (which is separated from its neighbor by tissue paper) contains about four grains. Dentists who use gold in this form usually teach the assistant to "roll" gold pellets of the proper sizes from this gold leaf. The most commonly used sizes are 1/64, 1/32, and perhaps 1/16—each fraction indicating what part of a whole "leaf" each pellet contains. Thus, to make 1/64 pellets, each leaf is first cut in half, each half into quarters, each quarter into eighths, each eighth into sixteenths, each sixteenth into thirty-seconds, and each thirty-second into sixty-fourths—and each sixty-fourth is carefully and loosely rolled into a pellet in such a manner that all edges are turned to the inside of the pellet. If done by an assistant with practice, a "drawer" section full of 1/64 pellets will have pellets which are all nearly identical in size (which is controlled by how tightly the pellet is rolled). These are used as *cohesive* gold.

The "leaves" of gold foil as purchased in books may also be used to prepare cylinders of *noncohesive* gold. These are generally prepared as one-half and one-fourth cylinders. Experienced operators will use noncohesive gold to build up the larger part of the bulk of a gold-foil restoration, especially in work in the posterior part of the mouth or in large gingi-

val restorations, then complete the restoration with cohesive gold.

Gold foil may also be purchased as ready-prepared gold-foil cylinders of various sizes, supplied in small bottles.

The outstanding feature about pure gold foil is that it can be condensed by hammering (malleting), building up one pellet upon another—actually cold-welding—directly in the tooth which has been prepared to receive the restoration. It is precise, exacting work.

Cohesive gold foil is probably used most commonly by gold-foil operators. In order to cold-weld, this prepared pellet or cylinder must be annealed (heated to a cherry red) before placing it in the preparation, ready for condensing with an instrument called a gold-foil condenser (plugger).

Mat gold is furnished in sheets from which pieces fitting the size of the cavity may be cut, inserted, and condensed. Usually restorations filled with mat gold are completed with gold foil for a denser surface.

Another form of pure gold is furnished in small pellets which are actually pure gold powder of almost microscopic fineness, compacted into small, round pellets and then wrapped in gold foil. The pellet is placed into the cavity preparation following annealing. Due to its density, about one-tenth as many pellets are required to restore a given area as gold-foil cylinders. This powdered form of gold is free from surface impurities, and its cohesiveness permits each pellet to bond molecularly to that already placed as it is condensed in the cavity. To protect the pellets from possible contamination by gases in the air, *the stopper of the vial should be tightly replaced after each use.* As with gold-foil cylinders, these pellets should be annealed by holding them in the clean blue flame of the alcohol lamp until the pellet turns dull red, *but no longer.* After cooling for three or four seconds, the pellet can be carried to the cavity preparation as directed by the dentist.

A nichrome spear foil carrier is used for this purpose. It is made from a piece of 16-gauge nichrome wire which has been sharpened, smoothed, shaped to resemble an explorer, and mounted in a broach holder.

Annealing Gold

Annealing is a very important step in cohesive gold work.[1] Since it is performed by the dental assistant, it is important that she know exactly what is desired and what the operation is meant to accomplish. As an operation, it is simplicity itself, but its consequences are basic and far-reaching. If it has been done improperly, even a restoration that is apparently successful will eventually be a failure.

Annealing is a cleansing operation. When gold is absolutely pure and clean, it is inherently cohesive—that is, capable of uniting molecularly throughout the mass of foil. Its laminae (layers of individual foil sheet) will stick together on mere contact. Due to this characteristic, it is possible to weld it in the cold state, instead of using a welding torch such as is used to weld metals in repair shops.

The purity of gold is easily destroyed, however, and when impure, it either cannot cohere at all or does so imperfectly and cannot be welded successfully. Even exposure to the air can make it impure.

Gold may be contaminated by exposure to air because the atmosphere usually contains gases which attach themselves to the surface of the gold foil by molecular attraction. The gases deposit a film of salts on the surface of the gold, and it cannot cohere. Therefore, gold must have its surface thoroughly cleaned just before use. Consequently, it is subjected to annealing which drives off all volatile impurities (those which will evaporate, especially under heat)—leaving it clean.

---

1. This section adapted from materials supplied through the courtesy of Coe Laboratories, Chicago, Illinois.

Protecting Gold

Gold must be protected from the gases which will permanently injure it. Since these gases are present in the dental office, extreme care must be used in storing and using gold. One way to protect gold from these gases is to coat it with a film of alkaline salts. This protective film, usually of ammonia, is placed there by the manufacturer to prevent deleterious gases from condensing on the foil. The ammonia is then driven off by annealing.

Purpose of Annealing

Annealing drives off all surface atmospheric moisture and whatever film has been formed by the protective alkaline gas in combination with gases that may have settled afterward.

Proper annealing means heating gold foil long enough, at a given temperature, to volatilize *all* moisture and gases, cleansing *all* its surface; avoiding injury to the foil in the process; and guarding it against all contamination, from the start of its annealing to its condensation in the cavity.

Underannealing is to be avoided. It leaves impurities on the foil, which prevent its thorough condensation and thus cause the restoration eventually to pit and flake. *Overannealing* is to be avoided no less. It scorches the foil, shriveling the fine edges and rendering it generally harsh and unworkable—with the same harmful consequences as those of underannealing. Scorched foil will not burnish properly. *Contamination* of gold foil during or after annealing may be as harmful as contamination before annealing.

In general, gold foil can be annealed by either of two methods: (1) piece by piece in an open flame or (2) in bulk, on a tray or some other suitable receptacle. Each has its advantages and disadvantages, and either is capable of giving satisfactory results.

PIECE-BY-PIECE ANNEALING The method of annealing piece by piece consists in picking up individually each piece of gold foil, of whatever form, heating it directly in an open flame, and placing it in the cavity.

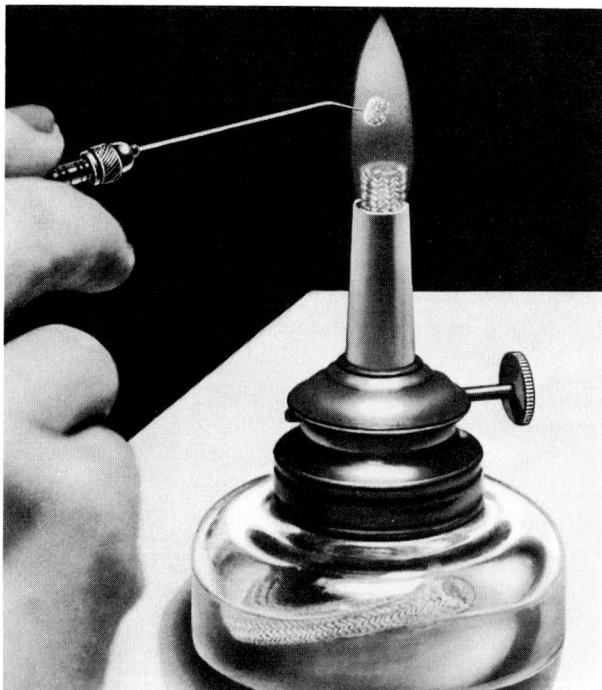

Courtesy Morgan-Hastings & Co.

Fig. 34.41. Annealing gold foil in the alcohol lamp.

The instrument best adapted for carrying the foil is one with a fine, smooth point. Whatever the instrument, its point should be non-oxidizing, and it should pick up the foil so as neither to crush it nor to cover any portion of it. And obviously it should be cleaned just before use. Simply scrub it with a stiff nailbrush dipped in alcohol, and then dry it throughly with a towel.

The foil is passed through the flame at the tip of the *inner* cone—neither close to the wick nor through the upper portion of the outer cone. Either of the latter may contaminate it with carbon. It is *passed through* the flame—

not held—at a rate that will bring every particle to a *dull red*. If kept in the flame until it shows a bright glow, it is liable to be over-annealed before it can be withdrawn. Heating it to a dull red usually takes no longer than a second or two. The exact length of time depends on the size of the piece and the intensity of the flame. Gauging it is entirely a matter of feel, which comes with experience. If a piece comes out of the flame looking the least bit shriveled, it is doubtless scorched and is best discarded.

Every annealed piece, in all open-flame annealing, is carried from the flame direct to the cavity. This has the important advantage of precluding all possible contamination of the foil *after* annealing, whether by atmospheric moisture or gases or by substances that can contaminate it on contact. A common procedure is as follows:

While malleting an annealed piece with one hand, the assistant picks up another piece with the other. When the condensing of the former is finished, she then anneals the latter and carries it to the cavity. And so on until the restoration is completed. On reaching the cavity, the foil should have cooled sufficiently not to cause any painful reaction.

Bulk Annealing   A more controlled means of annealing can be achieved by the use of an electrical device designed expressly for the purpose of annealing in bulk. Electric annealers vary, but they all have in common, principally, an outer metal shell housing a heating element, a tray over the latter to hold the gold foil, and a lid that fits over the tray. They all operate directly from an ordinary electric outlet.

Place as many pieces of gold foil on the tray as it will hold loosely—without any two pieces touching each other. To prevent their sliding and sticking together, the tray of a recent electric annealer provides individual compartments for each piece of foil. The current is

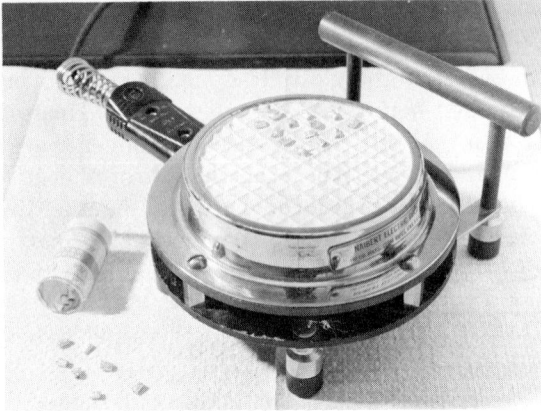

Fig. 34.42. Gold foil and electric annealer

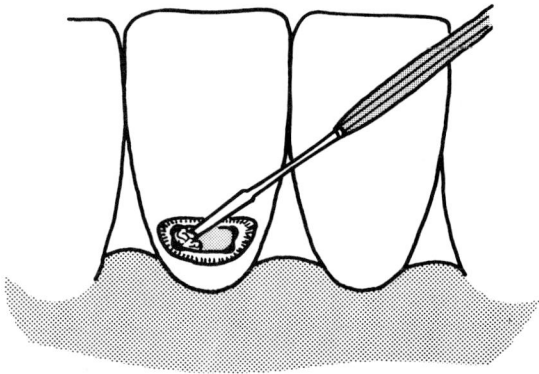

Fig. 34.43. Condensing alloy in cavity

for the tray to cool before annealing the next batch. Laying out foil on a tray that is hot is extremely difficult.

Annealed foil that remains after the restoration is completed is left on the annealer for the next restoration. Such foil cannot be returned to its usual container because it would stick together and could not be separated. Reannealing does it no harm. There is, of course, the hazard of its being contaminated by gases that are irretrievably deleterious. Since the only protection from them is given by the lid that fits over the tray, even though not altogether foolproof, it is important to replace the lid *tightly* as soon as the annealer is not in use. If the tray does not have individual compartments for each piece of foil, there is the further hazard that even a slight jarring of the annealer may cause some pieces to slide and stick together.

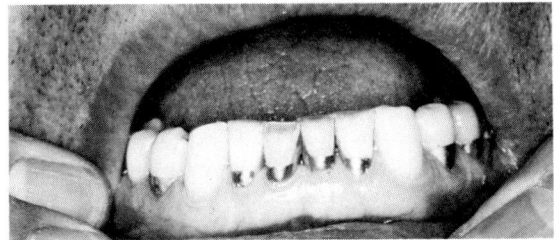

Fig. 34.44. Gold-foil restoration

turned on *after* the foil is in place and *with the lid off.*

It is advisable to keep the annealed foil warm until it is used. For this purpose some electric annealers have a rheostat which permits the current to be regulated downward. But even one which has no rheostat, provided that its maximum temperature does not exceed 700 degrees Fahrenheit, may be left on—full —without any hazard of overannealing. In the latter case, however, it is necessary that the current be turned off altogether in ample time

NONCOHESIVE GOLD FOIL. Noncohesive gold foil in the form of ropes or cylinders is used by many experienced gold-foil operators. This type of foil is not annealed before use.

Casting Alloys

Cast-gold restorations are not formed inside the mouth as the pure gold fillings are; they are made to conform to a specific shape outside the mouth and are then placed either in or on the tooth which is to be restored. If this casting is cemented into a tooth, it is known as an *inlay*, and the term to describe it is *intra-coronal*. If the casting is cemented on part of the tooth or covers the entire crown of the tooth, it is known as a *crown* or *onlay*, and the term to describe it is *extracoronal*.

In order to produce these shapes or forms so that they will accurately fit the tooth which has been prepared, a rather complicated and precise procedure is required. The purpose of this procedure is always the same—the production of an accurate casting which will properly fit the prepared tooth.

The casting gold alloys are generally composed of varying parts of four metals: gold, silver, copper, and platinum. Small additions of other metals, such as zinc, are possibly used by certain manufacturers in adjusting the properties of the particular casting gold designed for a certain purpose.

The most surprising fact is that gold, silver, and copper can be combined to form an alloy which is much stronger than any one of the three by itself. While this does not seem possible, it is correct. Many metals, when alloyed or combined with other metals, make an alloy which has completely different properties than are exhibited by the metals alone.

Improper handling of gold alloys can result in changes in the properties of the alloy. This is best shown in the method of cooling Type C golds after casting. (These gold alloys usually contain a certain amount of platinum, a white metal, which results in an alloy which is less yellow than those of the softer golds, Types A and B.) If the Type C gold is quenched (that is, submerged in water) immediately after casting, the result is a softening of the alloy. If, instead, the casting is allowed to cool on the bench top or in the casting machine for eight to ten minutes after casting and before quenching in water, the result is a hard alloy as Type C golds are designed to be.

The Type A golds are the softer gold alloys. These are designed for use where the restora-tion will not have much stress placed on it, such as gingival (Class V) inlays. The Type B golds are designed for greater stress, such as Class II inlays, three-quarter crowns or full crowns alone, or those which support one end of a short bridge. The Type C golds are designed for thin three-quarter crowns or full crowns, or those restorations supporting long bridges—restorations which will receive a great deal of stress in relation to their bulk.

The *ten tenets as applied to gold* are shown on the summary found in figure 34.1.

Summary

Biomaterials are materials directly associated with living tissues; in dentistry they are usually used in the mouth.

The environment of the oral cavity is restrictive because the oral cavity is constantly moist and is subjected to rather extreme changes of temperature and acid. Restorative materials may be placed under the stress and abrasion of masticatory forces.

Standards for certified dental materials are maintained by the American Dental Association and the National Bureau of Standards.

Ten tenets for a satisfactory filling material have been established. See the summary chart for each dental material.

The restorative materials of dentistry include dental cements, silver amalgam, gold, and gold alloys.

It is important that you understand the procedures used in mixing and using each of these materials.

Zinc oxide-eugenol cement is used for temporary covers for crown and bridge work, for sedative treatment, for bases under metal restorations, and for capping exposed pulps.

Zinc phosphate cements are used for bases under fillings and for cementing inlays, crowns, bridges, and jacket crowns.

Silicate cement is not mixed like the zinc phosphate cements. Mix it thick and mix it quickly.

The filled, unfilled, and composite plastics are similar in some ways to the silicate cements.

Silver amalgam is an alloy. Extreme care must be used in mixing the proper proportions of mercury and alloy when preparing an amalgam restoration.

Gold may be used in several forms. In the pure form, gold is used to make gold-foil restorations.

Annealing is a cleansing operation, and the foil will adhere to other gold when it is pure; thus, contamination of gold foil must be avoided. Proper annealing means heating gold foil long enough to volatilize all moisture and gases, cleansing all its surface, avoiding injury to the foil in the process, and avoiding contamination from the beginning of the process until it is condensed in the preparation in the tooth. Foil may be annealed by one of two methods: piece by piece or in bulk.

Noncohesive gold foil is used by some experienced operators. It is not annealed before use.

Another form of cohesive gold for dental use is composed of pellets of pure gold wrapped in gold foil. It is so dense that about one-tenth as many pellets are required to restore an area as gold-foil cylinders.

Casting alloys of gold are used to make a specific shape of restoration outside the mouth. This restoration is then cemented into place in the mouth. It may be an inlay, a crown, or a bridge.

Gold alloys are classified as Type A, Type B, and Type C. Type A is the softest of the three and is used for restorations where there is little stress; Type B golds are designed for greater stress; and Type C golds are used for restorations which will receive a great deal of stress in relation to their bulk.

Study Questions

1. What materials are included as restorative materials in dentistry?
2. Describe the procedures for mixing each of the following:

   > zinc oxide-eugenol
   > zinc phosphate
   > silicate cement.

3. What is an exothermic reaction? Which cement is more likely to need care to prevent this reaction? What would you do to prevent such a reaction?
4. Compare unfilled, filled, and composite plastics.
5. What is silver amalgam?
6. What happens during amalgamation?
7. Discuss making the strongest amalgam restoration.
8. Why is excess mercury deposited in a receptacle specifically for mercury?
9. Discuss the purpose of polishing amalgams and when it is done.
10. What is done with excess amalgam?
11. How can gold be used in restorations?
12. Discuss welded gold restorations.
13. Discuss protection of gold.
14. Discuss the uses of cast-gold alloys.
15. What is the difference between *intracoronal* and *extracoronal*? What other terms are used?

Bibliography

AMERICAN DENTAL ASSOCIATION. *Guide to Dental Materials.* 3rd ed. Chicago: American Dental Association, 1966.

JENSEN, JAMES R. "Anterior Restorative Materials." *Puerto Rico Dental Journal. Revista Odontologica de Puerto Rico* 1, no. 2 (August 1969): 9-13.

————. "A Place for Composites." Unpublished research paper.

————. "Materials for Anterior Restorations." Unpublished research paper.

35 | *Impression Materials*

Special Techniques

Restorations which are constructed outside the mouth require special techniques. Upon completion of the preparation for an inlay, a three-quarter crown, a full crown, or any multiples or combinations of them, it is necessary to construct a wax replica of that portion of the tooth which has been removed. This wax replica is later used to construct the gold inlay or crown and is technically called a *wax pattern*. It does not resemble a dress pattern; that is, it is not a flat piece of wax. It is a sculptured form. It is a pattern in that the inlay or crown will be an exact duplicate of the wax form.

Some dentists do make a *direct* wax pattern, that is, a wax pattern made directly in the mouth of the patient. Direct technique is usually limited to the less complicated patterns, such as patterns for occlusal inlays. It is possible to make direct patterns for all individual restorations constructed in gold should the dentist so desire. If a direct wax pattern is made, no impression is needed.

The majority of dentists, however, use an *indirect* method; that is, a wax pattern is made on a model, or duplicate, of the patient's tooth or group of teeth. With this method of constructing the wax pattern, the dentist must first make an impression of the prepared tooth in the patient's mouth so that a die or reproduction of the portion of the tooth left in the mouth can be made by one of several methods.

465

The die, or exact copy of the prepared tooth in the patient's mouth, is used to construct a wax replacement of the missing part of the tooth. The wax is molded onto the die until all the angles and surfaces are filled accurately. Then wax is added until there is enough wax so the outside of the tooth can be carved to fit properly with the existing teeth in the patient's mouth. (The inlay must properly mesh with the existing surfaces of other teeth in the area.) The wax model must be accurately formed (*a*) where it joins the remaining tooth structure and (*b*) where it touches other teeth.

When the dentist is positive the wax model is accurate, it is mounted on a tiny rod or post, called a *sprue pin,* and embedded in dental casting investment, which is plaster mixed with silica. (See chap. 37 for a detailed explanation.) When the investment has hardened, the base and sprue pin are removed, leaving a communicating hole through the investment to the wax model (usually called a *wax pattern*). This invested pattern is then placed in an oven where the heat burns out all the wax, leaving a void (hole) in the investment which is the identical shape of the wax model.

Hot, melted gold (called molten gold) is then forced through the hole left by the sprue pin into the hollow which is shaped like the wax pattern. When the gold cools and hardens, it produces a casting shaped exactly like the wax pattern. The investment plaster is removed, and the casting is cleaned, polished, and cemented to the tooth.

This brief, nontechnical explanation of the process of making a cast-gold restoration outside the mouth should help you understand the overall procedure. Now let us consider the process in more detail, beginning with the making of impressions.

If we regard a prepared tooth or group of teeth as an *original* or *positive* shape, the impression which is taken of an individual tooth or a group of teeth, or of any dental situation

for that matter, is a *negative* shape. If you leave an imprint of your hand in a section of modeling clay, that imprint is a negative shape of your hand. If into this imprint or impression you pour or place a soft mix of plaster, permit it to harden, then remove the plaster, this plaster will again have the same curve as the surface of the hand which you pushed into the clay originally. This plaster "model" is a positive copy of the surface of your hand.

The same is true of an impression taken for dental purposes. In order to complete the purpose for which the impression was taken, a positive form must be made from the impression. This positive is known as a *cast* when it involves an entire arch, but more specifically it is known as a *model* or *working model* if a dental restoration is to be constructed upon it. If the impression is of a single tooth for the construction of an inlay or crown, or if the impression is of a quadrant or full arch which contains teeth involved in multiple restorations, the individual tooth model is known as a *die.* In the case of quadrant or full-arch impressions, we shall see later on that it is possible to have the dies removable from the model. This means that the individual die may be lifted from the model and replaced to a definite position and relationship by means of some form of notching or keying. This ability makes it much easier to "wax-up" the pattern required for all gold castings.

The direct and the indirect methods of making a wax pattern have already been mentioned. A third method, the *indirect-direct* method, is also used by some dentists. In this method, the pattern is made on the model or die and is then rechecked directly in the patient's mouth prior to proceeding with the laboratory work.

Impressions for Cast-Gold Restorations

Many dentists carve wax patterns in the mouth on the prepared tooth. This direct method eliminates two intermediate steps, involving two extra materials, which could contribute to inaccuracies in the final fit of the restoration. Although the direct method can be simply performed with greater accuracy, most dentists and technicians prefer to work from models because this method permits greater use in contouring, carving, and manipulating the materials involved.

Impression compound is a thermoplastic material, the properties of which are governed by the American Dental Association's Specification No. 3. It is furnished in cakes and sticks. The most common use of this material is for taking full-mouth impressions for den-

tures; but it is also used for impressioning single teeth for full-crown restorations.

First, the material must be softened. For individual tooth impressions, it is possible to soften it carefully in an open flame, but a controlled temperature compound heater is usually used for larger impressions. In order to confine the material, the dentist will select a copper band of the proper size, shape it to fit the gingival margins of the prepared tooth, fill the copper band with impression compound, position it on the tooth, and force the softened material under pressure to the tiny recesses at the gingival margin. The impression must then be cooled. A stream of air from the

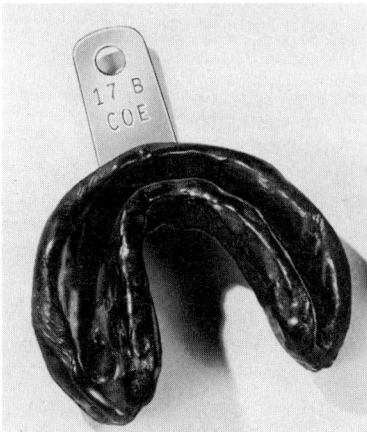

Courtesy Coe Labs., Inc.

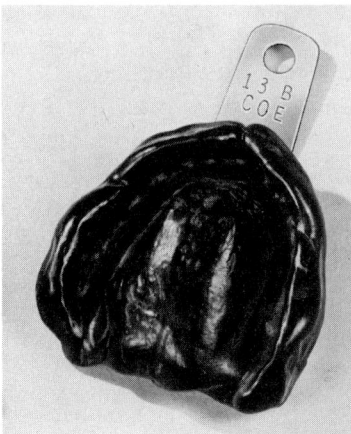

Fig. 35.1. Preliminary impression in modeling compound.

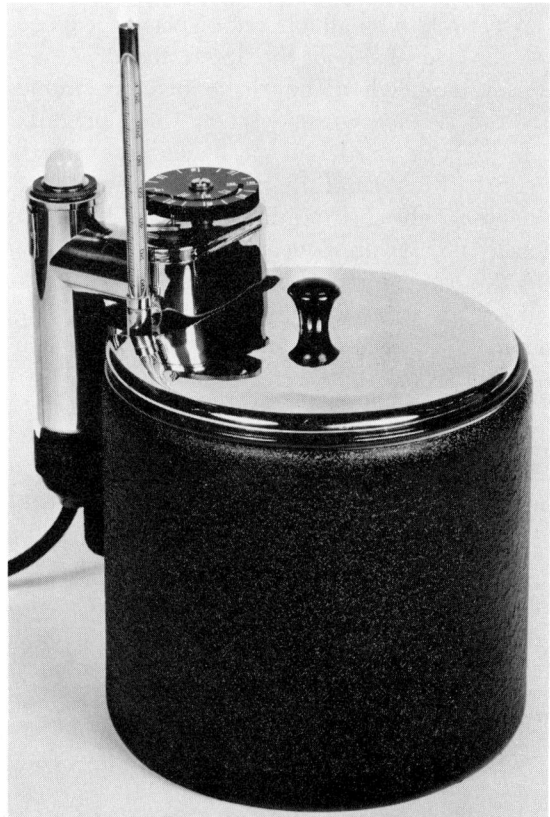

Courtesy Kerr Mfg. Co.

Fig. 35.2. Thermostatic compound heater

air syringe or cold water from the water syringe is used. The dentist then removes the copper band containing the impression material. He checks it for accuracy. Impression compound is an excellent material for accurate single-tooth impressions; however, it is rigid and cannot be drawn over undercuts in the preparation or contours of the tooth. For that reason it has limited applications for inlay impressions.

Impression plaster is another material which has been used for impressions in prosthodontics. Like impression compound, it is rigid and therefore has little application where cast-gold restorations are involved. It is used sometimes in making *bite registrations* which are records of the relationship of the upper arch to the lower arch. A small amount of plaster is placed on the buccal side of the upper and lower posterior teeth when they have been positioned as the dentist wishes. When this portion of plaster has hardened on each side of the mouth, it is carefully removed, trimmed to include only the required area, and used to position casts previously made so they will be in the same relationship on an articulator as the teeth were in the patient's mouth. (See chap. 33 for a discussion of the use of an articulator.)

Rubber-base Impression Materials

The rubber-base impression materials differ from modeling compound and impression plaster in that they are elastic in nature. They are rubbery. The two types of rubber-base impression materials differ in chemical makeup and in the manufacturer's choice of color for the finished product, but otherwise they are similar in texture when set. The silicone-base material is perhaps used somewhat more widely than the polysulfide type.

These materials are supplied in tubes. One tube contains the base material; the other tube contains the catalyst, or material which causes the mix to set. Usually these are of different colors, which make it possible to see more easily when you have a smoothly uniform mix.

Two general consistencies are usually available from any manufacturer—one heavier-bodied for tray use, one lighter-bodied for syringe use.

The tray material is used alone in impressions for full dentures, and at times for copper-band impressions of individual teeth. The syringe material is used together with the base material when taking impressions for multiple restorations or partial denture impressions. The technique of preparation and use is illustrated in this chapter.

No special treatment of the rubber surface is required before pouring models in the rubber-base impression materials. This material is dimensionally more stable than the next group of materials to be discussed.

Hydrocolloid Impression Materials

The original hydrocolloid made its appearance prior to World War II. In its final set form it resembles chocolate-colored gelatin with somewhat more density and toughness. This set condition can be changed to fluid again by heating the material. It is therefore a *reversible* hydrocolloid, that is, it can be changed from solid to liquid and back again by heating and cooling it.

(There is also an irreversible hydrocolloid material which remains solid once it has set.)

The primary function of the reversible hydrocolloid is taking impressions for restorative dentistry and taking impressions of inlay and crown preparations. It is also used in prosthetics. Although it is a very accurate material, the special heaters, tempering baths, and water-cooled trays make its manipulation more intricate; and consequently it is less popular than the rubber-base impression materials.

The original reversible hydrocolloid is changed from solid to fluid by heating the material in a hydrocolloid conditioner (fig. 35.4). Boil the material for eight to ten minutes. It will then have acquired a consistency somewhat like thin molasses. At this stage and at this temperature, it is much too hot to place in a patient's mouth. For this reason, the conditioners have tempering baths which permit the material to cool to about 105° Fahrenheit over a period of minutes prior to loading the impression tray and inserting it into the patient's mouth. When seated properly, the circulating water is turned on and the tray is chilled. The resulting impression is extremely accurate when properly taken; however, unless it is properly managed, hydrocolloid is extremely susceptible to dimensional changes through loss of water by evaporation. Therefore, models should be poured as soon after the impression is taken as is possible. Storage, when absolutely necessary, should only be in an atmosphere of 100 percent humidity—wrapped in a thoroughly wet towel or stored in a humidifier designed for the purpose. Even such storage should not be permitted for extended periods of time.

Read the directions for the proper use of the hydrocolloid available in the office in which you work. There are some variations in temperatures, in treatment with a fixer after the impression is taken and before the model is poured, in the length of time a model may be permitted to remain in the impression, and in the treatment recommended for the combined impression and freshly poured model.

As with the rubber-base materials when used for full-mouth or quadrant impressions of multiple preparations, the reversible hydrocolloids reproduce detail most accurately when a preliminary thinner mix is either painted on the area concerned or is injected with a type of syringe made for the purpose. If syringes are used, they are loaded, sealed from contact with external water, and prepared in the conditioner just as are the full tubes of normal material for tray use.

As with the rubber-base materials, the purpose of the thinner material is to eliminate air

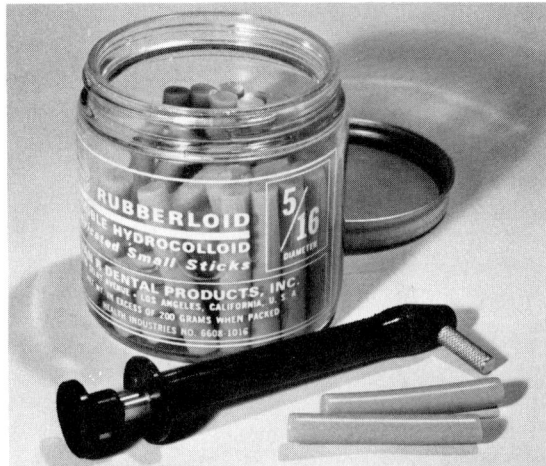

Fig. 35.3. Hydrocolloid syringe and material

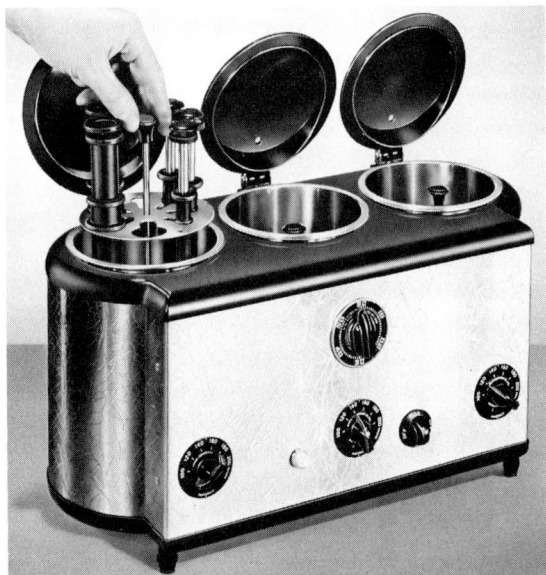

Courtesy Hanau Engr. Co.

Fig. 35.4. Hanau hydrocolloid conditioner

in undercuts present in the area to be covered by the tray, as well as to provide the ultimate of fine detail in the impression.

The reversible hydrocolloids are made of agar-agar, a product obtained from seaweed. At the time of its development, most of the desirable seaweed was to be found off the coast of Japan. With the opening of World War II, this seaweed was no longer available from the previous source, and a search was begun for a substitute impression material.

This search resulted in the development of an *irreversible* hydrocolloid impression material, more commonly known as the *alginates*. This material is prepared in powder form, is mixed with water at a specific temperature (usually 70°) in a mixing bowl for one minute, and does not require a water-cooled tray. The resulting impression paste has little application in restorative dentistry, but it is sufficiently accurate for preliminary impressions in partial-denture and full-denture construction. Since it also forms a gel, as do the reversible hydrocolloids, it is susceptible to the same dimensional changes and handling characteristics. Models should be poured immediately, or proper storage should be instituted for brief periods only. The irreversible hydrocolloids are easy to work with and therefore are very commonly used in dental offices.

However, most offices will use either the rubber-base impression materials or the *reversible* hydrocolloids for impressions of multiple restoration procedures.

The elastic impression materials, in general, do not lend themselves to making amalgam dies. The very dense die stones which have been developed provide a technique for making models with removable dies which has been found entirely satisfactory; but as with all dental procedures, preciseness and care must be used if a good result is to be obtained. A material must always be used in the manner for which it is designed.

Summary

Restorations which are prepared outside the mouth are made by taking an impression in the mouth and then working with a model outside the mouth.

Materials which are useful for impressions are

1. impression compound, used by dentists for a preliminary impression for full dentures and for individual full-crown preparations;
2. impression plaster, which has been used in prosthodontics;
3. rubber-base impression materials which are elastic in nature. They are supplied as pastes and are dimensionally more stable than hydrocolloid materials;
4. hydrocolloid impression materials which are both reversible and irreversible. The irreversible hydrocolloids are easy to work with and are commonly used in dental offices for full-mouth impressions but are not accurate enough for dies for gold castings. The reversible hydrocolloids are used, as are the rubber-base impression materials, for impressions involving multiple restoration procedures.

Study Questions

1. Distinguish between direct and indirect wax patterns.
2. Explain an impression and its use.
3. What is a die?
4. Describe briefly the process of making a gold restoration outside the mouth.
5. Describe the use of

    a. impression compound.
    b. impression plaster.
    c. rubber-base impression materials.
    d. both kinds of hydrocolloid impression materials.

6. Discuss the uses of rubber-base impression materials, reversible hydrocolloid materials, and irreversible hydrocolloid materials.

36 | *Models and Dies*

Restorations which are constructed outside the mouth are the subject of three chapters: thirty-five, thirty-six, and thirty-seven. The second skill to be learned is making a model or wax pattern from the impression we learned to take in chapter thirty-five.

Dies on which to fabricate (make) wax patterns for cast-gold restorations may be made of artificial stone or amalgam. Amalgam is used only occasionally for individual copper-band compound impressions. The artificial stone or die stone is a material similar to plaster but is much more dense, providing a hard, smooth surface which will withstand the manipulation necessary when carving wax patterns. Although plaster can be used in preparing study models, it is too porous and weak to be used for dies.

Artificial Stone and Plaster

Artificial stone and plaster[1] are supplied in almost any amount, by weight, from five-pound cans to hundred-pound barrels. Do not purchase larger quantities than can be used in a period of two or three months and, naturally, no more than the dental office is equipped to store.

Plaster is most commonly supplied in white. Die stones are supplied in several contrasting

1. This section adapted from materials supplied through the courtesy of Coe Laboratories, Chicago, Illinois.

colors, varying with the particular brand or use intended. The color coding of these materials quickly indicates which material has been used to pour a given cast.

Both die stones and plaster are made from a similar variety of natural gypsum. The gypsum is mined, crushed, and fed into kilns where it is heated to drive off some of the water of crystallization to form what is called a *hemihydrate*, which is then prepared in a powder form and packaged.

The rough, irregular, and porous particles of plaster require a relatively large amount of water for mixing when compared to the more regular shape of die-stone particles. The artificial stones require about half as much water for mixing as does plaster. Although the final product is stronger when less water is used, you must have sufficient water to separate the particles and wet them thoroughly in order to manipulate the mix and pour a cast

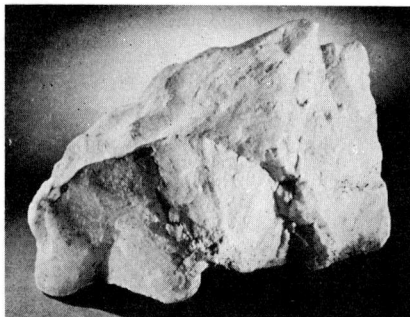

Fig. 36.1. Natural gypsum rock as it is mined.

Courtesy Coe Labs., Inc.

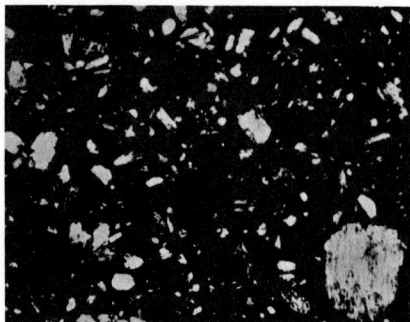

Fig. 36.2. Photomicrograph of plaster particles.

Courtesy Coe Labs., Inc.

from it. The water added replaces that driven off when the gypsum was heated. In addition, the particles are porous, and water must penetrate and fill these pores. Therefore, an excess of water must be present. The effect is somewhat the same as if many small sponges were stirred under water. The final product of the reaction is gypsum. In other words, when water is added to the hemihydrate, the original calcination reaction is reversed—and gypsum, the original product, is again attained. It is by no means as dense as the product mined from the ground, however, because excess water is necessary for the mixing. It is obvious that the final gypsum product must be porous in order to contain this excess water. It should now be evident that the less water used in mixing a gypsum material, the stronger the final product will be. The less amount of excess water, the denser the gypsum and, consequently, the greater its strength.

Since plaster is chemically the same as dental stone, why is stone so much stronger and harder when it has set?

The particles of hemihydrate used in the dental stone show a fairly smooth and regular surface, and they are quite free from porosity. Therefore, when the dental stone is mixed with water, much less excess water is required to separate the particles since they are neither porous nor rough.

In contrast to model plaster—which requires approximately 60 cubic centimeters of water per 100 grams of plaster for mixing—stone can be easily mixed with 28 cubic centimeters of water per 100 grams of the powder. In fact, as little as 25 cubic centimeters of water per 100 grams of stone can be used, although the mixture is very thick and requires vibration to make it flow. Very strong, hard casts can be obtained with this heavy mix.

Special die stones have particles which are slightly larger in size. The larger-size particles are more easily displaced by the water and therefore require less water to make a mix of the same consistency.

You should note that a relatively slight difference in the water content of the mix with a dental stone results in a considerable difference in the strength of the final product. In certain instances, an *increase* in water content of as little as 1 cubic centimeter per 100 grams of stone may result in a *decrease in strength* of as much as 1,000 pounds per square inch. While this difference in strength is not as great in mixing plaster, it does make a noticeable difference to mix plaster with as little water as possible.

When plaster is used, you can judge reasonably well the proportion of water to powder after some familiarity with the "feel" of mixing correctly proportioned mixes. Such guesswork should not be used in the case of stone.

Unless the amounts of water and powder are being properly measured, the chances are that the resulting cast will be deficient in strength, hardness, and accuracy—with possibly critical and costly consequences.

Fortunately, most die stones are prepackaged. Therefore the powder is already weighed, and only the correct volume of water must be measured and added.

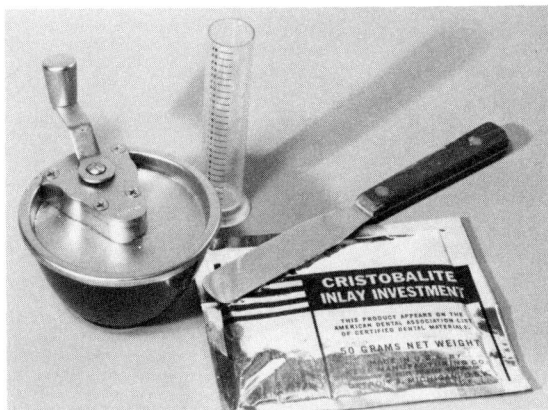

Fig. 36.3. Premeasured powder, mixing bowl, and measuring cup for water.

A word of caution should be given concerning the use of a stone in connection with the hydrocolloid technique. The hydrocolloid is apt to soften the surface of the stone when the latter is allowed to set in contact with it. This effect can be definitely minimized if certain precautions are observed. For example, if a "fixer" is required by the manufacturer, it should *always* be used according to the directions supplied.

Another precaution is to be sure that there is no water clinging to the impression when the cast or die is poured. The surface of the hydrocolloid can be dried by blotting it with an absorbent, *but under no circumstances should it be dried by an air blast.*

A third precaution is to separate the impression from the stone cast or die approximately one hour after it has been poured. If it is separated too soon, its surface will not be hard; and if it is allowed to set too long in contact with the hydrocolloid, it will also be softened. If it is absolutely necessary to leave the stone in contact with the impression for a prolonged period, the impression should be immersed in water after the stone attains its first set. However, the best method is to separate at the end of an hour as previously stated.

All stones may lose their properties if they are not stored properly. *By all means*, store them in a dry place. Since they are *hygroscopic*, they absorb moisture to a degree. Once they take up moisture, a deterioration sets in. The first evidence of deterioration is an increase in setting time. Later, a longer setting time is observed, and finally a stage is reached when the stone will not set at all.

Such changes may be slow and not easily observed. An increase in the setting expansion and a decrease in strength may occur before any change in setting time is evident. Therefore, the can of stone should be kept *tightly shut* at all times, and it should always be stored in a clean, dry place. Before every use shake up the contents while still in the container.

Mixing Artificial Stone

To prepare artificial stone for pouring a cast, the following materials are required:

1. Plaster bowl.
2. Plaster spatula.
3. Water measure (50 cc. graduate is convenient).
4. A common teaspoon.
5. Scale for weighing.
6. Waxed paper cups for weighing.
7. Six-inch-square glass slabs for each cast.
8. Artificial stone.
9. A vibrator (if available).
10. A pan of water deep enough and large enough to hold the poured impressions (not required for impressions taken in modeling compound).
11. The impression which is to be poured.

For the average single-arch impression, 42 cc. of water will be ample. This amount of water is poured into the mixing bowl.

With a spoon, place sufficient artificial stone from the storage bin or can into the paper cup on the scale to weigh 150 grams. Sift this powder into the water in the mixing bowl by using the spoon. When all the powder has been sifted into the mixing bowl, place the bowl with its contents on the vibrator and vibrate for five to ten seconds. Then spatulate the contents of the mixing bowl until a uniform, creamy mixture is obtained. Again vibrate the bowl with its contents for ten to fifteen seconds. If no mechanical vibrator is available, rapidly jar the bowl on the laboratory bench for one minute.

For special care, rubber bowls should be rinsed with water, then inverted and shaken before the measured amount of water is placed in the mixing bowl. The surface of a rubber bowl will require a certain amount of water

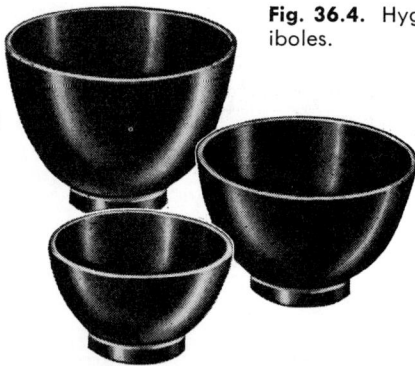

Fig. 36.4. Hygienic flexiboles.

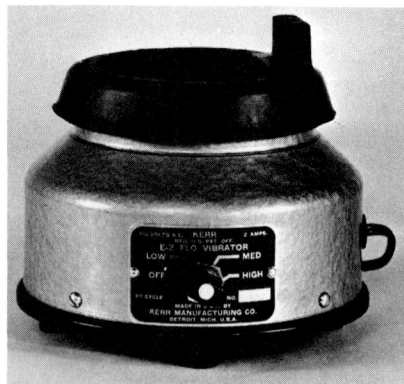

Fig. 36.5. Kerr E-Z Flo vibrator.

Courtesy Kerr Mfg. Co.

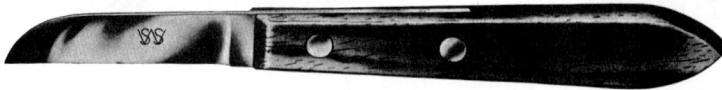

Courtesy S. S. White Co.

Fig. 36.6. Office knife, 5A.

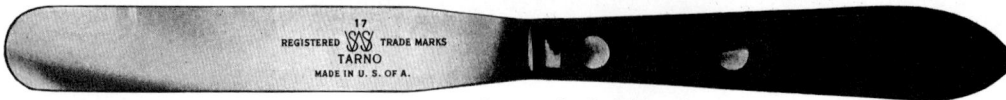

Courtesy S. S. White Co.

Fig. 36.7. Plaster spatula, No. 7.

just to wet it, and in working with stone, this may make a definite difference in the amount of water available for mixing with the stone.

Special forms of artificial stone are often used to make special types of casts and dies for indirect crown, bridge, or inlay construction. Specific instructions for mixing these special types accompany the material when purchased. These directions should be followed explicitly to secure the required results.

Mixing Plaster

The transition (change) of the soft mixture of plaster with water to a hard, set material is a controllable process. That is, the time required for the transition may be altered by various means. Cold water used for the mix will delay setting; warm water will hasten it. Adding a pinch of table salt will hasten setting, as will the addition of powder made by grinding previously set plaster. Spatulation helps hasten the setting, other conditions being the same.

Mixing bowls used for preparing plaster and artificial stone are frequently made of rubber to facilitate removing hard plaster. Bowls made of a resin material are easier to maintain and use.

A plaster or laboratory spatula is used to spatulate both materials. Spatulas which have become sharp-edged from long use should be discarded because of the tendency to cut the bowl, making the removal of old plaster or stone difficult.

To prepare plaster for pouring a cast, the following materials are required:

1. Plaster bowl.
2. Plaster spatula.
3. Water measure (100 cc. graduate is convenient).
4. Plaster.
5. A common teaspoon.

6. Six-inch-square glass slabs, one for each impression to be poured.
7. A vibrator (if available).
8. A pan of water deep enough and large enough to hold the poured impressions (not necessary when pouring impressions taken in modeling compound).
9. The impression which is to be poured.

For an average single-arch impression, 60 cc. of water will be ample. This amount of water is poured into the plaster bowl. To begin with, use the coldest water available in order to provide the greatest amount of time possible in which to work. The reason for measuring the water is simple economy. There is no object in wasting dental materials at any time. With a little care, a more accurate amount of material may be used with less waste.

Generously heap a teaspoon with plaster from the storage bin or can. Shake the plaster smoothly and rapidly off the spoon into the 60 cc. of water. Repeat until the water has absorbed all it will apparently take. This quantity of water will need approximately one-half cup of plaster to make a mix of moderately heavy consistency.

The spatula is then used to stir the mix smoothly, with as little air as possible incorporated into the mix. Spatulate until the mix of plaster is thoroughly smooth. Add more plaster, if required, to make the mix just heavy enough so that it will not drop off the spatula when a spatulaful is lifted above the bowl and turned over.

This point should be reached without wasting time. If you spatulate a thin mix long enough, it will begin to thicken—it will be starting its initial set. This stage is too late to pour the cast well.

When the mix is at the desired consistency, place the plaster bowl on the vibrator and vibrate well to remove as many entrapped air

• MODELS AND DIES

bubbles as possible. If no mechanical vibrator is available, rapidly jar the bowl on the laboratory bench for one minute. The material is then ready for use. (See "Pouring Casts.")

Plaster is available in two types: *Natural-setting* is used for the pouring of models in the laboratory. Setting time is between fifteen and twenty minutes. *Quick-setting* is used for some purposes in taking impressions directly in the mouth. Setting time is from three to five minutes. Either flavored or plain plaster is available.

The timing involved in preparing plaster of the quick-setting variety for an impression in the mouth is extremely important, as is the method by which it is spatulated and handled prior to the impression. These details are best learned by practice if this type is used in your office.

Boxing Models

In addition to the use of specific amounts of plaster or artificial stone, economy of both time and material is accomplished, whenever possible, by what is called *boxing* an impression. Boxing an impression is simply the enclosing of the impression and its supporting tray with sides made of waxed sheets or strips to enclose the plaster or artificial stone which forms the base of the impression. Boxing wax strips are available for this purpose. This particular wax is soft, pliable, and sticky enough so that two ends which meet can be "stuck" together with finger pressure.

The trimming required to reduce the overall size of a poured cast is reduced by the use of this procedure, and since the material used is confined within the box, less plaster or artificial stone is required to make an adequate base for the cast.

Any impression the dentist has trimmed enough to expose the outer surface of the tray in which it was taken can usually be boxed successfully. Care must be taken with ma-

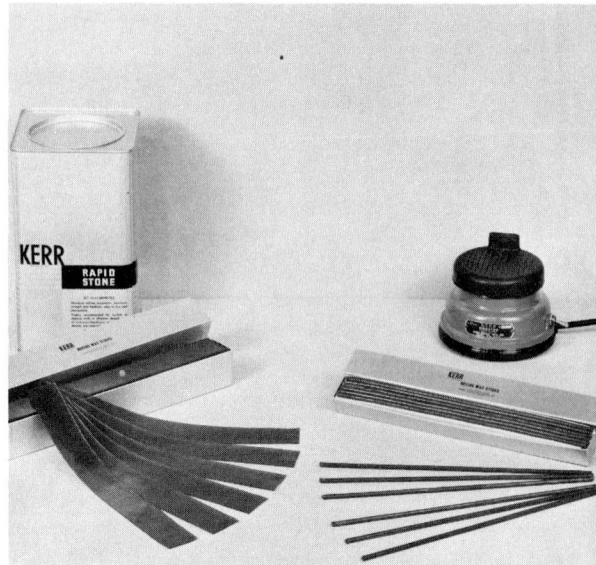

Courtesy Kerr Mfg. Co.

Fig. 36.8. Material for boxing and pouring impressions.

terials such as hydrocolloid and alginate to prevent distortion of the impressions. Impressions taken in modeling compound will not distort during the application of boxing wax.

An upper impression requires boxing material around its outer periphery only. This is easily accomplished. To hold the boxing material in place, it is *luted* (sealed to the tray with a warm instrument) with care to avoid damage to the impression material through the use of too much heat.

A lower impression is in the shape of a **U** and requires more effort to box well. The open section between the two arms of the **U** must be fitted with a piece of boxing material, which must then be well luted to the tray. Then another piece of boxing material is wrapped around the periphery of the tray, luted to the tray, and luted to the section which closes the opening between the arms of the **U**.

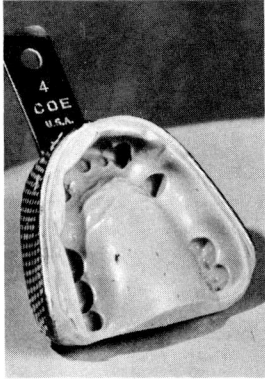

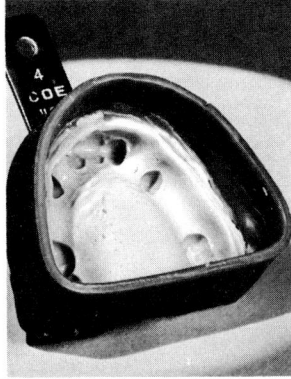

Courtesy Coe Labs., Inc.

Fig. 36.9. Alginate impression before boxing.

Fig. 36.10. Alginate impression boxed ready to be poured.

Pouring Models

Impressions taken in impression plaster must be coated with a film of some material which will aid in separating the cast from the plaster impression material. The impression may be coated with tincture of green soap or with a commercial separator, made for this purpose, applied shortly before the impression is poured.

When an impression is boxed and the material of choice has been prepared, the model is ready to be poured. The vibrator is turned on. A small quantity of the plaster or stone is picked up on the end of the plaster spatula. If the impression is an upper, the first addition of plaster or stone is made on the palate area while the impression tray is held snugly in contact with the vibrator plate. For a lower impression, the material is added at one or the other end of the **U**-shaped arch—the *heel* area. The plaster or stone will flow off the spatula even when mixed to a very heavy consistency.

Applied in small quantities to the palatal portion of the impression, the material will flow from the higher portion of the impression into the lower portions. When the impression

has been partially filled with the plaster or stone, the remaining mix may be applied at the edge of the boxing material and allowed to flow down into the boxed impression until a satisfactory amount to provide a base for the impression has flowed in. The object in flowing the cast material into the impression is to prevent trapping of air in the lower portions of the impression, especially when teeth are present on the cast, as well as to free any air bubbles which remain in the mix of plaster or stone.

If no mechanical vibrator is available, the cast material may be flowed into an impression by the use of a serrated instrument handle drawn across the handle of the tray much like a violin bow is used on a violin. The serrations will create sufficient fine vibration to aid the flow of material.

Impressions taken in alginate or hydrocolloid materials must be treated according to the manufacturer's instructions upon completion of the pouring process. These materials otherwise absorb water from the plaster or stone, resulting in a soft, chalky surface on the finished cast.

The poured impressions should be given ample time to set thoroughly before separation is attempted. The average time required for the material used in your office will be indicated on the container in which it is supplied. The recommendations of the manufacturer should always be followed to insure the best results with the product. Excessive time is not recommended.

If boxing is not possible with an impression, the low portions of the impression are filled with the cast material, using the vibrator as indicated above. When the impression has been filled to as high a level as possible, the remaining plaster or stone is placed in the center of a six-inch-square glass slab in the form of a mound. Care must be taken not to trap air. The filled impression is inverted over this mound of plaster or stone and gently seated until the periphery (edge) of the impression has been adequately covered with the cast material. All excess material is removed from the slab with the plaster spatula. After six minutes on the laboratory bench, the impression with tray, cast material, and glass slab is gently submerged in water and left until set. (Impression materials, such as the alginates, require this form of treatment.)

Separating Models

Separation of casts from alginate or hydrocolloid impressions is easily accomplished. The boxing material is stripped from the base of the cast. Hold the tray firmly in one hand, and with the other hand grip the base of the cast and gently but firmly start the cast at one edge to permit air to enter between the cast and the impression material. If teeth are present on the cast, care must be taken to prevent breakage by not removing the cast at too great an angle. Once started, the cast should be lifted directly out of the impression.

If the impression is taken in modeling or impression compound, it is best inserted (after thorough setting is accomplished) *in* the compound heater set at a temperature of five degrees less than is required to prepare the impression compound for use. Care should be taken not to leave the poured impression in the water at this temperature for any longer time than is required. After five minutes' immersion at the proper temperature, gently try separating the cast from the impression. If the compound is still too firm to allow separation, replace it in the compound heater and repeat the trial each minute thereafter. Five to ten minutes is usually sufficient time. If watched properly, the compound will leave the cast very cleanly. If left in the bath too long, the compound may stick to the cast to some extent. While the cast is still warm from the heat of the bath, this remaining impression compound may be removed by "picking" it off with a piece of stick compound which has been softened in the flame of the laboratory burner.

If a compound heater is not available, a pan of water may be used for the same purpose to separate casts from impressions taken in modeling compound. Greater care must be exercised to prevent overheating the compound.

Immediately after separation, the casts should be trimmed and the patient's name written on the cast with an indelible pencil to provide a definite identification.

Trimming Models

Properly boxed impressions will provide casts which require little if any trimming. A *model trimmer* consists of a rotating disc, with a very gritty surface, attached to a motor and provided with some means of wetting the disc as it rotates. These are available in a large laboratory size and in a small dental-office size. The harder the material used to form the cast,

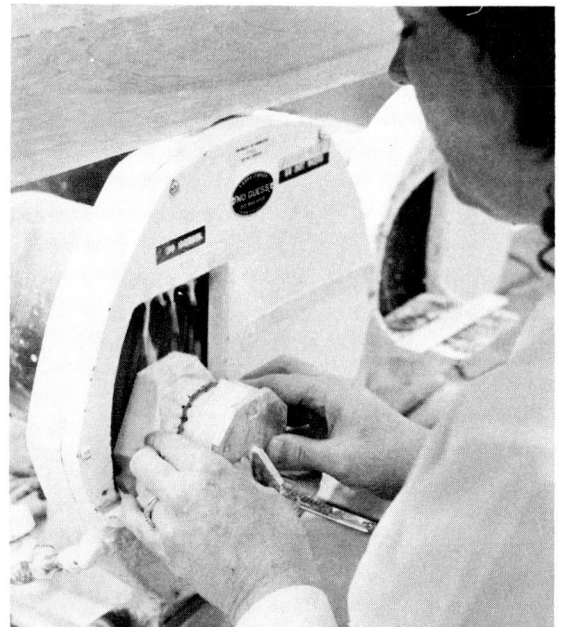

Fig. 36.11. Dental assistant using a model trimmer

the more desirable it is that any excess be avoided which will require trimming. Final finishing can be done with sandpaper after the cast is thoroughly dry.

Orthodontic Models

An orthodontic model[2] as used for record purposes is considered to be made up of an *art* portion (the actual base of the cast) and the *anatomical* portion. The art portion should consist of approximately one-third the total height from occlusal plane to bottom of the cast, the anatomical portion making the balance, or two-thirds the total height.

1. Trim base of the lower cast (fig. 36.12).
   a. The cast should be wet.
   b. The base should be trimmed parallel to the occlusal plane.
   c. Art portion, one-third total height; anatomical portion, two-thirds total height.
2. Trim heel of the lower cast (very important) (figs. 36.13-36.16).
   a. Use a divider to measure equidistant from midline at anterior teeth to an arc passing one-fourth inch behind the last molar (whichever molar is farthest back).
   b. Sight through the central grooves of the bicuspids and molars and make a mark intersecting the arc just scribed by the divider.
3. Trim heel of upper cast (figs. 36.17-36.18).
   a. Place upper and lower casts together, with teeth in occlusion.
   b. Mark upper cast to correspond to heel of lower.
   c. Heel of upper is trimmed separately until the marks are approached.
   d. Casts are again placed in occlusion for the final cut to minimize danger

of damaging the occlusal surfaces through handling.

4. Trim top of upper cast parallel to base of lower (figs. 36.19-36.21).
   a. For this cut, also, it is best to trim upper cast separately. Since casts are wet, the teeth are easily damaged.
   b. To mark cast for this cut, place casts in occlusion on a flat surface. Scribe a line two and one-half inches from the flat surface on which you have placed the casts, all the way around the upper cast.
   c. Final cut may be made with the teeth in occlusion.
5. Trim sides of the lower cast to a 55° angle with the heel (figs. 36.22-36.24).
   a. Check the angle with a hand instrument set for the purpose.
   b. Cut is made to within three-eighths inch of the bicuspid teeth.
6. Trim sides of the upper cast to a 63° angle with the heel (fig. 36.25).
   a. Check angles with a hand instrument set for the purpose.
   b. Make cut to within three-eighths inch of the bicuspid teeth, or to base of mucobuccal fold.
7. Trim front of lower cast to a curve (fig. 36.26).
   a. This rounded section should extend distally to the center of the lower cuspid on each side.
8. Trim front of upper cast to a point (fig. 36.27).
   a. The point should coincide with the median line of the upper teeth.
   b. Each cut extends distally to the center of the upper cuspid.
   c. The angle formed by these two cuts will vary, since it depends on the shape of the upper arch of this particular individual.

2. Photos for this section through courtesy of Dr. L.W. McIver, Minneapolis, Minnesota.

TRIM BASE OF LOWER   **TRIM HEEL OF LOWER**

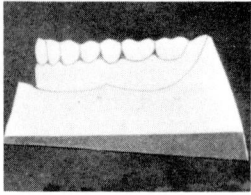 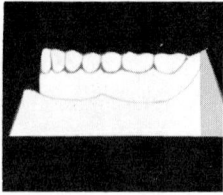 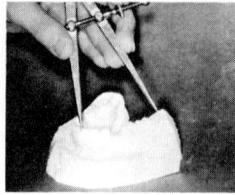 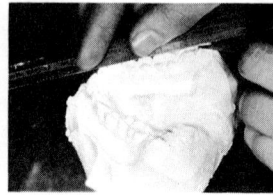 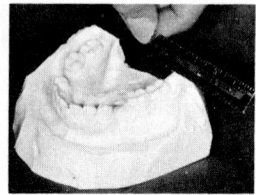

Fig. 36.12   Fig. 36.13   Fig. 36.14   Fig. 36.15   Fig. 36.16

TRIM HEEL OF UPPER   **TRIM TOP OF UPPER**

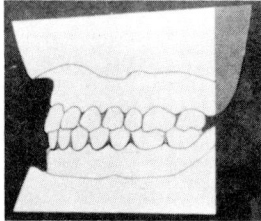 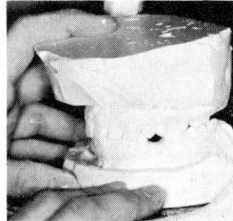 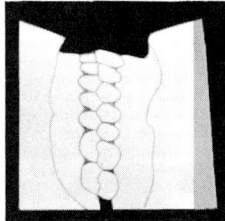 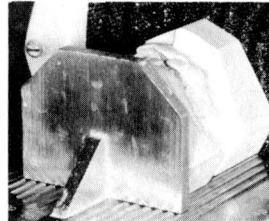 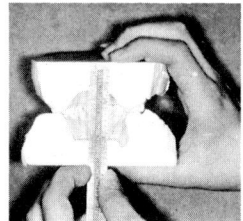

Fig. 36.17   Fig. 36.18   Fig. 36.19   Fig. 36.20   Fig. 36.21

TRIM SIDES OF LOWER 55°   **TRIM SIDES OF UPPER 63°**

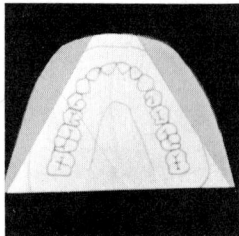 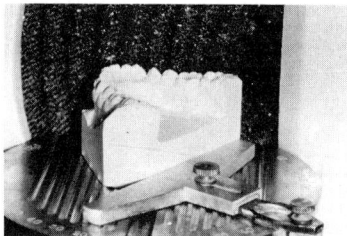 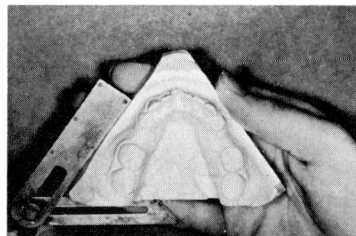 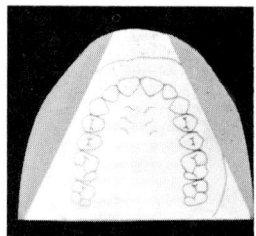

Fig. 36.22   Fig. 36.23   Fig. 36.24   Fig. 36.25

TRIM LOWER FRONT ROUND   **TRIM UPPER FRONT POINTED**   **TRIM HEEL POINTS TO 1/2" 125°**

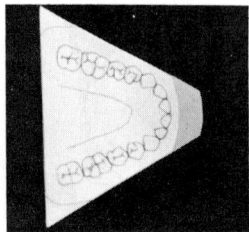 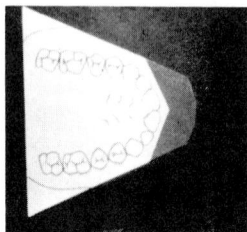 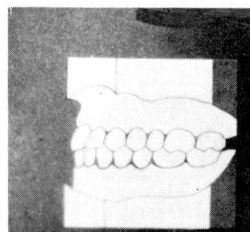 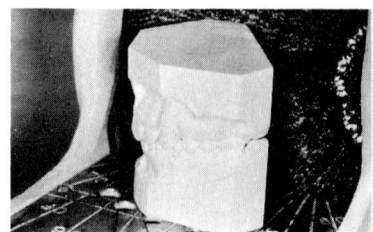

Fig. 36.26   Fig. 36.27   Fig. 36.28   Fig. 36.29

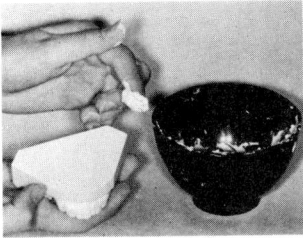

Fig. 36.30

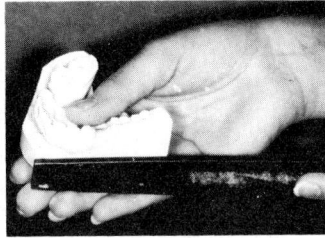

Fig. 36.31

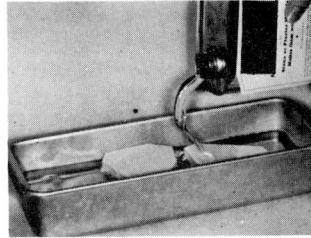

Fig. 36.32

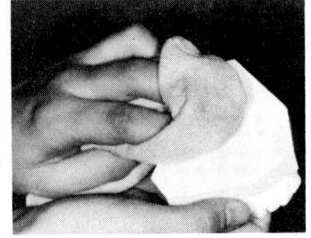

Fig. 36.33

9. Trim heel points to a plane one-half inch in width, at an angle of 125° with the heel of the casts (fig. 36.28-36.29).
   a. Casts are placed in occlusion for this cut on each corner.
10. Finishing the casts (figs. 36.30-36.33).
    a. Fill all holes by working soft plaster into the cast with your finger.
    b. Use a file to smooth the art portion of the cast.
    c. Let the casts dry thoroughly.
    d. Soak for thirty minutes in soap solution or other cast-finishing solution.
    e. Shine the casts by rubbing with a chamois or soft flannel.

Articulating Working Models

If an upper and a lower cast are to be mounted in their proper relationship, they are to be *articulated*. Some method of positioning is provided at the time the impressions are taken, usually by placing small pieces of softened wax in the mouth. The patient is asked to close with the pieces of wax in position. The wax registers the position of the upper teeth in relation to the lower teeth. When the wax is inserted between the upper and lower casts, and the teeth are fitted into the indentations, the cast will be in the same relationship as the upper and lower arches were when the patient registered their position in the wax in his mouth.

While the casts are retained in this position, they may be mounted in an articulator to provide a record of the relationship.

Denture Models

Denture models are of two types: full-denture models or partial-denture models. Full-denture impressions, then, will be impressions of *edentulous* ridges—the ridges without teeth present. Partial-denture impressions may include any number of teeth, *dentulous*. Study models may be poured in plaster, and working models are generally poured in artificial stone of the type preferred by your dentist.

Full-denture impressions can be boxed in the same manner as other impressions. Care must be taken, however, to include all the area desired for the construction of the denture. Since no teeth are present, the limits of the cast are dictated by other anatomical landmarks.

Either the dentist or the dental assistant (where state law permits) takes impressions with alginate for study models.

Study models made from these impressions are used to form a special tray to be used in taking the final impression. This special tray may be made from baseplates provided for that purpose. When the tray is prepared, the dentist proceeds to make the final impression of the edentulous ridge areas, frequently with a zinc oxide impression paste. The final cast is poured in these impressions in the same

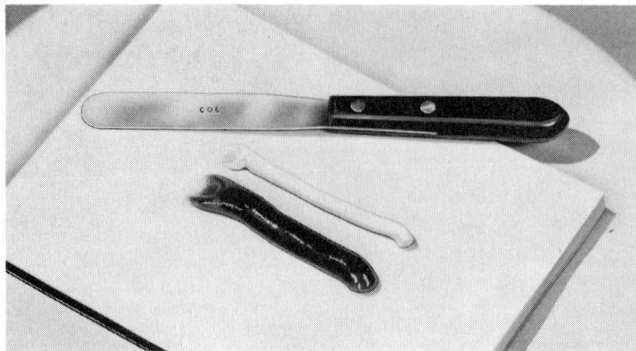

Fig. 36.34. Portions of Coe-Flo placed on mixing pad.

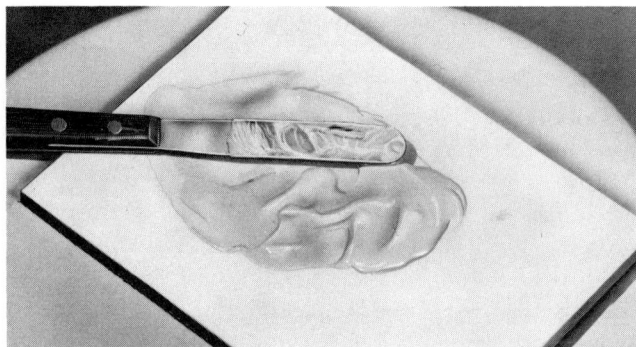

Fig. 36.35. Coe-Flo uniformly mixed in 30 seconds

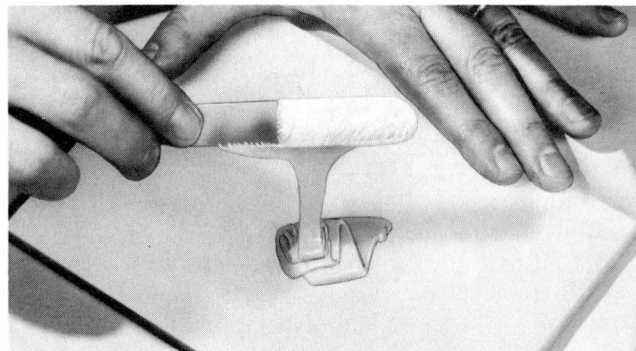

Fig. 36.36. Coe-Flo ready to place in primary impression.

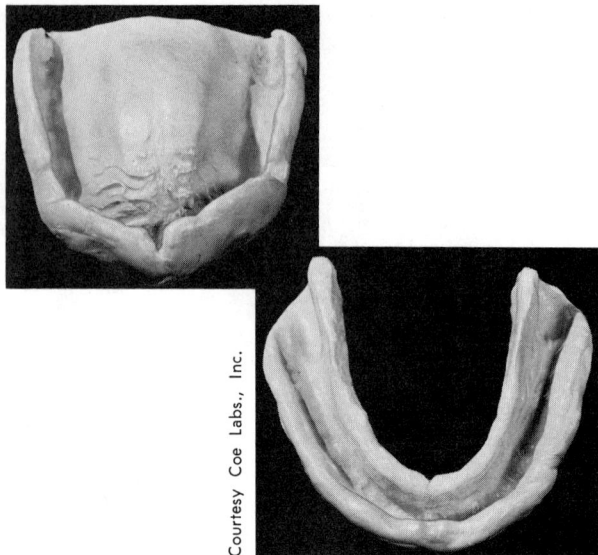

Fig. 36.37. Primary impressions finished in Coe-Flo ready to be boxed and poured.

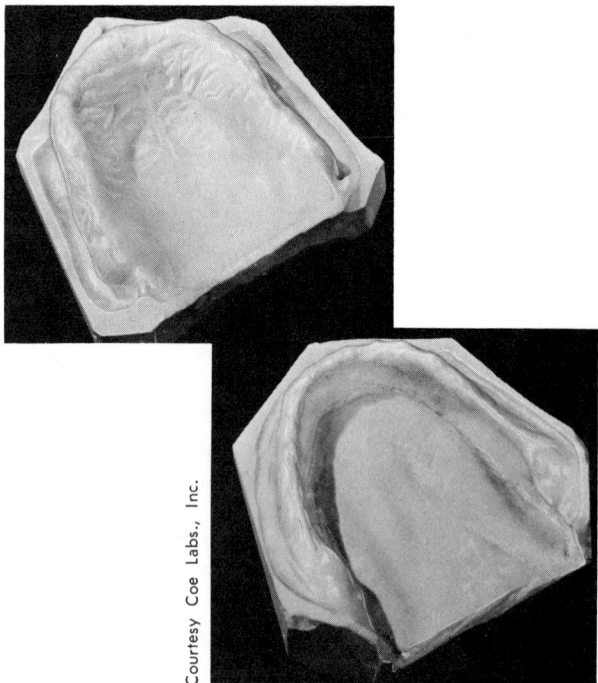

Fig. 36.38. Finished casts poured in Coecal

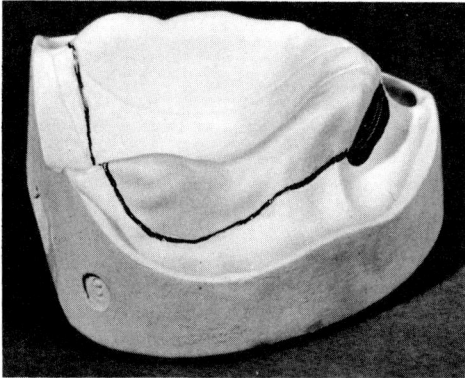

Fig. 36.39. Making an individualized impression tray. This is a cast of upper tissue area with outline indicating desired denture coverage. Note anterior undercut filled with red wax.

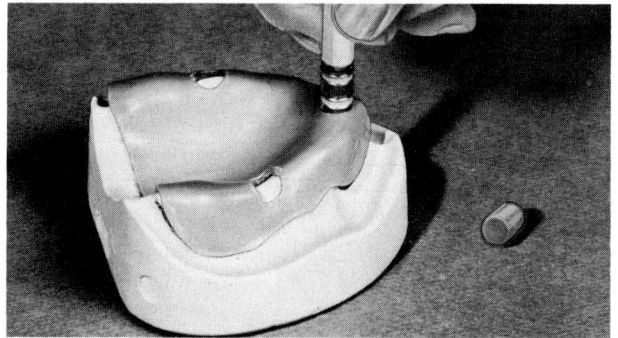

Fig. 36.40. Wax spacer adapted over cast, showing method of cutting holes to provide "stops" in the individualized tray. After eraser is removed from pencil, metal ferrule is slightly heated before use.

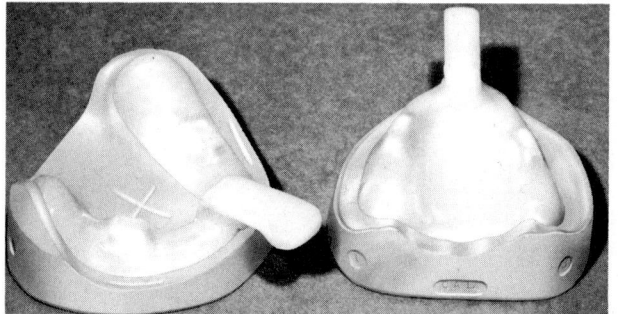

Fig. 36.41. Completed lower and upper individualized trays adapted to casts, showing handles attached.

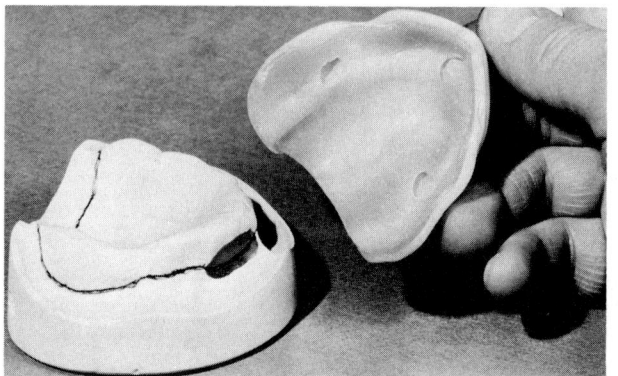

Fig. 36.42. Completed upper tray separated from cast but still containing the wax spacer. Note formation of "stops." Spacer must be removed from trays before the impression paste is applied.

manner as with any other impression material; no coating is required over the zinc oxide paste. To separate, the cast and impression are immersed in water at about 160° for ten minutes, after which separation is easily accomplished because the zinc oxide paste and the base material will be softened to some degree to facilitate peeling it from the cast and tray. Remember to mark the casts with the patient's name immediately after separation and trimming.

Casts for partial dentures must be separated very carefully from the impression material, especially if isolated teeth are present in the arch. These can be very easily fractured during separation unless the cast is withdrawn from the impression in a line parallel to the long axis of the teeth. Trial bases may be constructed for partial denture procedures, particularly if more than half the teeth are missing from the arch involved. If less than half the teeth are missing, the dentist very frequently will arrange some form of bite registration at the time the impressions are taken.

Trial Bases

Trial bases are then constructed for the full-denture cases. First, a base of *baseplate* gutta-percha is made to fit the cast much the same as the finished denture is to be constructed. The baseplate gutta-percha is warmed in the flame of a gas burner and carefully molded to the cast. The excess around the periphery of the baseplate gutta-percha is trimmed with a scissors or hot knife blade when the baseplate is in a softened condition.

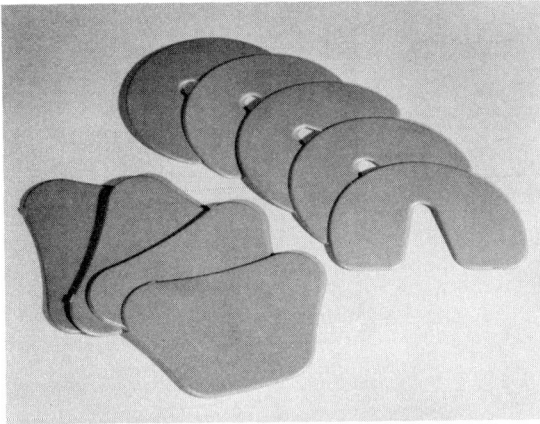

Fig. 36.44. Occlusal wax rims

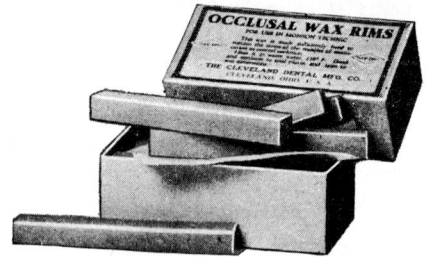

Fig. 36.43. Trial baseplates

Bite Rims

A wax *bite rim* is next applied to the baseplate gutta-percha. Wax bite-rim material is supplied in 4½-inch bars of wax about ½ inch square in cross section. These are softened in warm water. (The softening temperature is usually about 125° unless otherwise stated on the box in which the wax rims are supplied.) They are then molded into a curve corresponding with the curve of the dental ridge on the cast. Melted wax is used to fill in the spaces and angles between the baseplate gutta-percha and the wax bite rim until a smooth contour is established. When well filled in, the wax surface may be "flamed" slightly and wiped with a dry towel to produce a shiny, smooth surface.

In some dental offices the upper trial base is constructed with a wax bite rim, and the opposing lower rim is built up in modeling compound. When using modeling compound for this purpose, care must be exercised to prevent burning your fingers. Keep your fingers moistened when working with warm modeling compound to prevent burns and to prevent the modeling compound from sticking to your fingers.

After dentures are processed by the commercial laboratory, they are frequently remounted in the articulator to recheck articulation of the teeth. If the original mounting has not been preserved by the laboratory (using a *split-cast* technique in processing), then a new base to hold the finished denture must be made. Since most dentures will have some areas which are *undercuts,* they could not be removed from a plaster base which is poured directly into the denture. To facilitate removal from these temporary bases, the tissue side of the denture is lightly coated with Vaseline; then all the undercut areas are filled in with wet pumice or wet cotton patted to place with the finger. When the plaster base is made over this preparation, the denture can be easily removed when desired and is easily cleaned.

Dies or Positives of the Impressions

The Amalgam Die

Impressions taken with impression compound in a copper band are usually impressions of a full-crown preparation. This may be used to construct an amalgam die, a positive of the impression made of the same material as the amalgam restoration your dentist uses every day.

The excess impression material is carefully trimmed away. The impression, in the copper band in which it was taken, is then embedded in a larger rubber ring filled with semi-firm plaster to provide a solid support against the pressure of condensing the amalgam into the impression.

The amalgam material is prepared as for an amalgam restoration. Use a very wet portion of amalgam and carefully fill the impression. Use small pieces of amalgam and condense them with the shaped end of an orangewood stick. Care must be exercised not to damage the inner surface of the impression.

When the coronal portion of the impression has been filled, greater pressure may be applied in condensing the amalgam. Excess mercury is removed whenever possible as the condensing proceeds. The final addition of amalgam is made with the amalgam wrung out as dry as possible.

The amalgam die is allowed to set, preferably overnight, before separation is accomplished. The plaster matrix can be broken away from the copper band and the "root" portion of the die. The impression material can be warmed very cautiously in a flame or in the compound heater, and the amalgam die can be withdrawn from the impression.

The Stone Die

The rubber-base impression materials *can* be used to construct an amalgam die, but it is preferable to use a die stone made for the pur-

pose. An individual tooth impression of this material, either in a copper band or in a tray, is first wrapped either with a section of sheet boxing wax, softened and molded around the tray or band, or with a strip of very heavy tinfoil. In either case, the wrapping should be deep enough to provide for forming a "root" for each prepared tooth.

The special die stone is then prepared according to the manufacturer's directions and either vacuumed to remove entrapped fine air bubbles or vibrated onto a piece of paper towelling and squeezed to remove excess water, as well as to reduce the likelihood of bubbles.

An individual tooth impression may be completely poured in one section. A quadrant impression or full-arch impression can be prepared as illustrated to provide the removable individual dies of the prepared teeth. (See figs. 36.49-36.130.)

Model Kryptex Die

Model Kryptex, a material very similar to synthetic porcelain, is sometimes used for individual dies. It is mixed on a glass slab to a heavy consistency. The die is boxed with plaster, wax, or tinfoil. Small pieces of Model Kryptex in a puttylike consistency are packed firmly into the impression. Vibration is helpful.

Model Kryptex and silver amalgam when used for dies are preferably used in an impression taken in an inelastic material such as modeling compound. The die stones are preferably used with the elastic impression materials.

Electroplating

Many dental offices perform another operation in the preparation of dies before they are used for constructing the wax pattern. This additional operation consists of giving the impression a coating of copper by electroplating processes. It is considered an effective way of securing a better working surface on the die.

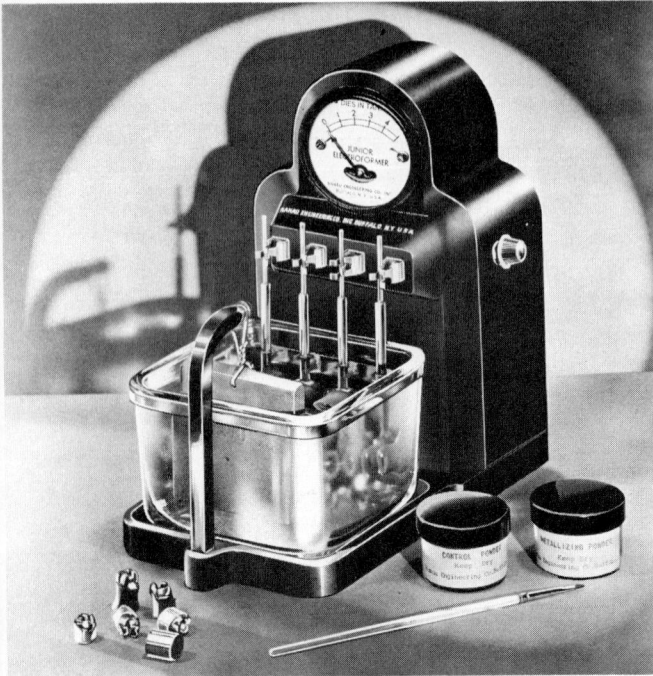

Courtesy Hanau Engr. Co., Inc.

Fig. 36.45. Hanau junior electroformer for plating dies with copper.

When the amalgam, stone, or other material is then packed into the impression after the impression has been electroplated with copper, it is allowed to set hard in the usual manner. Upon separation, the copper shell which has been deposited in the impression forms the outer surface of the die. The thickness of the copper is controlled by the length of time the impression is plated and the amount of current used during this period of time. The process is always begun at a slow rate, which can be increased once the initial film of copper has been deposited, until the thickness has reached the point preferred by the dentist. Copper-plated dies are used very well with a light coating of Kerr's Microfilm as a separating medium.

Lubricating the Die

The amalgam die is coated with Kerr's Microfilm or similar separating media. A die of artificial stone may be soaked or vacuumed in a mixture of fifty percent glycerin and fifty percent water, dried, and then given a light coating of Kerr's Microfilm. These surface coatings facilitate removal of the wax pattern after it has been shaped on the die and is to be sprued. Without such a coating, the wax pattern is almost impossible to remove without fracturing. The lubricant used should be water-soluble—never use machine oil. It should be a thin lubricant—and do not use too much. An oily lubricant, or too much of any kind of lubricant, can result in a rough casting.

Copings

After the dentist has made individual dies of crown preparations in the construction of a bridge, he may decide to make copings for the abutment teeth. A coping is made as a thimble which fits over each crown preparation. It is placed in the mouth over the crown preparation to check the gingival fit. When the dentist is satisfied that the gingival fit of each coping is accurate, he places the copings over each crown and takes a plaster impression, embedding them in the plaster. The impression is

Fig. 36.46. A plaster impression taken with two copings in position on the prepared teeth.

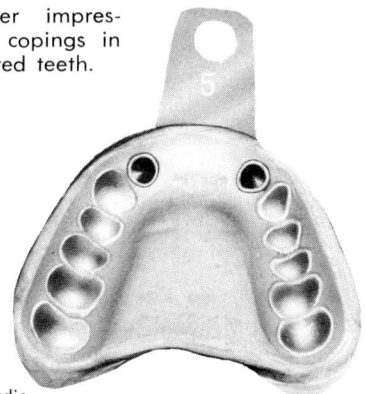

Courtesy Kramer Dental Studio

Fig. 36.47. The opposing arch impression taken in modeling compound or alginate.

Courtesy Kramer Dental Studio

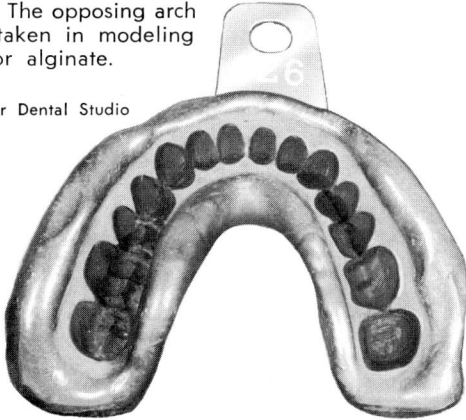

Fig. 36.48. A wafer wax bite taken to assist in mounting the upper and lower casts in their proper relationship before actual crown and bridge laboratory work is begun.

Courtesy Kramer Dental Studio

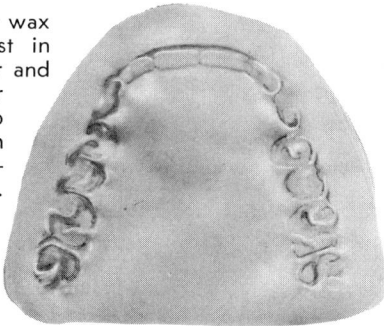

allowed to set and is then removed from the mouth as any other plaster impression would be. Now the individual dies of the crown preparations which were previously made are set in the copings in the impression, and a working model is poured. When the model is separated, the dies will be in their proper relationship because the copings will have held them accurately in place.

Indirect and Fixed Bridge Technique

An indirect inlay and indirect fixed bridge technique is illustrated on the following pages. Those portions of the procedure which are performed by the dentist are also illustrated in order to present a complete technique. (All photographs in this series courtesy of the Kerr Manufacturing Company, Detroit, Michigan.)

Tray Impression for Single or Multiple Inlays

This series begins with figures 36.49 and continues through figure 36.67, page 490.

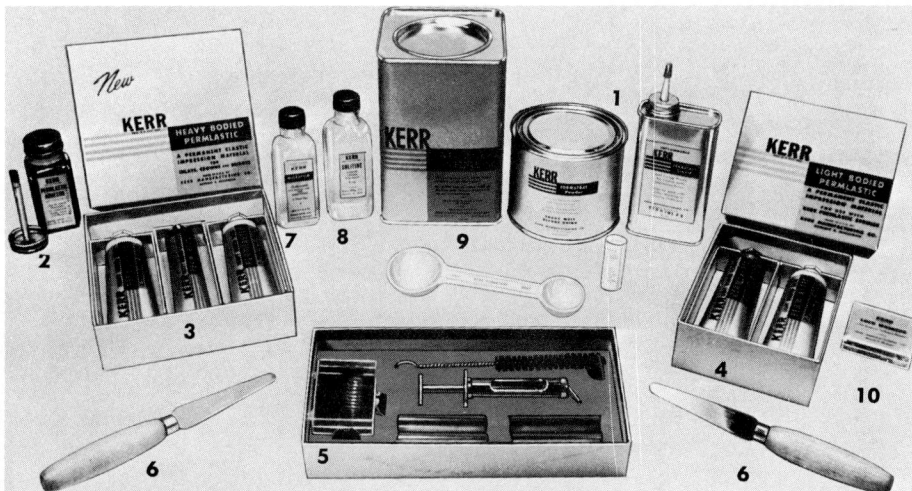

Fig. 36.49. The armamentarium used in the Permlastic inlay and fixed bridge technique. (1) Formatray, a plastic tray-making material. (2) Permlastic adhesive. (3) Heavy-Bodied Permlastic. (4) Light-Bodied Permlastic. (5) Permlastic Syringe. (6) Spatulas. (7) Microfilm. (8) Solitine. (9) Vel Mix Stone. (10) Lock washers.

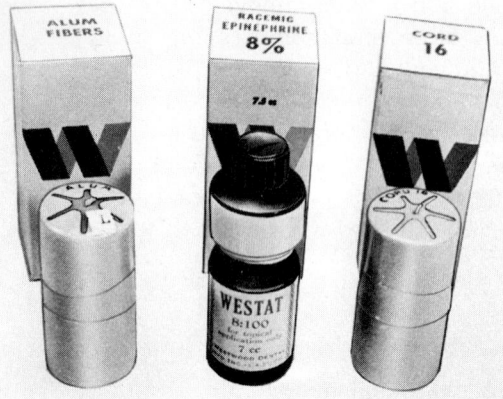

Fig. 36.50. Subgingival margins of the preparations in the mouth must be exposed. A tissue retraction kit for this purpose is available.

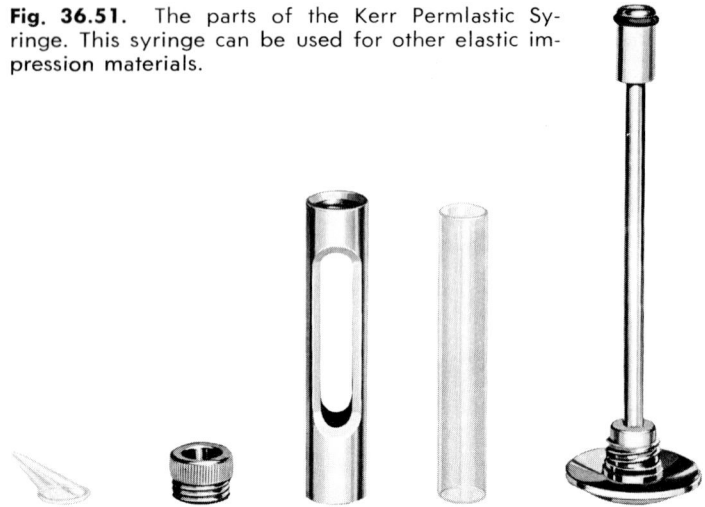

Fig. 36.51. The parts of the Kerr Permlastic Syringe. This syringe can be used for other elastic impression materials.

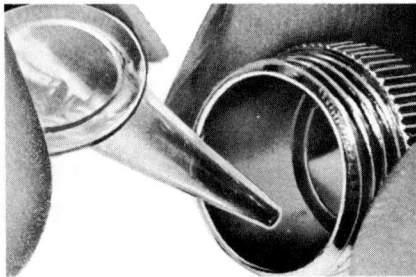

Fig. 36.52. To assemble the syringe for use, first insert the plastic tip into the tip retainer. Screw retainer into metal barrel.

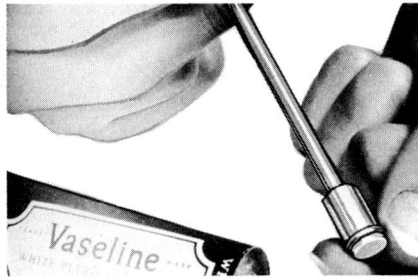

Fig. 36.53. Lightly lubricate the rubber ring washer with white petroleum jelly.

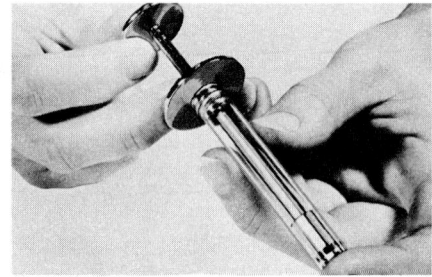

Fig. 36.54. Insert plunger into plastic sleeve and push forward until plunger is flush with end of plastic sleeve.

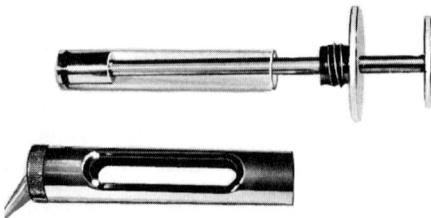

Fig. 36.55. Prepared syringe is set aside until Light-Bodied Permlastic has been mixed.

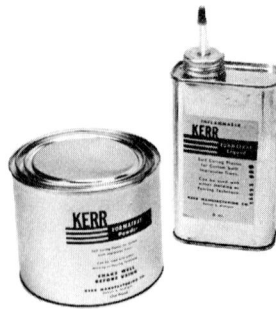

Fig. 36.56. Kerr Formatray, powder and liquid used to make the impression tray.

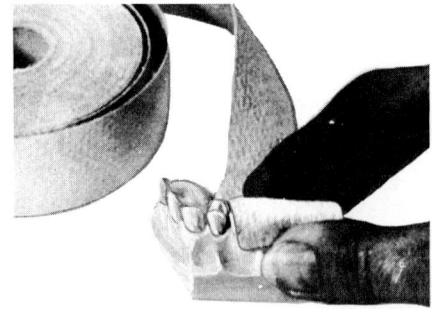

Fig. 36.57. Asbestos is used as a spacer.

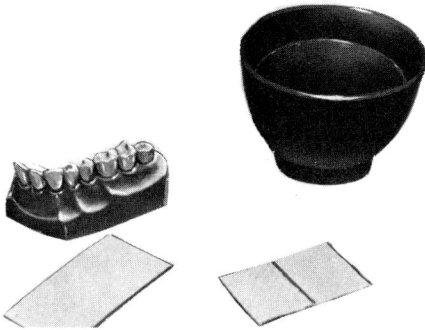

Fig. 36.58. Cut two pieces of asbestos

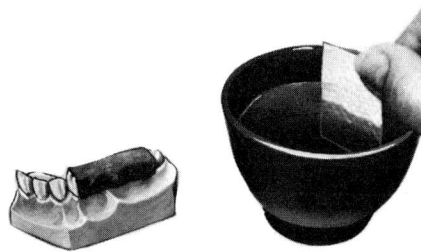

Fig. 36.59. The short piece is moistened and folded (as marked in photograph). Place over the teeth.

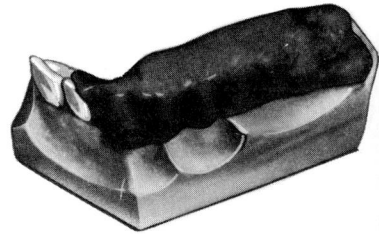

Fig. 36.60. Second piece is moistened and adapted lengthwise.

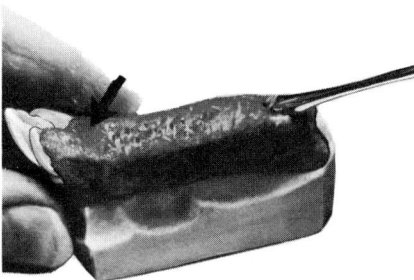

Fig. 36.61. Remove asbestos from two small areas to provide stops to prevent tray seating too far when actual impression is taken.

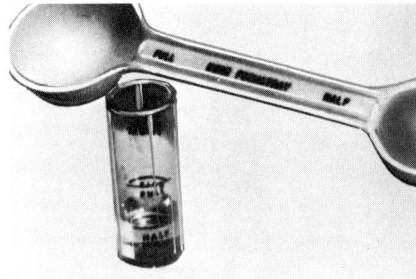

Fig. 36.62. Use one-half measure of powder and liquid. (Fill to the lower blue line in the measure.)

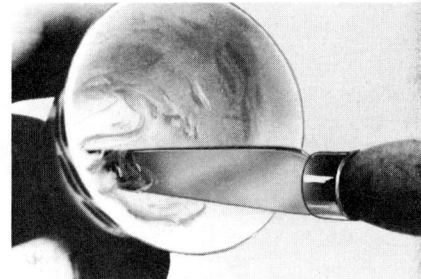

Fig. 36.63. Combine powder and liquid in a 30-second mix.

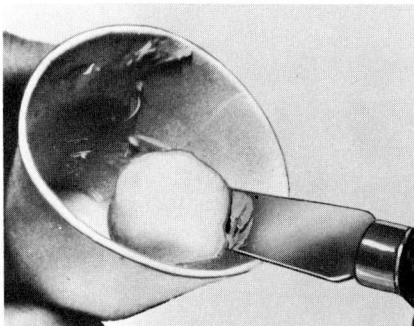

Fig. 36.64. Allow to stand until nonsticky (two to three minutes).

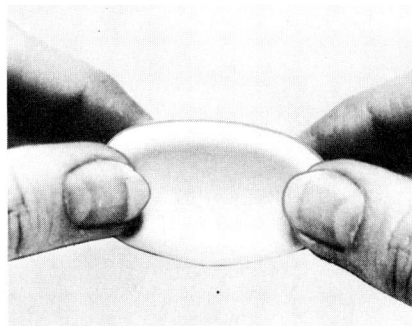

Fig. 36.65. Preform to approximate size.

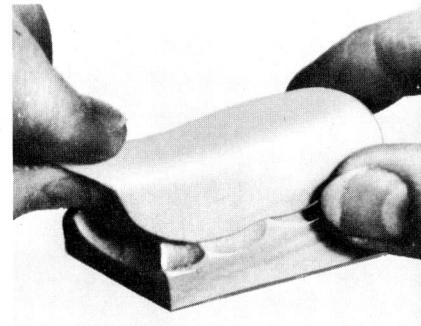

Fig. 36.66. Adapt Formatray over asbestos and form a handle.

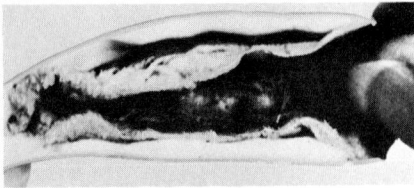

Fig. 36.67. Remove tray in seven to ten minutes. Strip out asbestos.

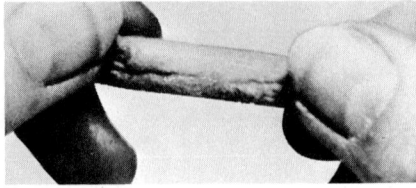

Fig. 36.68. Form asbestos into roll and save (see 36.72).

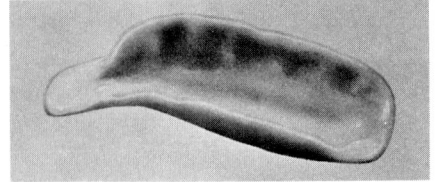

Fig. 36.69. The finished, custom-built tray has been brushed free of any remaining asbestos.

Making the Impression in the Custom-made Tray *(Figs. 36.71-36.85)*

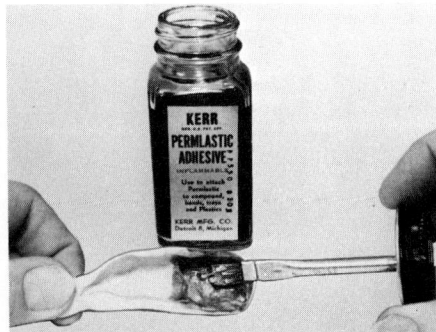

Fig. 36.70. Apply Permlastic Adhesive lightly to all inner and peripheral surfaces. Permit adhesive to dry.

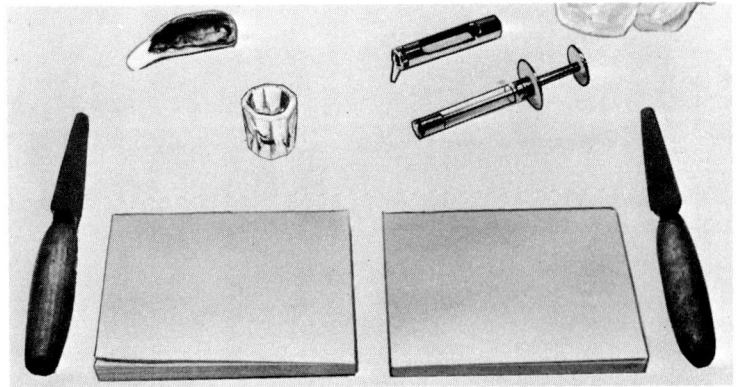

Fig. 36.71. With syringe and tray now prepared, lay out Permlastic mixing pads, spatulas, and dappen dish.

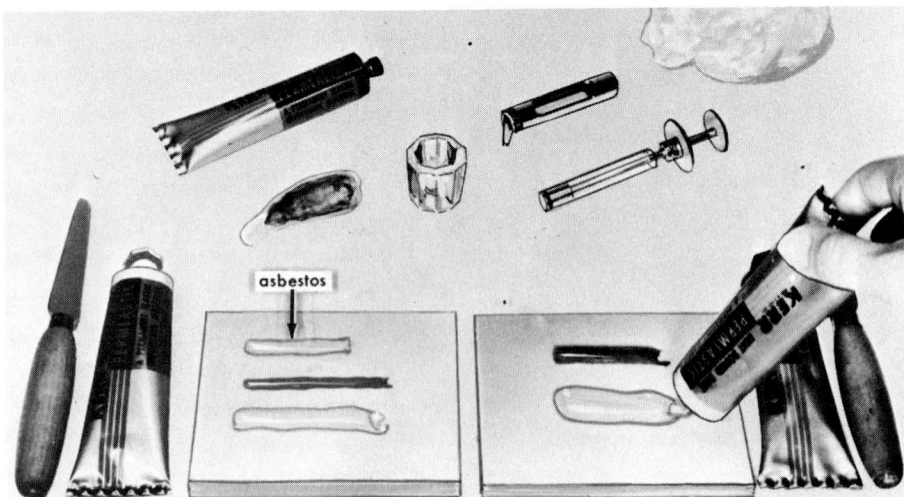

asbestos

Fig. 36.72. Heavy-Bodied: The length of asbestos roll formed from the tray spacer (plus one-half inch) serves as a guide for the length of Heavy-Bodied Base and Catalyst to be extruded.
Light-Bodied: Extrude equal lengths each (one and one-half to two inches) of Base and Catalyst.

Fig. 36.73. Mix Light-Bodied Permlastic, Base and Catalyst, in 45 to 60 seconds. Complete loading of syringe so that over-all time does not exceed one and one-half minutes from beginning of mix.

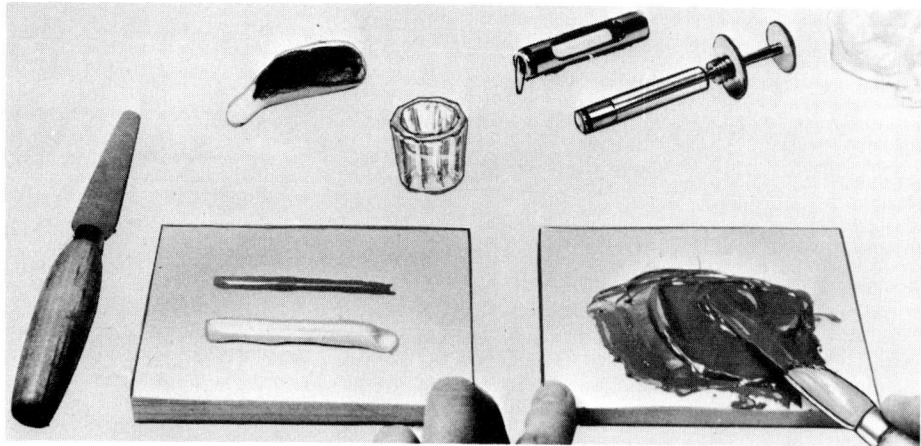

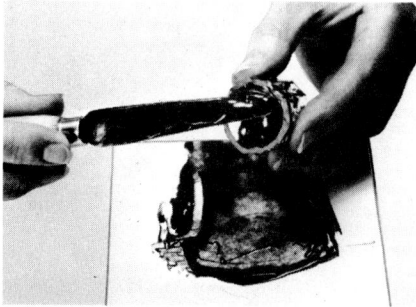

Fig. 36.74. Transfer entire mix of Light-Bodied Permlastic from mixing pad to dappen dish.

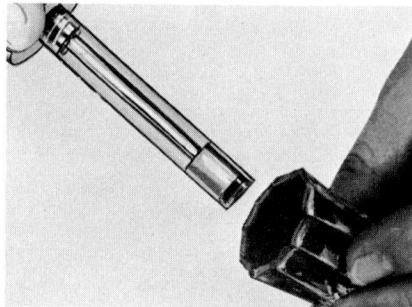

Fig. 36.75. Insert plastic sleeve of syringe with plunger into filled dappen dish.

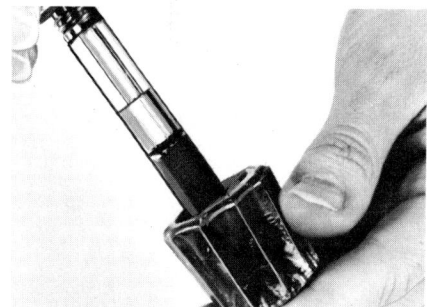

Fig. 36.76. With locking disc forced against plastic sleeve, draw plunger back slowly to fill sleeve.

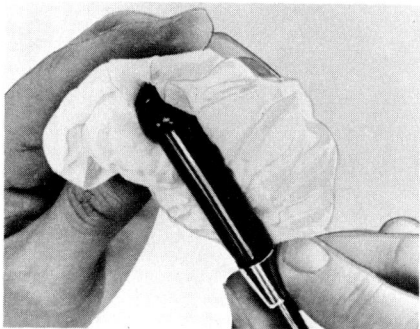

Fig. 36.77. Grasp plastic sleeve at locking disc end and wipe opposite end (which was in the dappen dish) free from all Permlastic.

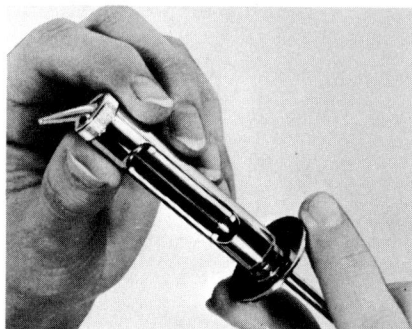

Fig. 36.78. Place filled plastic sleeve into metal barrel of syringe and screw locking disc down as far as possible. **Tighten securely.**

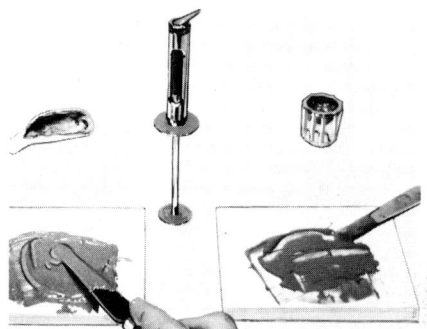

Fig. 36.79. Mix Heavy-Bodied Permlastic, Base and Catalyst, for approximately one minute.

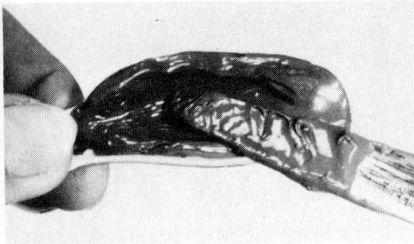

Fig. 36.80. The dentist may have his dental assistant spread Heavy-Bodied Permlastic over all adhesive-covered surfaces of the tray, using remainder of mix to fill tray. Effort is made to prevent trapping air in the material.

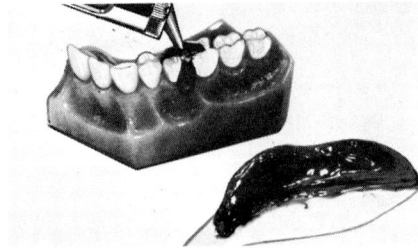

Fig. 36.81. While the dental assistant is preparing the tray, the dentist will dry the prepared teeth, and with the syringe, inject Light-Bodied Permlastic into all preparations. He over-fills preparations and injects material into the subgingival crevices. Care is exercised, again, to prevent trapping air.

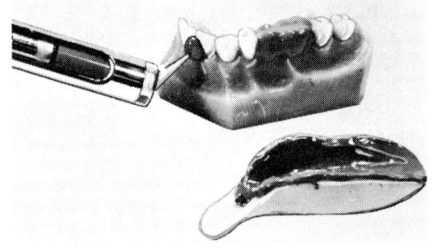

Fig. 36.82. The last small amount of Light-Bodied Permlastic is ejected, by the dentist, between teeth in an area not involved in the impression. This material provides a means of checking for set.

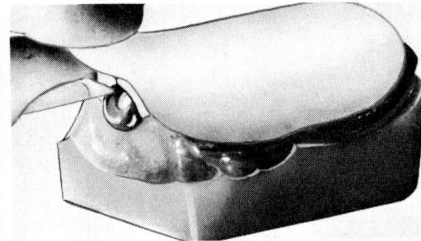

Fig. 36.83. The dentist immediately seats the tray with a slight rocking motion.

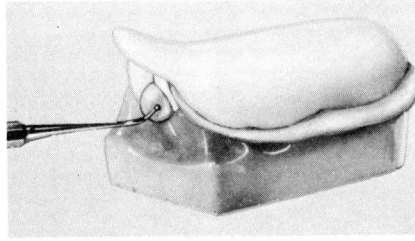

Fig. 36.84. Approximately ten minutes after beginning the mix of Light-Bodied Permlastic, the small specimen amount is checked for set, and the tray is removed from the mouth.

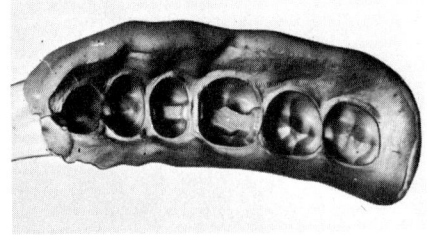

Fig. 36.85. Rinse the impression. Blow dry before pouring the model.

Alternate Reline Impression Technique

An alternate technique may be used. The Permlastic Reline Impression Technique is illustrated and described in figures 36.86-36.102.

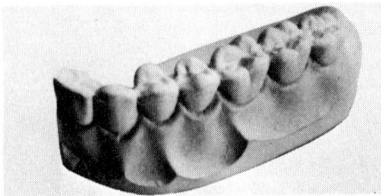

Fig. 36.86. After the Formatray tray has been completed, as illustrated in figures 36.57 through 36.70, the model used for making the tray is cleaned of any wax or asbestos.

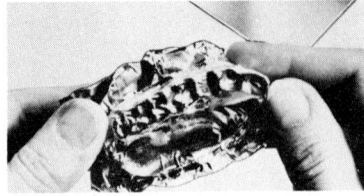

Fig. 36.87. A sheet of .002 tinfoil is pressed over the model with no attempt at close adaptation.

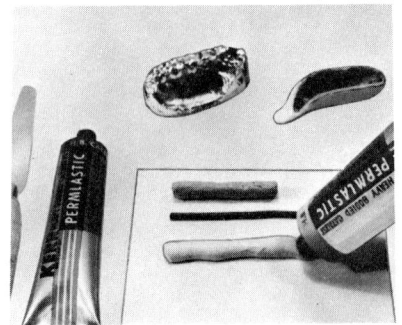

Fig. 36.88. Heavy-Bodied Permlastic is extruded onto the mixing pad. The length of asbestos roll formed from the tray spacer (plus one-half inch) serves as a guide for the length of Base and Catalyst to be extruded.

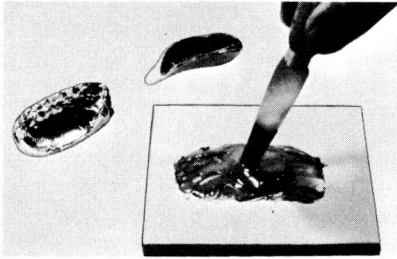

Fig. 36.89. The Heavy-Bodied Permlastic Base and Catalyst is mixed in a stirring motion with the tip of the spatula for approximately one minute.

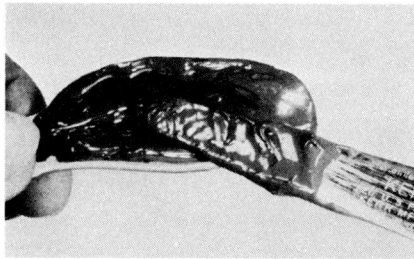

Fig. 36.90. The dentist may have his dental assistant spread Heavy-Bodied Permlastic over all adhesive-covered surfaces of the tray, using remainder of mix to fill tray. Effort is made to prevent trapping air in the material.

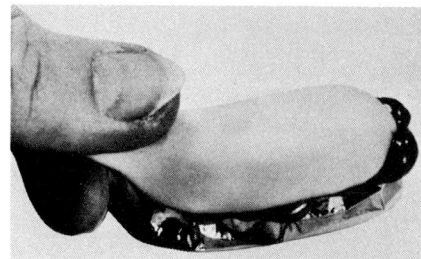

Fig. 36.91. Seat tray over tinfoil-covered model.

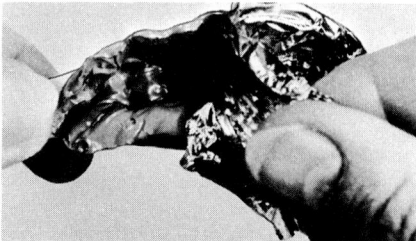

Fig. 36.92. After the Heavy-Bodied Permlastic has set approximately fifteen minutes, remove the tray from the model and strip tinfoil from the impression. This is the primary impression.

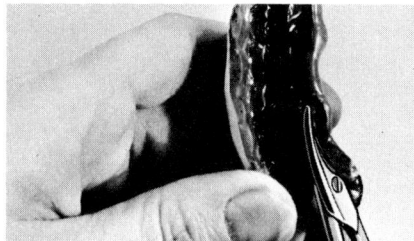

Fig. 36.93. The Heavy-Bodied Permlastic is trimmed from the periphery of the impression. It is now ready for completion, after the preparation of the involved teeth is accomplished in the patient's mouth, either at this appointment or a later one.

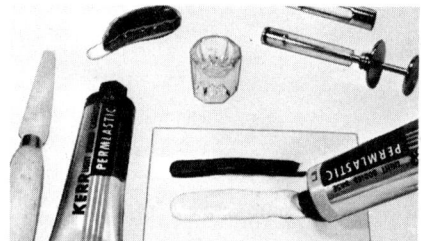

Fig. 36.94. The dentist is now ready to complete the impression. Extrude equal lengths of Light-Bodied Permlastic Base and Catalyst onto the mixing pad. Approximately three inches of each for an impression involving one quadrant.

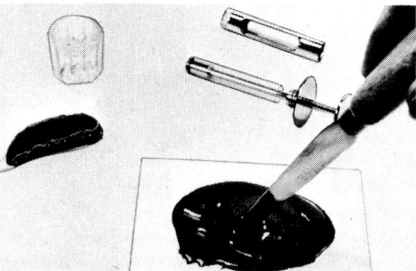

Fig. 36.95. Mix Light-Bodied Permlastic Base and Catalyst within 45 to 60 seconds.

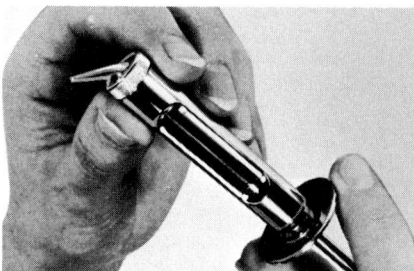

Fig. 36.96. Fill syringe with part of the mix as illustrated in figures 36.74 through 36.78.

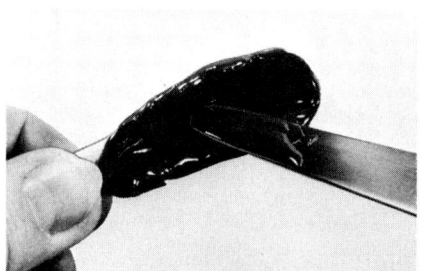

Fig. 36.97. Spread the remainder of the mix of Light-Bodied Permlastic over the entire surface of the Heavy-Bodied Permlastic primary impression.

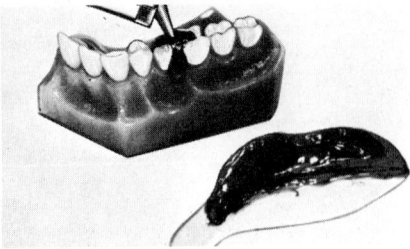

Fig. 36.98. The dentist will have dried the prepared teeth and with the syringe injected Light-Bodied Permlastic into the preparations, over-filling them, and also injected material into the subgingival crevices.

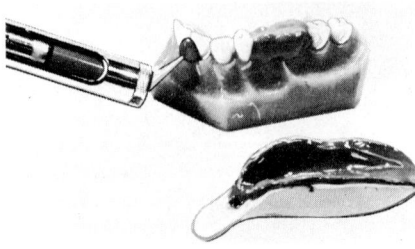

Fig. 36.99. The last small amount of Light-Bodied Permlastic is ejected, by the dentist, between teeth in an area not involved in the impression. This material provides a means of checking for set.

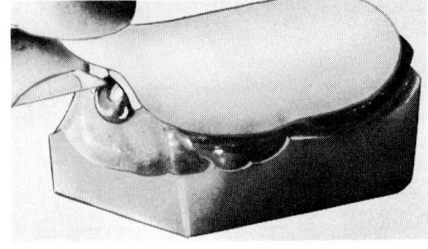

Fig. 36.100. The dentist immediately seats the tray with a slight rocking motion.

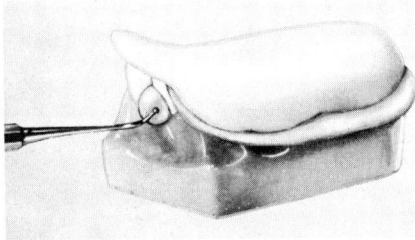

Fig. 36.101. Approximately ten minutes after beginning the mix of Light-Bodied Permlastic, the small specimen amount is checked for set, and the tray removed from the mouth.

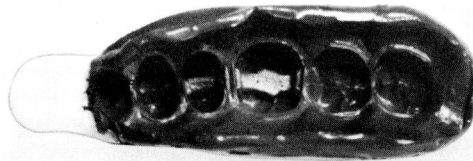

Fig. 36.102. Rinse the impression and blow it dry before pouring.

Pouring the Model (Figs. 36.103-111)

Models and dies can be poured in Vel Mix stone; or the Permlastic impressions can be electroplated, using the Kerr Silver Plating kit. The following will illustrate only the stone model technique.

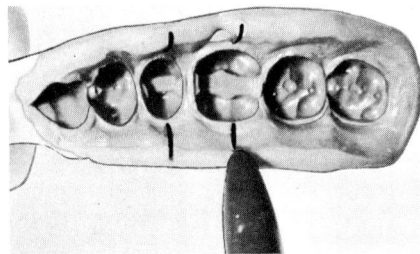

Fig. 36.103. With ball-point pen or pencil, draw guidelines on the impression for locating the prepared teeth and positioning dowel pins.

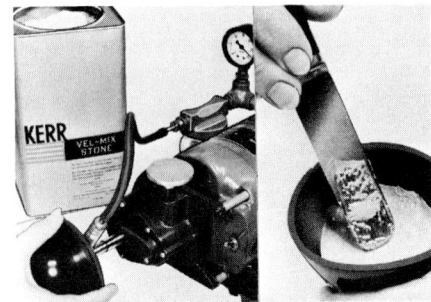

Fig. 36.104. Mix enough Vel Mix stone to fill impression three to five millimeters above the gingival of the teeth. Vacuum mixing is recommended, but mix can be completed by hand spatulation.

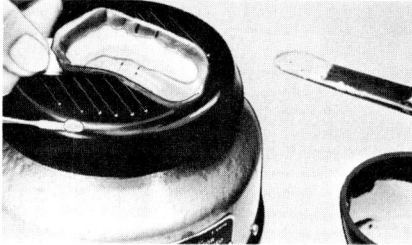

Fig. 36.105. Pour impression, using medium vibration. Make small additions of mixed stone until impression is filled three to five millimeters above teeth.

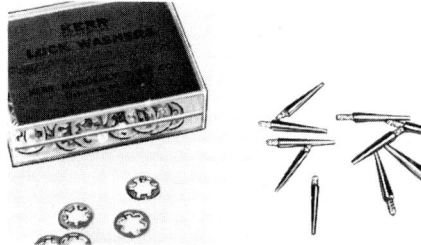

Fig. 36.106. Dowel pins are used to produce individual removable dies. Lock washers provide necessary anchorage between the two pours of stone.

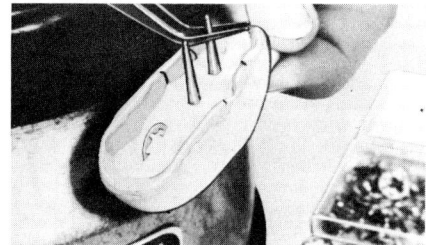

Fig. 36.107. Rest hand on vibrator with switch on low. Line up dowel pins with markings on impression and set into the soft stone. Set lock washers in sections which are not to be separated.

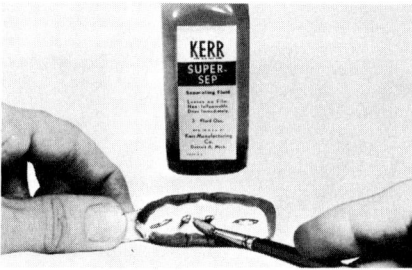

Fig. 36.108. Permit first pour of stone to set, then apply one or more coats of Super Sep over areas of dies that are to be removable.

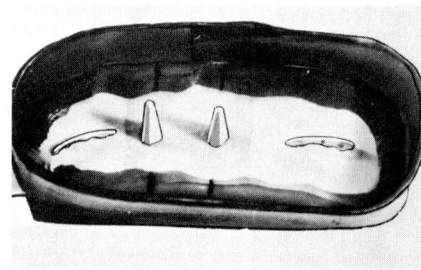

Fig. 36.109. Box impression preparatory to final pouring.

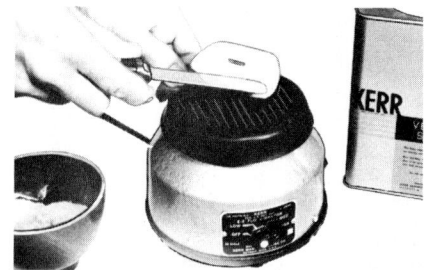

Fig. 36.110. Place a piece of utility wax across the ends of the dowel pins (to assist in locating them later). Make a second mix of Vel Mix stone and complete the pouring of the model.

Cutting the Removable Dies and Completing the Castings (Figs. 36.112-36.121)

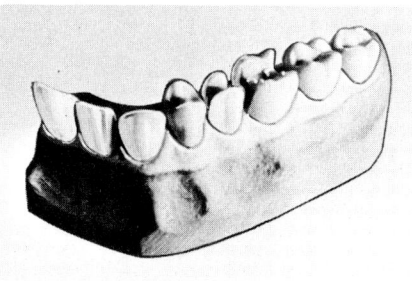

Fig. 36.111. Allow the second mix of stone to set, then separate the model from the impression.

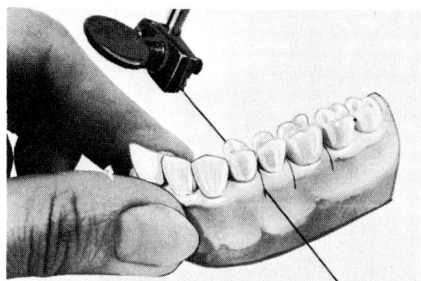

Fig. 36.112. Use a 2/0 gauge saw blade to cut through first pour of stone. See next figure for angle of cut.

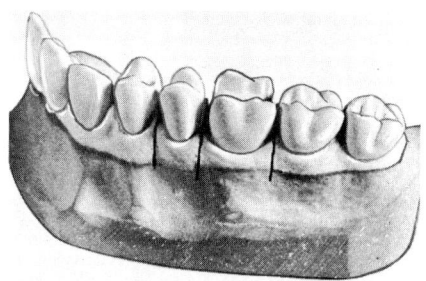

Fig. 36.113. Cuts must be either vertical or converging at the base of the first pour of stone to permit withdrawal of dies.

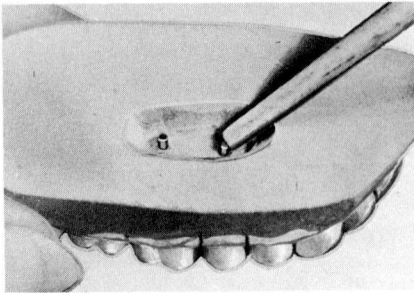

Fig. 36.114. Remove utility wax from ends of dowel pins. Tap dowel pins lightly to aid in removing the die from the model.

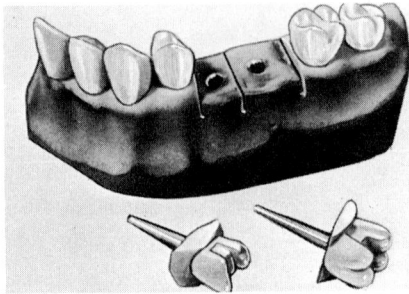

Fig. 36.115. The dies are now removed and ready for trimming.

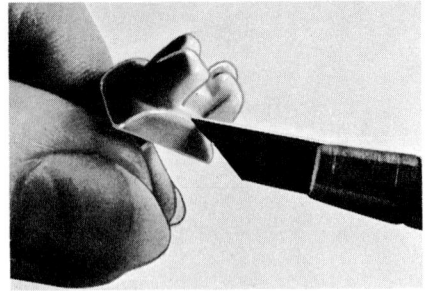

Fig. 36.116. Remove excess stone from gingival margins with a sharp blade.

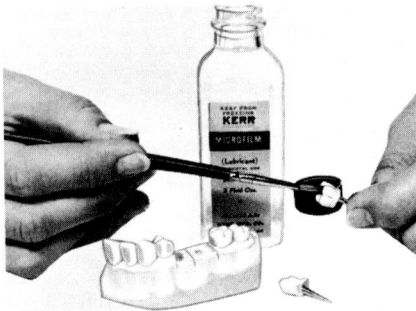

Fig. 36.117. Lubricate dies with microfilm.

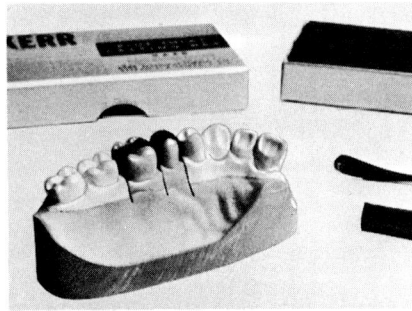

Fig. 36.118. Wax patterns on dies. Replace dies in model to establish contact areas. Occlusion is carved by manner of choice—either on opposing model, or a wax registration of the opposing teeth used as a part of the final wax-up.

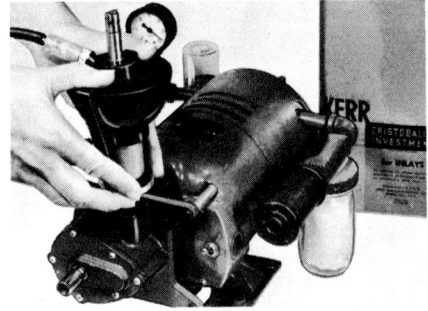

Fig. 36.119. Wax patterns are removed from dies, sprued and invested. Vacuum investing is preferred.

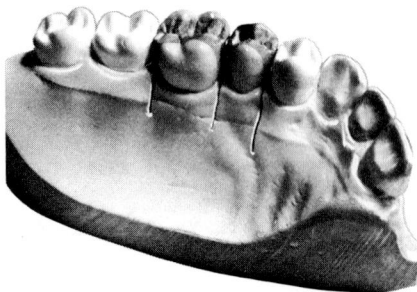

Fig. 36.120. Unpolished castings seated on stone dies.

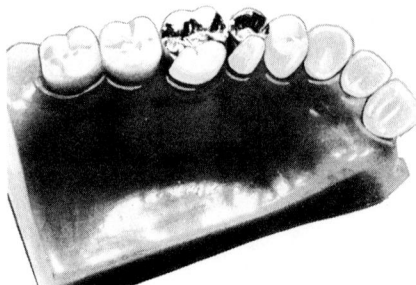

Fig. 36.121. Polished castings on model.

Fixed Bridge Impression Technique (Figs. 36.122-36.126)

Impressions for fixed bridges are taken in the same manner as those for single or multiple inlay impressions.

In constructing the bridge, however, it is sometimes desirable to keep the abutment teeth and the included ridge area of the model in one solid piece. (This is especially true in the most common bridge, that which replaces one missing tooth, a *three-tooth* bridge). To accomplish this goal it is necessary to make the teeth adjacent to the abutment teeth (beyond the bridge area) removable so that the wax patterns can be carved.

The accompanying figures illustrate pouring of the model for this method of bridge construction.

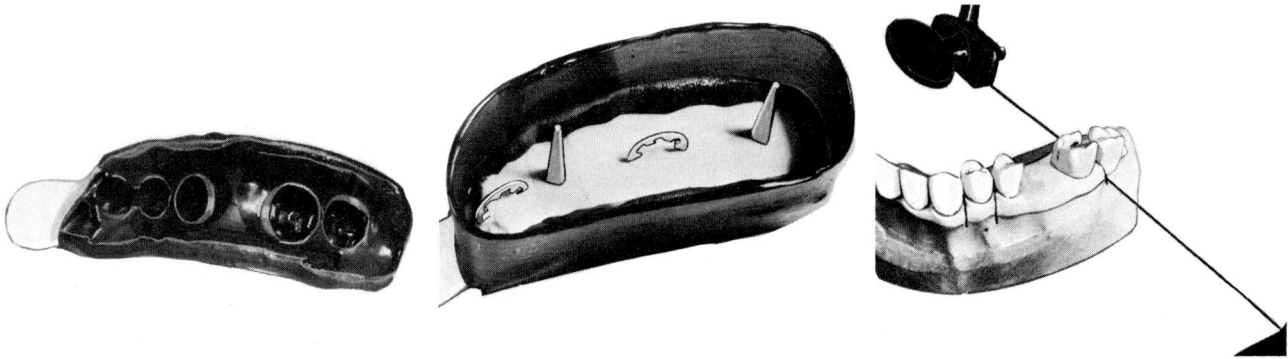

Fig. 36.122. Rinse and dry the completed impression. With ball-point pen or pencil draw guide lines to the teeth adjacent to the abutment teeth for the proper positioning of dowel pins.

Fig. 36.123. Prepare first mix of stone and pour model as illustrated and described in figures 36.105 through 36.109. Permit stone to set. Paint Super Sep over areas of teeth that are to be removable, and complete the pouring of the model.

Fig. 36.124. After stone is set, remove model from impression and section to enable removal of teeth adjacent to abutment teeth.

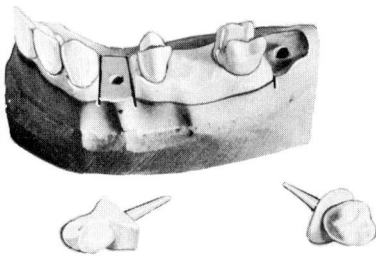

Fig. 36.125. Remove adjacent teeth, leaving entire bridge span attached to the main body of the model. Lubricate dies, wax, invest, burn out and cast the bridge according to your usual laboratory technique.

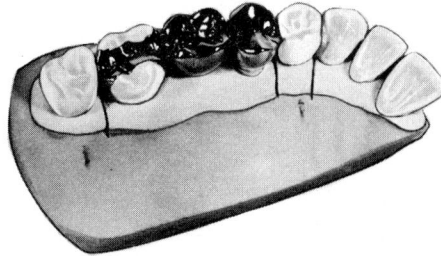

Fig. 36.126. Finished fixed bridge on Vel Mix stone model.

Copper-band Impressions
(Figs. 36.127-36.130)

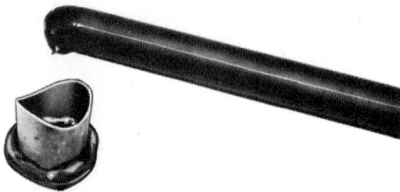

Fig. 36.129. Paint the inside of the band and reinforcing material with Permlastic Adhesive.

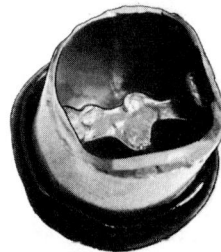

Fig. 36.127. Your dentist will select, festoon the band (trim the edge) to properly fit the gingival area of the prepared tooth. Reinforce the copper band by plugging one end with impression compound.

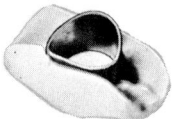

Fig. 36.128. Or the band can be reinforced by using Kerr Formatray.

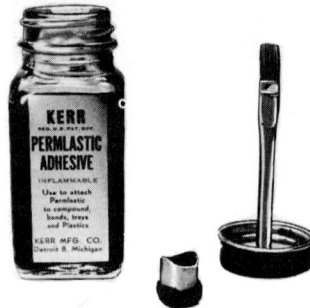

Fig. 36.130. Extrude one inch each of Base and Catalyst onto the mixing pad. Mix within thirty to sixty seconds. While your dentist is drying the tooth, load the band carefully so as to avoid air entrapment. When your dentist has completed the impression, blow it dry so he can inspect it. Pour the die according to your usual laboratory technique.

Emergency Denture Repair

One of the common denture emergencies is the breaking of the denture along the midline. The repair of this breakage can be accomplished as follows:

1. Lock the two halves into their proper relationship by placing short applicator sticks or wooden matchsticks across the arch, luting each end to the teeth with sticky wax. (The same process may be used if the denture is broken into more pieces, which occasionally occurs.)
2. Eliminate undercuts with wetted cotton or pumice.
3. Gently fill the tissue side of the denture with plaster. The line of fracture must be completely supported by plaster, however.
4. After the plaster has set, remove the pieces of the denture from the cast and wash them clean.
5. Widen the area of the fracture, using a vulcanite bur in a dental lathe or handpiece.
6. Cover the plaster which is in the area of the fracture with tinfoil, carefully burnishing it to place with a piece of cotton. An alternate method is to give the plaster a coating of *liquid foil* made for this purpose.
7. Reposition the pieces of the denture on the cast.
8. Now, by alternately adding repair powder and liquid, replace the area cut away through the fracture (fig. 36.131).
9. Thoroughly cure according to directions with the material you use. (The cure may be hastened by immersing the cast and denture in water.)
10. Trim and polish the repair area to create a smooth joint with the original denture parts.

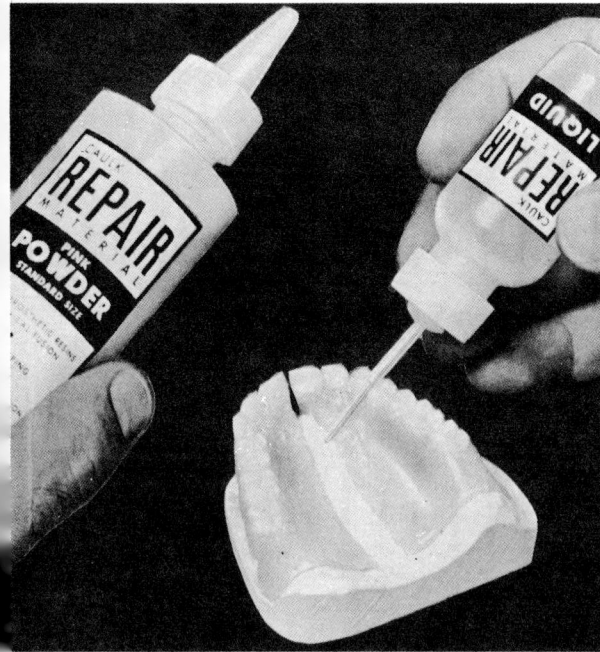

Fig. 36.131. Adding the powder and liquid to a denture fracture.

Summary

Two of the materials used to produce a positive cast or model from an impression are plaster and artificial stone. Each type of stone and plaster has specific uses in the dental office. They must be properly stored and carefully used. Be accurate in measuring water and powder when mixing them.

Directions for mixing plaster and stone vary and are given specifically in this chapter. Be sure you care for the bowls and spatulas when you are through with the mixing process.

A model may be boxed to conserve on plaster and make it easier to pour a good model.

Models should be properly poured, separated for trimming orthodontic models.

Models are mounted on an articulator to provide a working relationship for construction of inlays, crowns, bridges, and partial or full dentures.

Full- and partial-denture casts must be handled carefully. Impression trays and trial bases may be constructed for full-denture cases.

Single-tooth impressions are used to construct an amalgam die, a positive model of the impression of the tooth. Stone is also used to make a die, as is Model Kryptex. The die stones are preferably used with elastic impression materials; the amalgam and Model Kryptex dies are used with inelastic materials such as modeling compound.

Some offices also electroplate the impression. It gives a better working surface on the die.

There are several materials which can be used to lubricate the die so that it will permit the wax pattern to slip off without fracturing when it has been completed.

It is possible to make custom trays for impressions for both single and multiple inlays and bridges. Some four techniques for different procedures are illustrated, in addition to pouring models with removable dies.

You may frequently make emergency repairs of dentures with laboratory supplies available in your office.

Study Questions

1. Explain the uses in the dental office of artificial stone and plaster.
2. Describe the difference in mixing artificial stone and plaster.
3. Explain boxing—its process and purpose.
4. Describe the steps in preparing models.
5. Describe the preparation of orthodontic models.
6. Define *die*.
7. What materials are used to make a die?
8. What is the purpose of copings?
9. Describe four techniques for constructing custom trays.
10. Describe an emergency denture repair.

37 | *The Basic Principles of Casting to Dimension*

The process of constructing restorations outside the mouth includes three important stages. In the last two chapters we have learned to take an impression of an area in the mouth after it has been prepared for the restoration; then we learned to make a wax model or pattern, invest it, and burn it out. The hardened investment material now contains a hole shaped like the inlay or crown which is to be made of gold alloy.

The next process, to cast the gold alloy into the hole in the investment material, is the subject of this chapter.

Successful Casting Technique

A successful inlay casting technique[1] must produce accurately fitting inlays. To do this it must utilize the dimensional changes of the wax, investment, and gold in such a manner that the shrinkages and expansions balance out, with the net result that the casting is neither smaller nor larger than the wax pattern which was originally made to fit the preparation. There are a number of ways they

1. This section "Successful Casting Technique," through the courtesy of J. M. Ney Co., Hartford, Connecticut, with modifications.

can be made to counterbalance each other. Theoretically, it should be possible to measure exactly the amount of shrinkage or expansion of each material and the effects on these dimensional changes of variations in manipulative procedure and, solely with the aid of these data, to select a combination of materials and technique that would invariably produce the required accuracy. From a practical standpoint, the problem is not so simple as this, and a certain amount of "cut and try" is necessary. Nevertheless, a basic understanding of the properties of the materials used and of the effects of variations in manipulative procedure does make it possible to establish a satisfactory technique with a minimum of experimentation and to standardize the various steps so that consistent results will be obtained.

The principal shrinkage to be taken into account is the casting shrinkage of gold which, in common with most materials, expands when heated and contracts when cooled. Since the gold must be liquid to cast, the mold is filled with expanded metal which shrinks as it cools to room temperature. Unless compensated by an expanded mold, the casting will be too small. The casting shrinkage of gold alloys was studied at the National Bureau of Standards, and the results were published in Research Paper No. 32. It was found that in every case the net casting shrinkage was less than the free thermal contraction of the metal from its solidifying temperature to room temperature. This was thought to be due, at least in part, to the fact that at very high temperatures the metal was quite weak and might actually be weaker than the investment, so that if there was any interlocking between the casting and the investment mold, the cooling metal would be held and stretched by the investment and thus prevented from shrinking its normal amount. This suggests that thin castings and those which, because of their irregular shape, would be well locked in the investment mold might

show somewhat less shrinkage than bulky castings or those with fewer irregularities. This may explain why bulky castings appear to require more compensation than thin ones, and one-surface inlays more than two- or three-surface inlays. It may also explain why the tests made at the Bureau of Standards on gold rods 0.12 of an inch in diameter and 3¼ inches long, cast under dental laboratory conditions, showed a net linear casting shrinkage of 1¼ percent, while more recent tests made on much shorter and bulkier rods, cast in abnormally weak investment molds, showed shrinkages ranging up to about 1.6 percent. There is also evidence that casting golds with varying compositions have slightly different casting shrinkages, but these differences appear to be so small as to be of little practical significance.

Other factors which might make the casting too small include possible shrinkages of the impression and die materials in the indirect method, and thermal contraction of the wax pattern. Impression materials, for instance, have relatively high rates of contraction on cooling which can result in serious inaccuracies if uncontrolled. However, if the compound, hydrocolloid, or rubber-base impression material is used with a very careful technique, the impression can be made to fit the preparation at a temperature low enough to minimize the effect of its normal shrinkage on cooling. Similarly, the impression should be guarded against temperature changes during the interval between removal and completion of the die.

If the die is to be made of amalgam, avoid an alloy that shrinks on setting and use one that has a very slight setting expansion. Most of the gypsum-base die materials have a small setting expansion, which is desirable. If the impression is copper-plated before the die is poured, the setting expansion of the die material has no effect on the size of the die. Wide variations in the temperature of the plating solution will, of course, cause corresponding variations in the size of the impression being plated.

Pattern waxes also have high rates of thermal expansion and contraction so that if the pattern is made to fit the preparation at one temperature and invested at a lower temperature, shrinkage will be produced. Such shrinkage can be avoided by investing the pattern at the same temperature at which it was made or compensated for by providing additional expansion of the mold. The thermal expansion of the wax and the setting expansion, hygroscopic expansion, and thermal expansion of the investment are the principal compensating means available for offsetting unavoidable shrinkages.

Inlay wax has a high rate of thermal expansion so that if the pattern is made to fit the preparation at approximate room temperature, and then invested at a higher temperature, a relatively large expansion will be introduced. This was one of the earliest methods used in compensating for the casting shrinkage of gold. Unfortunately, it presents a number of practical difficulties, chief of which is the fact that when a wax pattern that has been formed to the preparation and chilled under pressure is reheated, it not only expands but also tends to warp due to the release of internal strains. Although progress has been made toward overcoming this fault, the danger of warpage still appears to be a real hazard; and consequently, thermal expansion of the wax pattern as a major means of compensation has been largely abandoned.

The setting expansion of investments varies from brand to brand and also with the water/powder ratio. Generally speaking, the thicker the mix, the more the expansion. The amount of the setting expansion for various water/powder ratios is usually published by the manufacturer and may run as high as 0.5 percent. While this type of expansion does affect the size of the mold, it is doubtful if the full theoretical amount is effective in compensating casting shrinkage. In the case of full and three-quarter crowns, MOD inlays, and similar patterns, there is a tendency for the wax pattern to restrain the setting expansion of the investment. In order for this expansion to take place unrestrictedly, the wax pattern should move uniformly with the investment. This could occur theoretically if the heat evolved by the setting investment were just enough to expand the wax thermally as much as the investment itself expands due to its setting reaction, but it seems doubtful if this exact balance is achieved. Therefore, the wax pattern will be stretched by the force of the expanding investment or the investment will be compressed by the resistance of the confining wax pattern. What actually takes place is probably a combination of three things: (1) some thermal expansion of the wax due to the heat of the setting reaction, (2) some stretching of the wax by the force of the setting reaction, and (3) some compression of the investment by the resistance of the wax pattern. Consequently, the full amount of the setting expansion will rarely be effective in expanding the mold, and the degree to which it is effective may vary depending upon the type of pattern and the physical characteristics of the wax and investment used. There is also a tendency for the metal inlay ring to restrain the setting expansion radically and force it to take place toward the open ends of the ring, causing distortion. However, the use of a liner of asbestos paper or similar material to serve as a cushion and permit free expansion in all directions can eliminate this effect.

Hygroscopic expansion of the investment occurs when the investment sets in contact with water, and for some investment compositions it is much greater than ordinary setting expansion. The exact mechanism of this expansion is obscure, but it is known that the amount varies with the formula of the investment, the water/powder ratio, the temperature of the water in which the investment is immersed, the amount of time after mixing at which it is immersed, and the length of time it is kept immersed. The usual procedure is to invest the pattern and immediately immerse the ring in water at approximately 100°F. and allow it to stay there until the investment has set. A commercial investment especially designed for this technique is stated by its manufacturer to have an "effective hygroscopic expansion" of about 1.4 percent after thirty minutes' immersion at approximately 100°F., after which there is no further change. However, there is some uncertainty as to how much of this expansion is actually effective in enlarging the mold, because the same factors that tend to restrict ordinary setting expansion are also operative here, though to a much more limited extent. The temperature of the water bath will expand the wax pattern, but the amount of this expansion is ordinarily much less than the hygroscopic expansion so that the difference will be reflected in stretching of the wax and compression of the investment. Although the softened wax offers less resistance to stretching, it seems probable that it would still have sufficient strength to compress the investment to some extent, especially in the early stages of the setting reaction. To be considered, also, is the possible danger of warpage of the pattern due to the higher temperature of the wax and the release of internal strains as previously described. While the exact amount of the enlargement of the mold by hygroscopic expansion is indefinite, it is certain that if an additional 0.8 to 0.9 percent thermal expansion were added by heating to approximately 1300°F., the mold would be overexpanded, and the casting would be too large. For this reason the mold is cast at a lower temperature, usually about 800° to 900°F., at which the thermal expansion of the investment is only about 0.3 percent. At this relatively low temperature, a much longer time would be required to carbonize and eliminate the wax by burning it out in the usual manner. This problem is met in one of three ways: by heating the ring rapidly while the investment is still wet so that the water in the investment will boil and flush out the wax; by flushing out the wax by placing the ring in a pan of boiling water; or by removing the wax with a suction device made for the purpose. Properly controlled, the hygroscopic technique yields excellent results in the form of well-fitting castings with smooth surfaces.

Thermal expansion of investment is perhaps the most easily and accurately controlled of the various expansion means available for compensating the casting shrinkage of gold. Again, the amount will vary over a wide range, depending upon the type of investment, the water/powder ratio, and the temperature at which the casting is made. It may be as much as 1.35 percent. Data on the thermal expansion for various water/powder ratios over the commonly used range of temperature are available from most investment manufacturers. Since the metal ring and the investment do not expand at the same rate when heated, it is advisable to line the ring with asbestos paper or similar material to serve as a cushion which will allow the investment to expand freely. If this is done, the maximum thermal expansion should be fully effective in enlarging the mold.

Most of the investments intended for this technique are heated to approximately 1300°F. to develop thermal expansion which, combined with the usable setting expansion, will completely compensate for the average 1¼ percent casting shrinkage of gold. There is one type of investment which develops sufficient thermal expansion at 800° to 900°F. so that the mold may be cast at that temperature or at 1300°F., depending on the wax elimination technique followed.

From the foregoing discussion it is clear that in spite of the great advances in the common fund of knowledge on this subject and the enormously improved materials and techniques that have been provided, there are still factors common to all inlay techniques that are not completely understood and provided for. Inlay casting is not yet an exact science. Nevertheless, enough is known of the properties of the materials used and the effects of variations in manipulative procedures to enable the operator to make enlightened choice of materials and techniques and, with some experimentation, to make such adjustments in his procedure as may be necessary to meet his individual requirements.

For efficient and practical operation, a standardized technique should be adapted to the need and equipment of the office and made "routine." With the various steps in the technique standardized as far as possible, it will be reasonable to expect consistently satisfactory results. Furthermore, it will be relatively easy to detect and correct any errors that might creep into the technique.

Inlay castings that come out too small or too "tight" indicate that more compensating expansion is needed. If the operator is presently using a "low-heat" technique, a study of the curve in figure 37.1 will show what would happen if the burnout temperature were increased. Assuming the investment has a thermal expansion curve as shown in figure 37.1 and the burnout temperature was about 800°F., we see that the thermal expansion of the mold is less at that temperature than at any other between 600° and 1650°F. Increasing the burnout temperature to 1000°F. or over would increase the amount of expansion. Referring to figure 37.3 (the thermal expansion curve of another widely used investment), we see that thermal expansion is also increased as the mold temperature is increased.

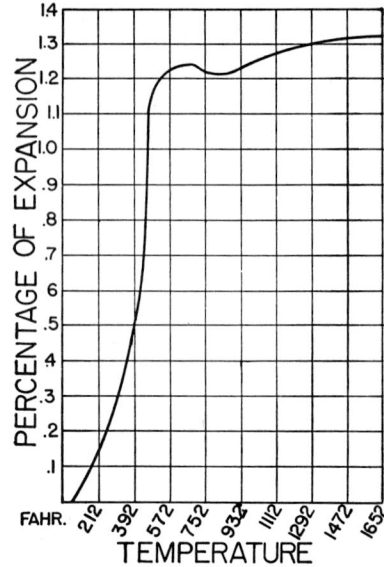

Fig. 37.1. Thermal expansion curve of Cristobalite inlay investment.

Courtesy Kerr Mfg. Co.

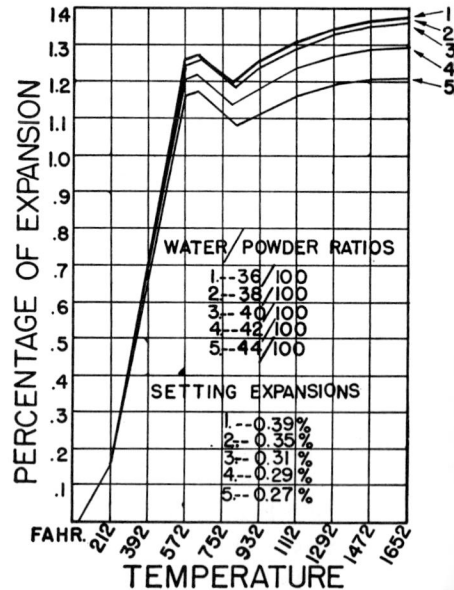

Fig. 37.2. Thermal expansion of Cristobalite inlay investment, using different water-powder ratios.

Courtesy Kerr Mfg. Co.

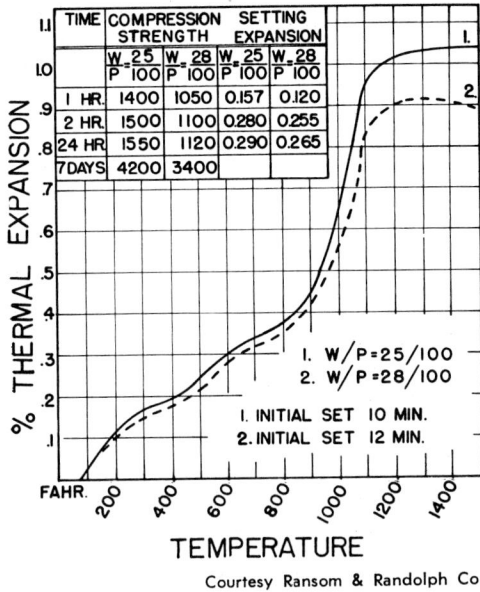

TIME	COMPRESSION STRENGTH		SETTING EXPANSION	
	W=25 P=100	W=28 P=100	W=25 P=100	W=28 P=100
1 HR.	1400	1050	0.157	0.120
2 HR.	1500	1100	0.280	0.255
24 HR.	1550	1120	0.290	0.265
7 DAYS	4200	3400		

1. W/P = 25/100
2. W/P = 28/100

1. INITIAL SET 10 MIN.
2. INITIAL SET 12 MIN.

Courtesy Ransom & Randolph Co.

Fig. 37.3. Physical properties of Ransom and Randolph gray investment.

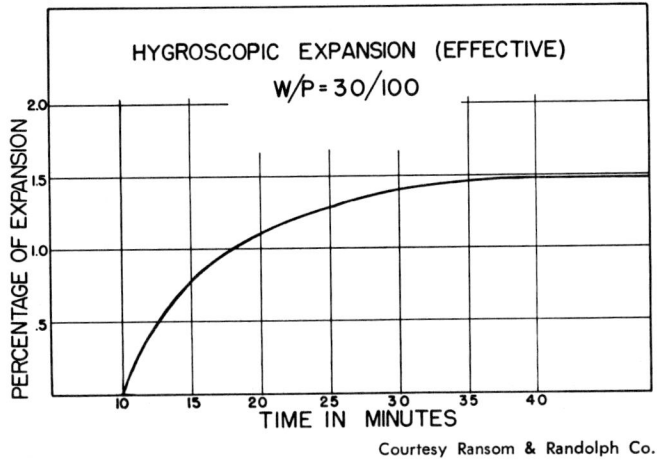

Courtesy Ransom & Randolph Co.

Fig. 37.4. Effective hygroscopic expansion of Ransom and Randolph hygroscopic investment.

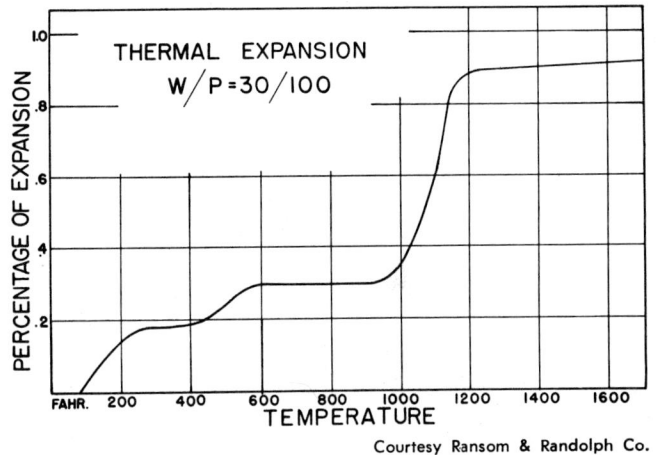

Courtesy Ransom & Randolph Co.

Fig. 37.5. Thermal expansion of Ransom and Randolph hygroscopic investment.

Both figures 37.2 and 37.3 illustrate another method of gaining mold expansion—by decreasing the water/powder ratio. The thicker the mix, the greater the thermal expansion at any temperature. It is true, furthermore, that the thicker mixes produce greater setting expansion.

Figure 37.4 shows the hygroscopic expansion curve of an investment developed especially for this technique. As can be seen, the greater the length of time—up to thirty minutes—that the investment is allowed to set in water, the greater the expansion. The expansion may also be increased by using a thicker mix, by increasing the temperature of the water bath, or by immersing the investment sooner after mixing.

Figure 37.5 shows the thermal expansion of this same investment, and it is evident that the expansion can be increased by raising the burnout temperature up to 1400°F. Between about 950° and 1200°F. this investment expands very rapidly so that a small variation in temperature causes a relatively large variation in the size of the mold. To avoid this wide and hard-to-control variation, it is preferable to cast either below 950° or above 1200°F. It should be noted, however, that heating the mold to temperatures above 1350°F. is inadvisable since the plaster binder in the investment tends to break down at these excessive temperatures, liberating corrosive sulphur compounds which attack the cast metal.

If inlay castings are overexpanded and "loose," less mold expansion is required, and the adjustments in the technique would be just the opposite of those described for increasing expansion.

Description of Step	CRISTOBALITE INLAY INVESTMENT (Kerr Mfg. Co., Detroit, Mich.)	
	Control Technique Kerr *Control Powder* added to Cristobalite in definite proportions will produce controlled reduction in expansion where desired.	*Low Burnout Technique* Cristobalite Only
Preparation of Inlay Ring	Line with single thickness of asbestos, lapped, and ⅛″ short at both ends. Moisten thoroughly.	Line with single thickness of asbestos, lapped, and ⅛″ short at both ends. Moisten thoroughly.
Water Temperature	Room	Room
Mixing Ratio	Proportions under Control Technique are automatically delivered by Kerr Scale.	15-17 cc. water to 40 gms. investment. When mixing, add investment to water.
Mixing Technique	Hand spatulate; vibrate bowl 30 sec. then mechanical mixer 30 sec. (or use vacuum equipment as directed.)	Hand spatulate; vibrate bowl 30 sec. then mechanical mixer 30 sec. (or use vacuum equipment as directed.)
Investing Pattern	Paint carefully with camel's hair brush. This painting may be blown off and pattern repainted. Do *not* dust with dry investment.	Paint carefully with camel's hair brush. This painting may be blown off and pattern repainted. Do *not* dust with dry investment.
Filling Ring	Fill inlay ring with same mix and insert painted pattern with slight wavy motion.	Fill inlay ring with same mix and insert painted pattern with slight wavy motion.
Setting Time	Allow to set 30 min. or longer.	Allow to set 30 min. or longer.
Wax Elimination and Burnout	Place flask into furnace preheated to 850-900°F., sprue hole down. Raise temperature to 1200-1350°F. in 30-45 min. Cast into red hot mold. *or* Flask can be placed into cold furnace and heated to 1200-1350°F. Longer time is required.	Place flask into furnace preheated to 850-900°F. Cast in approximately one hour and after discolored investment has regained a white color.

Courtesy J. M. Ney Co.

Fig. 37.6. Condensed step chart for thermal expansion technique for Cristobalite inlay investment (based on procedures recommended by the investment manufacturer).

Description of Step	R & R GRAY INVESTMENT (The Ransom & Randolph Co., Toledo, O.)	
	Single-mix technique is suggested for all two-surface inlays and ¾ crowns for anteriors.	*Double-mix* technique is suggested for M-O-Ds, ¾ crowns for posteriors, full crowns and single occlusal inlays.
Preparation of Inlay Ring	Line with wet asbestos loosely placed in ring, lapped for half circumference.	No liner required.
Water Temperature	Room	Room
Mixing Ratio	14 cc. water to 50 gms. investment.	For first mix, 7 cc. water to 25 gms. investment.
Mixing Technique	Spatulate mechanically (or use vacuum equipment as directed).	Spatulate mechanically (or use vacuum equipment as directed).
Investing Pattern	Paint carefully with fine brush; vibrate gently to eliminate entrapped air.	Paint pattern, then dust with dry investment and vibrate gently until powder is absorbed. Repeat 3-4 times. Allow to set 5-10 min.
Filling Ring	Pour investment into ring and carefully vibrate painted pattern into filled ring.	Fill ring with second mix, made 16 cc. water to 50 gms. investment. Immerse painted pattern momentarily in water and insert in ring.
Setting Time	Allow to stand for 10-15 min.	Allow to stand for 10-15 min.
Wax Elimination and Burnout	Heat invested ring until entire sprue hole shows dull red color (1200-1300°F.) Cast *immediately.*	Heat invested ring until entire sprue hole shows dull red color (1200-1300°F.) Cast *immediately.*

Courtesy J. M. Ney Co.

Fig. 37.7. Condensed step chart for thermal expansion technique for R & R gray investment (based on procedures recommended by the investment manufacturer).

Description of Step	R & R HYGROSCOPIC INVESTMENT (The Ransom & Randolph Co., Toledo, Ohio)	BEAUTY-CAST INLAY INVESTMENT (Whip-Mix Corp., Louisville, Ky.)
Preparation of Inlay Ring	Line with one layer asbestos ⅛″ short at crucible end.	Line with single thickness of asbestos ⅛″ short at both ends of ring to provide investment seal; then wet.
Mixing Ratio	15 cc. water to 50 gms. investment.	15 cc. water to 50 gms. investment. No change in W/P ratio is necessary when using vacuum equipment.
Mixing	Spatulate mechanically (or use vacuum equipment according to directions).	Add powder to water, hand spatulate to wet, then spatulate mechanically 50 turns. (If vacuum equipment is used, follow manufacturer's instructions.)
Investing Pattern	Paint with fine brush; vibrate gently.	Paint with brush; vibrate with serrated instrument on crucible former.
Filling Ring	Place ring around painted pattern and fill, gently vibrating.	Place ring around painted pattern and fill slowly, using spatula; vibrate to place.
To Obtain Hygroscopic Expansion	Immerse immediately in water bath at approx. 100°F., water covering the ring.	Immerse immediately in water held within 2° of 100°F.
Setting Time	Allow to remain in water for 30 min. or longer.	Let set for at least 30 min. under water.
Wax Elimination and Burnout	Place wet ring at 800° to 950°F. Heat 45 min. or longer, depending on size of pattern. Cast immediately. *or* Place ring in water and heat to boil. Discontinue heating and with rubber bulb (e.g. chip blower) or with manufactured wax evacuator, remove the wax. Place wet ring in furnace at 800° to 900°F.; heat 30 min. Cast immediately.	Place ring in furnace and bring to 900°F. in 40 min. *or* Burnout directly in a hot furnace at 900°F. for at least 40 min. Cast any time thereafter. If a good grade of inlay wax is used, it is not necessary to eliminate the wax with boiling water or any other method before burning out.

Courtesy J. M. Ney Co.

Fig. 37.8. Condensed step chart for two hygroscopic techniques (based on procedures recommended by the respective investment manufacturers).

Wax Patterns

The waxing-up of the pattern is accomplished by the use of the gas burner, wax spatula and carvers, and inlay wax. Inlay waxes are specially compounded to burn out of the mold cleanly, leaving no residue harmful to the casting of the gold into the form left by removal of the wax.

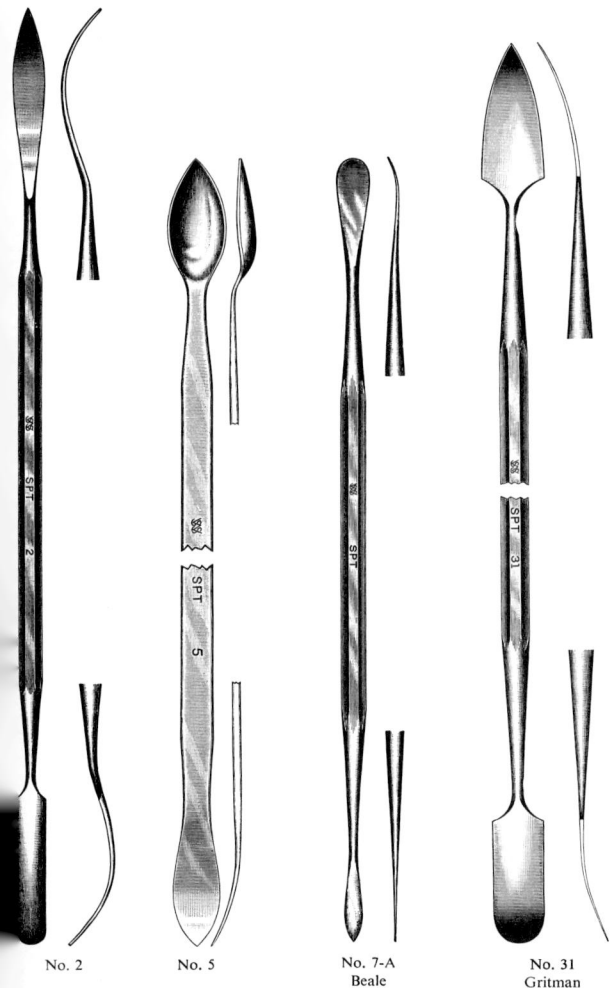

| No. 2 | No. 5 | No. 7-A Beale | No. 31 Gritman |

Courtesy S. S. White Co.

Fig. 37.9. Wax spatulas

With a hot spatula, inlay wax is melted, run into the preparation, and pressed against the walls of the die with the fingers to insure adaptation. It is essential that all grooves and angles in the preparation be reproduced in the wax, and a convenient way to insure this is to flow a thin film of *soft* wax into the cavity first and then build up the remainder in the harder inlay wax. Pressure must be applied continuously to prevent the wax from shrinking from the margins as it cools, and this pressure applied to the hard wax effectively forces the softer wax into all corners of the die.

The pattern is built up to approximate shape, removed from the die, and its inner surface is checked for accuracy. If satisfactory, it is replaced, the die is seated in the model, and the contacts and occlusion are established. The contact areas on the model, if present, should be lubricated and the wax pattern softened with a hot spatula to permit the excess to be squeezed out as the die is seated. If it is undersize, the contacts should be built up by adding wax. The occlusion is established by closing the articulator or by the marks established on the wax registration and adjusting the wax to the bite. The die is then lifted from the model, and the carving is completed. Remove all surplus wax and carefully create the proper contours and occlusal carvings, using as one guide the general shape already developed in the pattern through the articulation of the waxed die.

Check all margins carefully and replace any missing portions, using a hot spatula, but do not flow wax beyond the margins as it may get into an undercut area and cause distortion of the pattern when removed from the die.

Smooth the pattern by polishing the wax with a piece of soft cloth, rubbing the surface gently toward the margins. It is advisable to make a final check under a magnifying glass with a good light.

Since the wax pattern is the basis of every gold casting, much of the hard work in finishing and polishing can be eliminated before the casting is made by paying particular attention to the waxing procedure. Obviously, it is much easier, faster, and less costly to shape, smooth, and finish a wax pattern than a gold casting, and any additional effort spent in perfecting the pattern will be rewarded later on by a considerable saving in time and gold.

Spruing the Pattern

The method adopted for spruing the wax pattern is much more important to the success of the inlay than is generally realized. Although the fundamental principles are simple and easy to follow, many inlays are ruined by failure to carry out this primary step correctly.

Thickness of Sprue

A very common error, which results in *shrink-spot* porosity or pitted castings, is the use of *too thin* a sprue. When molten metal is cast into a mold, the outer surface of the casting cools fastest and freezes first, forming a shell of solid metal around a molten center. As the metal continues to cool, this shell increases in thickness, and finally the thinner sections freeze solid while there is still molten metal at the center of the thicker sections. If the sprue is thinner than the casting proper, it will solidify completely while the bulkier casting is still partially molten. The molten metal in the casting continues to cool and shrink, and since no more metal can be supplied from the button because the sprue has already solidified, this shrinkage produces voids or pits known as *shrink-spot* porosity. This type of porosity is not a peculiar defect of the inlay golds or of dental alloys generally. It has to be provided for in all foundry practice and is a simple demonstration of the fact that metals in their solid state occupy less space than when they were fluid. Consequently, if a solid

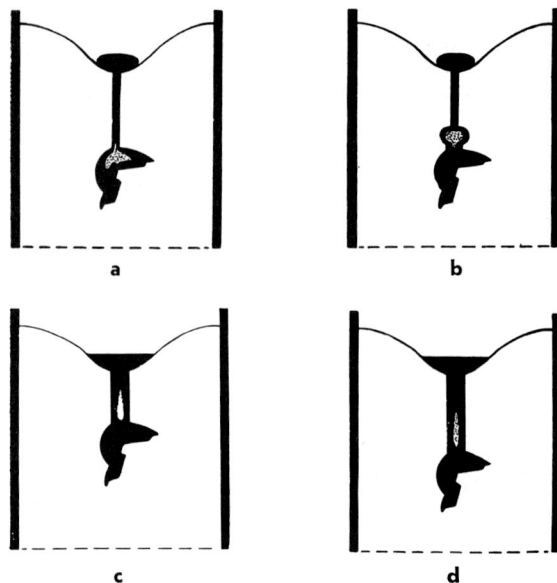

Courtesy J. M. Ney Co.

Fig. 37.10. Results of various methods of spruing the pattern: (a) incorrect spruing—thin sprue freezes before the casting, causing "shrink-spot" porosity; (b) correct spruing for air-pressure castings—by adding a reservoir to the thin sprue, the "shrink-spot" porosity is concentrated harmlessly outside the casting; (c) incorrect positioning—pattern too far from end of ring, resulting in casting with rounded margins; (d) correct positioning and spruing for centrifugal castings—pattern placed 1/4 inch from bottom of ring for sharp margins; thick sprue used to prevent porosity in casting.

metal is required to occupy the same space that it filled in its fluid form, it can do so only if it adds to its volume by "acquiring" porosity.

To avoid this type of defect, the sprue should be thicker than the pattern so that the inlay will freeze first and the sprue will remain molten to feed additional metal to the inlay until it has frozen solid. In centrifugal casting, the use of a thick sprue is practicable; but in pressure casting, if the sprue opening into the crucible is thicker than fourteen gauge, molten metal is likely to slip down and block off the sprue before casting pressure is applied. However, a reservoir added to the sprue will get around this difficulty and will concentrate the shrink-spot porosity harmlessly outside the inlay. The reservoir should be thicker than the thickest part of the pattern and placed as close as possible to the pattern, never more than one-sixteenth inch away. The very short length of sprue between the reservoir and the pattern should be thickened with wax. Such a reservoir is conveniently made from the end of a stick of inlay wax cut off about one-eighth inch long, or by wrapping a one-eighth-inch strip of sheet casting wax around the sprue.

Attaching the Sprue

Shrink-spot porosity will also occur when a bulky section of a casting is separated from the sprue by a thinner section. Naturally, the thinner section freezes first and so prevents the sprue from feeding additional metal to the bulky section as it solidifies. For this reason the sprue should always be attached to the thickest part of the pattern. When there are two bulky sections separated from each other by a thin section, as in an MOD with heavy mesial and distal legs connected by a thin occlusal isthmus, it is helpful to attach a sprue to each bulky section.

The wax pattern must be securely attached to the sprue so that it will not break away and be lost during investing, but forcing or melting the sprue deeply into the pattern may cause serious distortion. To avoid such distortion and yet assure firm attachment, place a small amount of sticky wax on the pattern and insert the sprue into the sticky wax.

Mounting the Pattern on Crucible Former (Sprue Base)

In mounting the sprued pattern on the crucible former, it should be adjusted so that there is not more than one-fourth inch separating the bottom of the casting ring from the nearest part of the wax pattern. The reason

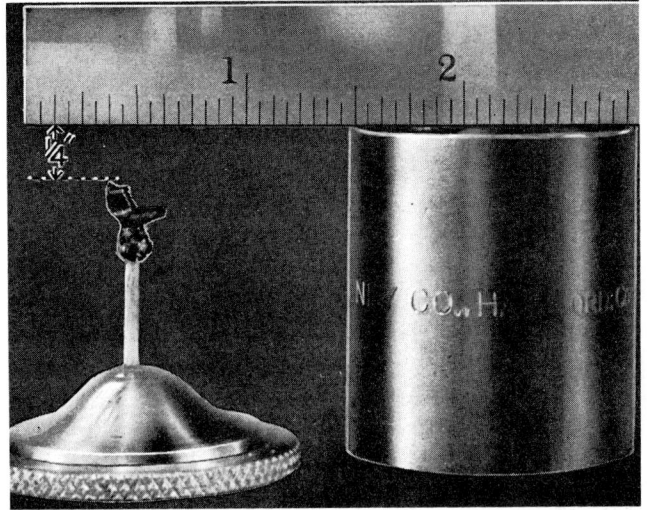

Courtesy J. M. Ney Co.

Fig. 37.11. Correct spruing and positioning of pattern for pressure-casting, using Ney crucible former and heat-resisting Ney inlay ring.

for this is that the air in the pattern chamber is of necessity forced out through the investment as the molten metal enters, and if the bulk of investment is too great, the escape of the air may be so slow that the gold will freeze before the mold is completely filled. This is one of the principal causes of incomplete castings with rounded or short margins.

The crucible former should be clean and free of old investment or other debris. This debris could produce a rough crucible, or the loose particles might be flushed into the pattern chamber with the gold and cause a defective casting. It is also advisable to lubricate the crucible former lightly with a thin oil or with Vaseline to prevent the investment from sticking. If the crucible former is rubber, this lubrication is not necessary.

The shape of the crucible former is also an important factor. A very shallow flat-bottomed crucible does not concentrate the gold over the sprue hole, and much of it may remain in the crucible instead of being forced down the sprue, resulting in an incomplete casting. When a centrifugal casting machine is used, this type of crucible may cause spilling of the gold. A deep, steep-walled crucible is satisfactory for centrifugal casting, but if used for pressure casting where the gold is melted directly in the investment crucible, the gold at the bottom is not readily reached with the blowpipe flame, and melting is difficult. The crucible former illustrated is flared at the top for easy access of the flame and has slightly steeper walls at the bottom to concentrate the gold over the sprue hole. Consequently, it gives excellent results with both centrifugal and pressure casting machines.

Two Methods of Investing

Introduction

Investing of wax patterns may be accomplished in either of two ways: (1) by hand or mechanical spatulation of the investment material, beginning the application of the investment to the pattern by painting with a small brush, then vibrating the balance of the investment material into the casting ring, or (2) by mixing the investment material under vacuum and investing the wax pattern also under vacuum.

The actual casting of gold into the prepared mold is also commonly done in either of two general ways: (1) by use of a simple centrifugal casting machine, or (2) by casting with vacuum casting equipment. It should be mentioned that casting has been done using air under pressure to force the gold into the prepared mold—a method which is not often found in use today.

Either method of investing wax patterns—investing without vacuum or investing under vacuum—may be followed by the use of a simple centrifugal casting machine to make the casting.

Vaccum investing, however, can be and often is used together with vacuum casting equipment.

1. Investing the Pattern (Without Vacuum)

The particular investment material which your dentist desires you to use, the technique to be followed in investing the pattern, the equipment available in your office for this purpose, and the technique for burning out the pattern—all are factors which will dictate the method you will use in the dental office in which you are employed. There are several investments, several techniques of investing a pattern, several methods of burning out a pattern, and several methods of casting gold. Some of these techniques will be discussed.

First, a technique depending chiefly on the thermal expansion of the investment to compensate for the casting shrinkage of the gold will be outlined here. This technique requires the use of a high-expanding investment, a number of which are available. Each should be handled according to the instructions supplied by its manufacturer.

Lining the Casting Ring

In this technique it is advisable to use an asbestos paper lining in the inlay ring. The investment and the metal ring do not expand at the same rate when heated, and the asbestos lining serves as a cushion which allows the investment to expand freely and tends to prevent distortion or cracking of the mold due to this unequal expansion. The ring with liner should be dipped in water to moisten the asbestos.

Cleaning the Pattern

Just before investing, the pattern should be thoroughly cleaned with a half-and-half mixture of green soap and hydrogen peroxide, then rinsed in room-temperature water, and thor-

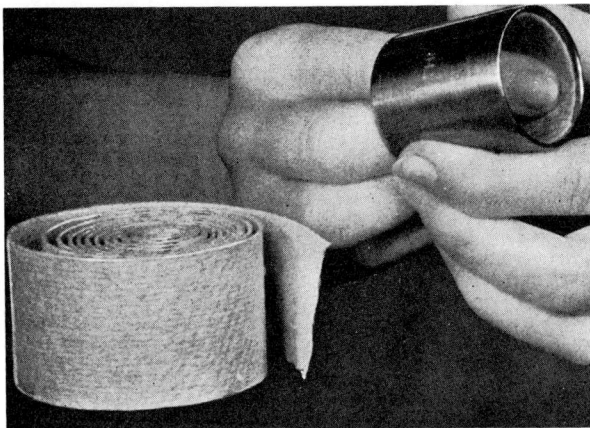

Fig. 37.12. Lining the inlay ring with asbestos paper to cushion the unequal expansion of investment and ring.

oughly dried. This procedure is essential in obtaining castings that are free of surface bubbles and nodules. If the pattern is not clean, the investment will not adhere readily to the wax surface, and a rough casting is quite likely to result. If it is desired to use one of the wetting agents available for reducing surface tension, it should be applied to the pattern at this time, carefully following the manufacturer's directions.

Mixing the Investment

In mixing the investment it is advisable to use a good mechanical spatulator because this method produces a smoother mix, freer from entrapped air bubbles, than hand spatulation. Air bubbles in the investment are likely to collect on the wax pattern and, when cast, produce a rough surface and prevent the inlay from seating. It is also important to use the exact proportions of investment powder and water recommended by the manufacturer. Too thin a mix may have insufficient expansion and is likely to crack during the burnout, causing fins and rough surfaces. Too thick a mix is dif-

ficult to apply to the pattern and may result in damaged margins and entrapped air. Prior to the mix, wet the rubber bowl and then shake off any excess moisture.

Painting the Pattern

Paint the pattern carefully with the investment mix, being sure to carry it into all grooves and angles. A good method is to apply the investment with a small brush held lightly against a vibrator. As the brush is vibrated, the bristles work their way into all corners and cover all areas of the pattern thoroughly with investment, eliminating any air that might be entrapped in the investment. After the first coat has been applied in this manner, the bulk of the investment may be gently blown off the pattern and the process repeated as an additional precaution to assure thorough painting and a smooth casting.

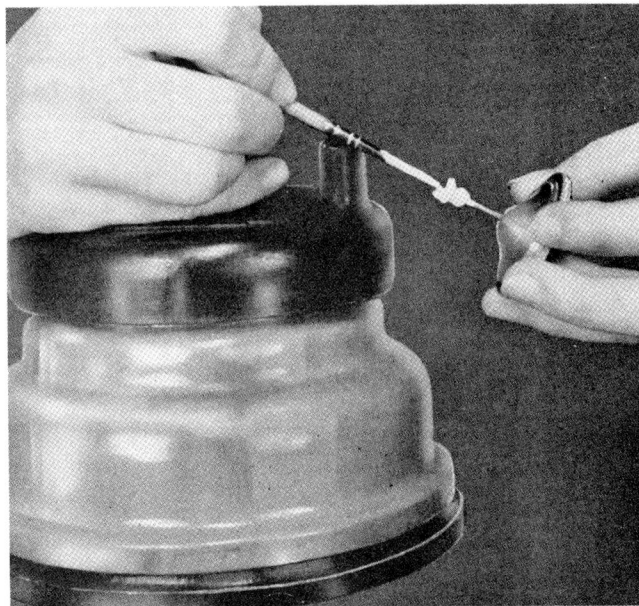

Courtesy J. M. Ney Co.

Fig. 37.13. Painting the pattern. The brush is held lightly against a vibrator.

Filling the Ring

After the painting is completed, it is sometimes suggested that the invested inlay be dusted lightly with dry investment powder to absorb excess water, as well as to harden the mass so that it will hold its shape while investing is completed. The ring is now seated over the invested pattern and onto the crucible former and is filled to overflowing with the balance of the mixture. Pour the investment so that it runs down the side of the ring, filling it from the bottom up to avoid trapping air or washing the painted investment off the pattern.

2. Vacuum Investing

Introduction

Vacuum investing of wax patterns results in some differences in technique even before the actual investing is done.[2]

For purposes of standardizing, it is recommended that a fifty-gram ring (an inlay casting ring which will contain a 50-gram mix of investment material) be used for all casting.

2. This section, "Vacuum Investing," is through the courtesy of Torit Mfg. Co., St. Paul, Minnesota.

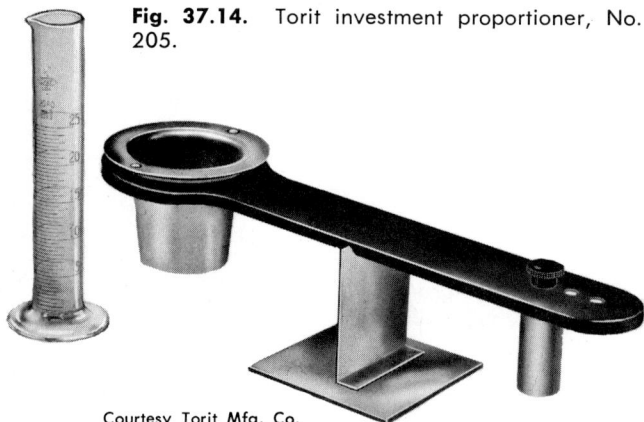

Fig. 37.14. Torit investment proportioner, No. 205.

Courtesy Torit Mfg. Co.

In addition to the fact that it will not cool down as fast as will a smaller ring when removed from the burnout oven for casting, it is also unnecessary to be constantly changing the balance weight on the casting machine to balance different size rings.

When vacuum investing, it is advisable to use a thinner mix of investment and water than is usually recommended. For example, using straight cristobalite (no control powder), the proportion 21 cc. to 23 cc. water to 50 grams investment is good—with silicate investments such as R & R Gray, 16 cc. to 17 cc. water to 50 grams of investment. The difference in amount of water used might be explained by the fact that less air will remain in the finished mix, and the difference is filled with water. Also, during the vacuum process some moisture is undoubtedly lost through evaporation under the low-pressure condition.

Many dentists prefer to eliminate the use of asbestos liners in the casting ring for most castings, since it has been found that expansion is greater under vacuum investing because practically all air is drawn out of the investment. Air forms tiny voids, creating cushions into which expansion is partly dissipated. With practically all air eliminated, the mass of investment is more dense. Expansion is then greater because the grains of investment are compressed closer together and the expansion is not dissipated into tiny air voids. If additional expansion is desired on any particular case, one may readily obtain it by immersing the casting ring in a pan of 90° to 100° water immediately after removing the ring from the vacuum unit (the hygroscopic technique). The higher the temperature of the water, the greater will be the expansion obtained.

The crucible former—or sprue base—used in vacuum investing is formed of rubber in order to seal one end of the casting ring. Spruing position and thickness of sprue are the same as in the method discussed in earlier pages, if casting is to be accomplished in a simple centrifugal-type casting machine.

The Barr Vacuum Investing Unit

One of the typical methods of vacuum investing is accomplished through the use of the Barr vacuum investing unit. This unit accomplishes the *double vacuum method,* that is, the investment is mixed under vacuum and the ring is filled under vacuum (fig. 38.17).

Using the Barr unit, the procedure is as follows: (1) The casting ring with rubber sprue base and sprued wax pattern is inserted in the investment ring holder; (2) The correct amount of water for the investment being used is measured into the plastic bowl of the unit;

(3) The correct weight of investment material is added to the water in the plastic bowl of the unit; (4) The casting ring in the investment ring holder is inverted over the mixing bowl; (5) The vacuum bell is placed over the mixing bowl, the vacuum pump is turned on, and

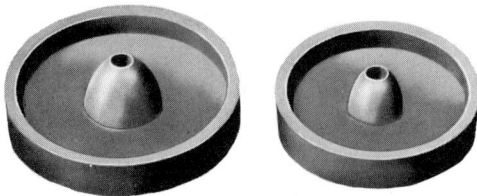

Courtesy Torit Mfg. Co.

(above) **Fig. 37.15.** Rubber sprue bases by Torit.

(below) **Fig. 37.16.** The Barr investing unit by Torit.

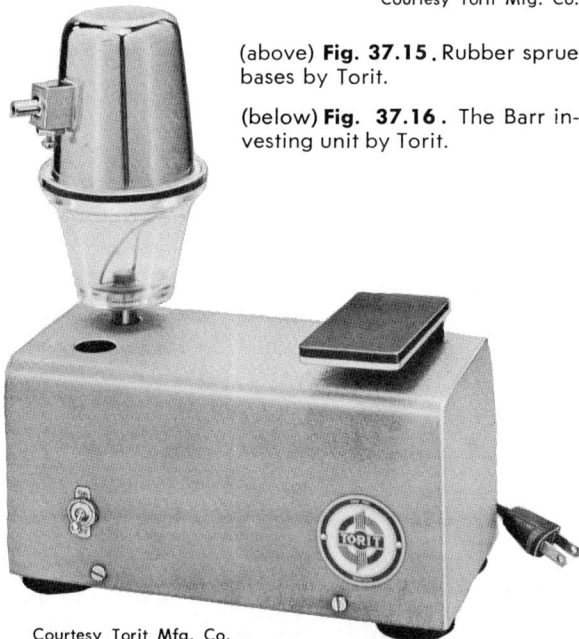

Courtesy Torit Mfg. Co.

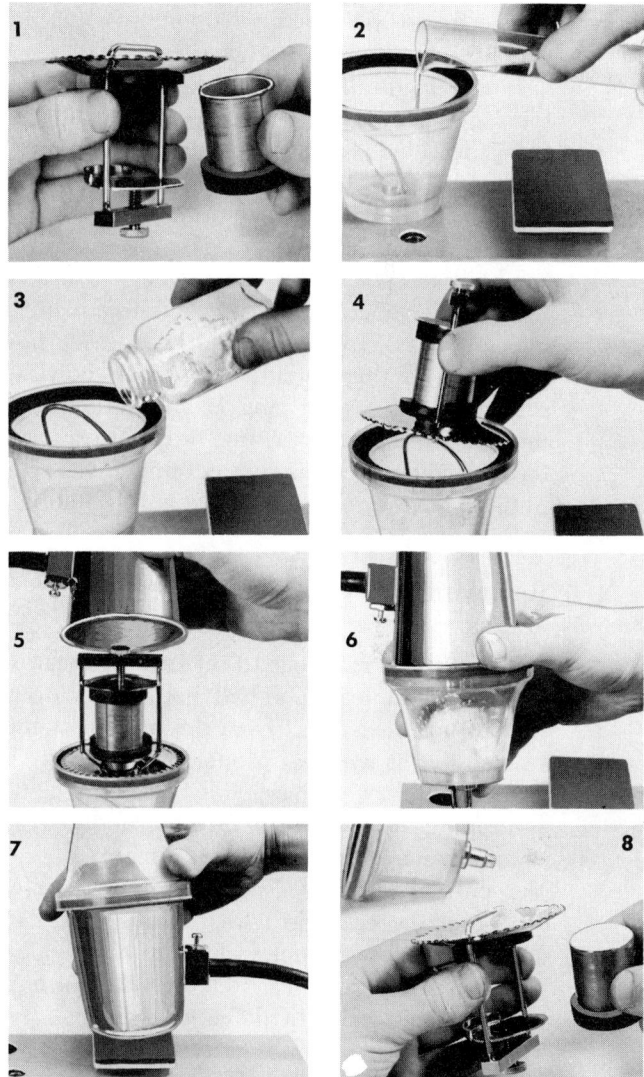

Courtesy Torit Mfg. Co.

Fig. 37.17. The Barr vacuum investing procedure as described in the text.

when twenty-nine inches of vacuum is reached, the vibrator and mixing unit are switched on; (6) The entire assembly is lifted from the holding socket on the case, and the shaft is inserted into the mixer shaft opening and held for sufficient time to thoroughly mix the investment (20 to 30 seconds); (7) The entire unit is removed from the motor drive opening, is placed over the vibrator pad on its side, and the investment is vibrated into the casting ring while the unit is slowly raised to a vertical position; (8) The filled casting ring is removed from the mechanism after releasing the vacuum.

If a bell-jar type of vacuum system is used, the investment is mixed in air, is placed under the bell jar (still in the mixing bowl), and is held under vacuum until the investment bubbles and rises (vacuum should be released immediately at this point); the mixing bowl is removed, the casting ring is vibrated full of investment, and the casting ring with an extension collar is again placed under vacuum until the investment rises and begins to bubble.

Removing the Crucible Former and Sprue

Allow the investment to set until it is hard, usually for at least one-half hour. Then trim the surplus investment from the bottom of the ring so that it will seat properly in the casting machine. Remove the crucible former by gently rapping the base. Trim off any rough edges or overhanging ledges of investment around the periphery of the crucible and carefully flush out the crucible with running water to remove all loose particles of investment which otherwise might be carried into the pattern chamber and cause a defective casting. The sprue is heated over a flame to loosen it from the invested wax pattern and is then removed with tweezers or pliers, being careful to use a straight pull and not to drag or break the surrounding investment.

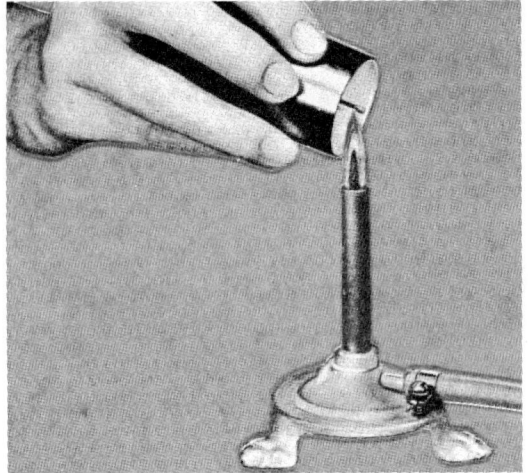

Courtesy J. M. Ney Co.

Fig. 37.18. Heating the sprue to loosen it from the invested wax pattern before removal.

Burning Out the Mold

There are numerous methods of burning out the mold, but since the technique described employs a high-expanding investment, a so-called high-heat burnout is used. The method requires the use of a heating device capable of heating the mold uniformly to a temperature of 1300° to 1350°F., or a dull red, and provided with means for controlling both the rate of heating and the final temperature. An experienced and careful technician can obtain good results with simple equipment, but it should be remembered that the burnout is one of the most important steps in the entire technique. Failure to carry out this operation correctly, through carelessness or lack of adequate equipment, is a frequent cause of defective castings. The following paragraphs describe the most common errors and a method of avoiding them.

Too Rapid Burnout

One common defect, usually traceable to incorrect burnout technique, is a casting with

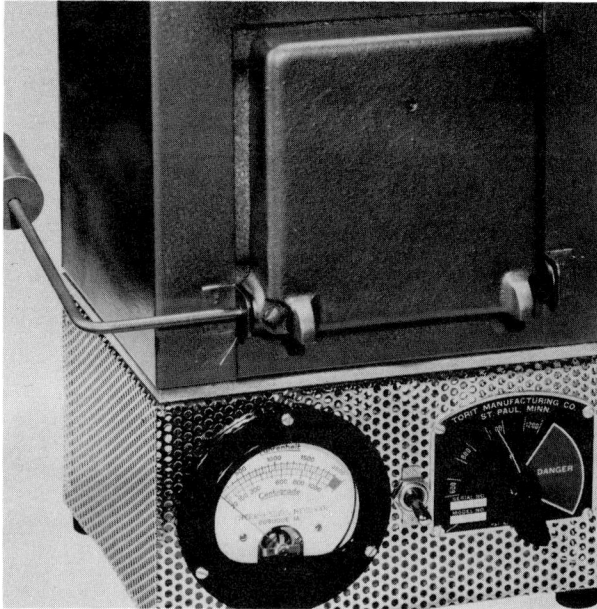

Fig. 37.19. Torit electric furnace

"fins" or "feathers" caused by cracks in the investment around the pattern which become filled with the cast gold. This condition frequently results from starting the burnout before the investment has had time to set thoroughly, while it is still too weak to stand heating without cracking, or from too rapid

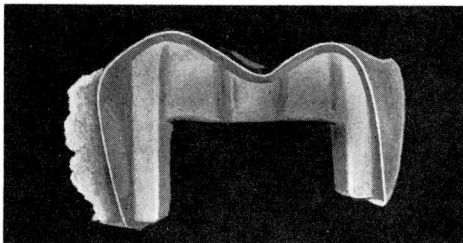

Fig. 37.20. Casting with "fin" from cracked investment, caused either by starting the burnout before the investment had completely set or by too rapid heating.

heating during the initial stage of the burnout. It may also be caused by mixing the investment too thin.

Overheating the Mold

Black or badly discolored castings that *do not clean up* readily when pickled are also the result of incorrect burnout technique. Many technicians believe that any discoloration of the surface of the casting as it comes out of the investment indicates some fault either in technique or in the materials used, but this is not necessarily true. Most casting golds oxidize at high temperatures, and it is therefore natural for some surface oxidation and discoloration to take place as they cool in the investment. This normal oxidation is easily removed by pickling and does no harm. However, the black casting that does not clean up in acid pickle is not normal and indicates an error in the burnout—usually that the investment mold was too hot when the casting was made.

The binder in most investments is plaster or some similar form of gypsum which chemically is calcium sulphate. At high temperatures the calcium sulphate slowly decomposes and gives off sulphur or sulphur compounds which readily combine with most base metals to form metallic sulphides. If the investment mold is cast at a temperature high enough for this reaction to occur, the sulphur combines with certain metals in the casting gold, especially copper and silver, forming a surface film of sulphides. This type of discoloration usually can be removed by boiling in nitric acid pickle, which is a better solvent for the sulphides, or by repeatedly heating the casting to a dull red and exposing it to air and then pickling it in sulphuric acid. The heating and exposure to air break up the sulphides and form oxides which are dissolved away in the ordinary pickle.

It is usually possible, though troublesome and inconvenient, to salvage an inlay that has been badly discolored by casting into an over-heated investment mold. However, there is another serious consequence of this error in burnout technique. The sulphur given off by overheated investment attacks the metal inlay ring, the heating element of electric furnaces, and other metal parts, causing rapid deterioration. This is a frequent cause of abnormally short life of inlay rings and the metal parts of heating devices.

Incomplete Wax Elimination

Black castings that will not pickle-clean easily may also be caused by incomplete elimination of the wax pattern as a result of heating the mold to too low a temperature for too short a time. Under these conditions a thin layer of carbonized wax remains in the pattern chamber and sticks to the surface of the casting, causing it to be quite black. Since carbon is insoluble in acid, pickling will not clean up the casting. This type of discoloration can be removed by holding the casting in the flame of a Bunsen burner, which burns off the carbon or oxidizes the metal underneath it, and then pickling to dissolve the oxides.

Frequently, incomplete wax elimination will have an entirely different result. The wax residue combines with the oxygen of the air in the pattern chamber to form carbon monoxide gas, which is a reducing agent. This gas prevents oxidation of the surface of the cast gold, with the result that the inlay comes out of the investment bright and shiny. However, when this occurs, the formation of the gas is likely to be so rapid that enough back pressure is created to slow up the entry of the gold so that it freezes before the mold is completely filled. This causes incomplete castings with margins rounded or short. Consequently, inlay castings which are abnormally shiny should be looked on with suspicion and carefully checked for margin deficiencies.

A Practical Burnout Technique

The foregoing description of several common burnout errors readily suggests the simple precautions necessary to avoid them:

1. Do not start the burnout until the investment has thoroughly set.
2. Heat the mold slowly at first, at least until the investment is dry.
3. Heat the mold to a high enough temperature and for a long enough time to completely eliminate the wax, being careful at the same time not to allow it to get too hot.

To observe the first precaution, allow the investment to set for at least one-half hour, or longer if a very slow-setting investment is used. If allowed to stand overnight, it is advisable to soak the ring in water just before starting the burnout to prevent roughness on the surface of the casting.

When starting the burnout, place the ring in the cold oven of the electric furnace. If a gas furnace is used, see that the flame is turned low or that the ring is placed high above the flame. The heat should be regulated from time to time if necessary—the important point is that the rate of heating should be reasonably uniform and such that the investment mold reaches 1300° to 1350°F., or a dull red, in not less than one hour. The heating device must then be regulated to maintain that temperature for at least an additional one-half hour. Under no circumstances allow the mold to exceed this temperature and do not use a heating device not equipped with a rheostat, gas regulator, or other suitable means for obtaining this necessary temperature control.

To help eliminate the wax completely, the mold should be burned out with sprue hole down so that the wax can run out instead of soaking into the investment. The casting should be made as quickly as possible after the ring has been removed from the furnace to avoid a drop in temperature and consequent shrinkage of the mold.

Melting the Gold

The most widely used melting equipment is the blowpipe supplied with artificial or natural gas and compressed air. Where neither artificial nor natural gas is available, numerous substitutes may be used including hydrogen, bottled gases such as propane, and acetylene. In some localities the available natural gas used with compressed air does not produce enough heat to melt the higher-fusing inlay golds efficiently so that it is advisable to use oxygen in place of compressed air. Each of these fuels has its individual characteristics and requires its own method of handling, but all of them will give good results if used with care and understanding.

Gas-air Blowpipe Technique

Because it is widely used and because it is important to handle it correctly, the gas-air blowpipe flame is illustrated and described in detail. When properly adjusted, this flame has a dark blue inner cone near the tip of the blowpipe, a center cone of lighter blue, and an outer sheath of dark purplish blue. The dark blue inner cone consists chiefly of a stream of compressed air mixed with unburned gas. It is relatively cold and strongly oxidizing and, therefore, should not be directed against the metal being melted. The light blue center cone is the area of almost complete combustion and is, therefore, the hottest part of the flame and slightly reducing. This part of the flame should contact the gold and cover it as completely as possible for rapid melting and protection from oxidation. The purplish outer sheath is made up of the products of combustion, burning gas, and oxygen absorbed from the surrounding air. It is cooler

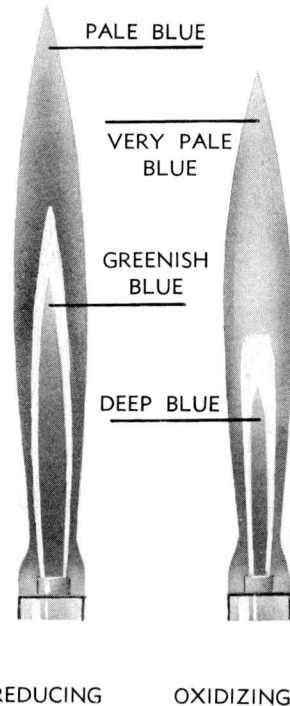

Fig. 37.21. The gas-air blowpipe flame. The pale blue part of the flame is the wrong part to use. Incompletely burned gas from melting area absorbs oxygen from surrounding air; this part of the flame is slightly oxidizing. The greenish-blue part of the flame is the correct part for melting. Rapid but not quite complete combustion; hottest part of the flame, slightly reducing. The deep blue part of the flame is the wrong part to use. It is a mixture of unburned gas and compressed air; coldest part of the flame; will oxidize hot metal.

If at all possible, use a reducing flame. Never have a noisy, hissing flame. To get a reducing flame, turn on the gas first, then add air, or oxygen, until the yellow has **just** disappeared. Notice that the reducing flame is pale blue on the tip while the oxidizing flame is **very** pale blue.

Courtesy J. M. Ney Co., with modification.

than the center cone and oxidizing in its effect and should not be used in melting.

The effects on the molten metal of the three principal parts of the flame can be graphically demonstrated. Simply hold the blowpipe close to the button of gold so that the dark blue inner cone touches the metal and note the rapid formation of a scum of oxides. Then withdraw the blowpipe slowly until the light blue center contacts the metal, noting that the oxide film disappears and the metal becomes noticeably hotter and more fluid. As the blowpipe is withdrawn until only the purplish blue outer flame touches the gold, the oxide film reappears, and the metal seems to become more sluggish. It is helpful for the beginner to actually carry out this experiment with the blowpipe to become familiar with the characteristic appearance of molten gold when the flame is being used correctly and incorrectly. The experienced technician often moves the blowpipe back and forth slightly to be sure that he is using the correct part of the flame.

Two Methods of Casting

1. Without Vacuum

When using a pressure machine, the casting gold should be placed on the side of the crucible so that as it melts, it runs down and fills the crucible from the bottom. This minimizes the risk of having unmelted gold at the bottom of the crucible which would block off the sprue hole and prevent the molten metal from entering the mold. When a centrifugal machine is used, the gold and the fire-clay crucible can advantageously be preheated with

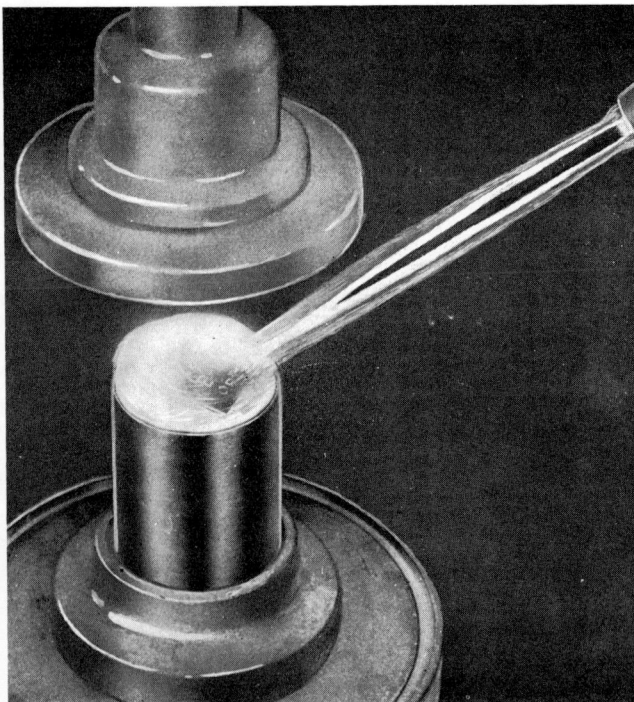

Courtesy J. M. Ney Co.

Fig. 37.22. Melting gold for pressure casting. The nuggets are placed on the side rather than in the bottom of the crucible to minimize the possibility of incomplete melting.

the blowpipe or in the burnout furnace before the ring is placed in the casting machine to save time in melting and avoid unnecessary cooling and possible shrinkage of the mold before casting.

2. Vacuum Casting

Vacuum casting[3] requires some changes in the method of spruing wax patterns to the crucible former of the sprue base. The first is that it is advisable to sprue patterns about one-half inch away from the top of the casting ring (instead of one-fourth inch recommended for conventional casting) to provide strength in the investment to prevent the vacuum in the casting machine from pulling the investment out of the back of the ring.

A relatively small sprue may be used for almost any inlay or crown pattern, such as a sixteen-gauge size. The sprue may be attached to any convenient part of the pattern, without consideration for such factors as thickness or the position in relation to the whole pattern, which are otherwise very important when casting. It is recommended, however, that you do use a sprue of near-normal size and position it with some consideration.

The back of the ring, that end opposite the crucible former, should be finished without a hump—finished perfectly level across the ring.

When ready to cast, using a Torit casting machine No. 270 with centri-vac attachment, wind up the crossarm in accordance with directions furnished. The vacuum pump is a completely separate mechanism, connected to the casting machine by tubing. Turn on the vacuum pump. Remove the burned-out casting ring from the furnace and place it in the casting machine. Proceed to melt the metal in the crucible.

Less heat is lost from the casting ring in this interval, since the heat from the blowpipe is

3. This section through the courtesy of Torit Manufacturing Co., St. Paul, Minnesota.

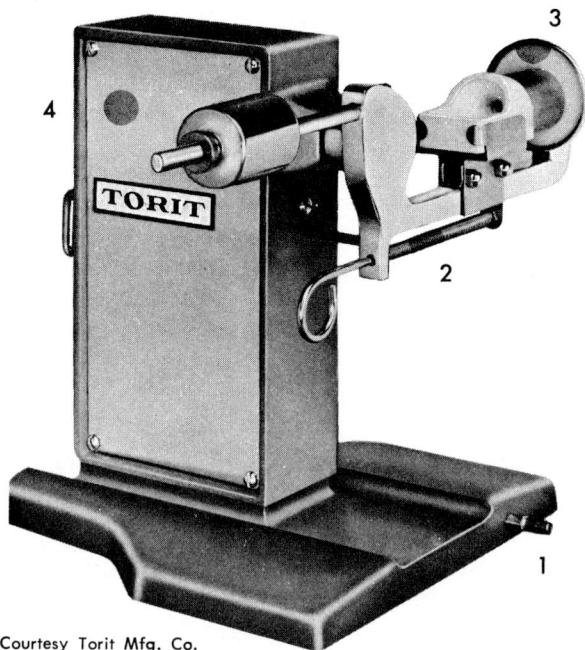

Courtesy Torit Mfg. Co.

Fig. 37.23. Torit vacuum casting machine, No. 270. (1) To vacuum pump; (2) One-piece cast aluminum arm with stainless-steel vacuum tube cast within; (3) Air and gases drawn out of casting ring here; (4) Internal steel drive shaft permits vacuum to draw from arm.

being drawn through the casting ring by the vacuum pump.

When the metal is ready for casting, the crossarm is released by the trigger. The molten metal flows into the mold by centrifugal force and is also aided by the fact that it does not have to force air out of the mold as it enters. The vacuum also speeds the flow of molten metal into the mold and thus helps eliminate premature solidification of the metal.

Fluxing

Regardless of how carefully the blowpipe is handled, some oxidation of the metal will nearly always occur during melting. For this rea-

son it is important to protect the gold with a good casting flux. Ordinary borax, frequently used for this purpose, is unsatisfactory. Although it forms a covering and protects the metal to some extent, it also dissolves and slags off any oxides that may be formed. The oxidizable metals present in casting golds—principally copper and a small amount of zinc—are important indgredients added by the manufacturer in the exact amounts required to give each alloy the desired properties. If any part of these metals is lost by being oxidized and then dissolved in the borax, the balanced formula of the alloy will be upset and its properties impaired. For best results it is essential to use a reducing flux (such as Ney's casting flux) which not only forms a protective covering, but also contains an effective reducing agent to convert the oxides back to clean copper and zinc, returning them to the molten button and thus retaining the original composition and properties of the alloy. This flux should be applied as soon as the gold starts to turn red and is hot enough for the flux to stick to it. More flux should be added just before casting.

Cleaning Residue Buttons

Before reusing sprues and residue buttons cut from previous castings, they should be thoroughly cleaned of investment and surface oxidation. The most satisfactory method is to melt down the button on a clean charcoal block with liberal applications of *casting flux* and then plunge the hot button into sulphuric acid pickle. Asbestos and fire clay blocks are unsuitable for this purpose because it is practically impossible to keep them free from small beads of metal that become entangled in adhering flux and contaminate metal subsequently melted. A charcoal block, however, is easily scraped clean just before using, and in addition, the charcoal has a valuable reducing action which, in combination with the reducing action of casting flux, breaks up the metallic oxides and converts them back to clean metal. The flux slags off adhering investment; and if a great deal of investment is present, it is advisable to remove the slag with a clean slate pencil during the melting operation. When the hot button is finally plunged into pickle, the sudden cooling crazes and cracks off the glasslike flux, and the acid dissolves any surface oxidation.

Correct Casting Temperature

It is, of course, essential that the gold be completely melted before an attempt is made to cast, otherwise it will not flow freely into the mold. It is also important to avoid heating the metal to unnecessarily high temperatures, since such temperatures promote excessive oxidation and absorption of gases and tend to produce rough castings that are weaker and more brittle than normal. A practical method of judging the right casting temperature is to shake the crucible slightly and cast when the metal rolls freely.

Heat Treatment

Soft and medium-hard golds are not affected by heat treatment, but the hard and extra-hard types can be hardened appreciably by slow cooling or left in a softened condition by rapid cooling. If the inlay is not to be soldered subsequently (which would destroy the effects of a previous heat treatment), these hardening or softening treatments can be carried out conveniently and effectively by regulating the time the casting is allowed to cool in the investment after casting. For softening, the mold should be plunged in water one to two minutes after casting; for hardening, it should be allowed to cool for three to six minutes before quenching. Plunging instantaneously, while the casting is very hot, may cause serious warpage, but air-cooling to room temperature will do no harm. However, investment is removed more easily if the ring is plunged while still warm.

Pickling

After removing the casting from the ring, brush away adhering investment and boil the casting in acid pickle to remove surface oxidation. Sulphuric acid pickle is preferred for this use because it is a very effective solvent of oxides, and its fumes are not as objectionable as those of hydrochloric or nitric acid. The pickle should consist of approximately equal parts of acid and water; and in making up the solution, the acid should always be poured into the water. If water is poured into sulphuric acid, it will boil violently and may splatter and cause serious burns.

The acid should be hot for rapid and effective pickling. It is common but definitely poor practice to heat the casting and plunge it into cold acid to speed up the pickling. Because the resulting sudden and uneven cooling may cause serious warpage of the inlay, this procedure should be avoided.

Pickling solutions should be stored in glass-stoppered bottles and kept clean at all times. One of the possible causes of discoloration of a gold casting in the mouth is a contaminated pickling solution. After a period of use, any pickling solution will have base-metal salts dissolved in it. If iron or *any other metallic* tweezers are used in handling the inlay, and if the tweezers are in contact with the inlay while it is immersed in the acid, then base metal can very easily be thrown out of solution by an electrolytic action, and the surface of the casting may be contaminated.

For example, after some use, an acid pickle will contain dissolved copper salts, among others, and a thin copper plating can be given the inlay if it is handled in acid with metal tweezers. This copper "flash" is extremely difficult to entirely remove from the casting, even with thorough polishing. Therefore, when the inlay is placed in the mouth, the copper discolors, and this discoloration is frequently mistaken for tarnish of the gold.

To avoid this complication use two pickling dishes and discard the tweezers. Place the inlay in one dish, cover it with acid, and boil. When the pickling is completed, pour the *acid only* into the second dish, leaving the inlay in the first dish. Flush this dish out with plenty of running water and then remove the inlay.

Because metal ladles also contaminate the acid, it is preferable to use a nonmetallic dish (such as the Ney pickling dish which is made of sillimanite, a porcelainlike material which is highly resistant to acids and to thermal shock). When the pickle becomes dirty and discolored from the dissolved flux and oxides or investment, it should be discarded and a fresh solution made up. After the casting is removed from the pickle, it should be dipped in a solution of ordinary soda and water to neutralize the acid.

Finishing and Polishing

Before attempting to seat the casting on the die or tooth, the inner walls should be carefully checked. Any nodules or surface roughness that might interfere with seating should be removed with a small, sharp bur. The sprue is then cut off with a separating disc, and the inlay is checked for marginal fit, occlusion, and contact. The method of carrying out these steps depends on whether the direct, indirect, or a combination of these techniques is being followed. The casting is then ready for final finishing and polishing.

The importance of a smooth, highly polished outer surface cannot be overemphasized. It is common knowledge that natural teeth acquire deposits of solid matter from the saliva, but the fact that the same deposits also form on inlays, fillings, and other hard-surfaced objects in the mouth is frequently overlooked. These deposits become stained and discolored and are frequently mistaken for "tarnish." Rough, poorly polished surfaces hold the saliva and greatly accelerate the formation of deposits; while smooth, highly polished surfaces allow the saliva to wash across freely and tend to remain clean and bright. While such deposits can usually be removed from accessible areas of gold inlays by thorough cleaning with toothbrush and dentifrice, it is obviously a much better practice to minimize the *cause* of their formation by giving the inlay a high polish.

A practical method of obtaining a high polish is to start with a heatless stone, followed successfully by a sandpaper or separating disc, rubber wheel, tripoli on felt cones and wheels, and, finally, rouge on a soft chamois buff. In each step, the coarser marks left by the previous abrasive should be completely removed before going on to the next finer abrasive. The polishing should be done toward the margins in order to spin them into closer contact with the cavity walls and to avoid nicking and injuring delicate margins. After the final polishing, the inlay should be boiled with a soapy cleaner and water to remove all traces of rouge and dirt.

If the technique is followed carefully, the inlay will have a smooth, high-luster surface with minimum tendency to acquire a deposit and become discolored. It should be remembered, however, that a good polishing job must be a thorough one.

Summary

A proper casting technique uses several ways of counterbalancing the normal shrinkage and expansion problems.

The principal shrinkage occurs in the change from liquid gold alloy to solid gold alloy. Impression and die materials may also shrink. Some die materials expand; pattern waxes and certain investment procedures can also cause expansion of the finished casting.

The variable factors can be controlled by a systematic approach to the entire procedure from beginning to end. Use a standardized technique.

The first step is to build a wax pattern. Since the wax pattern is the basis of every gold casting, much hard work in finishing and polishing can be eliminated before the casting is made by perfecting the wax pattern.

The method adopted for spruing the wax pattern is much more important to the success of the inlay than is generally realized. The thickness of the sprue is important. It is necessary to attach the sprue correctly. Directions for mounting the pattern on the crucible former should be followed meticulously.

There are two methods of investing—with and without vacuum. After the investing is completed, it is necessary to remove the crucible former and sprue. The mold is then burned out. There are problems with burnout technique which make it necessary to follow three precautions to avoid such problems.

In melting the gold it is necessary to learn to use the flame correctly.

Two methods of casting are without vacuum and vacuum casting. Follow the directions for the method which is used in your office.

Care must be exercised to follow directions accurately throughout all stages of casting and also through pickling, finishing, and polishing. A good polishing job must be a thorough one.

Study Questions

1. Discuss proper casting techniques.
2. Discuss shrinkage and expansion of materials.
3. How can the variable factors be controlled in casting?
4. Discuss the building of a wax pattern.
5. Why is the thickness of the sprue important?
6. Describe two methods of investing.
7. Discuss three precautions to take during burnout.
8. Describe two methods of casting.
9. What steps follow casting?

PART EIGHT | *RADIOGRAPHY*

—Radiography—Roentgenography—X ray—

—Names you will encounter in your studies, your conversations, and your practical work in the dental office—

They all refer to one and the same thing.

Dr. Roentgen discovered something unusual which he called X ray because its character is so puzzling. X ray has become of utmost importance. Since its original discovery, other scientists have renamed X ray to honor Dr. Wilhelm C. Roentgen, its discoverer. They call it roentgen ray.

In scientific communications we correctly refer to *roentgen ray*. In lay communication, that is, with patients in the office, it is correct to say *X ray*. Somewhere between X ray and roentgen ray, the term *radiograph* has also been developed, probably because it is radiant energy.

Regardless of which term you find in your readings—roentgenography, radiography, or X ray—each refers to the same subject.

It is the purpose of this section to acquaint the dental assistant with radiographs—their use, hazards, care, and techniques for processing.

Acknowledgement is made of the gracious consultations given in the preparation of this section by J. Donald Hauptfuehrer of the University of Illinois College of Dentistry, Department of Radiology.

38

Radiography: Elementary Knowledge... Theory

More Than the Eye Can See

When a dentist examines a patient's teeth to detect any carious lesions, he uses his eyes to see all the lesions on the exposed surfaces of the teeth. However, he cannot see the surfaces of the teeth which touch each other. If there are any carious lesions on these surfaces, the lesions will become unnecessarily large before they can be seen. Sometimes the caries reaches the pulp chamber of the tooth before it is discovered visually. In addition to dental caries, there are many other diagnoses which are made with the aid of the X ray.

It becomes evident that something more than the eye is needed to examine the mouth. Radiographs (X rays) have been developed and are used commonly for routine examination. Bitewing radiographs are frequently taken on each recall visit of a patient, or at least annually. These pictures show the surfaces of the teeth which the dentist cannot see with his eyes. If any caries is present, he can read it on the radiograph. A full-mouth radiograph is taken regularly for the well-educated and well-cared-for dental patient. The frequency with which this diagnostic measure is used is determined by the dentist. These radiographs show not only the surfaces of the teeth which touch each other, but the roots of all teeth in the mouth and the area immediately around the roots. If there is a cyst, impacted third molar, an abscess forming around a root tip, or some other abnormality, the radiograph is a diagnostic aid. The dentist can diagnose the problem and prescribe the necessary treatment with greater accuracy. If a tooth must be surgically removed, the radiograph is of vital importance to the oral surgeon prior to removal and, frequently, postoperatively (after removal).

Considering these facts, you can understand that complete diagnosis of conditions within the mouth cannot be made without the use of radiographs. It is one of the necessary tools of dentistry. *It can be a dangerous tool if improperly handled, however.*

Regulations governing the use of radiographs vary in different states. In some states the dental assistant may take the radiographs; in other states she may only assist the dentist by operating the timer. In most offices, however, it is the dental assistant who *processes* the radiographs, *mounts* them, and places them with the rest of the examination record of the patient.

Definition

A dental radiograph is a photographic record produced by the passage of X rays through the tissues of the mouth to a film. The dentist studies this photographic record as an aid to diagnosis.

It is important to make high-quality radiographs. The operators must understand what they are doing, and why, in order to achieve this essential high quality.

What Are X rays (Roentgen Rays)?

A roentgen ray is electromagnetic radiation produced when electrons strike a metal target in a vacuum tube. Like light, X rays are a form of radiant energy; they can be measured because they travel as a wave motion. (See fig. 38.1.)

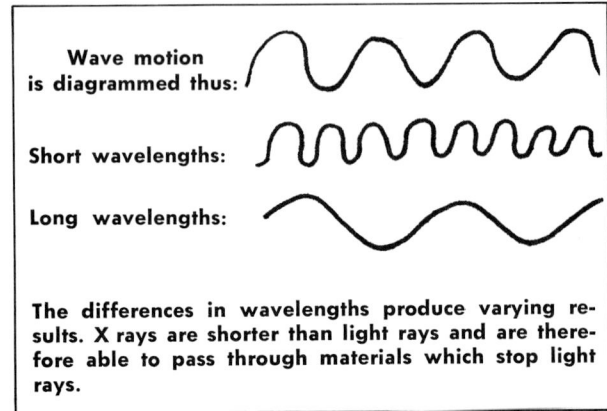

Wave motion is diagrammed thus:

Short wavelengths:

Long wavelengths:

The differences in wavelengths produce varying results. X rays are shorter than light rays and are therefore able to pass through materials which stop light rays.

Fig. 38.1. Schematic illustration of wavelengths

X rays penetrate materials which absorb or reflect light because they have such a very short wavelength (about 1/10,000 the length of light waves). X rays have the same properties as light rays, but they have them in different degrees; therefore X rays behave differently from light rays. Three characteristics of X rays are important to dentistry:

1. They penetrate many materials which either absorb or reflect light.
2. They can be seen on photographic film. (They can take a picture.)
3. *They can produce biological changes and even kill;* thus, we must be exceptionally careful in using X-radiation.

The Creation and Use of X rays

Electrons are minute particles of negative electrical charges which can be made to move rapidly. If electrons collide with a metal target at a high speed, X rays (or X-radiation) are produced. An X-ray tube is designed to be an

NEGATIVELY CHARGED
HOT FILAMENT
EMITTING
ELECTRONS

ELECTRON
PATHS TO
FORM A
BEAM

FOCUSING
CUP OR
REFLECTOR

FORMATION OF ELECTRON BEAM
BY FOCUSING DEVICE

AN ELECTRON SOURCE

The three requirements for the production of x-rays are all met in the x-ray tube. The cathode serves as the electron source. Electrons are emitted from the filament, a coil of tungsten wire, as it is heated to a high temperature. Because the filament gives off electrons in all directions, some means must be used to focus them on the target, directing their travel in a convergent stream across the x-ray tube. A reflector, or focusing cup, within the cathode structure, into which the filament is placed, focuses the electron beam much as light is focused by a flashlight reflector.

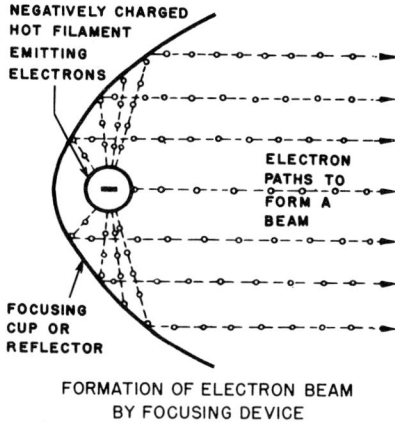

A TUNGSTEN TARGET

There must be a target for the electron beam to strike before x-rays are actually produced. In radiographic tubes the target proper is made of tungsten since it is a metal relatively efficient in x-ray production and one that will stand high temperatures without melting.

To help dissipate the large amounts of heat generated at the target, the tungsten is usually embedded in a large mass of copper. Copper conducts the heat away from the tungsten, dissipating it into oil, in the case of an oil-immersed tube.

FUNDAMENTALS OF AN X-RAY TUBE

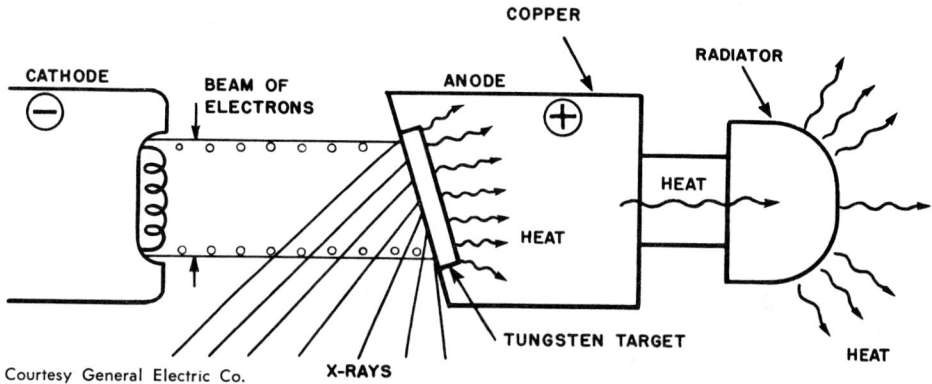

COPPER

RADIATOR

CATHODE   BEAM OF   ANODE
             ELECTRONS

HEAT

HEAT

HEAT

TUNGSTEN TARGET

Courtesy General Electric Co.   X-RAYS

Fig. 38.2. Schematic drawing of X-ray tube

efficient means of producing X rays. In an X-ray tube, the rapidly moving stream of electrons is directed against a metal target. When the electrons strike the target, they are stopped. A small portion of their energy is made into X rays; the rest is changed to heat.

In dental radiography, an X-ray tube is a sealed glass bulb from which all air has been pumped. It contains a *cathode* and an *anode*. The cathode is a filament of tungsten wire inside a focusing cup which directs the electrons to the target on the anode side of the tube. (See fig. 38.2.) The anode is a copper bar

with a tungsten button in it.[1] The button is called the target at which the stream of electrons is directed. There is an area on the tar-

1. The anode is made of copper because copper conducts heat well and helps absorb and remove the tremendous heat generated by the electrons when they strike the target. Remember that only a small portion of the electron energy becomes X rays; the rest is heat. Something must be done with the heat. It is a waste product to be dissipated. X-ray heads are either oil-cooled or gas-cooled. The oil-cooled tubes are completely immersed in oil, and the heat transfers from the copper bar to the oil. The gas-cooled tube is cooled by a similar process, using gas instead of oil. The heat is a waste product. Only the X-radiation is of use in radiography.

get, called a *focal spot,* which the electrons strike. The smaller the focal spot is, the better the detail of the X ray.

The number of electrons produced to form X rays is very important to good dental radiography. The number of electrons is determined by the heat of the cathode filament.[2] As the temperature of the cathode filament is increased, more electrons are produced. The number of electrons which form the stream is measured in *milliamperes,* which is an electrical term referring to the amount of electrical current being carried by the conductor (the copper wire). Thus, in X ray the milliamperage refers to the amount of current flowing to the X-ray head. If more current flows, the cathode filament becomes hotter. The hotter the cathode filament becomes, the more electrons are produced. The more electrons available, the greater the intensity of the X ray. Thus, when you adjust the milliampere control on the X-ray machine, you are watching the effect in the milliammeter of the increase or decrease in the number of electrons being hurled against the target. The milliammeter measures the amount of electrical *current* available. This really means that you determine with the milliammeter the current flow to be used in taking the photograph (which regulates *how many* electrons will hit the target).

Kilovoltage is another electrical term to be understood. Kilovoltage controls the *speed* at which the electrons travel, which is very important to the quality of the radiographs produced.

When the electrons travel at greater speed, the X rays produced are of shorter wavelength which gives them greater penetrating power.

2. One type of X-ray machine uses a heater in addition to the cathode. The cathode heats the heater. The heater produces the electrons. But regardless of its construction, either the heat of the cathode or the heat of the heater which is heated by the cathode produces electrons.

What do we mean by *penetrating power?* It simply means the ability to pass through an object. Thus, with greater penetrating power, the waves can pass through an object of greater thickness and density. The waves which pass through the object record the image on film; therefore, the X-ray waves which have the greatest penetrating power are most desirable in dentistry. The longer X-ray waves are *absorbed* by the tissue rather than being able to pass through it. (See chap. 39 "Safety," for a discussion of the longer waves.)

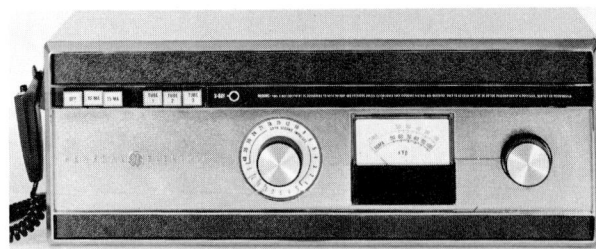

Fig. 38.3.   Controls for an X ray

Other factors which must be considered are the thickness and density of the object to be X-rayed. Obviously, two pieces of identical matter of different thickness will absorb X-radiation in different amounts. For example, a 2″ x 3″ sponge 1″ thick will absorb more water than a 2″ x 3″ sponge ½″ thick. Thus, thickness of the bone will determine the amount of X rays absorbed and the amount allowed to pass through. In addition, the density of the material will affect the absorption rate. Bone is denser than soft tissue. Some bone is denser than other bone. Thus, cortical bone (denser) absorbs more X-radiation and allows less to pass through than spongy bone. Spongy bone allows less radiation to pass through and absorbs more radiation than soft tissue. Soft tissue absorbs more than air spaces. Adult bones have greater calcium content and thus absorb more than the bones of young people, other considerations being equal.

The degrees of difference in absorption of X rays by the various tissues in the mouth give a radiograph its different shades of gray which make it an aid to diagnosis. The film is blacker—more exposed—where there is tissue; lighter where there are bones and teeth. The degree of darkness varies with the degree of denseness and thickness of the tissues through which the X ray must pass before reaching the film.

In technical discussions this degree of difference is spoken of as "an area-to-area variation in the intensity of the X rays which emerge from the subject." It simply means that the denser part of the bone lets less X rays through; therefore a variation in darkness on the X-ray film exists. It is called *subject contrast.* (The heavier the bone, the lighter the shade of the X-ray film.)

There should be subject contrast on a radiograph. However, if the equipment is not properly operated, the contrast can be so poor that the radiograph is unreadable or of such poor quality that diagnostic value is questionable.

To summarize, then, higher milliamperage produces a greater number of electrons, which means a greater total quantity of X rays. Likewise, decreasing the milliamperage decreases the quantity of X rays. The X-ray intensity of the image created on the film directly corresponds with the milliamperage setting. More milliamperage equals more blackness; less milliamperage equals less blackness, but over a range of milliamperage settings, *these various intensities of the parts of the image on the film will have an identical relationship to each other.* For example, let us assume that a given milliamperage setting is used to produce a film image which contains three different degrees of X-ray intensity as projected through the subject: one area is twice as dense as the second area, the second area is twice as dense

as the third. If the milliamperage setting is reduced and the X ray of the subject is repeated, the overall intensity of this film image will be lighter, but the three areas will be as before: one area will be twice as dense as the second area, the second area will be twice as dense as the third.

The kilovoltage setting controls the penetrating power of the X rays. Higher kilovoltage moves the electrons more rapidly. Faster-moving electrons mean greater penetrating power. Thus, the higher the kilovoltage, the more penetrating the X rays.

There are two additional effects which are not always desirable, however. (1) The entire range of X rays produced, if affected by the increase in kilovoltage setting, including the total production of "soft" or unused rays, will result in more radiation to the patient but no more effective exposure of the film. (2) Overall subject contrast is reduced when the kilovoltage is increased.

There is no universal agreement among dental radiologists on the ideal combinations of film, milliamperage setting, and kilovoltage setting to secure the best results. Distance (from target to film) is also a variable factor, depending on the particular technique your dentist wishes to use. Distance, milliamperage, and kilovoltage control the image intensity.

Geometry of Shadow

One objective in taking dental radiographs is to obtain as accurate an image of an area as possible. It is sometimes said that an X ray of a tooth is essentially the same as a shadow of the tooth. Sharpness and size of the radiographic image are two factors which contribute to the accuracy of the image. Thus, the smaller the focal spot and the nearer the film to the object being photographed, the more accurate the picture. If one tooth is farther from the film than its neighbor, the shadows of the teeth will be magnified in direct relation to their relationship to the film. If you will place a single light bulb in a holder about six feet from a wall, this principle can be more easily understood. Consider the light bulb as the target in the X-ray tube, and the wall as the X-ray film. Hold your clenched fist (the tooth) between the light source and the wall—first six inches from the wall, then a foot from the wall. When your fist is six inches from the wall, the shadow (the radiographic image of the tooth) is smaller than the shadow of the fist held one foot from the wall. In other words, the tooth closer to the film will show on the film as a smaller shadow than the tooth farther from the film. The difference in size can be figured mathematically if you know the difference in distance from the film. (See fig. 38.4.)

We have mentioned that the distance from the target to the film is a variable factor, depending on the X-ray technique used by your dentist. The eight-inch target-film distance has been used for many years and is still commonly used. "Long cone" techniques using target-film distances of sixteen inches are used for purposes of obtaining more true radiographic images, but due to problems of dental office design, the additional cone length is not always as convenient to use since there is limited space for maneuverability of the X-ray head.

You should understand the manner in which distance affects the radiographic image, however, not only because eight-inch target-film distance and sixteen-inch target-film distance techniques are used for periapical and bitewing films, but also because different dis-

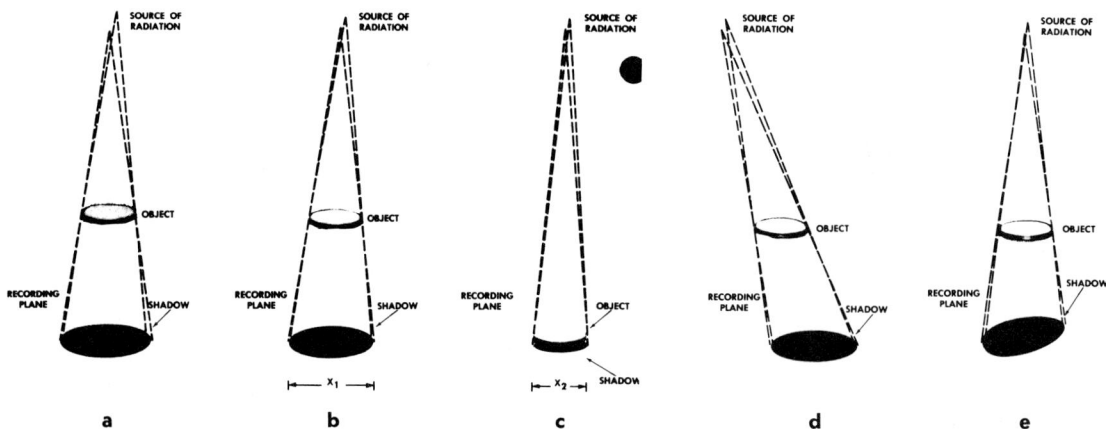

Courtesy Eastman Kodak Co.

Fig. 38.4. Diagrams showing geometrical effects on image sharpness: (a) Unsharpness caused by a large focal spot and long object-recording plane distance. (b) Improvement in sharpness produced by a small focal spot. (c) Superior result of a small focal spot and minimum distance between the object and recording plane. Notice also the enlargement (X_1) caused by the distance of the object from recording plane as compared to the more accurate size (X_2) produced when the object is close to the plane. There is a true enlargement in (d) because the object and recording surface are parallel even though the source of radiation is not vertically above the object. Distortion results when the object and the recording plane are not parallel (e).

tances are used for other dental X-ray procedures. An occlusal film packet may be used for a radiograph of the maxillary incisor region, a radiograph of the maxillary cuspid-molar region, or a radiograph of the maxillary arch. Each of these uses a distance of nine inches. The corresponding radiographs of the mandibular areas use a distance of ten inches. Sheet films, with intensifying screens, may be used for large-area radiographs of the mandible or of the temporomandibular articulation at distances of fifteen inches or greater. When necessary, even lateral headplates can be made at distances of seventy-two inches, using a dental X-ray machine.

It is necessary to know that distance also affects the intensity of the X rays reaching the film. The relationship of intensity to distance is known as the *inverse-square law*. This law states that the intensity of the radiation varies inversely as the square of the distance from its source. For example, let us say that the correct exposure at eight inches is one second. For the second area to be photographed imagine that it is physically impossible to place the X-ray machine head so that the distance is still eight inches. It has to be sixteen inches away. You can have the same intensity of X rays reaching the film if you will leave the milliamperage and kilovoltage settings exactly the same and increase the exposure time by the square of the increase in distance. Sixteen inches is twice as far away from the source (target) as the original eight inches; therefore, the exposure is two squared (2 x 2), or four times the exposure at eight inches, making the new correct exposure four seconds. A change in distance from target to film does not alter the subject contrast. The same is true in changing milliamperage. A change in kilovoltage, however, *will* result in a change in subject contrast, together with a change in the intensity of the X rays.

The factor of distance of the object from the film is important because it affects the quality of the X-ray photograph which your dentist must read for accurate diagnosis of the conditions within the mouth. If the film is placed close to the object to be X-rayed and in a plane parallel to it, the image is more likely to be accurate. If the object to be photographed is not parallel to the film, it will be distorted because part of it is farther from the film.

Accurate image formation is obtained by observing five rules:

1. The smallest practical focal spot is used. Usually this is controlled by the manufacturer of the dental X ray, and you don't need to think about it.
2. The longest focus-film distance which is practical is used.
3. The film is placed as close as possible to the area to be photographed.
4. The central ray of the X ray is directed as nearly at a right angle to the film as possible. The position of the film in the mouth will affect somewhat the possibility of using a right angle. You simply can't change the anatomy of the head of an individual, and often it will be impossible to aim at a perfect right angle.
5. The film should be parallel to the area being photographed insofar as it is practical.

Recording the Image

Photography is really the basis for radiography. A special film is used, but the essentials for photography—radiant energy, photosensitive film, and a chemical process which makes an invisible image visible and lasting—are present, as well as the object to be photographed.

Gelatin containing a silver compound forms an emulsion which is found on one or both sides of a base. This base and emulsion sand-wich is actually the X-ray film.

The emulsion is exceedingly sensitive, and whenever X rays are absorbed by it, a physical change occurs which is so fine that special chemical solutions must be used to make this change visible. The special chemical solution is called a *developer,* and it causes the exposed grains of silver compound to change to tiny masses of black metallic silver. Since the un-exposed grains are unaffected, the silver par-ticles suspended in gelatin make the visible image on the film.

Exposure

A radiograph is obtained when the film has been *exposed* to the area to be recorded by having X-radiation pass through the area to the film, thus physically changing the silver in the emulsion coating on the film.

The intensity of the X-radiation and the length of time the rays act on the film deter-mine the darkness of the image on the film. When the area to be X-radiated is dense, the time the X rays are allowed to penetrate the area must be increased, while the time neces-sary for penetrating an area where the bone is less dense is of shorter duration. For example, the lower incisor area takes the least amount of time for exposure, while the upper molar region takes the greatest amount of time.

Every manufacturer of dental film provides a table of exposure for their film which you can follow when exposing radiographs.

Sensitivity

The rapidity with which film responds to exposure is known as *sensitivity.* When little exposure is needed, the film is very sensitive and is known as high-speed film.

All dental film manufacturers make a regu-lar film and a high-speed film. One of the ad-vantages of high-speed film is that less X-radiation is used to make a photographic rec-ord, thus decreasing the X-ray dosage of the personnel and patient. Another advantage is that there is less chance that the patient will blur the image by moving.

Learn to produce the radiographic results which your dentist desires with the equipment he has available for your use.

Summary

X rays are necessary to complete diagnosis in dentistry. They can be dangerous and there-fore must be properly used.

A dental radiograph is a photographic rec-ord produced by the passage of X rays through the tissues of the mouth to a film.

Three characteristics of X rays important to dentistry are the following:

1. They penetrate many materials which either absorb or reflect light.
2. They can be seen on photographic film.
3. They can produce biological changes and even kill; thus, we must be exceptionally careful in using X ray.

We need to understand the construction of an X-ray tube and its correct operation. Vo-cabulary to understand includes milliamperes, kilovoltage, penetrating power, subject con-trast, geometry of shadow, exposure, and sen-sitivity.

Study Questions

1. What value are X rays in dentistry?
2. Give three important characteristics of X rays which must be considered when using them.
3. Define or explain these terms:

cathode	kilovoltage
anode	penetrating power
focal spot	subject contrast
milliamperes	geometry of shadow
exposure	sensitivity
emulsion	

4. Discuss "an area-to-area variation in intensity of X rays which emerge from the subject."
5. Give five rules for accurate image formation.

Bibliography

Eastman Kodak Co. *X-rays in Dentistry*. Rochester, N.Y.: Radiography Markets Division, Eastman Kodak Co., 1969.

General Electric Co. *Dental X-ray Generation and Radiographic Principles*. Milwaukee, Wis. Medical Systems Department, General Electric Co., n.d.

YALE, SEYMOUR H. "Radiology." In *Current Therapy in Dentistry*, vol. 4, edited by Henry Goldman et al. St. Louis, Mo.: C. V. Mosby, 1970.

39

Radiography: Elementary Knowledge... Safety

Potential Dangers of X ray

The potential danger of X ray, both to the personnel operating the equipment and to the patient whose teeth are X-rayed, must be thoroughly understood, and necessary precautions must be taken for the complete protection of all persons in the dental office. The use of X rays in dentistry contributes to the total radiation exposure of humans. This exposure must be kept within "safe limits" since the effect of radiation is cumulative over a period of time; that is, the dose you will receive tomorrow adds to the dose you received today, and they add to the amount you received yesterday to build a total X-radiation dosage.

Since the use of radiographs is *essential* to diagnosis in dentistry, it is important to continue using them. Proper precautions will result in adequate protection. But you must *know* how to eliminate the dangers to yourself and others and be careful to see that you *do eliminate them*.

Many pioneers in the field of radiology died because the dangers of X-ray radiations to the unprotected operator were not understood.

Today, detailed information for the protection of personnel is available in NCRP Report Number 5, available from the National Council on Radiation Protection and Measurements. The report is titled *Dental X-ray Protection* and is listed in the Bibliography with information concerning its purchase.

What are the risks to the patient and office personnel from an overdose of X-radiation? Repeated doses of X-radiation build up the effect of X rays on the tissues of the body. When the radiation goes beyond the limits which the body tissues can tolerate, the tissues begin to break down. A "burn" is the first symptom. Continuation of the breakdown will eventually result in death when it is a vital organ or fluid which is affected. X-radiation is also known to cause biologic changes by affecting the reproductive organs of certain humans, which in turn affect the unborn children. Some of the tissues of the body are radiosensitive, which means that these cells are very sensitive to X rays. Cells of the blood, hair, skin, nails, and reproductive organs are some of the tissues most sensitive to X-radiation. However, any tissue may be injured by overexposure. You have only to think what would happen to you if the cells of the blood were overexposed to X-radiation and began to break down. Continued breakdown would result in the inability of the blood to function at all.

One of the first symptoms of overexposure is radiation dermatitis. It looks somewhat like sunburn. If the erythema, or reddening of the skin, is not heeded, further stages of the condition include scaling of the skin, a loss of hair, brownish pigmentation, stiffening of fingers, cracking of tissue over joints, longitudinal splitting of the nails, piling up of outer layers of the skin, and sores which fail to heal. These may become chronic and may eventually become cancerous.

Hazards

What are the hazards and how can we eliminate them?

Primary Beam

The first hazard, obviously, is the direct roentgen beam itself. It comes from the X-ray head. This beam is needed to photograph the area which your dentist wishes to study. The head of the machine is aimed at the patient's face. Most of the rays enter his tissue and record the desired image on the film. However, anything in front of that tube receives the rays. The finger which holds the film in position receives as much dosage as the rest of the area. Therefore, it is a hard-and-fast rule that never, *never* does the assistant or dentist —or anyone else habitually exposed to working with radiology—*ever* hold that film in place.

Formerly the patient was asked to hold the film in place. However, the NCRP recommendations of 1970 suggest that film holders are available which eliminate the need for the patient to hold the film packet in place. Some of the holders help reduce the dosage of X ray to the patient.

Should your dentist not employ film holders, and a patient is unable to hold the film for any reason, a relative or friend should hold the film—*not* the dental assistant.

The roentgen rays from the focal spot on the target of the X-ray machine are primary beams and are most dangerous for repeated exposures.

It is important to understand where the X-ray beams are traveling in order to remain out of their path.

X rays radiate from their source in all directions. Since they are needed in only one direction to take the picture, the X-ray tube is designed so that the X-radiation can escape only through one opening—a sort of window in the tube housing. The X rays which escape through this opening are of different wavelengths and penetrating power.

We speak of the X rays "escaping" in only one direction. Obviously something must be able to stop the rays from traveling. Generally, lead is used. It is found in the X-ray tube housing to keep the X rays from escaping anywhere but through the one opening designed for the purpose.

The primary beam (the greatest number of X rays) leaves the target of the machine in a cone-shaped path. The size of the cone increases as the distance from the target increases. The plastic cone of the X-ray machine does not limit the beam; it only aids in visualizing the field due to the open-end cone.

Closed-end plastic cones are conceded to be a source of secondary radiation. In some states open-ended metal or lead-shielded cones are required by law.

X-ray machines which are currently being sold now have a lead-lined or metal-lined cone which contains the X rays more effectively, permitting the rays to travel only in the desired direction.

Studies indicate that an operator should stand six feet from the machine, in an area between ninety and forty-five degrees from the central ray, as illustrated in figures 39.1 and 39.2, to be in the safest position while the machine is in operation.

Scattered Radiation

Scattered radiation is a danger to be considered carefully in any dental office. Scattered radiation is of two types: leakage and secondary.

Leakage radiation. Some of the X rays have bounced off the target in the X-ray tube in all directions. Modern tubes and heads of X-ray machines are protected, but where leakage from the head of the X ray occurs, it must be considered dangerous to the operator.

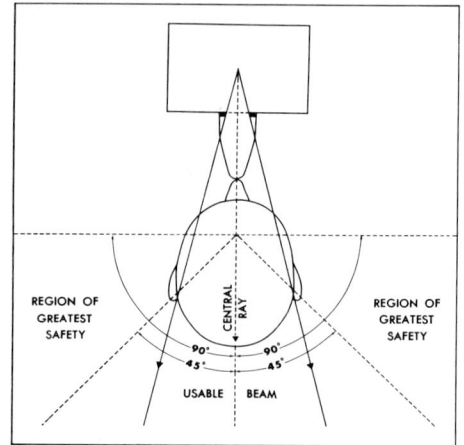

Fig. 39.1. Diagram illustrating the 2 positions of greatest safety during the projection of the central incisor region. They are located on each side of the patient's head at an angle of 45 to 90 degrees to the central ray.

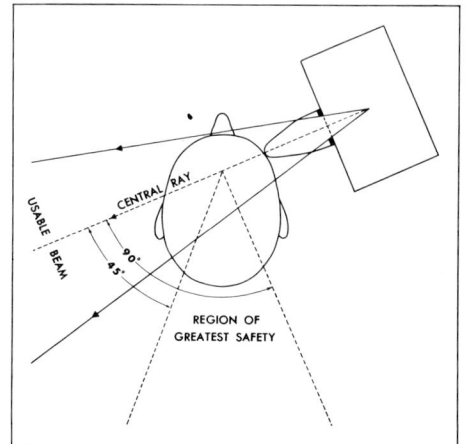

Fig. 39.2. Diagram illustrating the position of greatest safety for all projections except for the central incisors. It is located 45 to 90 degrees to the central ray, but the operator must stand behind the patient's head.

(Fig. 39.1 and 39.2 are reprinted with the permission of Doctor Albert G. Richards, Professor of Dentistry, University of Michigan, Ann Arbor, Michigan. They are from an article "Sources of X-radiation in the Dental Office" written by Doctor Richards in *Dental Radiography and Photography*, vol. 37, 1964, no. 3, published by Eastman Kodak Company, Rochester, New York. The article is highly recommended for study.)

Secondary radiation. This radiation is "new radiation which is created by primary radiation acting on or passing through matter."[1] Secondary radiation, then, is the radiation which is emitted in all directions from the patient's head as he is being radiographed.

A lead apron is required in some states to be placed over the patient during radiography. The apron is used to protect the patient from

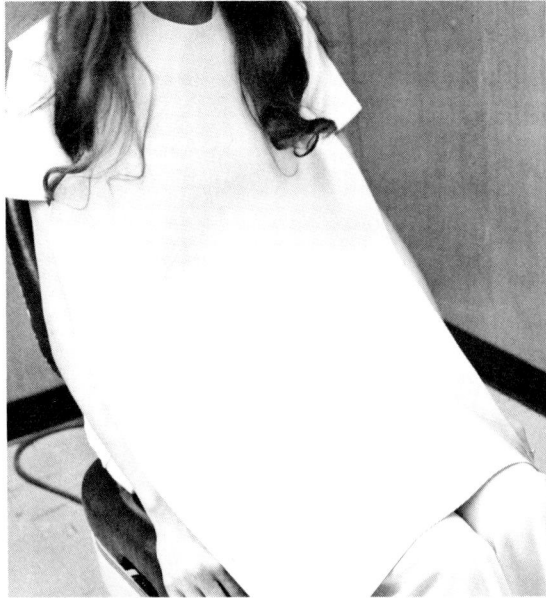

Courtesy Rinn Corp.

Fig. 39.3. A patient protective apron to be used during filming of radiographs.

the secondary radiation which is emitted from his head during filming. The primary beam from the X-ray machine is very well controlled and strikes only the area of the mouth at which it is aimed. It is the secondary radiation, the new radiation created by the primary radiation as it passes through the area of the mouth, which is dangerous to the patient—or *anyone else in its path.*

1. Carl O. Boucher, ed., *Current Clinical Dental Terminology,* p. 304.

Protection

Everyone in the dental office can be protected from overdosage by observing a few safety rules. The NCRP report states that the exposure of persons other than the patient can be limited by a combination of three measures:

(*a*) increasing the distance of the individual from the source,
(*b*) reducing the duration of exposure, and
(*c*) using protective barriers (shielding) between the individual and the source.

The bulletin further states that protective shielding and distance are the factors most easily controlled in the dental office. Protective shielding includes that which is built into the X-ray machine and barriers used in the office, such as thick concrete walls, lead-lined walls, or movable lead shields.

The patient can be protected by techniques of radiography and by careful record of the total exposure of the patient, with determination to eliminate any unnecessary use of X ray. (If the patient has had a cumulative dosage which is dangerously high, the necessity of radiographs versus the health hazard without them is a decision which the dentist must make.)

Although everyone can be protected from overdosage, uncertainty frequently exists about the dosage the personnel are receiving. Scattered radiation and the individual's lack of awareness of his own habit patterns are factors affecting the dosage received. One way to be certain that an individual employee is not receiving a dangerous amount of X-radiation in the course of a day's work is for the office to subscribe to a film-badge service.

The service provides a film badge for each employee to wear. (See fig. 39.4.) Each week the badges are collected, and the service determines the amount of radiation and the energy level of the radiation. The energy level indicates whether the radiation is gamma or X

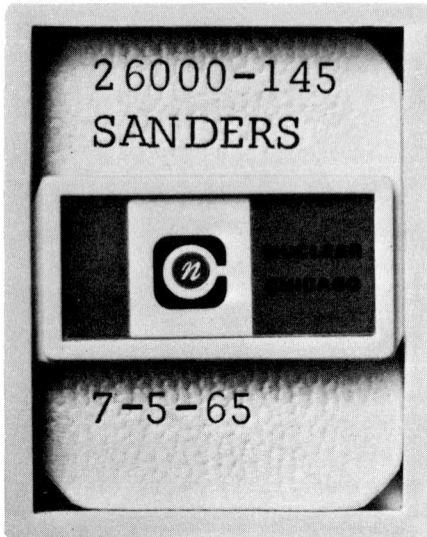

Courtesy Nuclear Corp.

Fig. 39.4.   Film badge

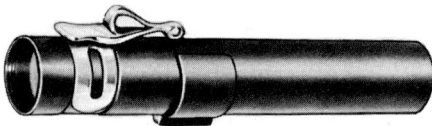

Courtesy Rinn Corp.

Fig. 39.5.   Radiometer to be worn by office personnel. Another method of measuring exposure to X-radiation.

ray. The service also determines whether the radiation passed through lead, plastic, copper, or aluminum. Thus the service tells you the *amount* and *type* of radiation to which you have been exposed. If there is leakage radiation in your office, it will be easy to recognize that your X-ray machine needs some attention.

Today, in some areas, legislation compels any owner of a radiation source to monitor the amount of radiation reaching personnel. (An X-ray machine is a radiation source.) Where passed, this legislation means that each dentist must provide film-badge service or some equivalent method of verifying the X-radiation dosage he and his staff receive.

Some persons believe that a paper clip or penny attached to a film packet worn in a pocket is a method of determining the exposure to X-radiation. (The film is developed at the end of a week. If there has been too much radiation leakage, the penny or paper clip will show on the film.) Actually, this method is ineffective because it doesn't tell the *amount* of exposure nor the type of radiation.

The rules, then, to protect everyone in the office from an overdose of deadly X rays are these:

1. Use of the fastest available film to cut the amount of time the deadly rays are in operation in your office.
2. Use lead protection whenever possible: walls, aprons, or shields.
3. Use a long cord for the controls or have the controls in another room.
4. Never hold the film for a patient.
5. Never have your hand on the tube housing or pointer cone while the machine is filming the patient.
6. Stand at least six feet away from the patient in the proper area of the room. (See figs. 39.1 and 39.2.)
7. Wear a film badge.

Summary

The potential danger of X ray must be thoroughly understood, and necessary protection should be afforded all persons who come in contact with X ray.

Symptoms of overdose of X ray must be recognized.

Hazards to be memorized:

1. Direct roentgen beam
2. Scattered radiation
   a. Leakage radiation
   b. Secondary radiation

Seven rules should be observed to protect everyone in the office from an overdose of X ray.

Study Questions

1. Describe the potential dangers of X ray.
2. What precautions must be taken in the dental office against dangers of X ray?
3. List and describe the hazards in the use of X ray.
4. Describe the symptoms of X-ray overdose.
5. What are the seven rules to be observed to protect the office personnel and patients from an overdose of X ray?

Bibliography

BOUCHER, CARL O., ed. *Current Clinical Dental Terminology.* St. Louis, Mo.: C. V. Mosby Co., 1963.

NCRP. *Dental X-ray Protection.* Washington, D.C.: National Council on Radiation Protection and Measurements, 1970. This booklet can be purchased for $1.50 from NCRP, P. O. Box 4867, Washington, D. C. 20008.

40

Radiography: Elementary Knowledge... Dental X-ray Machine and Dental Film

The Dental X-ray Machine

If you ever have a chance to visit the Smithsonian Institution in Washington, D. C., please do treat yourself to a trip through the dental section. There you will see early dental equipment—including an ancient X-ray machine with its high-tension wire strung out in the open. One look at it and you can really appreciate the handsome, efficient machines in use today.

A specific type of X-ray machine is used in the dental office. It is usually labeled 40 to 70 or 100 kvp which means that its voltage range is 40,000 to 70,000 or 100,000 volts. This high range is necessary for dental radiology. The machines used for medical radiology and therapeutic or industrial radiology are quite different in construction and voltage. Some are low-voltage machines, but some may use 3,000,000 volts.

We are concerned with only the dental X-ray machine. Its basic electrical parts are a high-voltage circuit, a low-voltage circuit, an X-ray tube, a control circuit, and a timer.

Not all dental offices have the latest equipment. You may find that the X-ray machine in your office is not of the very latest type. Some machines operate with a narrow, fixed range of kilovoltage (usually a fixed kilovoltage of 65, a milliamperage of 10, and target-film distance of 8 inches). The newer machines have adjustable kilovoltage controls. The selection is usually from 40 to 70 or 100 kilovolts, a milliamperage range of 5 to 15, and timers which permit exposures of extremely short duration. The new equipment also allows the use of either an eight-inch or sixteen-inch target-film distance. There will be two meters to check: the kilovoltmeter and the milliammeter.

The dental X ray has a high-tension transformer which steps up the 110-volt alternating current (which your office receives from the electrical outlet) to the desired 40,000 to 100,-000 volts necessary for radiography. There are two circuits involved in the transformer: the primary circuit is connected through a control device called the voltage compensator or auto-transformer; the secondary circuit is connected to the X-ray tube terminals. The auto-transformer is a manual control which you turn to the voltmeter reading you want.

Another transformer, the filament or step-down transformer, is used to provide current for the filament. It reduces the line voltage to about twelve volts which heats the tungsten filament in the cathode to produce the electrons.

The Tube

We have already described the dental X-ray tube and its operation in the production of radiographs. (See pp. 528-530.)

The Head

Recent developments in head construction of X-ray units have changed the appearance—and safety—of the head. Formerly, the closed-end cone was all plastic, and plastic acts as a source of secondary radiation. The new heads have a cylinder-shaped cone rather than a pointed one. The cylinder contains metal which prevents scattered radiations from escaping. (One leading manufacturer advertises the head cylinder as lead-lined acrylic; another as lead and stainless steel.)

The purpose of the cone is to allow the operator to align the beam accurately with the area to be radiographed. The new cylindrical cones are designed to accomplish this necessary function even though they are not shaped to a point as the older-model cones are. Diaphragms and filters are used to further restrict the X-ray beams and block scattered radiation. It is conceded that some operators find it more difficult to see angulation with open-ended cones, but compensation is possible with film holders and specific training.

Adaptations for older machines are available. The pointed cone is discarded, and the replacement cylindrical cone is attached to the X ray (fig. 40.1).

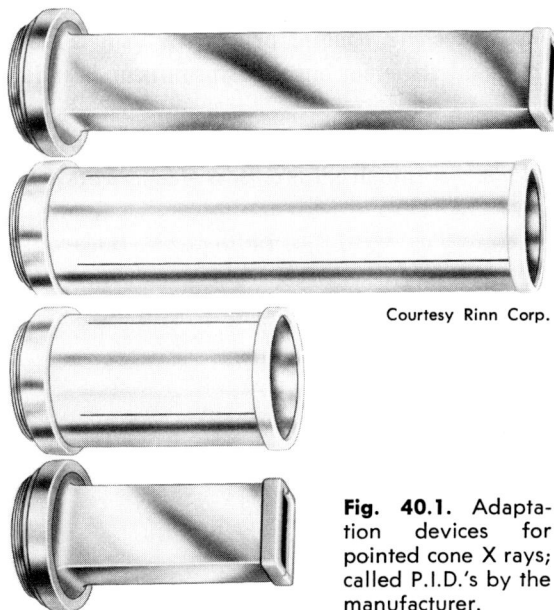

Courtesy Rinn Corp.

Fig. 40.1. Adaptation devices for pointed cone X rays; called P.I.D.'s by the manufacturer.

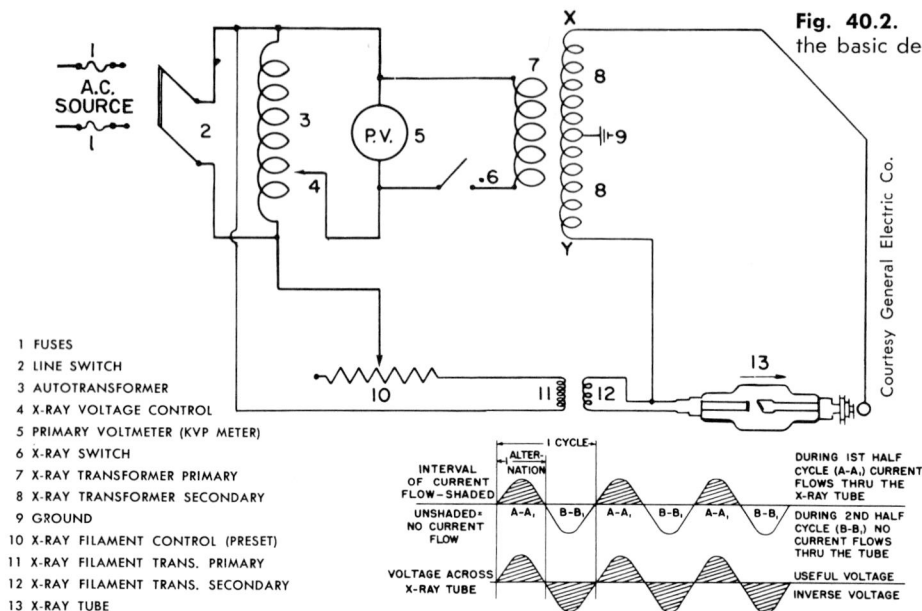

Fig. 40.2. Schematic drawing of the basic dental X-ray unit.

Courtesy General Electric Co.

1 FUSES
2 LINE SWITCH
3 AUTOTRANSFORMER
4 X-RAY VOLTAGE CONTROL
5 PRIMARY VOLTMETER (KVP METER)
6 X-RAY SWITCH
7 X-RAY TRANSFORMER PRIMARY
8 X-RAY TRANSFORMER SECONDARY
9 GROUND
10 X-RAY FILAMENT CONTROL (PRESET)
11 X-RAY FILAMENT TRANS. PRIMARY
12 X-RAY FILAMENT TRANS. SECONDARY
13 X-RAY TUBE

A basic x-ray unit consists of the three types of transformers, the x-ray tube and several additional devices. The circuit is shown above. For explanatory purposes the basic circuit is separated into the filament circuit, the high-voltage circuit and the timing circuit.

The Timer

The X ray has a timer on it which allows you to set a pointer at the desired number of seconds or fractions of a second for exposure and then push a button. The timer automatically allows the machine to produce X rays in the amount of time for which you have set the indicator. It increases markedly the accuracy of the time factor in radiograph. The only errors with such a device are caused by faulty equipment or inaccurate setting of the timer indicator by the operator. The directions with the X-ray machine which your dentist owns will explain what to do if you have made an error in setting the timer.

Operating the Machine

As with all work in the dental office, an orderly routine is important in operating the X-ray machine.

1. Turn on the switch. Warm-up may be required for some machines. Some manufacturers recommend turning the machine on in the morning and off at the end of the day.
2. Check the milliammeter setting to see that the current is reaching the machine.
3. Check the kilovoltmeter setting.
4. Set the timer to the desired number of seconds or fraction of a second.
5. When your doctor signals you that he is ready, press the release button and hold it depressed. The timer will count off the seconds or fraction of a second.
6. Observe the milliammeter during the exposure. If it is not operating, the photograph will not appear on your film. Usually the required milliammeter reading is ten.
7. When you have finished the series of radiographs for one patient, turn off the machine if so instructed.

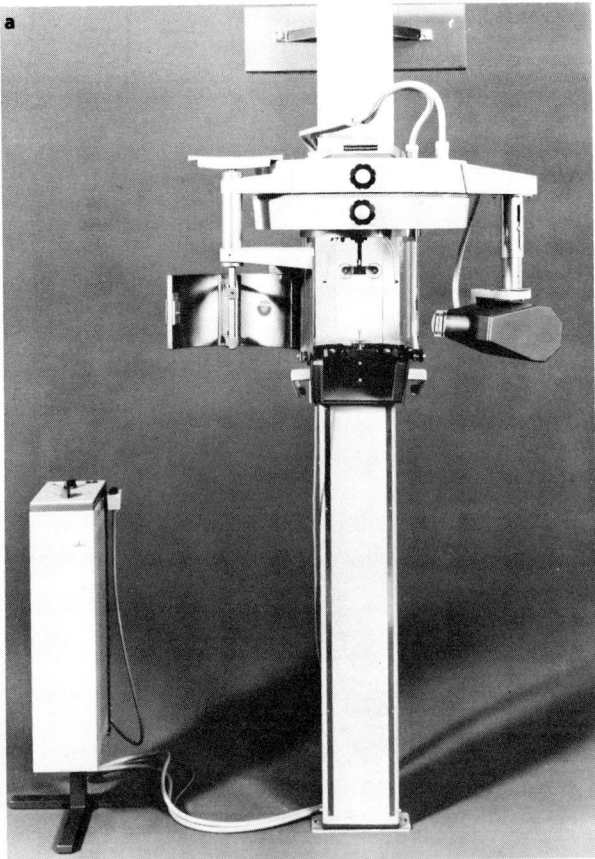

The Panoramic X ray

The panoramic X ray is used for a generalized overview of the oral cavity. The patient sits or stands with his chin on a chin rest (fig. 40.3a). The tube and film move around his head, recording an X ray of the oral cavity on one large sheet of film contained in a cassette

Fig. 40.3. (a) Orthopantomograph—panoramic X-ray unit. Patient positioning standing up, sitting down, or even in a wheelchair. Vertically adjustable; 6" x 12" size radiogram, including both T M joints and sinuses without center blur due to its continuous rotation. With the aid of the built-in 3 major rotation axis, image is completely distortion-free. (b) Orthoceph. Panoramic X-ray machine with cephalometric attachment permanently mounted on it. Vertically adjustable. Cephalostat timer built in the control box. Combination of the Orthopantomograph and cephalostat.

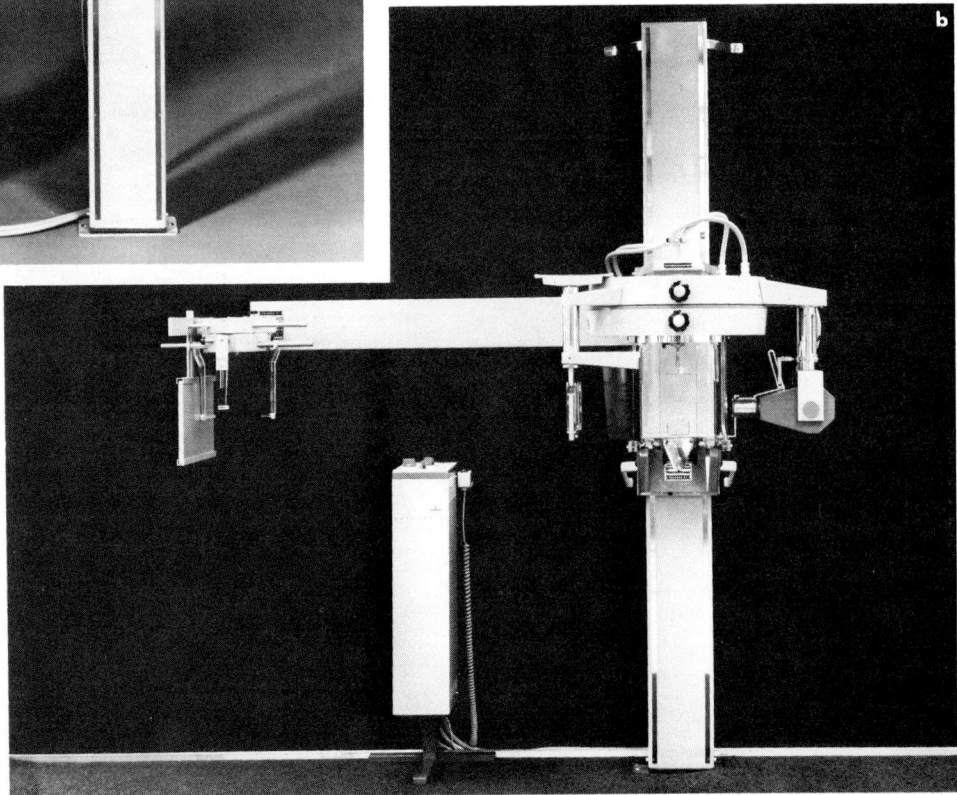

Courtesy Siemens Corp.

mounted in the machine (fig. 40.5). Because the film is outside the mouth and far from the X-ray source, the detail is relatively poor in some areas. A theoretical curved plane is in focus, and the rest of the area is out of focus. The result is a radiograph with some areas in excellent focus and others out of focus.

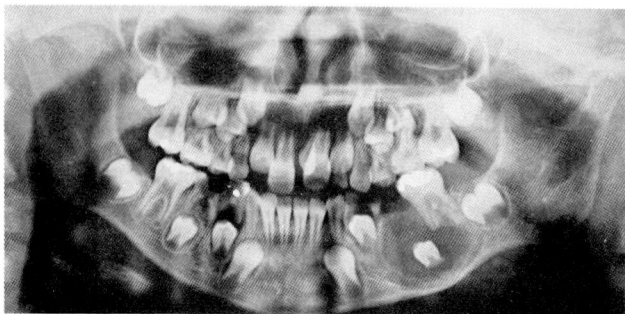

Fig. 40.4. Radiogram made with the Orthopanto-mograph. Advantages: (1) Less radiation exposure; it takes 13 seconds. (2) Uses 5″ x 12″ or 6″ x 12″ film due to 3 axis rotation system; 6″ x 12″ film shows upper and lower jaw, T M joints, and sinuses. (3) Patient can stand or sit in normal chair or wheelchair. (4) Occupies one square foot of floor space with no chair required.

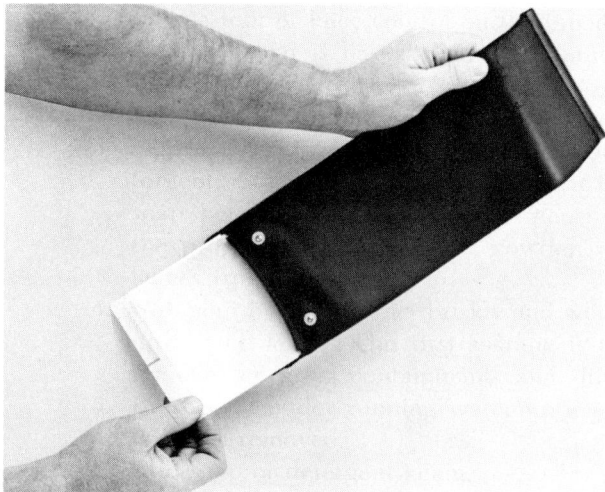

Fig. 40.5. A panoramic X-ray cassette for film

The panoramic is intended as a survey-type film which enables the dentist to see more anatomy. It is a screening view. The periapical film may still be necessary for operation. If a dentist uses the panorama approach to roentgenographic study, the usual procedure is a panorama view and posterior bitewings. If anything on the panorama indicates the need, individual periapical films are made of those areas.

One of the advantages of the panorama is that the radiation dose is less than for a full mouth taken on individual periapical films. In addition, the problem of holding films correctly, either with bite blocks or by the use of the patient's finger, is eliminated. Film confusion is lessened because films are identified in the cassette. Films need not be mounted, thus a tedious, time-consuming, and difficult job is eliminated.

Dental Film—Intraoral and Extraoral

Two general classes of film are used for dental radiography. They are *intraoral* and *extraoral*. In this usage, *intra* means "inside" and *extra* means "outside": inside the mouth, outside the mouth.

Intraoral radiography is the type most commonly used by the general practitioner of dentistry. This technique allows the examination of teeth, surrounding tissue, and some limited examination of the maxillae or mandible.

There are three types of intraoral film: periapical, interproximal (or bitewing), and occlusal. *Periapical films* are used to examine the entire tooth and its surrounding tissues. *Interproximal films* examine the surfaces of the teeth which touch each other and the tissues and bones in those areas. We call them bitewing X rays in the dental office. *Occlusal films* are used for areas of the maxillae or mandible to discover pathology, root fragments, unerupted teeth, fractures, and other conditions.

In addition to providing total oral cavity view with the panograph machine, other types of extraoral radiographs are used to give the dentist additional information which he may need for certain conditions. They are used for further examination of the mandible and maxilla and, in addition, of the temporomandibular joints and articulation and the facial bone and profile. These radiographs may be used in the study of injury, bone disease, presence of foreign bodies, development of the jaws, and presence of abnormalities. Orthodontists use facial profile radiographs (cephalometry) to measure bone structure and unerupted teeth, record conditions of the patient, and later to observe changes due to treatment or growth. They may be used in prosthodontics to record the relationship of the soft tissue of the face and the natural relationship of the teeth prior to their removal in order that the prosthetic devices may restore as much natural appearance as possible—and that the patient may be allowed to see that the natural appearance has been restored.

Film Description and Management

Dental film itself is composed of an emulsion, that is, gelatin containing a silver compound coated on a tinted base which is made from a cellulose derivative. The base is about 0.008 inch thick. It is stiff and flat to the degree necessary for proper manipulation. If the base is coated on both sides with emulsion, it provides maximum film speed, which means less radiation for patient and operators. Speed means shorter exposures. Shorter exposures also have an added advantage: the patient is less likely to move and blur the image; therefore less retakes are needed with faster film.

Standardization is occurring in film production. All manufacturers now put the film speed on the outside of the package. Perhaps film speed will be standardized and classified by number in the near future. The correct number for the speed of the film can be used on all film packets. In addition, film size could be standardized.

The large sheets of emulsion-coated base which is to become dental film are cut to the size used for one of the several types of dental films. It is then either made into a packet for the intraoral work or packaged for extraoral use.

Intraoral Film

Periapical film is manufactured in three sizes: No. 1, or standard film, is about 1¼" x 1⅝"; child's film, or No. 0 or 00, is about ⅞" x 1⅜". Some manufacturers make an in-between size for older children (6 years to 11 or 12 years of age) which is about 15/16" x 1-9/16". Standard periapical film is used for older children and adults. It usually shows three or four teeth and the surrounding bone and tissue, including the apex of the root. Children's film is used for small children.

Bitewing film is made in three sizes: No. 1 for anterior teeth, No. 2 for bicuspid or molar teeth, and No. 3 for bicuspid and molar teeth. One manufacturer has a film which is twice as long as a normal periapical film. It is used to replace two films of the regular size for bitewing use.

A tab or flap is used with bitewing film to hold it in proper position for these X rays. The tab fits between the lower and upper arches and is held firmly in place by the patient when he closes his teeth as the film is placed.

Occlusal film is about 2¼" x 3" and is used to show larger areas which cannot be seen on a periapical film. The film is held in place in the mouth, much like a cracker, by gentle pressure of the teeth.

Extraoral Film

Extraoral film is usually a 5" x 7" or 8" x 10" sheet. The 5" x 7" size is used for the lateral jaw technique; the 8" x 10" size is used for posteroanterior views. Sometimes a larger size is also used for these views.

The film is supplied in boxes of various sizes. Each film is placed between a folded sheet of black paper. All the films are wrapped in lightproof paper which usually has a tinfoil backing and are then placed in a cardboard container and sealed. This container must not be opened except in a darkroom which is equipped for safely handling such film. In order to use this film, a film holder can be made of cardboard to hold the film in a lightproof container while exposure is made.

If it is desirable to reduce the time exposure and still use the same emulsion, a cassette is used instead of a film holder. It is usually an aluminum case in which two intensifying screens are placed.

An *intensifying screen* is a device which helps obtain the image on the film in a shorter period of time than is possible with X-ray film alone. A screen is a smooth cardboard or plastic sheet coated with tiny fluorescent crystals mixed in a suitable binder. X rays can make certain substances give off visible light. These substances are phosphors. Two of them, calcium tungstate and barium lead sulfate, both of which give off blue light, are used to make intensifying screens. Each fluorescent crystal which absorbs X-ray energy gives off blue and ultraviolet radiation. The intensity is directly related to the intensity of the X rays in that part of the image. Therefore the differences in intensity of the X ray are transformed into differences in intensity in the blue and ultraviolet light. The film is highly sensitive to this light. It means that the light helps make the image faster than the X-ray beam alone can make it. Usually there are three types of intensifying screens: (1) fast for high intensification, (2) average for balance between speed and definition, and (3) "slow" for better image sharpness. Average screens usually are used for extraoral radiography. These screens, placed in

the cassette, must contact the surface of the film perfectly, and the cassette must be lightproof.

Suitable marking equipment is needed to identify the X rays and the side visualized. This is important since an X ray may be used as evidence. The question may arise as to how your dentist knows that this particular film is actually an X ray of the patient involved in the court action. A code number or actual printing of a patient's name on the X ray will remove any doubt. No method is available for intraoral film marking as yet.

Panographic Film

The panographic film is placed in a cassette with an intensifying screen. One manufacturer uses a wrap-around film cassette which is a lighttight vinyl envelope. Another manufacturer uses a flat metal box as the cassette.

Care of the intensifying screen is important because anything which affects the screen also affects the film image. The screens must be protected from damage and dust. Chemicals dripped into the cassette can leave a stain on the screen which will block the X ray. Be certain the cassette and screens are clean at all times. Screens may be cleaned with a *damp* (not wet) sponge or with alcohol.

Getting Acquainted with the Actual Film

For all practical purposes, the periapical film will acquaint you with dental X-ray film. To the layman, an X-ray film is a white paper-covered object which is placed in his mouth when an X ray is to be made. To the dental personnel, this packet consists of the outer wrapper which is sometimes in two pieces, a piece of black paper, a thin sheet of lead foil, the film itself (the emulsion-coated base), and another piece of black paper.

Take a packet apart. See and feel each part. Close your eyes and learn to distinguish the various pieces by touch so that you will recognize them when you develop X rays in the darkroom. The larger 5″ x 7″ or 8″ x 10″ film will feel the same as the periapical-size film itself. Thus you can discern its texture from the wrappings in which the larger films are packaged just as you differentiate the periapical, occlusal, or bitewing films from their wrappings.

Protecting the Film

Film must be protected from the X rays which escape in the dental office during the filming of a patient's mouth. Thus it is kept in a film storage box which is lined with lead to protect the film.

There are two commonly used types of storage boxes. One is approximately ten inches long, six inches wide, and four inches deep, with a removable lid. The other type is a wall-mounted metal container which will hold more than one package of periapical film stacked vertically. Individual films are removed from the bottom of the film "safe," and provision is made for refilling as needed. (See fig. 40.6.)

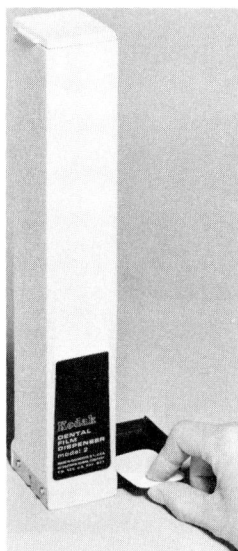

Courtesy Eastman Kodak Co.

Fig. 40.6. Film dispenser

In the first type of storage box mentioned, more flexibility is available for storing different sizes of films. The various sizes of film used in the office may be kept separate from each other by the use of cardboard boxes within the film storage container.

It is also important that the film exposed during radiography of a patient be stored in a lead container in order that stray radiation does not spoil the radiograph already recorded on the film.

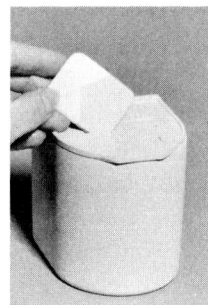

Fig. 40.7. Receptacle for exposed film. Film is placed in this protective container until all radiography for the patient has been completed.

Summary

The parts of the X-ray machine with which you should be especially familiar are the tube and the timer.

There are seven steps in operating the X-ray machine which should be memorized.

The panograph X ray automatically records a full-mouth roentgenogram of a patient who is resting his chin on a chin rest. The full-mouth X ray appears on one sheet of film. Less exposure time is required than for the individual periapical films. However, detail may not show as clearly in all areas. The panograph may indicate the use of a periapical film for a particular area.

Two general classes of film are used for dental radiography. They are intraoral (inside the mouth) and extraoral (outside the mouth).

Three types of intraoral film are periapical, interproximal, and occlusal.

Extraoral radiography is used to give the dentist added information which he may need for certain conditions.

Dental film is composed of an emulsion coated on a tinted base. High-speed film is more desirable since it means less exposure to X rays and less danger of the patient moving and blurring the image.

Films are made in various sizes. You should be familiar with the sizes used in your office.

Extraoral film is usually a sheet 5″ x 7″ or 8″ x 10″. This film is sometimes used in a cassette instead of a film holder.

An intensifying screen helps obtain the image in a shorter period of time than is possible by the film alone.

Extraoral film should be marked with an identifying number or name.

It is wise to get acquainted with X-ray film by taking a packet apart.

Film must be protected both before and after exposure from the radiation which will be found in the dental office during the exposure of other films. There are lead-lined containers for used and unused film.

Study Questions
1. Discuss the X-ray head as it is manufactured today.
2. What is the purpose of a timer?
3. Describe the operation of a standard X-ray machine.
4. Describe a panoramic X ray and state its purpose.
5. Discuss the different types of film and their purposes.
6. How is film protected? From what must it be protected?

41 *Radiographic Techniques... Intraoral and Extraoral*

Quality Radiographs

The quality of radiographs depends on the skill with which they are produced. A poor radiograph prevents or interferes with the making of an accurate diagnosis. Since the purpose of the radiograph is diagnosis, we should not expose human beings to dangerous X rays unless the results of the exposure will be radiographs of excellent quality.

This chapter is devoted to a discussion of the techniques which will produce excellent radiographs. Whatever part you play in their production (depending upon the laws of your state and the wishes of your dentist), it is imperative that you develop expert skills in the execution of your duties from proper preparation of the patient for X rays to hanging films to dry. While some states do not permit the dental assistant to take X rays, it is the belief of the writers that this function will be more broadly legalized as a function of the dental assistant.

Certain steps must be followed to secure good radiographs: It is necessary to select the correct film, properly prepare and position the patient, correctly place the film, see that it is properly retained, position the X-ray head, make the correct exposure, remove the film, and place the film in safe storage before the next film is exposed. Intraoral radiographs add one step after removal of the film: Wipe off all moisture; then place the film in safe storage before proceeding with the next exposure.

The patient should be routinely asked when he last had X-ray studies made; whether he has been exposed to X-ray or gamma-ray radiation for industrial, experimental, medical diagnostic, or therapeutic reasons. It may be that the patient has received his maximum dose of X-ray or gamma-ray radiation and that further exposure might produce detrimental results for which you might be held responsible.

The patient should remove such items as glasses, dentures, removable partial dentures, or removable bridgework. Any of these objects will produce shadows on the X ray. These shadows may obscure details which should be observed or may cause confusion in diagnosis.

Intraoral Procedures

The Relationship of the Patient to the X-ray Tube

The plane of occlusion of the teeth to be visualized on the radiograph should be parallel to the floor. The sagittal plane (vertical, midline plane) of the body should be perpendicular to the floor. Thus the spine should be straight—at right angles to the floor—and the occlusal plane of the teeth should be parallel to the floor.

Mouths vary, and it is sometimes necessary to make adjustments in the film techniques to accommodate the differences in individuals. Some mouths have narrow dental arches, some have high vaults.

Angulations, as indicated on charts of recommended X-ray tube positions, are now properly read on the angulation scales on the X-ray machine. Having the patient properly

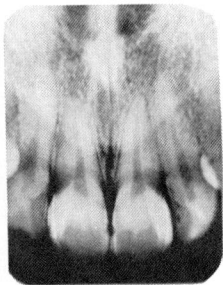

Courtesy Eastman Kodak Co.

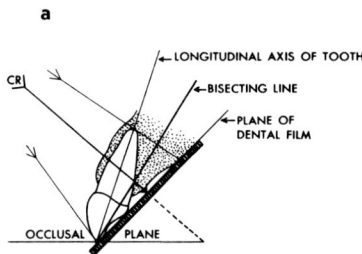

Fig. 41.1. Central ray—verticle angle. (a) Proper projection of central ray (right) results in images of correct proportion (left). (b) When central ray is projected from too low an angle (right), images are elongated (left). (c) When central ray is projected from too high an angle (right), images are foreshortened (left).

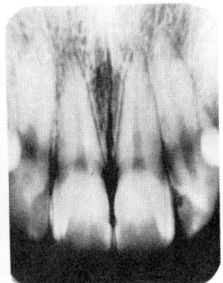

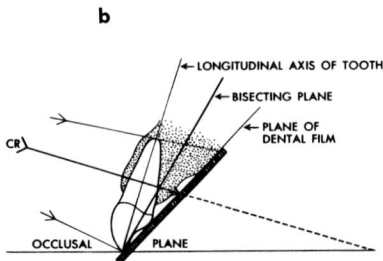

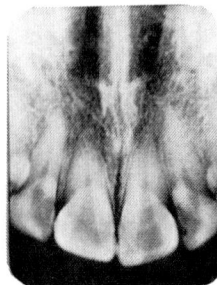

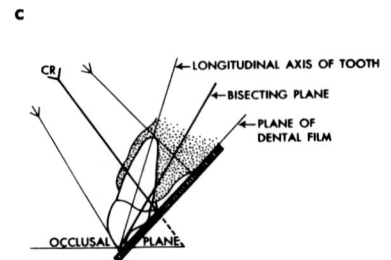

positioned makes these scales on the machine effective and useful. For example, if the patient is to have an upper central incisor radiographed, he is seated with the upper arch horizontal. The X-ray tube head is adjusted to a vertical angle of forty to forty-five degrees. The X-ray film is placed, any necessary adjustment is made in tube angulation for variation in vault shape, and the exposure is made.

If, however, the patient is seated with the upper arch sloping toward the distal twenty degrees (let us say), the tube-head angle would have to be increased to sixty to sixty-five degrees for an average range. If the exposure were made at the recommended angulation but with the patient incorrectly oriented to the tube head and no visual correction or adjustment made, the resulting X-ray visualization would be elongated to the point of worthlessness.

The general rule for the vertical angle of the central ray is that the central ray must be projected perpendicularly to a plane bisecting the angle formed by the longitudinal axis of the tooth and the plane of the film packet.

Ninety percent of the jaws are fairly symmetrical and can be photographed by the use of this rule. Individuals with a high vault may need to have the angle *decreased* about five degrees because the high vault causes the packet to be more nearly vertical in position. If the vault is low, the angle may have to be *increased* five degrees because the low vault causes the packet to be less vertical in position. When an individual's mandibular area is not symmetrical, it may be necessary to increase the vertical angle about five degrees when the teeth are buccally inclined or the mouth is shallow. If the teeth are more vertically positioned or the floor is deep, the angle is decreased about five degrees.

The central ray must also be correctly projected at a horizontal angle. The beam must pass through the spaces between the teeth without overlapping the adjacent tooth structures. (See fig. 41.2.) Thus the central ray must be positioned correctly both vertically and horizontally.

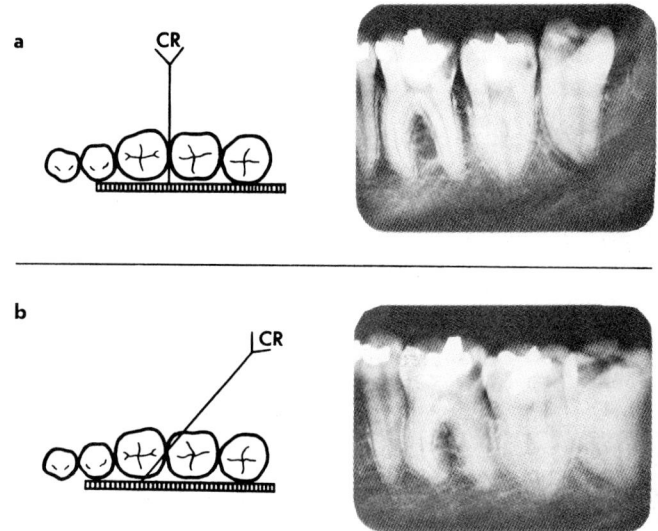

Courtesy Eastman Kodak Co.

Fig. 41.2. Central ray—horizontal angle. (a) When central ray is projected at correct horizontal angle (left), images are distinct, and overlapping is avoided. (b) When central ray is projected at incorrect horizontal angle (left), images are badly overlapped and blurred.

Periapical Short Anode-film Procedure

Average Angles

Figure 41.3 gives directional information for placing films properly in the average mouth. The average angles are a guide in placing films —which may then be varied if the mouth is nonsymmetrical.

Bending of Films

Whether or not a film should be bent when placed in a patient's mouth has been the subject of considerable discussion. It would seem that the films must be bent in order to permit the film to occupy the positions given in figure 41.3.

REGION	LONG AXIS OF FILM	CENTER OF FILM	ANTERIOR EDGE OF FILM	OCCLUSAL EDGE OF FILM	APPROX. VERT. ANGLE*
Upper Molar	Horizontal	Over 2nd Molar	Over Middle of 2nd Premolar	¼" Below Occlusal Surface	35°
Upper Premolar (bicuspid)	Horizontal	Over Interproximal Space Between Molars	2nd Incisor Region	¼" Below Occlusal Surface	45°
Upper Canine (cuspid)	Vertical	Over Canines		⅛" Below Nasal Edge	45° to 60°
Upper Incisors (centrals and laterals)	Vertical	Over Interproximal Space Between 1st Incisors		⅛" Below Incisal Edge	50° to 60°
Lower Molar	Horizontal	Over 2nd Molar	Over Middle of 2nd Premolar	¼" Above Occlusal Surface	−5°
Lower Premolar (bicuspid)	Horizontal	Over Interproximal Space Between Premolars	2nd Incisor Region	¼" Above Occlusal Surface	−35°
Lower Canine (cuspid)	Vertical	Over Canine		⅛" Above Nasal Edge	−35°
Lower Incisors (centrals and laterals)	Vertical	Over Interproximal Space Between 1st Incisors		⅛" Above Incisal Edge	−35°

*If the jaws are edentulous, it may be desirable to increase the above approximate angles by 15° in the upper and −15° in the lower. If a child's mouth is to be visualized, increase in the above approximate angles may be desirable.

Courtesy Weber Dental Mfg. Co.

Fig. 41.3. Table showing correct placement of films for best results in various regions of the mouth

The packet must not be bent so that the bend occurs over the center of the region of interest because the image will then be distorted. This distortion will make the film valueless for the purpose of interpretation.

In bending the film packet, great care must be taken so that the packet is not sprung. If this occurs, light may leak in around the packet and expose the emulsion. The packet must not be bent to such an extent that a crease is produced. The emulsion is extremely sensitive to pressure, and a sharp bend will result in increased pressure along a definite line. When the film is processed, a clear line will cross the film over the region of the bend.

Since there is plenty of depth or height in the molar region, no bend is necessary. However, in the bicuspid region the film must be bent at the anterior radicular edge away from the side of the film, which will be placed next to the teeth, so that the film may occupy the correct position in the mouth and not gouge into the anterior portion of the floor or the roof of the mouth. Since the cuspid occupies the corner of the arch, the film must be adapted to the curvature of the arch, and the anterior radicular edge of the film must also be bent away from the tube side of the packet. In the anterior region, the film must be gently curved in the long axis so that it will fit this region of the mouth.

Placement of the Film

The correct positioning of film in the patient's mouth is of utmost importance. The center of the film must be placed so that it is over the center of the region of interest. This might be the bicuspid region or it might be a single tooth, as, for example, the first molar.

When increased vertical angulation is necessary for the production of a shadow of a tooth equal in length to the tooth itself, the buccolingual diameter of the tooth will cast a shadow on the film which will add to the length of the shadow of the tooth. Therefore, in the molar and bicuspid region the occlusal edge of the film must be one-fourth inch below the occlusal plane of the upper teeth and one-fourth inch above the occlusal plane of the lower teeth so that the entire occlusal surface of the tooth can be visualized on the X ray. Since the anterior teeth do not have large buccolingual diameters at the level of the occlusal plane, the occlusal edge of the film need be placed only slightly above or below the incisal edge of the anterior teeth.

Figure 41.3 outlines the position for the film packet in order to produce a satisfactory X ray of each region of the mouth. It is important, in all regions of the mouth, to place the packet in such a way that the occlusal edge of the packet will be parallel with the occlusal or incisal edge of the teeth.

The anterior edge of the film is mentioned in figure 41.3 because it is frequently easier to place the anterior edge of the film over a certain tooth or region than to place the center of the film over the center of the region of interest. The vertical angulations are only approximate and over a long period time have been found to produce satisfactory X rays in the majority of instances. Occasionally, even though these angles are used, elongation or

foreshortening results. If unsatisfactory results are produced, this condition may be corrected by taking a second picture and increasing or decreasing the vertical angle in a positive or negative direction by at least fifteen degrees as described in the section of the geometry of shadows.

The placement of film must be deftly carried out so that the delicate structures of the mouth are not lacerated nor the patient's gag reflex stimulated.

Procedure for placing films in the upper molar region varies according to the side to be examined. For the upper right side, the film is carried in the mouth so that it is parallel with the occlusal plane. It is pushed back in the patient's mouth on the occlusal surface of the upper teeth until the posterior edge of the film contacts the tissue over the anterior border of the ascending ramus of the mandible. With your right hand, grasp the patient's left palm and guide his thumb so that it presses the film packet firmly against the roof of the mouth and the lingual surface of the teeth. If this procedure is carefully followed, no gagging will result.

For the upper left molar region, the same procedure is followed, except that the patient's right thumb is guided into the mouth to hold the film firmly against the lingual surface of the teeth and the roof of the mouth.

If the film is not back in the mouth far enough, grasp it between the thumb and forefinger and slide it back so that it occupies the position outlined in figure 41.3.

Placement of the packet in other regions of the upper jaw presents no appreciable difficulty, provided that the films are adapted to fulfill the requirements stated above.

Great care must be taken to have the patient relax the tongue and muscles of the floor of the mouth in order to place films for the lower jaw. To accomplish relaxation is frequently difficult. One way of teaching the patient is to insert one forefinger under the tongue and the other forefinger on the outside of the face underneath the floor of the mouth. Your forefinger then bounces up and down on the muscles of the floor of the mouth. The patient will know which muscles he should relax, and his cooperation is usually secured. The film packet is ready for placement following the attainment of a relaxed state of the floor of the mouth.

To place film for the lower right side, displace the tongue with your right index finger and place the film with your left hand. Remove your right hand and place the patient's left forefinger on the film so that it is held firmly against the molar teeth and gums. When placing film for the lower left side, the same procedure is followed except that the duty of each hand is reversed.

Wipe all moisture from each film packet as it is removed from the mouth.

The easiest and most direct technique for the retention of film is to have the patient use his thumb to hold the film against the upper teeth and use his forefinger to hold it against the lower teeth so that an exposure may be made.

Bite blocks are used with very satisfactory results. The film is inserted in a small groove in a block which is then placed between the teeth. The block is held steady by the pressure of the upper and lower jaws on it. This technique has some advantage over the finger-thumb method since the film does not slip as readily in a bite block.

The *long target-film technique* differs from the short target-film technique in three basic ways:

1. The distance between the target and the film is increased from approximately eight inches to at least sixteen inches. A special extension cone is used. The central rays of the X-ray beam are at the center of the cone.

2. The film is placed in the mouth so that the mean plane of the film and the tooth are as nearly parallel as possible. It involves the use of special film-holding devices. Because the film is more nearly parallel to the tooth, the vertical angles are much smaller than those used in the short target-film technique.

3. Contrast and penetration are controlled by increasing or decreasing the KVP setting on the X-ray machine.

In order to have an exposure time which is practical, ultraspeed film should be used. With sixteen-inch film-target distance and ultraspeed film, the exposure times become approximately equal to those used for techniques using the short film-target distance and intermediate-speed film.

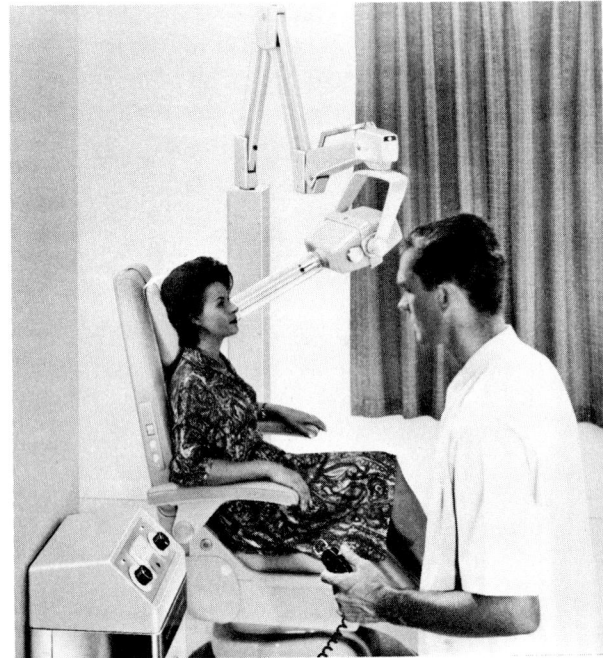

Courtesy General Electric Co.

Fig. 41.4. Periapical technique using a long anode-film (long cone) distance with the GE 100 dental X ray.

Periapical Long Anode-film (Long-Cone) Procedure

Since ultraspeed film is more sensitive to variations in exposure factors, it is desirable that the X-ray unit be equipped with a filament stabilizer whenever it is to be used with the extension-cone technique.

Bitewing Technique

Bitewing technique has very definite advantages, and also disadvantages. It is designed for the specific purpose of visualizing the coronal portion of the tooth. It is excellent for locating interproximal and occlusal caries. It may be helpful in studying the alveolar process and alveolar bone at the neck of the tooth. Since only the coronal portion of the tooth is visualized, any change in the apical structure cannot be seen.

The film is placed so that it is parallel with the long axis of the teeth. Special film designed for the bitewing technique may be purchased;

or a film for this technique may be made inexpensively by fastening an index tab to the "tube side" of the packet of a regular periapical-type film. When this method is used, be sure to use water—not saliva—to moisten the index tab. A paper loop is also available for this purpose.

For the molars, place the film so that the tab is on the occlusal surface of the lower teeth. Carry the film as far posteriorly as possible. Ask the patient to close carefully so that the teeth touch the tab, using the tongue to hold the film close to the lingual surface of the teeth. A vertical angle of +5 degrees and correct horizontal angle will produce a satisfactory result.

When X-raying the bicuspid area, the anterior radicular edges of the film must bend away from the tube side of the packet so that these edges do not dig into the roof or floor of the patient's mouth.

Bitewings in the anterior region are not especially valuable because the long axes of

Courtesy Eastman Kodak Co.

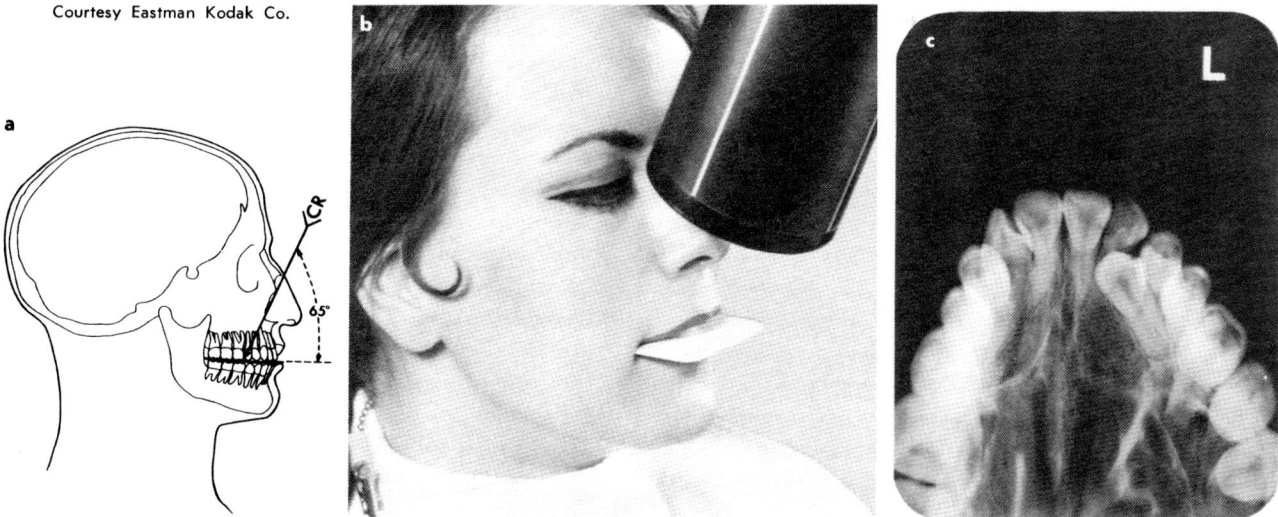

Fig. 41.5. Maxillary incisor region. (a) Projection of central ray (CR). (b) Placement of packet and cone. Insert occlusal packet with nonslip side toward upper arch; long axis coincident with median plane. Direct central ray at vertical angle of +65 degrees through bridge of nose, to center of packet. Patient slowly closes mouth and immobilizes packet with gentle end-to-end bite. (c) Resulting radiograph.

the upper and lower teeth are not parallel. Angulation which produces suitable X rays of the upper teeth produces elongation of the lower teeth, and vice versa. A good periapical film of the anteriors usually will produce better results.

Occlusal Technique

Occlusal films are used when the small periapical films do not permit complete visualization of the region which is to be inspected roentgenographically. Occlusal films are 2½″ x 3″ in size.

Insert the film in the mouth in much the same way as you would a cracker. The packet is held in the occlusal plane by gentle pressure of the teeth.

Extraoral Procedures

Extraoral radiographs often supplement the information which your dentist obtains from his periapical, occlusal, and bitewing radiographs. In some instances the extraoral radiographs are used without the intraoral examinations. (For example, the orthodontist uses

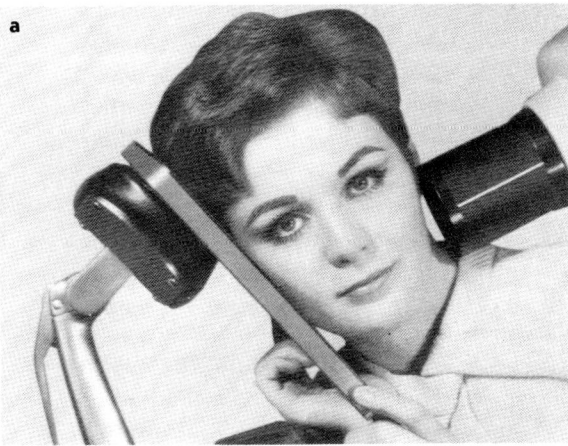

Fig. 41.6. Ramus of mandible. (a) Arm of dental chair on side to be examined lowered so that patient can sit sideways. Place film holder on the headrest and the chair back so that film is at +45 degrees with horizontal plane. Patient holds film holder in position with both hands at lower corners. Patient's cheek in contact with front of film holder; median plane of head slightly rotated until zygomatic arch is touching film holder; lower border of mandible parallel to its lower edge. (b) Projection of central ray. Direct central ray approximately +25 degrees through lower second molar area on side being examined, to center of film. (c) Resulting radiograph.

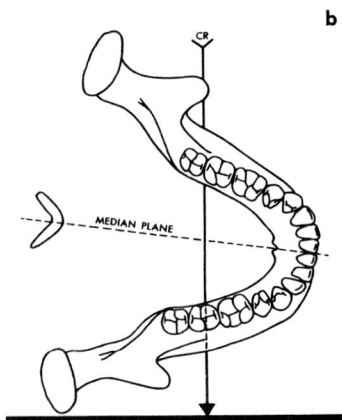

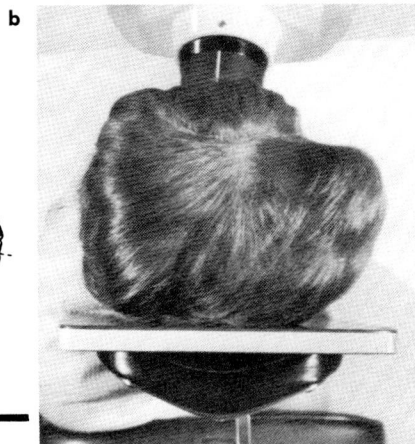

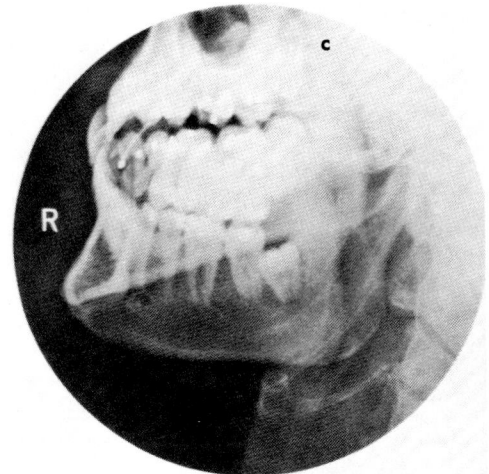

Courtesy Eastman Kodak Co.

facial profile radiographs to record changes due to treatment or growth.)

Extraoral radiography is used for examination of the mandible, maxilla, temporomandibular joints, and the facial profile. These radiographs are used more frequently by orthodontists, oral surgeons, and sometimes prosthodontists, in addition to institutions such as hospitals and clinics.

These films require special handling because their packaging is different from the film packet used for intraoral radiography.

Extraoral technique requires equipment in addition to that necessary for the intraoral technique. Various sizes of film are used. For the lateral-jaw technique, 5″ x 7″ film is used; for posteroanterior views, 8″ x 10″, or larger, film is used. See "Extraoral Film" for a description of these films.

The panograph is included as an extraoral radiographic technique. One panoramic X ray, the Orthopantomagraph, has an attachment which permits the combination of the panoramic and cephalometric X-ray procedures on the same machine.

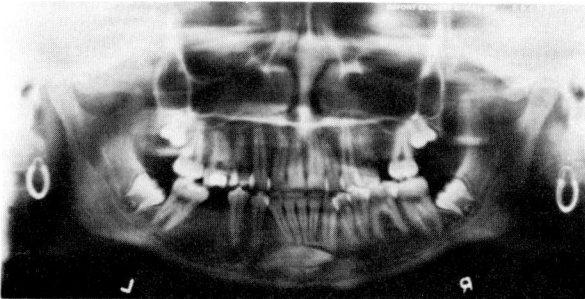

Courtesy General Electric Co.

Fig. 41.7. A panoramic film

Seven Steps for Better X-ray Exposures

1. Be certain that the patient's head is correctly positioned.

2. Remove the film from its storage box.
3. Place the film packet correctly.
4. Align the central X ray accurately.
5. Select the correct exposure from your chart.
6. Make the exposure.
7. Store the film in a safe box where it will not receive further radiation.

Summary

The quality of radiographs depends on the skill with which they are produced. A poor radiograph prevents accurate diagnosis. It is essential that the correct film be selected, the patient properly prepared, the films correctly placed, the correct time used for the exposure of the film, and proper care taken of the film after exposure.

Short-target techniques are commonly used in the dental office, but long-target techniques are also important and use of eight-inch and sixteen-inch techniques are to be encouraged.

Intraoral techniques include periapical, bitewing, and occlusal radiographs. Panoramic X-ray procedures produce an overview of the oral cavity for which a special machine is used. Some dental offices use the panorama and posterior bitewings for the routine dental examination, adding periapical films of doubtful areas. Other extraoral techniques are used to supplement information gained through the use of the intraoral techniques. In some instances the extraoral radiographs are used without intraoral examinations. The common uses for extraoral radiographs are examination of the mandible, maxilla, temporomandibular joints, and the facial profile. The extraoral radiographs are more commonly used by orthodontists, oral surgeons, prosthodontists, hospitals, and clinics.

The extraoral film receives special handling.

Check the seven steps for better X-ray exposures.

Study Questions

1. On what does the quality of radiographs depend?
2. What three basic differences are there between long target-film technique and short target-film technique?
3. List the types of intraoral film.
4. For what purposes is extraoral film used?
5. What dental specialties most commonly use extraoral film?

42 | *Processing of Film*

Changing the image on the film so that it can be seen is a process referred to as *developing* or *processing* the film. The process is accomplished by the use of chemicals, and at least the beginning stages must be performed in the dark. Thus the term *darkroom* developed as the place where exposed film is developed. Sometimes reference is made to the *processing room*.

Advances in technology have created the development of automatic processing in which the assistant places the film in an opening in a machine. The entire process is then automatically accomplished, with the finished film emerging from the machine minutes later.

Automatic Film Processing

The automatic developer is described as a mechanical link in a system designed to process dental X-ray films; it offers mechanical and chemical control of the process. It maintains solutions at proper temperatures and transports the film mechanically through these solutions at a specific speed, ending with a drying cycle Some processors may be equipped with a hood which eliminates the need for a darkroom.

We will describe *one* processor,[1] but the principles of operation are similar regardless

1. S. S. White Dental Health Products are to be credited with the description of the automatic processor. Adapted from their *Auveloper Catalogue* No. 2459.

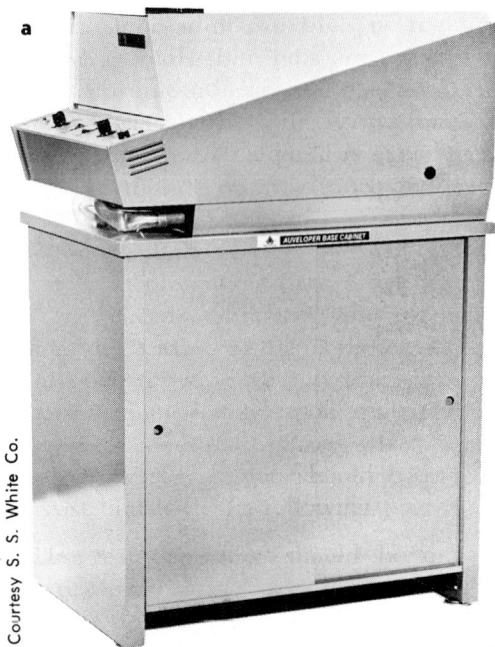

Courtesy S. S. White Co.

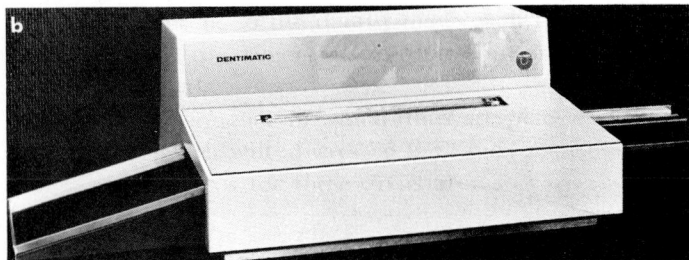

Fig. 42.1. (a) S. S. White processor described in text. (b) Siemens fully automatic processor: For dental films from the intraoral up to 8″ x 10″ cephalostat size. Built-in automatic replenishing system. (c) Siemens Procomat: Automatic developer for intraoral and occlusal film. No plumbing needed. Equipped with special light screening hood. 6-minute cycle.

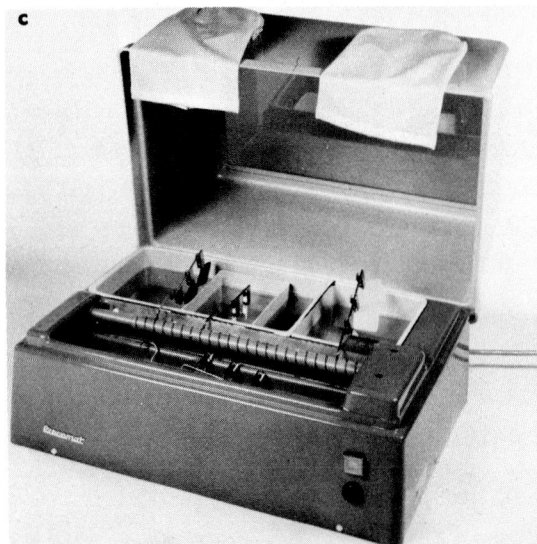

Courtesy Siemens Corp.

Courtesy Siemens Corp.

of the manufacturer. The developer consists of three sections: film loading section with an electrical control panel; film processing section with plastic tanks, solution recirculation pumps, the roller transport system, temperature control devices, and the replenishment system; and a film dryer section containing air heaters, a blower system, and the receptacle for processed, dry radiographs.

Automatic processing is desirable because quality radiographs can be made in less time. Drying time also is cut with automatic processing. The entire automatic process is less than ten minutes.

Chemicals for the automatic processor are not the same as those for hand processing. They are purchased especially for the automatic processor, and the manufacturer's directions for use must be carefully followed, both for original filling of tanks and for replenishment.

Hand Processing of Films

Inasmuch as many dental offices still use hand processing and darkrooms, it is important that the process be explained thoroughly.

The Darkroom or Processing Room

A darkroom must be exactly what its name implies—a place which can be made totally dark. This does not mean it cannot be painted in bright colors. It usually is a small, windowless room containing only the necessary special equipment for developing X rays. Order must be maintained so that it is possible to find what you need in very low illumination. It must be kept absolutely clean if high-quality processing is to occur. It must contain a minimum of the special equipment, but some darkrooms will contain very elaborate equipment. Figure 42.2 is a model processing room. Note the seventeen items which are listed for this particular room. Not all these items are actual

LEGEND

1 KODAK Darkroom Lamp with ML-2 Filter

2 Electric fan

3 Rack for drying films

4 Storage rack for intraoral hangers

5 Bulletin board

6 Exposure and Processing Chart for KODAK Dental X-ray Films

7 Drip pan

8 Shelf

9 Timer

10 KODAK Utility Safelight Lamp, Model C (fitted with opalized glass)

11 Gooseneck faucet

12 Loading area

13 Splashboard

14 Hot- and cold-water valves

15 8 x 10 dental processing tank

16 Utility sink

17 Supply cabinet for chemicals, cassettes, and other accessories

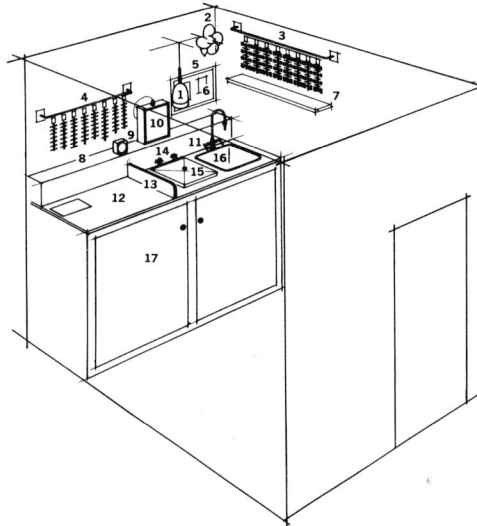

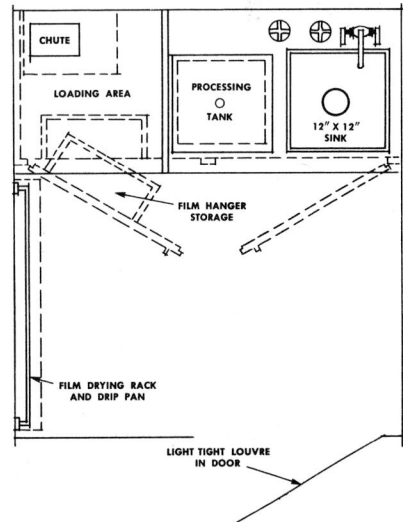

Courtesy Eastman Kodak Co.

Fig. 42.2. The components for a processing room

necessities, but they certainly help make the task easier. Let us look at the processing components which are necessities and at some which are "nice to have."

A normal electric light is necessary for use when films are not being processed, in addition to a darkroom lamp (fig. 42.2 [1]) which is necessary for use during processing. This allows some dim illumination of the room, yet will not affect the X-ray films being processed because the light rays which are harmful to film are filtered out. Counter-top safelight [10] for viewing wet films may also be used.

Racks for holding X-ray films [3] during processing and drying are necessary. The sizes your office uses will be determined by the types of radiographs your dentist takes.

A timer [9] is a necessity to time the development and washing of films.

A sink [16], equipped with hot and cold running water and a way of managing hot and cold water supply to processing tanks, is essential, as is a drain for the tanks.

A bulletin board [5] is convenient for posting your list of films and the developing chart [6] for the film which your office uses, but these lists can be taped on the wall if no bulletin board is available.

Some experts believe that it is better *not* to use an electric fan [2] in the darkroom because a fan stirs up dust in the room, and this dust may mar your films. An electric dryer is more desirable. However, proper cleaning can eliminate most dust.

The rest of this chapter is devoted to descriptions of the various items which are necessary for processing films, and the use and care of the facilities and supplies.

Care of X-ray Developing Tank and Solutions

X-ray developing tanks are generally made to hold one gallon of developer and one gallon of fixer in separate compartments, with a larger central compartment connected to the water supply line and to the drain. The tank may be made entirely of hard rubber, a hard-rubber shell with stainless-steel one-gallon inserts to hold the solutions, or entirely of stainless steel. The tanks generally are made so that the containers for the developer and fixer are removable from the tank shell for easier cleaning.

When solutions need to be changed, they are drained by removing the plug which faces the central compartment on each side—one for the developer compartment and one for the fixer compartment. This allows the used developer and fixer to escape down the drain in the central compartment.

Always use the same compartment that previously contained the developer for the fresh developer, and the other for fixer. If your tank has steel inserts which are removable, remove, clean, and replace only one at a time to prevent reversing their positions.

The compartments for developer and fixer, when emptied, are scrubbed with a stiff brush and a solution of a strong detergent; the interior of the main tank is also scrubbed; then all are thoroughly rinsed with clear water.

Seat the rubber plugs very firmly. The developer and fixer compartments may now be filled with their fresh solutions.

X-ray Processing Solutions

Proper preparation, use, and storage of X-ray developing and fixing solutions are of extreme importance in the production of quality radiographs.[2]

You know that when a film packet is exposed to X-radiation a change occurs in the silver salts in the emulsion. The change causes the

---

2. This section, "X-ray Processing Solutions," through the courtesy of A. Porter S. Sweet, D.D.S., F.A.A.O.R., formerly with X-ray Division, Eastman Kodak Company, Rochester, N.Y.

formation of a latent image (one to be developed). This image can be converted into a visible one by the chemical action of a *developer*. The film is then rinsed and placed in a *fixer* solution which prevents the developing action from continuing so that your picture does not become entirely black and unreadable. The fixer solution changes the undeveloped silver salt particles to another salt which is water-soluble and transparent. If the film is thoroughly washed, the white particles are washed off, and the film is transparent where it should be transparent. If you do not wash the film thoroughly, it becomes milky white again and is not transparent. Thus it is very important to wash the film thoroughly.

X-ray Developer

An X-ray developer, like a photographic developer, contains four kinds of ingredients:

1. The *developing agents* which free the silver from the silver halide crystals.
2. The *preservative* which prevents the developer solution from oxidizing in the presence of air.
3. The *activator* which softens and swells the gelatin of the emulsion and provides the necessary alkaline medium so that the developer can readily attack the silver halide crystals.
4. The *restrainer* which inhibits the fogging tendency of the solution. Like the activator, it also controls the rate of development.

MIXING DEVELOPER SOLUTIONS   When mixing developer solutions, the manufacturer's directions on the label *must be followed carefully* to obtain best results. Cleanliness is essential. Any chemicals spilled or splashed should be wiped up at once. Tanks must be kept in good condition by thoroughly cleaning after discarding old solutions. All traces of scum, dirt, and sediment must be removed.

Observe these general recommendations when mixing solutions:

1. In most instances, city water supplies are satisfactory. Chlorine produces no bad effects, but water should not be used that has a high calcium content or that contains metallic impurities or hydrogen sulfide. Temperature of the water in which the chemicals are to be dissolved should *never* exceed that recommended in the manufacturer's directions.
2. The container reserved for mixing the developing solution may be a clean crock, tank, or other suitable vessel of inert material. Stainless steel, hard rubber, glass, enameled iron, and glazed earthenware are satisfactory, but wood or reactive metals such as aluminum, galvanized tin, zinc, and copper are not suitable as either mixing containers or developing tanks. Stainless-steel tanks should have welded rather than soldered seams, for solder will react with the developer solution to fog the radiographs produced.
3. Water should always be poured into the container first and the chemicals added. When powdered chemicals are used, they should be added slowly with vigorous stirring.
4. When the chemicals are entirely dissolved, sufficient cold water should be added to bring the solution to the correct volume and temperature. Solutions should be at the optimum temperature of 68°F. (20°C.) before they are used.
5. Separate stirring spoons or paddles should be used for mixing developer and fixing solutions.
6. Tanks should be covered when not in use.

Containers

Experience has shown that a processing-tank unit, especially the gallon size, is best.[3] Such a unit is efficient: solutions will keep better in it than in smaller units, temperature control is easier, several full-mouth radiographs can be processed at the same time, and radiographs up to 8″ x 10″ can also be processed.

Development Difficulties

Development difficulties of various kinds may result if proper solutions and correct procedures are not used.

Lack of activity of a fresh developer solution may be the result of incorrect mixing or an error in dilution.

High activity occasionally occurs, although it is less likely than low activity. It may be caused by incorrect mixing, such as the use of too small a volume of water, or by too high a temperature.

Crystallization is due to insufficient dilution when mixing or storing solutions at too low a temperature. The first difficulty can be avoided by proper mixing; the latter can be corrected by raising the temperature.

Care of Solution

The solutions employed in developing X-ray films are most effective when used within a comparatively narrow range of temperatures. Below 60°F. some of the chemicals are definitely sluggish in action, which slows the action of the developer. Above 80°F. they work too rapidly. Within these limits, changes in temperature can be compensated for by varying the development time. A temperature of 68°F. is most practical from the standpoints of uniformity of chemical activity and time required.

After the temperature of the developer has been determined, the films should be left in the solution for the exact interval that is required. Consult the manufacturer's directions. Guesswork should not be tolerated. An accurate timer and thermometer should always be used.

One of the advantages of time-temperature technique is that it provides a definite check on the accuracy of the exposure used. If a radiograph is too dark after fixation, exposure was too great; if the radiograph is too light, the film was underexposed.

Agitation

When films are first placed in the developer, they should be agitated for a second or two beneath the surface of the developer in order to break loose any air bubbles that might be clinging to their surfaces. These bubbles would cause a round spot on the radiograph.

Replenishment

Not nearly enough dentists practice developer replenishment to maintain developer activity. They get along by increasing development time as the developer loses its activity. This is not a good procedure for two reasons: (1) It is inaccurate, for no one can judge how much activity has been lost and compensate by establishing a new time factor that will be accurate. Radiographs will therefore be of top quality only when the developer is fresh. (2) Even though sufficient time is allowed for development, there will always be a loss of quality near the end of the useful life of the developer. All this can be avoided by adding more developer as the level of the solution is lowered through use and evaporation. The replenisher solution should be mixed according to the directions on the container label.

3. A. P. S. Sweet and Charles Bridgman, "Radiodontic Processing Rooms," *Dental Radiography and Photography* 24 (1951): 1-7.

Discarding Developer

Developer solutions should be routinely discarded on schedule so that radiographic quality will stay high. Some try to "stretch" developer solutions by using them longer than they should. This is poor economy, for although a few pennies can be saved, the quality of the radiographs is bound to suffer. Developer used past its useful life will produce developer fog which greatly impairs the interpretive quality of the radiograph. Be safe. Discard developer on schedule. If yours is a busy office where many radiographs are processed every day, discard the developer every two weeks, even though you have replenished it. If fewer radiographs are processed, a three-week interval may be all right, but the developer should seldom be used longer.

Storage of Developer Solution

Developer is exhausted by use and by exposure to air, since both cause oxidation. For the latter reason, all air should be excluded from stored developer solutions.

One excellent method of storing developer is in six- or eight-ounce bottles. Each bottle is completely filled so that there is no air included in the bottle. There can then be no oxidation. When it is time to replenish the developer, one entire bottle of solution is added to the tank. The rest of the solution, stored in other six- or eight-ounce bottles, is not opened and thus remains fresh.

This method is far superior to storing all the solution in one large bottle which acquires more air each time the solution is poured from it to replenish the tank.

X-ray Fixer

An X-ray fixer solution also contains four kinds of ingredients:

1. The *clearing agent* chemically changes the unexposed silver halide crystals remaining after development.

2. The *preservative* prevents decomposition of clearing agent and assists in clearing the film.
3. The *hardening agent* shrinks, tans, or hardens the gelatin emulsion to prevent excessive swelling and softening.
4. The *acidifier* provides the necessary acid medium and makes possible the correct action of the other ingredients.

Clearing time is the interval between placing the film in the fixer and the disappearance of its initial opaqueness.

Fixing time is the total interval the film must remain in the solution to chemically change the undeveloped silver salts and to harden the gelatin. This should be at least ten minutes, but films should not be left in fixer solutions for prolonged periods or overnight, for the image itself will gradually lose density.

MIXING FIXER SOLUTIONS   When mixing fixer solutions, the manufacturer's directions on the label *must be followed carefully* in order to obtain best results. Cleanliness is absolutely necessary.

TEMPERATURE AND AGITATION   It is desirable that the developer, rinse water, and fixer be maintained at a constant temperature.

Fixing time is shortened and nonuniformity of the image prevented if films are agitated in the fixer. Thus a greater volume of the fixer solution is brought in contact with the films in a given period, and rinse water is more rapidly removed.

DISCARDING FIXER   The usefulness of the fixer solution comes to an end when it has lost its acidity or when too long a time is required to change the unexposed silver salts. Use of an exhausted fixer should be avoided in order to assure production of radiographs of good quality. A good rule is to discard the fixer solution at the same time that the developing solution is discarded.

Procedure for Developing X rays

Materials Required:

1. X rays to be processed correctly labeled with the patient's name.
2. Film holders for the number of X rays you are to develop.
3. A pencil.
4. Developer.
5. Fixer.
6. X-ray washing equipment.
7. Timer or watch with a sweep-second hand.

It is extremely easy to confuse the identity of X rays during processing and mounting. To exchange X rays of two different patients can be most embarrassing, if not dangerous. Be very careful to keep X rays correctly identified at all times.

Most dentists use a type of X-ray packet containing one piece of film, but some packets are available with two pieces of film. It is possible to take two identical X rays with such a packet. Discover just what film packets are used in your office before you begin to develop X rays.

X-ray film, while still wrapped in the packet, is not harmed by light. When unwrapped, however, it is sensitive to most kinds of light and must not be exposed in this manner anywhere but in a darkroom. This room is so designed that no light can reach the unwrapped film except the special illumination provided by a safelight designed for the purpose. This safelight, while very dim, will give you enough light to work after your eyes have become adjusted.

To Develop the X-rays

With the ordinary lights on in the darkroom, place the packets which you have to process —still wrapped in groups with the name of the patient written on the bundle—on the work top.

Place a pencil beside the films to be developed.

Place as many film holders as you need on the work top. The holder is usually a metal bar about twelve inches in length. The top end of the bar is curved to form a hook. A series of clips are arranged along each side of the metal bar. The individual films are attached to these clips. Another excellent type of holder has an arrangement of slots into which the film is placed.

At the top of the holder you may have noticed a white piece of plastic. The patient's name is written on this in pencil. If more than one patient's X rays are to be mounted on one holder, the names are written in the order in which the films are mounted on the holder.

The length of time for which the film is left in the developing solution is very important. On the bottle or can in which your developer is supplied to your office, you will find a recommended time-of-development scale. In general, the warmer the solution, the more quickly the film is developed. A floating thermometer should always be kept in the developer in order to indicate its exact temperature whenever you need to develop X rays. Find this temperature. Then, checking with the time-of-development scale, determine the length of time needed to develop the films you are about to do.

Developing solutions should not be used at temperatures in excess of seventy-eight degrees because the X-ray film may be damaged. If the temperature of the water in the central compartment is such that it cannot cool the solutions to less than seventy-eight degrees during the hot summer months, ice may be placed in it to accomplish this purpose. Do not put the ice directly into the developer or fixer. Unless it is confined in a plastic bag, the ice is placed in the central water compartment.

Fresh developing solutions are more active than solutions which have been used for a period of time. When first using a fresh solution, developing time should be exactly as recommended by the manufacturer at the temperature of your solution. As the solution gets older, when one-half minute more than the recommended time is needed to secure good development of the film, the solution should be discarded and fresh developer put in the tank. It should be changed every three weeks, or more frequently.

Turn on the darkroom safelight. Turn out the ceiling light in the darkroom. Pick up a package of films belonging to one patient. The patient's name and the number of films which are his have previously been written at the top of a hanger. If there are four, for example, these four films are mounted, two on each side, at the top end of the hanger. If the first pair of clips are quite close to the top end of the holder, never use them. They may be out of the solution when part has evaporated.

Separate a film from its wrappings, black paper, and foil. With forefinger and thumb open a clip, and with the other hand place an end of the film in the clip. Release the clip, then give it a firm squeeze to be certain that it has gripped the film securely. This is necessary to prevent the film from coming loose and dropping to the bottom of the X-ray tank while processing. If your holders have slots instead of clips, slide the film into the slots. Hold the film by its edges.

Do not place films on the lowest pair of clips unless the lower end of the hanger has been bent at a sharp angle to hold it away from the side of the tank when immersed. Unless this has been done, films placed on this pair of clips often develop improperly because they are held flat against the side of the tank, and the solution cannot circulate around them. Use the top pair of clips only if you are certain that your solutions are maintained at a sufficiently high level to insure complete immersion of the top films.

When the holder is loaded with film, hold it in one hand and plunge it up and down in the developer compartment three or four times before finally hooking the hanger over the edge of the tank. Place the cover on the tank.

Set the timer for the proper length of time. Since this is a matter of minutes, you can go on to the other duties until you hear the timer bell indicate that the films must be removed from the developer. Leave the room with safelight only. Close the door. When the timer rings, the films must be removed immediately to prevent ruining them by overdevelopment.

Reenter the darkroom, closing the door behind you. The safelight is on. Remove the cover of the tank. Lift the hanger out of the developer and dip it four or five times into the water in the central compartment. Shake off the excess water. Plunge the hanger four or five times into the fixer compartment of the tank, then hook the hanger over the edge. Replace the cover on the tank.

The room light may be turned on now. It does not need to be turned off again, provided the cover of the tank fits well and is not removed until fixing is completed. The manufacturer of the fixer you use gives the recommended minimum period of time for proper fixing of film. Somewhat longer periods of time, such as half an hour, are not harmful, provided the temperature of the solution is not permitted to become too high.

When *fixing* is completed, the film must be washed to remove all traces of fixing solution which has soaked into the film. Washing can be done in either the central compartment with the water running continuously or in a separate pan placed in the sink under an open faucet. If a pan is used, one end should be raised slightly, and the water should enter the pan at this end. If the washing is done in water which is circulating vigorously, one-half hour is sufficient; otherwise allow one hour.

Upon completion of washing, hold the hanger firmly and shake off all excess water, then hang where the film may dry undisturbed. Do not touch the film until all trace of water is gone. The hanger clip points will be the last areas to dry.

Ten Steps for Excellent Processing of Radiographs

1. Stir developer.
2. Check the developer temperature.
3. Select the correct developing time.
4. Open the film packets.
5. Attach films to correct hanger.
6. Set timer and develop films.
7. Rinse them.
8. Fix them.
9. Wash them thoroughly.
10. Dry them.

Summary

It is necessary to develop or process the exposed X-ray film. The processing can occur with an automatic developer into which the assistant places the exposed film and then removes it some minutes later; or the film can be hand-processed. Hand processing is subject to more error than automatic processing.

If hand processing is performed, a darkroom must be utilized. A darkroom is a place which can be made totally dark for the development of X rays. The special equipment necessary to develop X rays is kept in this room.

The mixing and the care of solutions used for the development of the radiographs are very important parts of dental assisting.

Learn to care for the solutions properly and to develop X rays carefully. Follow the instructions given you either in this chapter, by your dentist, or on the direction sheets which come with your X-ray developer and fixer.

Study Questions

1. Explain the purpose of processing film.
2. Describe automatic processing.
3. List the advantages of automatic processing.
4. Describe the steps in hand processing of film.
5. Describe the care of developer for hand processing.
6. Describe the care of fixer for hand processing.
7. What is the procedure for developing X rays by hand processing?
8. List the ten steps for excellent processing of radiographs.

43

Processed Film . . . Its Use, Care, and Storage

Now that you have learned to develop radiographs, what do you do with them when they are dry and hanging on their hangers?

When the radiographs are completely dry, they should be prepared so that the dentist can read the film for each patient.

Mounting Radiographs

The first step is to mount the radiographs so that the films are more easily seen in relationship to each other. Prepare yourself for this task by gathering a few materials at your desk. You will need an X-ray mount for each patient whose X rays are to be mounted. An *X-ray mount* is a cardboard, Celluloid, or both cardboard and Celluloid card designed with openings or slots to hold the X-ray films in an orderly manner. They are available in many different sizes and combinations to suit the individual dental office.

You will also want the X-ray hangers, with the patients' X rays *still clipped to the hangers,* and a pen or pencil to write the name of the patient and the date of the X rays on the mount.

Again, we repeat: it is extremely easy to confuse the identity of X rays during processing and mounting. To exchange X rays of two

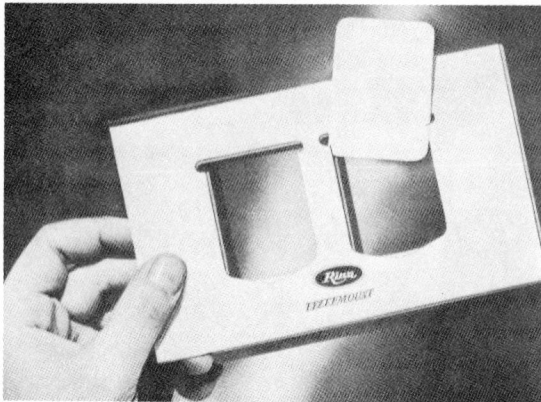

Courtesy Rinn Corp.

Fig. 43.1. Film X-ray mount. Rinn EEZEEMOUNTS. This type of mount is thinner than wire-stitched mounts and requires less storage space. Films are held in place on all four sides and cannot be accidentally dislodged.

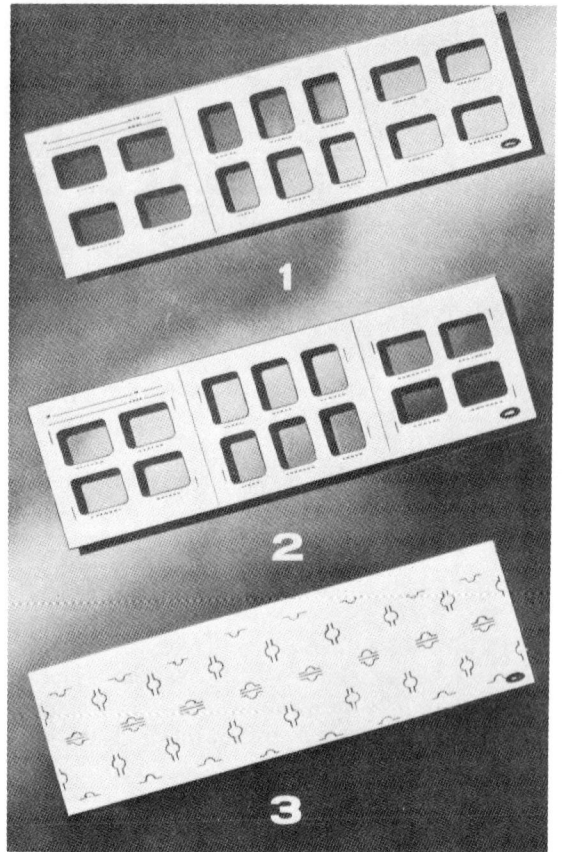

Courtesy Rinn Corp.

Fig. 43.2. Complete film X-ray mounts. These three types are all used for the same purpose, but the personal preference of the dentist is the factor which determines which type may be used. No. 1 is a frosted backing cardboard mount securely fastened with wire stitches. No. 2 is the clear backing mount, otherwise exactly like No. 1. No. 3 is an all-Celluloid mount with easy-opening notched tabs.

different patients can be most embarrassing, if not dangerous. Be very careful to keep X rays correctly identified at all times.

Remove from the hanger only those X rays belonging to one person. Mount them and write the patient's name on the mount, in pen or pencil, before removing the next group of X rays. The Celluloid tab on the hanger has each patient's films correctly identified. Following this procedure will help you keep that identification accurately.

Any group of X rays of a given patient are mounted in sequence; that is, each area shown in any one X ray is the neighboring area of the one mounted next to it.

Each X-ray film has a small, raised dot in one corner. When the film is mounted, this raised dot usually stands out on the side away from the face of the mount. (Some dentists prefer to reverse this mounting position, however.) Do not confuse clip marks from the hanger used in developing with the raised dot which the manufacturer places on the film.

Distinguishing Characteristics of Bitewing X rays

Examine a mounted set of bitewing X rays and learn to recognize these landmarks:

1. The slight curve upward from the cuspid area toward the molar area, formed by the biting (occlusal) surfaces of the teeth;

2. The upward curve of bone at the end of the lower arch;
3. The appearance of the area behind the upper molars as compared with the appearance of the area behind the lower molars.

Now dismount this set of X rays, mix them up, and turn them over thoroughly; then see if you can mount them correctly. Repeat this by remounting a set which you have not seen in the mount.

Distinguishing Characteristics of Complete Periapical X-ray Series

Compare a complete X-ray series with the bitewing X rays to recognize the same landmarks. Then learn these additional features:

1. The root differences between upper and lower teeth;
2. The way in which the root tips usually curve toward the back (distal) of the mouth;
3. The mental foramen in the lower bicuspid area;
4. The canal in the lower jaw through which the nerve and blood vessels pass;
5. The difference in size of upper anterior teeth as compared with lower anterior teeth;
6. The darkened area (sinus) usually visible above and between the roots of the upper bicuspid and molar areas.

Dismount this set of X rays, mix them thoroughly, and see if you can mount them correctly. Practice with several old complete X rays and have your work checked for accuracy.

X rays of a complete set of teeth are the easiest to mount correctly. With practice, you will soon be able to progress to mounting X rays which have few teeth visible to help you orient yourself.

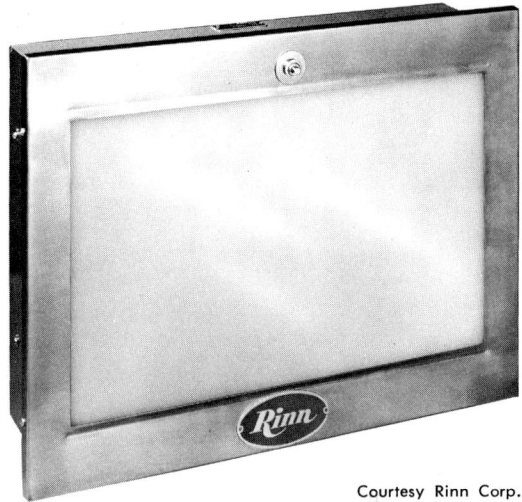

Courtesy Rinn Corp.

Fig. 43.3. Recessible X-ray viewer. The X rays are placed on the glass panel, and the illumination from behind makes it possible for the dentist to see all the details on the films for accurate diagnosis.

Panoramic X ray

Film sheets of panoramic X ray are often left unmounted, although there are mounts for them. The sheet of film can be stored in the patient's record envelope or in a separate X-ray envelope which is placed in a file for X rays. This envelope is the same size as the film and thus requires a special-size file drawer.

Filing X rays and Records

After your dentist has finished diagnosing the patient's dental needs from the radiographs which you have mounted, the films must be stored since they are a permanent part of the record of each patient.

Most dentists keep an X-ray film mount for each patient, with the current X rays in it. The method of filing these may vary, however.

The cardboard mount has lines on the upper border for the name of the patient and the date of current X rays. If the date is written in pencil, it can be erased and kept current through the years.

There are two commonly used methods of filing X rays in mounts. Some offices file them in a file drawer reserved for X rays only, either alphabetically by name or numerically by the patient's number. The mounts are filed as cards would be filed. For the alphabetical file, the name of the patient is written in ink, last name first, on the line provided in the upper-left-hand corner. The patient's number precedes his name if the office uses a numerical file. The penciled date is written on the next line.

The complete X-ray mounts are filed in one drawer, or at least under one set of alphabetical guide cards. The bitewing X-ray mounts are filed in another drawer, or under a separate set of guide cards.

The patient's mounts are removed from the file whenever he has an appointment and are returned to the file at the close of the appointment.

Some dentists prefer to keep the X-ray mounts in the patient's record envelope in accordance with the principle of having all records of the patient kept together.

In either case, when the X rays are no longer current (that is, when new X rays are taken), they are removed from the mounts and placed in an envelope. A coin envelope works nicely. The patient's name and the date of the X ray are written in ink on the outside of the envelope. These envelopes are usually kept in the patient's record envelope as part of the permanent record. The new films are then placed in the mounts.

Four Steps in Preservation of Radiographs

1. Mount the dry radiographs in proper mountings with accurate identification.

2. Have your dentist read them for diagnosis.
3. Keep them available during patient's visits.
4. File them properly when work has been completed.

Summary

Properly developed X rays are the first step to good diagnosis. Care should be taken in mounting the radiographs so that they may be read easily and correctly.

For properly mounting X rays you will need the following materials:

> Mounts for complete and bitewing X rays.
> X-ray hangers with patients' films still on them.
> Pen.
> Medium pencil.

Be careful to correctly identify all X rays.
Mount them in sequence.
Learn the identifying landmarks for both bitewings and full-mouth X rays.
Panographs are usually left unmounted.
Proper storage of X rays following use is desirable. They may be filed numerically or alphabetically in an X-ray file or kept in the patients' folders, depending on your dentist's preference.

Study Questions
1. Describe an X-ray mount.
2. Describe mounting periapical films.
3. Why must an X ray be positively identified?
4. Discuss the characteristics of bitewing X rays.
5. Discuss the characteristics of periapical full-mouth films.
6. Discuss panoramic X-ray storage.
7. Discuss two methods of filing periapical X rays.
8. What are the four steps in preservation of X rays?

PART NINE | # OPERATORY PROCEDURES

This section is devoted to a general discussion of work and conduct with adults and children in the operatory, followed by a series of basic requirements for most operatory procedures. Each dentist may vary his requirements for certain procedures, but the materials and instruments which are considered basic requirements are listed. Your dentist may wish to go through this section of your text and write in his preferred instrumentation and materials for each operation.

You can then memorize the instruments and materials needed for a particular operation and be certain that they are available whenever the dentist is likely to need them.

44 | *Conduct in the Operatory*

The appointments have been made, the case studies presented, the telephone answered—most of the jill-of-all-trades discussed—and now it is time to enter the operatory and actually assist at the chair.

Cleanliness

There are some ground rules to be observed first, however. We have mentioned *cleanliness*.

Let us reemphasize it now. Not that cleanliness is less important in the rest of the office, but it is mandatory in the operatory. Not just the operatory, either—but *you*. You must be clean to work here. Good grooming is essential, and this you will have accomplished routinely by now. Hands *must* be clean.

In the morning before you begin chairside assisting and again after lunch before you begin chairside assisting, it is wise to give your hands a thorough washing according to hospital standards.

Follow the directions given here (1) in the morning *after* you have given the office its morning cleaning but *before* you start chairside assisting and (2) on your return from lunch before you begin chairside assisting.

Preparation for Scrubbing

We learned in the section on microbiology that residue around soap dishes, water in which soap and brushes are left standing, and the residue on the dispensers of liquid detergent or soap cultivate the growth of bacteria. Thus at all times you should see that soap bars are set so that they drain dry. The dispenser for powder or liquids should be frequently scrubbed clean and brushes thoroughly rinsed. In addition, the wash basin itself must be scoured and kept shiningly clean.

Prepare the wash basin and soap so that they are clean and free from accumulations which encourage the growth of bacteria. This preparation can be made in the morning clean-up routine which precedes your preparation for chairside assisting.

Hospital scrub procedures require sterile brushes, which is a good idea. Your fingernail brushes can be autoclaved regularly.

Scrubbing Procedure

Once you are ready to assist at the chair, you can indulge in the thorough scrubbing of your hands as follows:

1. Turn on the water and adjust the temperature to be warm enough to clean well, but not so hot as to be uncomfortable. If you have a foot or knee control on the faucet, your problem is easier than with hand-operated faucets.
2. Wet your hands thoroughly.
3. Apply a generous amount of soap or detergent, either by rubbing the wet bar of soap between your hands or dispensing the proper amount of liquid, powder, or leaves from your dispenser.
4. Rub your hands together briskly and work up a good lather. This first soaping is to remove the gross contaminants and dirt.
5. Rinse well under running water until all lather is removed.
6. Add soap or detergent again.
7. Work up a good lather. Rub each side of each finger, massaging the lather between

the thumb and fingers of your other hand.
8. Rub between the fingers where they join the hand.
9. Rub well around the fingernails.
10. Use an orangewood stick to clean under each nail if you wish.
11. Use a nail brush to scrub the nails and cuticle of each finger.
12. Scrub the knuckles well.
13. Scrub the palms thoroughly.
14. Scrub the backs of the hands thoroughly.
15. Be sure to wash well above your wrists.
16. Rinse well with lots of running water. Be sure all the soap or detergent residue is removed from arms and hands and from under nails.
17. Dry thoroughly with a clean towel. Be sure to dry under your fingernails, too. Take time to do a good job.
18. Shut the water off. If faucets are hand-operated use your towel over your hand.
19. Set out a fresh towel.

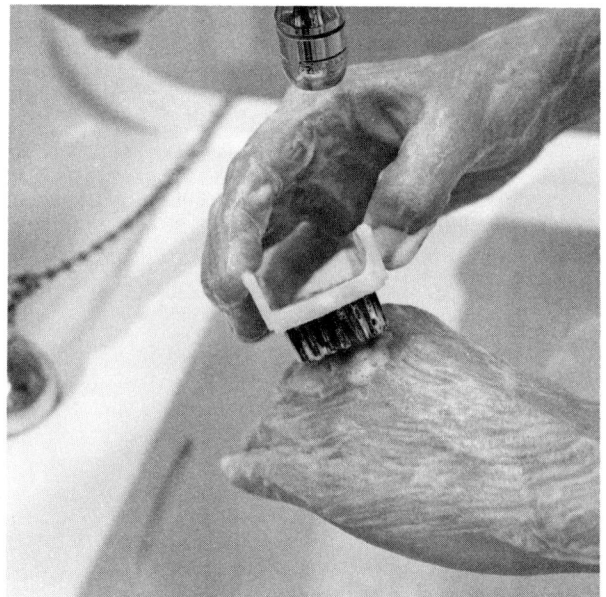

Fig. 44.1. Scrubbing the hands

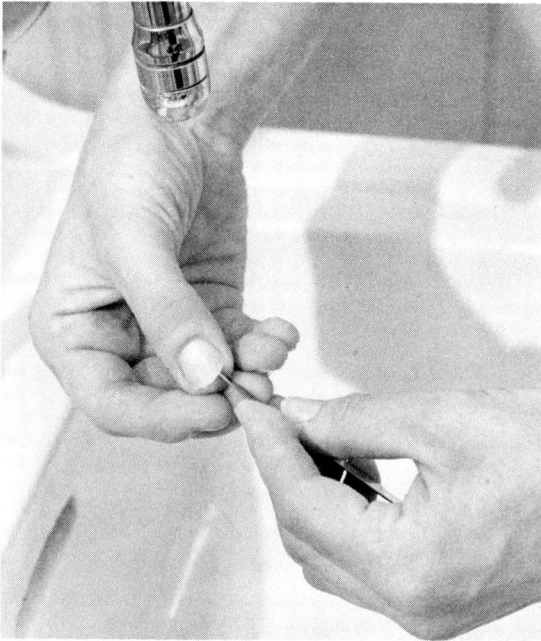

Fig. 44.2. Cleaning fingernails

You will notice that this is a *thorough* process—a time-consuming but necessary step. During the rest of the day it may not be necessary to wash your hands as thoroughly as you should at the beginning of the workday.

In between patients, when you touch your hair, face, or person, you usually do not deposit grime underneath nails nor in the crevices of the cuticle. If you have soiled some part of your hands and do need to disinfect them or cleanse them with a bacteria-destroying soap, a good sudsing, brisk rubbing, and thorough rinsing should suffice for almost all necessary washing after the first hospital-preparation procedure in the morning and again after lunch.

Some of the preparations on the market today actually remove bacteria from the skin and prevent the recontamination by bacteria for a few hours. The routine use of these products is better than ordinary soap.

General Rules for Conduct in the Operatory

1. No conversation should deal with any subject other than the patient, the work in hand, or dental education. The patient is not assumed to be interested in what your young sister, boyfriend, husband, or _____ said to you this morning or last night that was so funny.

2. Any message to the dentist while working on a patient should be indicated in a note held out of the patient's line of vision—just behind and to the left of the patient's head. If urgent, and beyond the scope of a note, indicate by note just the word "office" or "lab." The dentist will then go to the private office or laboratory as soon as possible to receive the message. Use this method only for urgent, confidential messages.

3. Be pleasant but never familiar with either the patient or the dentist.

4. Be sympathetic toward the patient.

5. Concentrate on the job you have to do.

6. Speak to and refer to the patient by name. The patient should not be referred to as *he* or *she* when the patient is present.

7. Keep your hands away from your person when working at the chair. If for any reason it becomes necessary to do otherwise, immediately wash your hands and return quickly.

8. When the dentist is with you at the patient's side, your contributions to any conversation should be a minimum. If the dentist leaves the chairside, you should take up the duty of conversation. If you also must leave the patient, ask him to excuse you. If any wait is involved for the patient, see that reading material is provided (preferably material related to dentistry).

9. Assistance at the chair is primarily to help the dentist perform his duties more rap-

idly. Whenever you must leave the chairside during operations requiring assistance, accomplish the task as quickly as possible and return.

10. Maintain a pleasant expression in the operatory. However, be sure that you do not laugh for any reason at a time when the patient is not ready or able to share a laugh with you.

Adjusting the Dental Chair

Learn to adjust the dental chair used in your office. Practice until you are skillful. Comfort of the entire body allows the patient to relax. Dentistry becomes less difficult for the comfortable, relaxed patient.

Most chairs have marks indicating the average position of the headrest, the height of the backrest, and the angle of the backrest to the seat. Ask your dentist to show you how these are used. Know how to make the chair as comfortable as possible.

Seating the Patient

Everything is in readiness for the patient. The patient's file is in its place, and the instruments are ready. The operatory sparkles with cleanliness and is attractive; you have viewed it from the patient's point of view. It is time to seat the patient.

The dental assistant should enter the reception room, rather than merely extend her head and shoulders through a doorway or service window. A hand extended to the younger child may be helpful.

"Will you come in, please, Mrs. Jones?"

"It's your turn now, Jimmy."

Your words should be carefully phrased to help the patient respond favorably to the trip into the operatory.

Lead the way to the proper operating room.

Ask men to remove jackets or to loosen neckties and shirt collars. Place women's purses or packages in a place visible to the patient but where they will not be in the way. A shelf for this purpose in each operatory is ideal and can usually be placed well toward the front, or on the front wall, about four feet from the floor.

Invite the patient to be seated and adjust the dental chair for his comfort.

Place the bib over the patient. The bib chain should not rest on bare skin at the neck unless unavoidable, and it should not be placed *over* a coiffure. If a full-length drape or throw is used, it is placed before the bib is put into position.

Give women a disposable tissue for removing lipstick. Often no words are necessary, but request removal of lipstick if the patient does not remove it.

If the patient is a stranger, introduce the dentist: "Mrs. Jones, may I present Doctor Smith?" Or, "Mrs. Jones, have you met Doctor Smith?"

Use the patient's name first. Pronounce the dentist's name clearly and distinctly.

Whenever possible, *listen* to patient-dentist conversation. Do so without being obvious to the patient. You may overhear an item you should note on the patient's record as a contact on the patient's next appointment. Pay attention to all sounds and words in the operatory. Awareness of everything occurring in the operatory is essential to good assisting.

Be fully prepared for all work scheduled for the patient's appointment.

Care of Patients' Dental Appliance

At an appointment for operative work or for prophylaxis recall to check a patient's remaining natural teeth, the patient is asked to remove his full denture, partial denture, or removable bridge after he has been seated in the dental chair. The dentist will make this request if he finds it desirable, although some patients will remove these appliances voluntarily when seated. Sometimes the dentist prefers to see the appliance while it is still in the mouth, and he then removes it after this examination.

The assistant should carefully take the appliance, rinse it under the cold-water tap, and place it in a bowl of water until the appointment is over.

Bring the appliance back to the patient *wet* and lying on a folded disposable tissue on the palm of your hand. Let the patient pick up the appliance.

Do not forget to return appliances. Patients very easily fail to remember the appliance is missing until they are out of the office. It is embarrassing for most patients to return and ask for their appliances.

Tray Setups

In many offices today all the instruments necessary for a specific dental operation are placed on a tray immediately after they have been sterilized. They are placed in the order of their use, neatly arranged. A storage section of a cabinet holds the group of trays. The number of similar trays for each dental operation will vary with the frequency of use. Each tray is labeled for quick identification.

When the day's work schedule indicates the next patient is to have a crown preparation, a tray for crown preparation is removed from the storage unit and set out on a special tray holder or on the work counter. In this way, change-over time between patients is kept at a minimum. The dental assistant simply removes the tray of used instruments and replaces it with a tray of sterilized instruments for the specific operation to be performed.

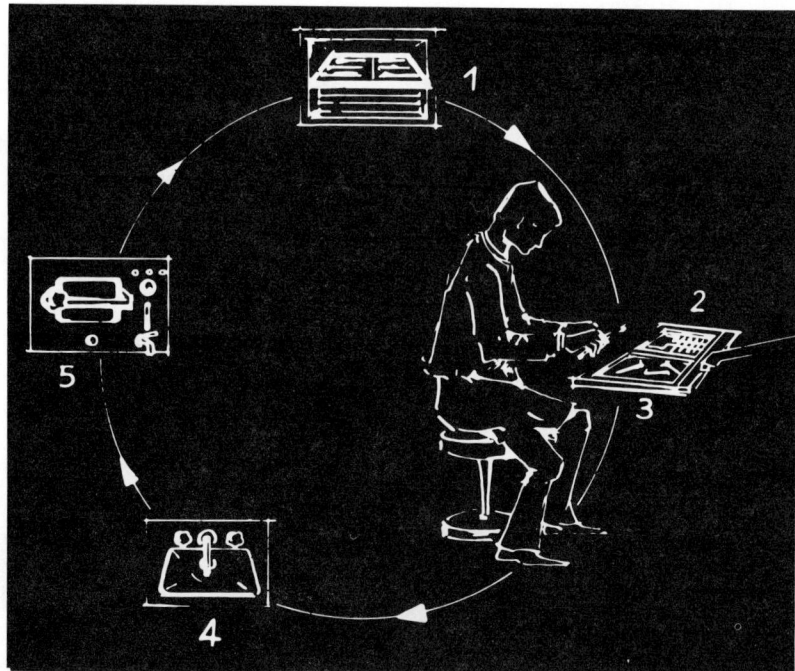

Courtesy Siemens Corp.

Fig. 44.3. Tray-System technique: (1) Removal of ready-to-use trays from cupboard; (2) Preparation of instrument sets for specific treatment; (3) Discarding of the used instruments; (4) Cleaning of the used instruments; (5) Sterilizing of the complete instrument sets in cassettes.

Some offices use a coding system with color and tapes. For example, all instruments to be placed on crown and bridge trays have a narrow blue ring painted or taped on them, operative instruments are ringed with green, and so on. If the office has more than one operatory, one ring indicates the first operatory, and two bands indicate the second operatory. The trays are also marked on the edge with one or two stripes of color.

It is also possible to indicate the sequence in which the instruments are used by the placement of the color bands. For example, let us say five instruments are used in a specific operation. The color band is placed at the top end of the first instrument used in the preparation, one-fourth inch farther down the handle of the second instrument, a half inch down the handle of the third instrument, etc. When the instruments are placed in proper order on the tray, the rings form a diagonal line across the instruments (fig. 44.4). The dental assistant knows immediately whether or not she has the instruments placed correctly. The same

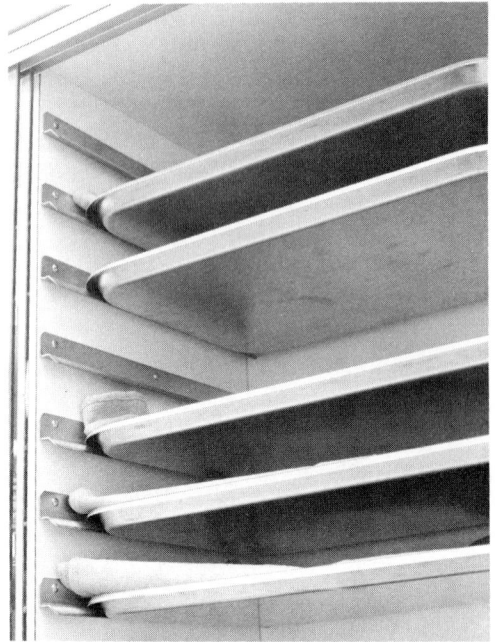

Fig. 44.5. Stacked trays in case

process can be used for operatory two by considering the two bands a unit.

The cleanup and sterilizing of instruments can be performed at a time when the day's schedule permits. The sterilized instruments and trays are then replaced in their proper storage units. If they have been labeled by color coding, tape writing, or banding, the dental assistant can quickly reassemble the trays and return them to the storage cabinet.

Washed-Field Techniques

In order to work effectively, the dentist needs a clear view of the field of work in the mouth. Proper evacuation of the debris and water used during operation is absolutely essential. Figure 44.6 illustrates a dental assistant using a good washed-field technique and the proper positioning for work in eight areas. The dentist is not shown in order to make

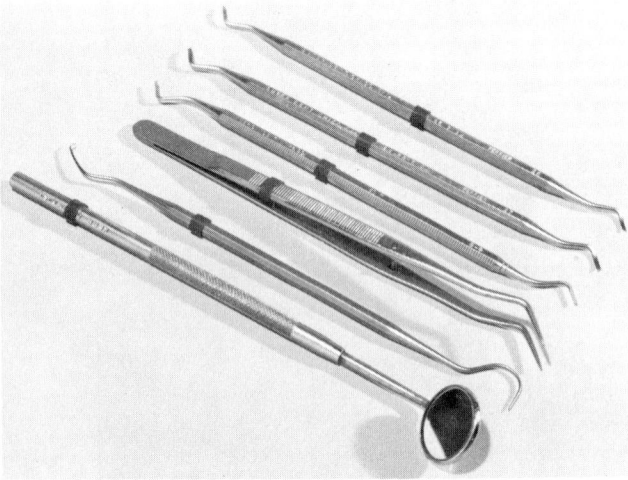

Fig. 44.4. Instrument handle identification

clear the position of the dental assistant and the equipment (fig. 44.6, pp. 584-586).

Assisting with Preparations

In dentistry, *preparation* is the term used to designate the shape a dentist makes in a tooth, with burs or other instruments, into or onto which the restorative material of choice is placed. The headings used in some of the following pages on operative procedures refer to the work associated with preparing a tooth to receive a restoration or crown of the particular type named.

The instruments required for a certain operation should be placed on the work surface (bracket table, cabinet top, or tray) before the operation is begun. A minimum number of drawers need be opened or instruments found once work has started. Keep all instruments lying in an orderly manner on the work surface. The "working" end of the instrument should always be visible. It is amazingly difficult to locate a particular instrument when it is lying tangled in a group of handles pointing in all directions. *You* keep the instruments in order. Place to one side the instruments which have been used and will no longer be required. Keep the instruments needed for the next step most conveniently placed.

Your dentist will endeavor to work in an orderly manner and to do each type of operation in the same sequence. Following orderly procedures will speed his operating time and will make it much easier for you to be of real assistance at the chair. There will be variations at times from a customary sequence, but over a long period of working together, even these variations take on a pattern of uniformity. You will be able to anticipate his needs and will always have the correct instrument in its proper working position for him.

Always observe which tooth is being prepared. The location of the tooth is the factor which accounts for most of the variation in procedure.

Study the sequence in which your dentist uses his instruments during each type of operation. Try to have each successive one held out to the dentist close to the front of the patient's chin. Have the other hand ready to receive the instrument the dentist has been using. Hold instruments so that the dentist can recognize which instrument you are holding and can take it from your hand *in the position required for use in the mouth.* When the handpiece is to be used, it is helpful to remove it from its hanger and bring it to the location at the front of the patient's chin. When its use is completed, it should be received from the dentist and restored to its hanger.

If the dentist wishes, the dental assistant should learn to place and remove carbide burs or diamond instruments used in the air turbines. The higher-speed cutting instruments, such as the air turbine, require less change of instruments than is required by the slower belt-driven handpieces.

Serving and Receiving Instruments

The assistant usually will work at the patient's left for right-handed dentists, her stool positioned four to six inches above the dentist's stool. Her work cabinet with instrument tray will be to her right, and the handpieces, evacuator, and three-way syringe will be to her left. If the standard dental unit is used, it may be necessary to rotate the cuspidor out of the way. She must remember to swing it back when the patient has need of it and whenever she finds it necessary to leave the chairside.

In this position she is ready to assist with keeping the field of operation clean and visible for the dentist. To do so she maintains the operating-light concentration on the field and uses low- and high-volume evacuation, water, and/or air. She is also prepared for the opera-

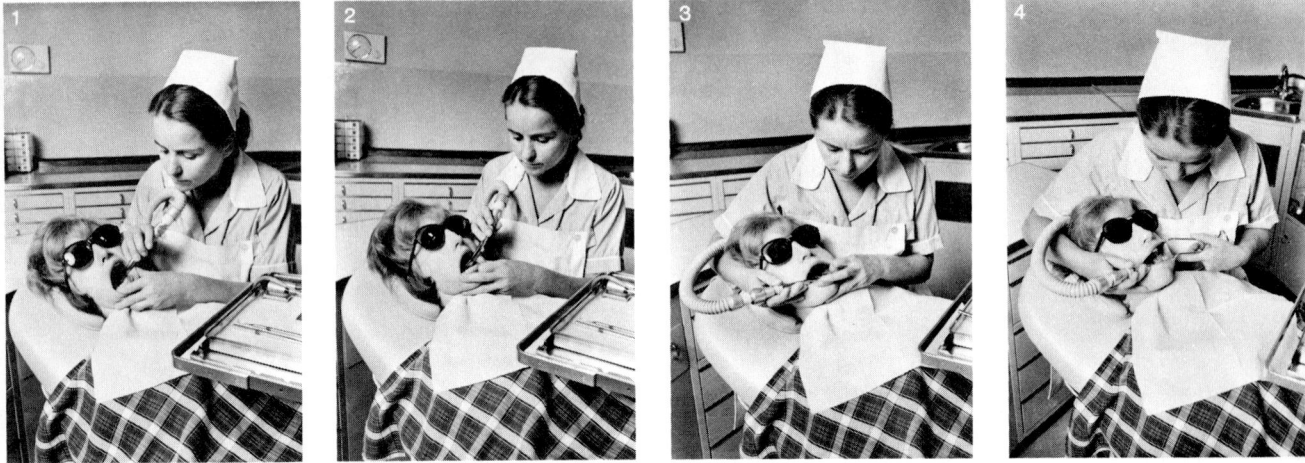

Right side of the mandible (fig. 1). The first picture illustrates the evacuation technique when the area between the right mandibular cuspid and the first molar is in direct view. The patient's head is supported by the pillow, and his head is turned slightly toward the dentist. The assistant must be able to see the tooth which is being prepared. Note the short evacuation tips in the photos. The left index finger lies in the oral vestibule, keeping the cheek approximately 1/2" away. The middle finger and the ring finger support the chin. The assistant should not support her left arm on the patient's chest, but rather should hold it close to her own body. The right hand leads the evacuation tip in a penlike motion, keeping the tongue and the floor of the mouth 1/2" away. By using short evacuation tips, the assistant can support herself comfortably and safely by holding her hand on the patient's head. She may also use her elbow to support herself on the back of the dental chair. The assistant must be especially careful to avoid pressure on the jaw and to avoid contact between the evacuation tip and the lip on the left side of the mandible. The assistant should not try to remove all the water during a tooth preparation. Rather, she should see to it that some water remains in the mouth at all times during the procedure. This is the only way in which coughing and foreign-body aspiration can be prevented. After the work is finished, the water which remains on the floor of the mouth and in the cheeks is evacuated. The assistant turns the patient slightly farther to the right with a little pressure so that the water collects on the right side. She uses her right hand to remove the tip from the patient's mouth and turns the tip so that its opening faces down. Then the tip is reintroduced into the patient's mouth and led across the teeth from the ascending ramus of the mandible to the front along the right side of the mandible. This permits the removal of all the water from the mouth.

Anterior mandibular area (fig. 2). To assure direct vision of the mandibular anterior area for the dentist, the assistant puts her left middle finger into the right side of the oral vestibule. The index finger and the thumb clasp the cheek on the left side and hold the lower lip away from the teeth. The evacuation tip is placed 1"-1 1/2" behind the anteriors and protects the tongue. The assistant's arms are supported as shown in fig. 1, which also demonstrates the position for evacuation of excess water from the angle of the mouth after the preparation is complete. The assistant may gain additional support by supporting her left hand on teeth 27 and 28 or on the mucosa through the tip of the middle finger. With preparations which involve the anterior mandibular teeth on the front side, e.g., in placement of cervical fillings, sufficient water may collect in the anterior vestibule that some escapes over the lip. The dentist need not interrupt his work if that occurs, if the assistant has learned to cope with this situation by moving her middle finger away from the tooth, pushing the cheek aside. This permits water to flow backwards away from the anterior vestibule. Attention must be given to place the assistant parallel to the dentist when work is being carried out in the right mandible or maxilla and in the anterior region of the mandible.

Left mandibular region (fig. 3). (From the cuspid to the first molar) The patient is again turned slightly toward the dentist. The assistant now places her chair slightly to the rear and behind the patient, rather than assuming a position opposite that of the dentist. The evacuation hose is not placed over the patient, but rather is found behind the patient. This makes it necessary that the hose be sufficiently long to be used without causing a strain.

The assistant cradles the patient's head in her arm. Her left hand props the mouth open, to afford a good view. All the fingers of the left hand have a part in this task. The index finger holds the angle of the mouth and is supported in the region of 24 and 25. The ring finger and the little finger are in contact with the chin. The thumb is used to hold the

Fig. 44.6. Washed-Field Technique

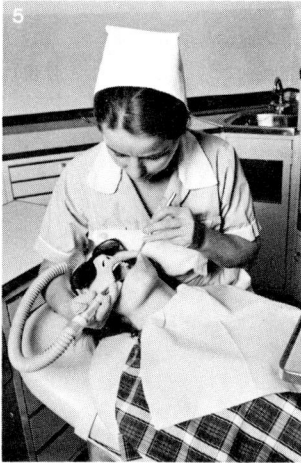

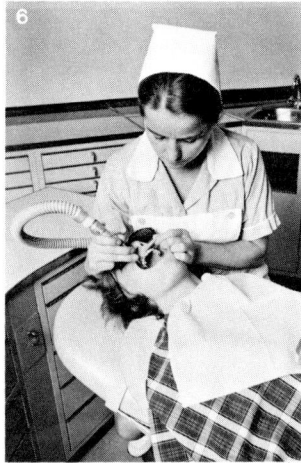

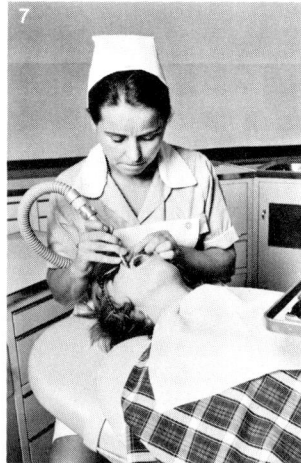

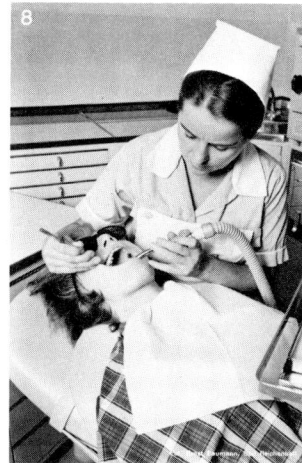

patient in the desired position, being supported by the application of constant pressure on the zygomatic arch. This position of the hand may be used to turn the patient's head toward the dentist if a better view is required by the dentist. The right hand guides the evacuation hose around the patient's head. The tip is placed linqual to 21-19 and moved along the path while being held in the manner of a pencil. The shield of the tip protects the tongue while the water is being removed partially. The tip remains in the area described even if water collects in other regions during the preparation. After the preparation is completed, the assistant removes any water which has collected at the deepest point in the right oral vestibule.

Molar region (fig. 4). The evacuation tip is held as in the previous figure. Care must be taken that the obturator of the tip does not exert pressure on the tongue, but rather that it is used to keep the tongue away from the jaw. The left hand is used to hold the mouth open with a dental mirror or with a cheek retractor, as shown in the illustration, rather than with the fingers. Note that the mirror should not push on bone if it is used! The assistant should take a short grip on the mirror so that she may use the cheek to support herself if necessary. Any water which collects in the right side of the oral cavity is removed after the work is completed.

Left maxillary molars (fig. 5). The patient is placed on the shoulder-neck rest. Usually this backward extension of the patient's head suffices to provide a good view for work in the maxilla. If the view is insufficient, the back of the chair is appropriately adjusted. The assistant is seated slightly to the rear of the patient. Almost all assistants must raise their chairs somewhat to have a truly good view of the maxillary molars. Because the tongue falls back upon the maxillary molars in many patients when they are placed in this position, the tip is used to hold the tongue away from

the teeth. It is advisable to support the back side of the evacuator tip on the left mandibular molars to provide more support for the assistant. This leads to a steady position of the tip, which is very desirable for the patient while he is being treated. The assistant's left hand is used to hold the cheek away from the teeth with a mirror. For most assistants this position is the most difficult of all those taken during any evacuation procedure, but it may be learned during the course of time.

Maxillary left premolar region (fig. 6). The assistant is seated slightly to the rear of the patient. The hose is led around the patient's head. The head is inclined toward the dentist. The evacuator tip is free to move in the region of the right angle of the mouth. The hose should not be permitted to block the dentist's line of vision, but should be directed towards the rear by the assistant. In this manner, water is evacuated from the region of the left maxillary premolars. The cheek is not retracted with a mirror because that instrument could easily slip. The fingers are used instead. If the assistant pulls too hard on the cheek, the patient eventually loses the position which is desired and the dentist loses his view. A useful tip: the assistant puts her flat hand on the patient's left cheek and uses her index and middle fingers to pull the cheek toward the hand surface. In this way, the assistant holds the patient on his right ear and simultaneously holds the cheek well and securely.

Maxillary anteriors (fig. 7). To provide a good field of view of the palatal side of the maxillary anterior teeth, the patient's chair must be raised and the back must be slightly lowered. When work is being done on teeth 7 or 8, the patient is inclined to the right; when 9 or 10 are involved, he is turned slightly to the left. The tip is held in the region of 2 or 3, with the opening toward the teeth. The assistant holds the lip away from the field with her left hand. The

Fig. 44.6 (Continued)

lip is not only held away, but it is used as a flap held between the index finger and the thumb to prevent water from splashing into the patient's nose. When the preparation is complete, the patient is turned slightly to the right and the tip is turned to permit removal of the remaining water from the mouth.

Right side of the maxilla (fig. 8). The assistant holds the evacuator in her left hand when the right side of the maxilla is the site of the operation. The short tip is held in the manner of a pencil in the right side of the mouth. The assistant may gain some support by resting the reverse side of the evacuator on the right mandibular molars and simultaneously resting the little finger of her left hand on the patient's chin. She must never press on the patient's tongue with the evacuator because that would expose the patient to the danger of aspirating water into the pharynx with air, causing him to gag. The cheek is retracted by the assistant, but the dentist may retract it as he does when working in the right mandibular quadrant. In that event, the assistant should not rest her right hand on the chair or hold the evacuator hose with both hands. Rather, she should place her index finger on the right cuspid and the thumb near the left cuspid so that she may assist in maintaining the patient's position as the dentist requires. Because some assistants cannot manage to turn the evacuator tip with the left hand, it is advisable to remove it from the mouth, turning it outside of the oral cavity, before removing the water which remains when the procedure is completed. The tip is then passed from the back to the front across the teeth of the right side of the mandible.

Courtesy of Prof. Dr. Fritz Schöen and Brigitte Gierl. Reprinted from Fritz Schöen and Brigitte Gierl, "A Rational Washed-Field Technique," in Quintessence International, vol. 2, Oct. 1971, p. 77.

Fig. 44.6 (Continued)

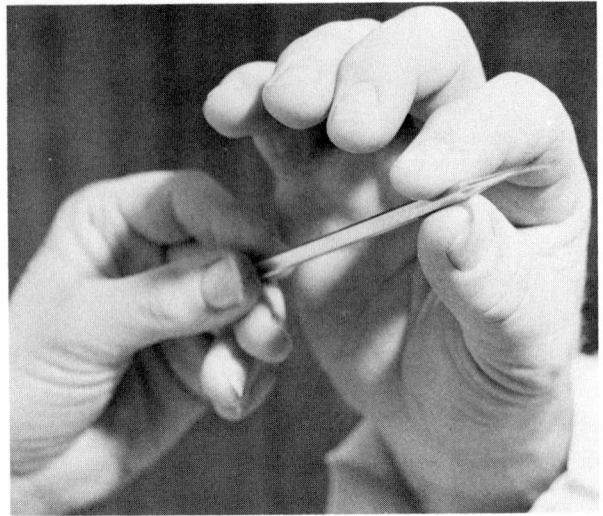

Fig. 44.7. Delivery—palm-thumb grasp

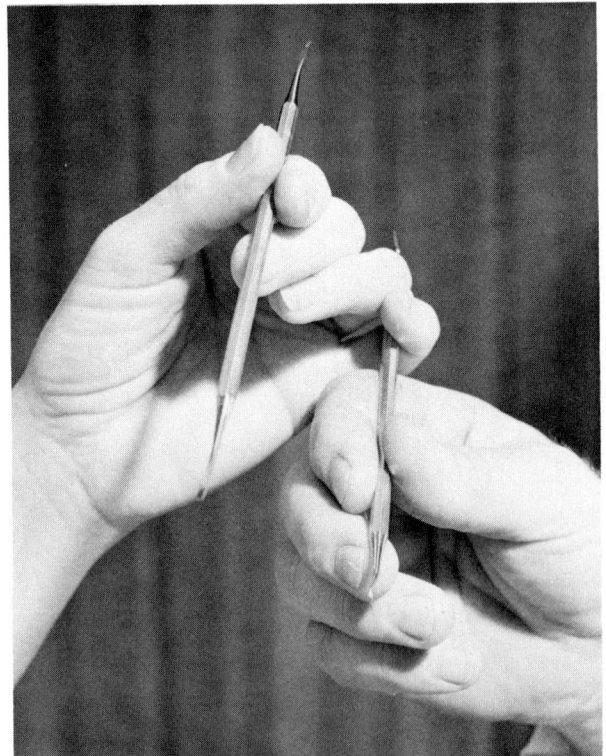

Fig. 44.8. Withdraw

tion at hand, passing instruments and delivering impression or restorative materials as needed, according to the preselected order prescribed by the dentist. The dental assistant is to minimize the interruption of the treatment procedures and be constantly aware of the patient's comfort during the operation.

Serving and receiving hand instruments at the dental chair, as well as serving and receiving other materials, requires the development of a pattern of movement on the part of the dental assistant. It follows, too, that the dentist must develop a pattern of instrumentation as well as a pattern of receiving and disposing of used instruments and materials. In addition,

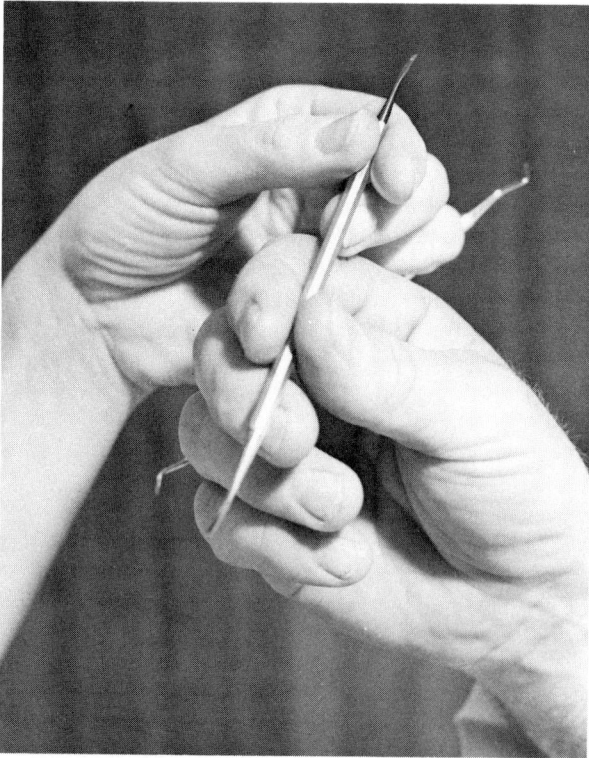

Fig. 44.9. Delivery—pen grasp

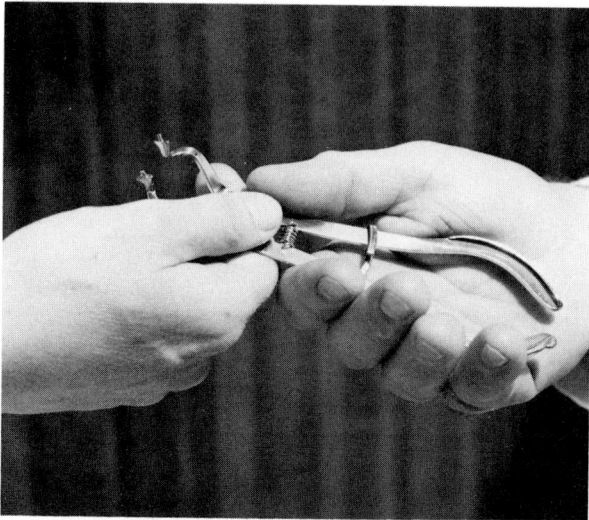

Fig. 44.10. Delivery—palm grasp

the dental assistant must be aware of each stage of the procedure and know what the procedure is meant to accomplish.

Assuming both dentist and assistant to be right-handed, the most effective direction of movement in serving instruments to the dentist is to serve with the left hand. Obviously, then, used instruments and other materials are received with the right hand. If you will imagine the field of operation as viewed directly from above (the top of the head would be at the 12 o'clock position on a clock, the chin at 6 o'clock, the patient's left ear at 3 o'clock, and the right ear at 9 o'clock), all serving should be accomplished within the range of 5 to 7 o'clock, at the patient's chin. Most serving will be done between 5 and 6 o'clock because this position will be the same distance from the dentist's eyes as the site on which he is working in the patient's mouth. His hands should not have to move more than six inches from the patient's mouth to receive instruments or materials.

While it may take a period of time before the dental assistant feels thoroughly comfortable serving and receiving in this manner, correct procedures will result in greater flexibility and speed when they have become habit. The pattern of movement is not cluttered with over-and-under hands and instruments. Nevertheless, there are some dentists who prefer to have the dental assistant serve with the right hand and receive with the left. It is possible to learn this pattern when required. *The most important point is that both dentist and dental assistant develop and use a given pattern and avoid the habit of using whichever hand seems more convenient at a given moment.*

The most common error of the dental assistant in the early stages of learning to serve and receive is the desire to dispose of a used instrument immediately when it is returned to her. Used instruments and materials should be momentarily retained by the assistant until an opportunity to dispose of them is afforded by the work in progress at the moment. If it becomes necessary to dispose of a used instrument or other material because of immediate need, the dental assistant should be able to do this without removing her eyes from the work in progress.

Remember: *Your purpose is to conserve the dentist's time and energy. Try to time your moves in such a way as never to delay progress of treatment.*

The dental assistant will find it most convenient to work while seated—if the dentist sits also. Otherwise, some assistants who stand use a low platform to elevate themselves to a satisfactory height. The platform should be large enough so that she can work comfortably without fear of stepping off and should be designed to fit in the space beside the chair where she will normally stand.

The assistant should watch for things which may be uncomfortable to the patient: wet chin, uncomfortable headrest, dry lips, saliva ejector pulling soft tissue, or pressure from evacuator tip pinching lips on teeth.

Many adults will appreciate the placement of a rubber bite block between upper and lower arches on the side opposite the operation when belt-driven older types of handpieces are used. It provides a very comfortable rest in long operations.

Dismissing the Patient

When work has been completed, the patient must be dismissed, i.e., taken from the chair to the reception-room door—graciously, unhurriedly—yet without preventing your dentist from continuing to the next patient. Most of this procedure becomes *your* job.

The dismissal begins at the chair when all dental procedures have been completed. When the dentist leaves the patient at this point, he should not be obligated to have any more con-

versation with that patient, unless he so desires. The assistant should plan to be present to take over promptly, and she will receive from the dentist any necessary information for future appointments.

If any debris is present on the patient's face, for example, some of the impression pastes which are difficult to remove, assist in removing it.

Return all possessions: dental appliances first, then packages or purses stored on the shelf, or suit coat if removed at the chair. Now show the patient to the powder alcove or mirror.

When the patient is satisfied with his appearance, proceed to arrange any further business which you may have with that patient. You should know the details of the patient's account and how it is being handled in the event that it is necessary to make new arrangements or change existing arrangements for the account. The patient may request information about his account.

Keep in mind the advisability of assisting elderly individuals whenever possible, and also mothers with small children.

Try never to let a patient leave the reception room without saying "Goodbye, Mrs. Jones" at the moment the patient is about to leave. If you must leave the patient before that moment, make the farewell definite and warm. The assistant should be standing in the reception room when these words are said, not inclining her upper body through the doorway showing her haste to return to other duties.

Assisting with Children

Some special emphasis should be given to chair assisting for young children. It is somewhat different from working with adults. Special attention to the psychology of the young child is most desirable if your office works with children. (See chap. 2, "Psychology and Public Relations.")

Dental work for children necessitates very efficient chairside assisting, as well as good management of appointments. One of the chief reasons for unpleasantness in performing dentistry for children arises from failure to start the child's relationships with the dental office at a sufficiently early period in the child's development. The recommendations given to parents officially by the American Dental Association in various forms of publicity have gradually lowered the recommended age level for the first dental appointment to age two. Activity of the American Society of Dentistry for Children has been largely responsible for this improvement.

Most children enter a stage of negativistic behavior at about two to two and a half years of age. If a direct suggestion is made to them, the answer is a vehement "No!" This is the period in which the child is trying to establish himself as an individual. He wants to assert himself, make his own choices, be a "person" in his own right. Unless he is a very phlegmatic child, he does not respond cooperatively to new experiences such as a visit to the dentist. As a common result, neither he nor the dentist enjoys the visit. On the other hand, if the child can be brought to the dental office prior to this stage in his behavior pattern, at the age of eighteen to twenty-two months, for a prophylaxis and examination visit involving the use of a revolving instrument on the teeth and an explorer and mirror in the mouth, he is usually more interested in the procedure than he is in objecting to it. Cases of rampant dental caries are thus observed at a more opportune time for treatment. However, the average youngster will require no treatment of a pain-producing nature. His experience is one of pleasant investigation and observation. Occasionally the child will shed tears at the beginning of the appointment, but

curiosity soon overcomes his fears. Frequently he is not willing to leave the chair at the conclusion of the appointment. Seen at frequent intervals thereafter, the youngster whose relationship with the dental office has been so advantageously begun rarely turns into the "problem" type of patient. His dental care is pleasant for him and for the dentist.

Many youngsters are first brought to the dental office because of pain. The dental assistant can be a greater influence in promoting cooperation than can the dentist. The young child's close association with his mother creates this preference in the child's mind. However, a child will not be led to believe that the assistant is sympathetic when actually she dislikes children. To be really successful in relationships with these young patients, the assistant must have a genuine liking for children.

Most dental offices which do have child patients have some arrangement to give the child a gift. The present is usually a small toy or novelty of some nature, given up to a certain age level.

The practice of using these toys or novelties as "rewards" for good behavior is not approved by child psychologists. The toy or novelty should be a present to the child from the dentist simply because the dentist likes the child. Properly used, such presents to children are a tremendous help in cultivating a pleasant attitude toward the dental office, but they should be presented impartially, without regard for behavior. The gift gives the child a pleasant memory of the office, regardless of the treatment he may have had in other respects. The uncooperative child very frequently will make an intense effort to be more cooperative at succeeding appointments when this procedure in handling gifts is used.

Care should be exercised in purchasing novelties for this purpose to select those which are least likely to be harmful in any way, dangerous for the child, or of danger to anyone around the child. Noisemakers of any kind are not appreciated by parents, although sometimes it is possible to give them with the admonition that they are to be used only out-of-doors.

When young children are in the dental chair, it is extremely important to be thoroughly set up before starting. The entire procedure should be completed as rapidly as possible and without interruption. Young children cannot hold their mouths open easily for any great length of time. The strain on them is lessened directly in proportion to the speed with which the operation is completed.

To most young children, the operatory is full of mysterious and unfamiliar equipment. If the child exhibits an apprehensive attitude toward the equipment, gently and slowly show the child the various parts, how they move, how they sound—with no effort made to explain their *use*. Touch his cheek with the evacuator tip, if one is to be used, to show its gentleness and yours. The child will frequently begin to ask questions at this point, and the conversation should then be led to things of interest to the child *outside* the dental office. The object of this approach is to de-emphasize the dental equipment as much as possible and to present a legitimate distraction.

Most children get along better without the presence of the parent in the operatory, although occasional youngsters will do better if a properly instructed parent is there. Most dentists prefer to have the parent remain in the waiting room.

Never leave a young child alone in the dental chair. When the dentist takes over at the chair, it is also your signal to keep silent in order that the child's attention may be given to the dentist alone. Keep a friendly expression always.

Everything done around a young child should be unhurried, calm, and performed with a friendly manner. All effort is directed toward giving the youngster the feeling that what is being done is as usual and commonplace as eating lunch at home. By your actions and words give the youngster the impression that he is expected to accept it as usual and commonplace, too.

You do not go into elaborate explanations, solicitous statements, or make apprehensive expressions when you are about to serve lunch to a youngster at home. If you were to do so, he would immediately begin to wonder what undesirable plans you had for him. The same is true of the dental office and its procedures. If the parent, the assistant, and the dentist are able to treat a dental appointment as a casual thing that calls for no unusual reactions, children are inclined to accept it as such.

Commonly, however, the child has heard (and remembered) little remarks made by adults in his presence concerning their dental visits or dental needs—sometimes dental pains. Perhaps the child has heard older children tell of the terrors of their visit to the dentist. When the day arrives that the child finds himself in the dental office, all these expressions and fears return, magnified a thousandfold because of the element of the unknown.

Children have vivid imaginations. However, if a child is properly approached, his imagination can be made an assistance in the dental office.

All the effort of the dental office should be devoted to giving or restoring the casual, friendly, "it's fun" attitude of the normal, well-adjusted child.

Oral Examination Technique

An oral examination is made of each new patient and also of regular patients at the time of their recall examination and prophylaxis appointment.

When the dentist is ready to proceed with this part of the examination, sit at the patient's left, facing the dentist, so that you may hear the dentist more easily. It is helpful to have the dental assistant aware of which part of the mouth is being examined so that she may assist in the prevention of charting errors due to incorrectly designating *left* or *right*.

Some dental offices use the patient's examination card to enter the notes of the examination, others may use a paper pad or clipboard with paper on which these notes are written for later entry on the patient's card. If a separate piece of paper is used, the patient's name and the date should be noted at the top for identification.

Record the information necessary to complete the charting. Remember to write legibly and accurately. Record every item the dentist mentions and indicate to him any need for slower dictation.

Summary

Cleanliness in the operatory is mandatory. Learn correct scrubbing procedures and use them.

Note the general rules for conduct in the operatory. The assistant is to *assist* the performance of dentistry and keep attention centered on the patient.

Learn to adjust the dental chair correctly and seat the patient properly. Pleasant attitude and concern for the comfort of the patient are essential.

Care for the patient's dental appliance and remember to return the appliance at the close of the appointment.

Tray setups, if used, will speed the setup and cleanup of the operatory.

Assisting with preparations is exacting work, and the dental assistant should learn the requirements for serving her dentist: maintain the correct lighting, keep a clear field of operation, and present instruments and materials as needed.

In serving and receiving instruments, the assistant should present the correct instrument in the position in which the dentist will use it. A pattern must be developed between the dentist and assistant.

The purpose of dental assisting is to conserve the dentist's time and energy.

Dismissal of the patient begins at the chair, with the dental assistant accepting the responsibility for the patient's appearance. She removes debris which would be difficult for the patient to remove. Dismissal continues through providing an opportunity for the patient's personal grooming, accepting payments for services, making new appointments, and ushering the patient out of the reception room. It may include helping with outer clothing.

Assisting with children is different from working with adults. Careful attention to the proper attitudes and remarks is essential.

Oral examination requires that the assistant make notes while the dentist examines the mouth. Charting is an important part of this examination and should be carefully learned according to the dentist's choice of method.

Study Questions
1. Detail correct scrubbing procedures.
2. What are general rules for operatory conduct?
3. Discuss the preparation of the patient for the dentist, beginning with the patient seated in the reception room.
4. What is important in assisting with preparations?
5. Describe serving and receiving instruments.
6. Describe dismissing the patient.
7. What is important to remember in assisting with children?
8. Describe *oral examination*.

45 *Chairside Assisting*

The Dental Assistant as Chair Assistant

The chairside assistant has become so important in dentistry that some students believe dental assisting *is* chairside assisting. *Four-handed dentistry* and *six-handed dentistry* have become common terms. In four-handed dentistry, an assistant is a second pair of hands, supplying the dentist with anything he needs.

In six-handed dentistry, a *floater* dental assistant is a second pair of hands for the dental assistant, serving her with anything which is not within easy reach. Some oral health care delivery teams are so well organized that the assistant to the dentist is served instruments by the floater so that she, too, keeps her eyes on the patient's mouth and is relieved of instruments she no longer needs.

If you are the chairside assistant, learn to be a second pair of hands which respond to the dentist's needs *in advance of his request.* That is, anticipate the next requirement and be prepared to serve him whatever he will need. The closer to his hands at the patient's chin you can have the instrument or material he needs, the less eyestrain he will experience, and the more rapidly he can complete his work.

In this chapter you will find specific instructions for each dental operation, including lists of materials and instruments necessary for each operation discussed. Do not be reluctant to list on the proper textbook page the materials and instruments *your* dentist uses for each operation. This alteration will make your book more valuable to you and your dentist. No two dentists work exactly alike, and some men prefer instruments not listed for these operations or may not use all the instruments listed here.

Basic Setup for Nonoperative Procedures

Materials required:

1. Mouth mirror

2. Explorer

3. Cotton pliers

4. For all specific procedures, such as removal of teeth, full-denture appointments, and postoperative treatments, certain additional instruments or materials will be required. See lists under the appropriate headings.

New Patient Examination Procedure Adult and Child

Adult

The patient will have filled out an Acquaintance Form. Make available a complete set of patient records, with the Acquaintance or Registration Form attached. *The basic setup for nonoperative procedures is required.* The material for a recall prophylaxis and examination is required. Films for full-mouth and bitewing X rays are usually required. Be prepared with the material for alginate impressions in case the patient has teeth missing or other conditions which would require study models. Pulp-testing equipment should be available. Read "Oral Examination Technique," chapter forty-four.

Child

The procedure is much the same as for adults. In many offices, however, full-mouth X rays of children are not taken until about the age of eight or nine. Bitewing X rays are the small No. 00 size for young children (under six years of age). The No. 0 size is often used from about six to eleven years of age.

The dentist frequently has the parent present in the operatory for this appointment. It provides opportunity for education of the parent, provided the behavior of the child is good.

Bitewing X-ray Procedure

Have the required films placed on the bracket table.

For patients twelve years of age and older, four films are required, together with the paper bitewing tabs. The box of paper tabs may be kept with the film in the film storage box.

For children under twelve years, two of the small films are used if the child's mouth is small. As soon as possible, many dentists begin to use four adult-size films or regular adult bitewing films. Bite tabs are available which the assistant attaches to the small films to make them into bitewing X rays for the young child. Service to the child is expedited if you prepare these films in advance and keep them in the film storage box.

Seat the patient.

Protect the patient from X rays.

In some dental offices you are expected to take the X rays.[1] If this is the case, always remember to wipe all moisture off each film packet immediately upon removal from the patient's mouth. In offices where the dentist takes the X rays, you should be prepared to assist him with the following procedures:

The X-ray machine should be in operating readiness.

While the dentist is placing the film in the patient's mouth, swing the X-ray head near the patient so the dentist may reach it easily.

Take the timer or exposure button in your hands.

The sequence in which films are placed in the mouth will always be the same.

Exposures for these areas are:

   Molar: _____ seconds
   Bicuspid: _____ seconds

When two films are used for small children, the sequence will always be: first, left side; second, right side.

   Exposure for both is   _____ seconds

When making exposures, watch for the signal from your dentist. He will teach you his signal system. Protect yourself and your dentist from X rays. Always be at least six feet away from the X-ray head when making exposures. Watch the dials of the X ray to see

1. Write Eastman Kodak Company, X-ray Division, Rochester, New York, for a complimentary copy of *X rays in Dentistry*. This booklet illustrates fully all positions for dental X-ray procedures.

that it is functioning properly. Your dentist will show you what these dials must indicate.

Upon completion of all exposures, hang up the timer and replace the X-ray extension arm and head in its customary out-of-the-way position.

Place the rubber-banded bundle in the film storage box until time is available to develop them.

Write the patient's name on the wrapper of the film immediately.

Complete X-ray Procedure

Seat the patient.

Protect the patient from X rays.

Films should be available, protected, in a film dispenser.

Fourteen films are used for a complete X ray—seven films for the upper arch and seven for the lower arch. The sequence of placing them in the mouth is always the same. The exposure time varies depending on the area of the mouth being X-rayed and the type of X ray used.

The sequence of film placement, together with the space for your dentist to enter the correct exposure for his X ray, is as follows:

Upper left molar area   _____ seconds
Upper left bicuspid area _____ seconds
Upper left cuspid area   _____ seconds
Upper central area   _____ seconds
Upper right cuspid area _____ seconds
Upper right bicuspid area _____ seconds
Upper right molar area   _____ seconds
Lower right molar area   _____ seconds
Lower right bicuspid area _____ seconds
Lower right cuspid area _____ seconds
Lower central area   _____ seconds
Lower left cuspid area   _____ seconds
Lower left bicuspid area _____ seconds
Lower left molar area   _____ seconds

Protect yourself and your dentist from X rays *before* you depress the timer button.

Wipe all moisture from film packets immediately after removal from mouth, or as soon as possible.

When all X rays have been taken, write the patient's name on the exposed film. Place the rubber-banded bundle in the film storage box until time is available to develop them.

Panoramic X-ray Procedure

Materials required:

1. Cassette

2. Two screens

3. Film sheet

4. Lead apron or other protection from X ray for patient

Insert film and screens in cassette prior to patient's arrival.

Protect the patient with proper shielding.

Insert the cassette in the machine.

Set the controls.

Protect yourself.

Expose the film.

Release patient.

Remove cassette from machine.

Toothbrushing Demonstration Procedure

Materials required:

1. Basic setup for nonoperative procedures

2. Large hand mirror—be sure that it is clean and free from fingerprints

3. Full denture for demonstration of brushing

4. Toothbrush for demonstrating on denture

5. Toothbrush for demonstrating in the patient's mouth and for presentation to the patient upon departure

This demonstration is often given to a new patient at the time of his initial appointment for examination as an aid in gauging his interest in and appreciation of dental care. It is commonly performed at the final appointment of a patient who has undergone any major amount of operative or restorative work. Frequently, regular patients are taught proper brushing procedures on their recall prophylaxis and examination appointment. The demonstration may be given by the assistant. If this is the procedure in your office, you should understand fully just what the dentist wishes you to teach the patient. (See "Personal Oral Hygiene.")

Basic Setup for Operative Procedures

Materials required:

1. Mouth mirror

2. Explorer

3. Cotton pliers

4. Air and water syringes

5. Medicaments available

6. Syringe and ampules of anesthetic

7. Air turbine prepared for use or contra-angle (miniature type for children)

8. Cotton rolls and cotton-roll holders or rubber dam

9. Burs and diamond instruments available as required (short-neck burs for miniature contra-angles)

10. A square of gauze or a disposable tissue inserted in the right-hand clip of the bib-holder for use by the dentist in removing debris from the instruments

11. Saliva ejector

12. High-volume evacuator prepared for use if needed

13. Topical anesthetic if needed

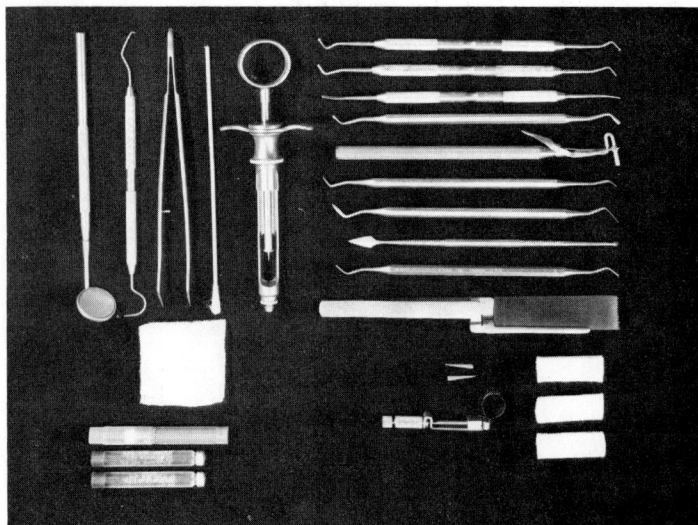

Fig. 45.1. Cavity preparation tray

Periodontic Procedures

Diagnosis Tray

Material required:
1. Basic kit
    a. Mirror
    b. Explorer
    c. Probe
2. U15 scaler and all curettes
3. Saliva ejector
4. Gauze sponges, 2" x 2"
5. Disclosing tablets
6. Spool of dental floss
7. Toothbrush
8. Napkin chain
9. Handpiece
10. Proper contra-angle for prophylaxis

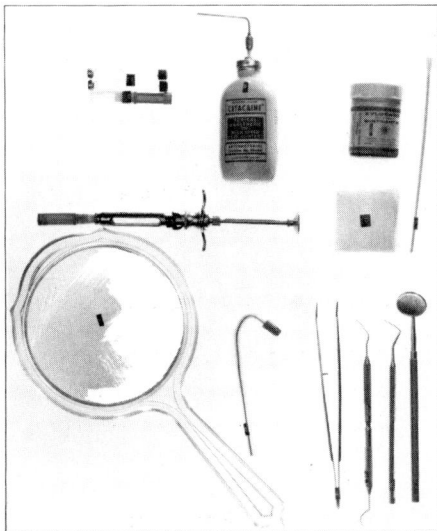

Fig. 45.2. Periodontic tray: diagnosis

Periodontic Procedures (Continued)

Prophylaxis Tray

Materials required:
1. Basic kit
    a. Mirror
    b. Explorer
    c. Probe
2. U15 scaler and all curettes
3. Sharpening stone
4. Disclosing tablets
5. Prophylaxis angle
6. Prophylaxis cup
7. Prophylaxis paste
8. Dental floss
9. Napkin chain
10. Handpiece
11. Saliva ejector
12. Topical anesthetic

Periodontic Procedures (Continued)

Instrumentation Tray

Materials required:

1. Basic kit
   a. Mirror
   b. Explorer
   c. Probe
2. U15 scaler with curettes
   a. Gracey's 1 & 2, 9 & 10 (or 7 & 8), 13 & 14
   b. McCall's 13s & 14s, 17s & 18s
3. 2″ x 2″ gauze sponges
4. Sharpening stone
5. Napkin holder
6. Handpiece
7. Proper contra-angle for prophylaxis
8. Saliva ejector
9. Topical anesthetic

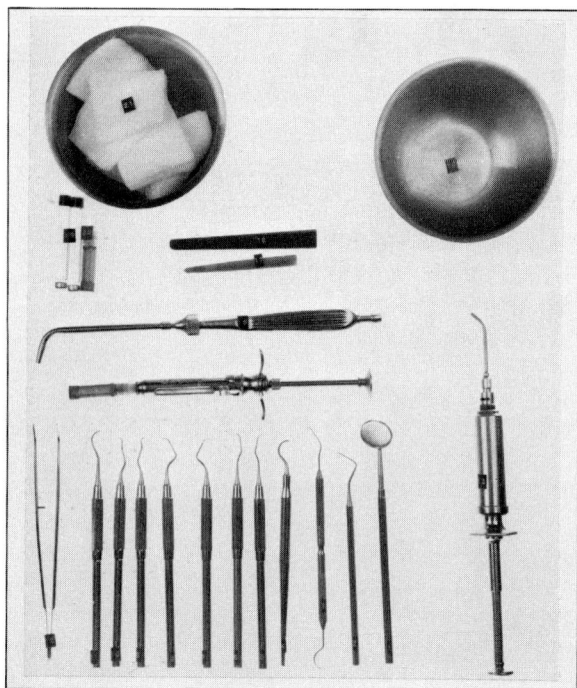

Fig. 45.3. Periodontic tray: instrumentation

Periodontic Procedures (Continued)

Occlusal Adjustment Tray

Materials required:

1. Mirror

2. Set of green stones for straight handpiece (Nos. 19, 22, 48, 23)

3. Burlew wheel

4. Midget or regular pumice-impregnated rubber polishing cups, tips, and points

5. Occlusal wax and pencil

6. Articulating paper holder (Miller)

7. Red or green typewriter ribbon or articulating paper

8. 2″ x 2″ gauze sponges

9. Napkin holder

10. Handpiece

11. Proper contra-angle prophylaxis

12. Saliva ejector

Periodontic Procedures (Continued)

Surgery Tray

Materials required:

1. Mirror
2. Explorer
3. Probe
4. U15 scaler
5. Bard Parker handle and No. 15 blade
6. Knives
7. Periosteal elevator (No. 7 spatula)
8. Curettes—Gracey's 1 & 2, 9 & 10, 17s & 18s
9. Sharpening stone
10. Needle holder
11. Suture scissors
12. Burs
    a. No. 8 round, straight handpiece bur
    b. Fl and F3 diamond stones

13. Stainless-steel bowl
14. Water bulb
15. Topical anesthetic
16. Topical anesthetic syringe with long and short needle and ampules of local anesthetic
17. Two or three sterile cotton-tipped applicators
18. Aspirator handle and 2 tips
19. Jones clamp and section of sterile rubber tubing with connector
20. Sterile napkin chain
21. Handpiece
22. Proper contra-angle for prophylaxis
23. Saliva ejector

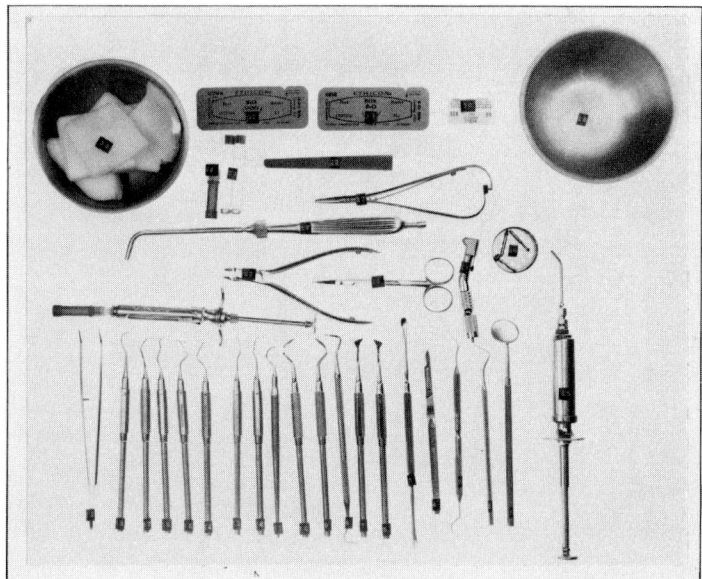

Fig. 45.4. Periodontic tray: surgery

Periodontic Procedures (Continued)

Postoperative Tray

Materials required:

1. Mirror

2. Explorer

3. Probe

4. Suture scissors

5. Cotton pliers

6. Handpiece

7. Proper contra-angle for prophylaxis

8. Saliva ejector

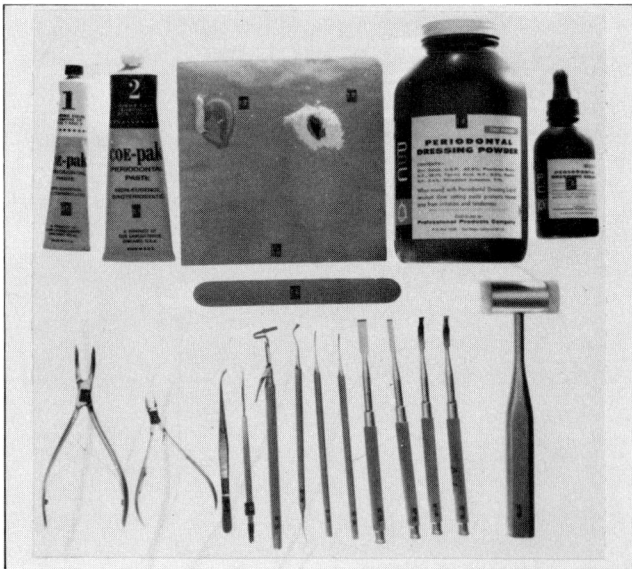

Fig. 45.5. Periodontic pack tray

Periodontic Procedures (Continued)

Pack Removal Tray

Materials required:

1. Mirror

2. Probe

3. U15 scaler

4. Handpiece

5. Proper contra-angle for prophylaxis

6. Saliva ejector

Pulp-testing Procedures

Materials required:

1. Basic setup for nonoperative procedures. At times, this procedure is required during an operative appointment, in which case the instrument setup is already complete.

2. Pulp tester. Some pulp testers are individual portable types. Others are part of the dental unit and require no assembly of components for use. The most recent type can be operated by the dentist alone.

3. Ice cones. Ice cones are made by filling used anesthetic ampules with water and freezing. When ice is needed for pulp testing, the stick of ice is removed from the container.

This procedure is used to gain information about the vitality of a tooth. In general, it is the application of a small electrical current to the tooth, increased slowly until the patient gives evidence of feeling the response in the tooth being tested. When the full degree of current is applied without response in the tooth, the tooth may be nonvital, or no longer alive.

The dentist applies the electrode to the tooth, using toothpaste as an electrolyte contact. The assistant gradually increases the amount of current through the tester, either by operation of a slide on the instrument or by rotation of a knob for that purpose on the dental unit. If the pulp tester used in your dental office is a separate unit, a manual is available which illustrates its assembly and correct use.

For a complete examination, the dentist will test each tooth in the mouth. The pulp tester may also be used in testing an individual tooth, in which case the dentist will usually test other teeth corresponding to the tooth in question in order to discover the usual range of response to be expected and then proceed to test the questionable tooth.

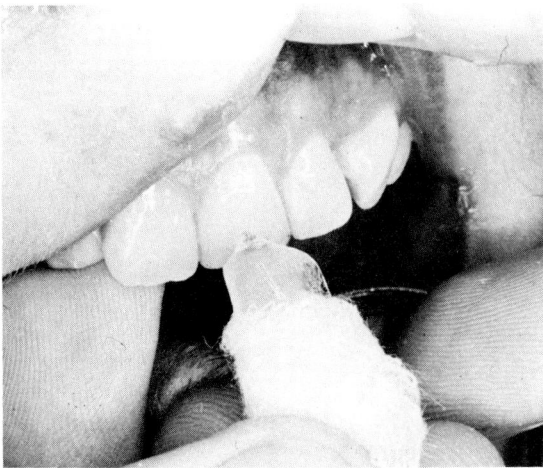

Fig. 45.7. Pulp testing with electric pulp tester

The patient will be instructed to raise a hand or give a signal of some kind to indicate that a response is felt. As the assistant is increasing the current slowly, she should watch or listen for this signal of response. Note the figure at which the pointer rests at the moment the signal is made. Speak this number clearly to the dentist and return the slide or knob to zero.

The slide or knob controlling the degree of current should be carefully and slowly moved to increase the current at a rate which would cover the scale consistently in ten to fifteen seconds. If a patient is highly sensitive, much care should be exercised in increasing the current very slowly. Too rapid increases in current are highly unpleasant to the patient.

The pulp tester is returned to its case or its receptacle on the dental unit.

Electric pulp testers cannot be used through restorations, especially teeth with full metal or porcelain crowns. In such cases, ice is used to provide a thermal shock when contacting the tooth or restoration. Like the electric test, the response is positive or negative. No *degree of vitality* can be judged from either test.

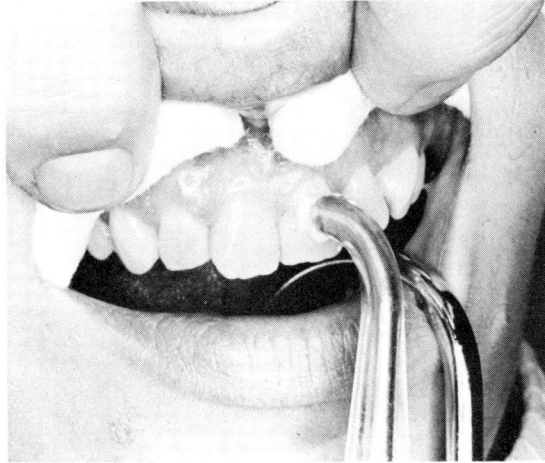

Fig. 45.6. Pulp testing with ice

Rubber Dam Application

Materials required:

1. Rubber dam
2. Rubber-dam frame
3. Rubber-dam punch
4. Assorted rubber-dam clamps
5. Rubber-dam clamp forceps
6. Dental floss
7. Plastic instrument
8. Saliva ejector
9. Vaseline or tissue lubricant

Amalgam Filling Procedure

Materials required:

1. Basic setup for operative procedures

2. Double-ended chisels

3. Double-ended hatchets, right and left

4. Double-ended gingival margin trimmers, right and left

5. Excavators, right and left, large and small

6. Amalgam carrier

7. Amalgam pluggers, hand type; automatic type, if used

8. Amalgam carvers

9. Amalgam burnishers

10. Matrix holders, Tofflemire or others

11. Matrix bands, molar medium and bicuspid medium

12. Wedge material, or separators

13. Curved crown and bridge shears for adjusting bands when necessary

Be ready to assist at the chair by the time the dentist is ready to work on the preparation of the tooth. Some time may be available while the dentist is making the injection of local anesthetic or waiting for it to become effective. Make use of such minutes to perform other duties.

Keep used instruments and other items in position for reuse as the work progresses by keeping trays neat.

An appointment for finishing and polishing these fillings should be made. Twenty-four hours are required before an amalgam filling is considered ready for finishing and polishing.

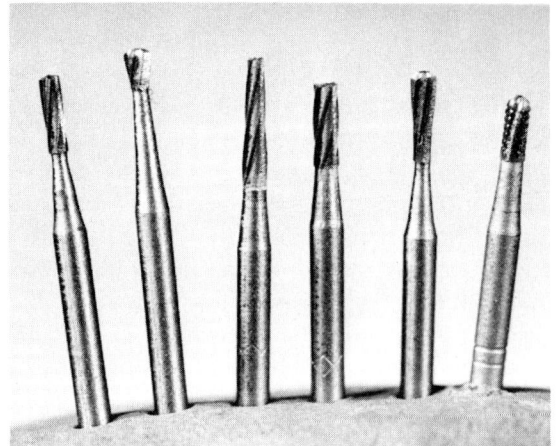

Fig. 45.8. Assortment of burs used in amalgam cavity preparation.

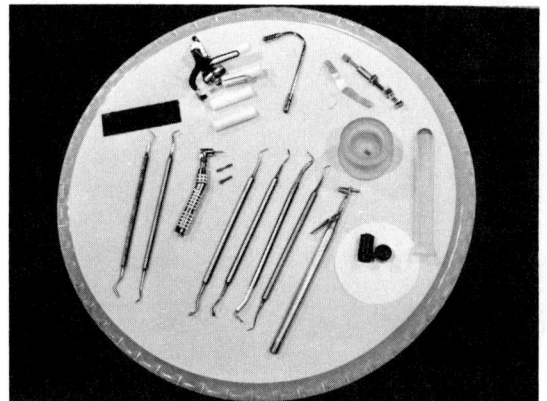

Fig. 45.9. Tray for placing amalgam

Polishing (Finishing) Amalgam Restorations

Materials required:

1. Basic setup for nonoperative procedures
2. Prophylaxis right angle and rubber cup
3. Polishing brush on mandrel
4. Fine sandpaper discs and mandrels, straight and angle
5. Contra-angle for item 4
6. Finishing burs in bur block
7. Cotton rolls and left and right lower holders as required
8. Dappen dish of prophylactic paste for coarse polishing
9. Dappen dish of half-and-half dry tin oxide and whiting for final polish
10. Large hand mirror for patient's use

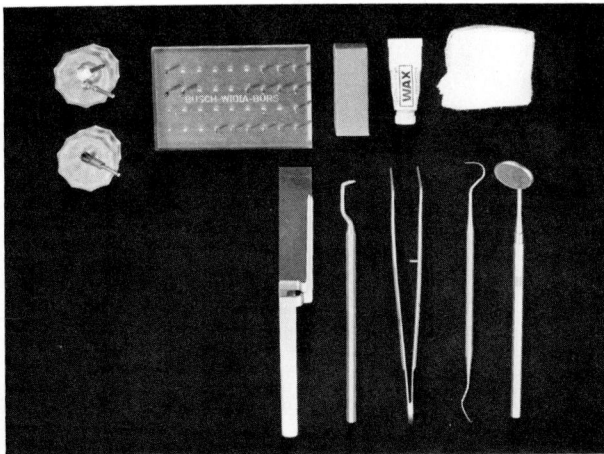

Fig. 45.10. Restoration polishing tray

Silicate Cement Filling Procedure

Materials required:

1. Basic setup for operative procedures
2. Chisels
3. Stellite plastic instruments for placing synthetic mix
4. Plastic strips, one for each preparation
5. White petrolatum or cocoa butter to coat filling upon removal of strip
6. Glass slab cooled to 65°-75°F.
7. Stellite spatula, broad, also cooled as above
8. Color guide for silicate cement
9. Silicate cement powders and liquids
10. Clamps or matrix retainer to hold plastic strips in position during setting time

Practice selecting the proper shade. The shade guides should be moistened by touching them to the inner side of the patient's cheek, and the tooth should be kept moistened. Lips should be held in normal position. Verify the shade with the dentist, then have only the necessary powders on the work surface. Bottles, powders as well as liquids, should be kept tightly closed except when material is being removed from them. Unused powder is not to be returned to the stock bottle.

By properly timing the procedure, the assistant can place the material on the glass slab, proceed to mix, and have the mix completed at the moment the dentist is ready to place it in the tooth. The dentist can best indicate by a signal when this moment arrives.

Hold the glass slab with the prepared mix just in front and to the left of the patient's chin so that the dentist may easily reach it with the stellite instrument he uses for placement of the material into the preparation. If your dentist prefers to time the setting, you do so, using a watch and indicating to him when the proper period has passed. Other dentists prefer to have the assistant roll up the excess material, hold it tightly between thumb and forefinger, and indicate when the material cannot be dented by the thumbnail.

The slab and spatula should be cleaned by immediately placing them under the cold running water, rubbing the surfaces with the fingers to remove any material remaining from the mix. Also be sure to remove, in this same manner, any material remaining on the instrument used to place the mix. You will then be ready for another mix, if more than one preparation has been made.

Silicate cement fillings are generally left for final finishing until a subsequent appointment.

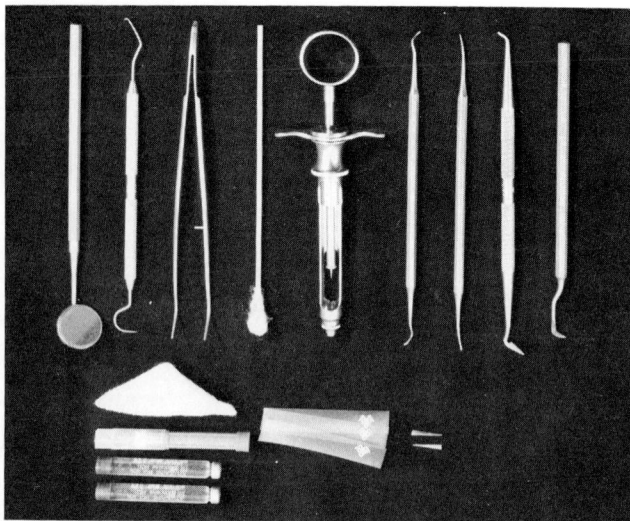

Fig. 45.11. Tray for silicate cement

Polishing Silicate Cement

Materials required:

1. Basic setup for nonoperative procedure

2. Fine sandpaper or cuttle discs with mandrels

3. White petrolatum or cocoa butter for lubrication of discs and filling

4. Contra-angle handpiece

5. Fine cuttle finishing strips

Plastic or Composite Filling Procedure

Materials required:

1. Basic setup for operative procedures

2. Chisels

3. Cement-base materials

4. Sable brushes, one straight, one angle

5. Glass slab for powder

6. Dappen dish for liquid (sometimes glass slab is used)

7. Correct shades of powder

8. Shade guide

9. Liquid for use with the acrylic powder

The above listing is used for the *brush-in* method of placement. If the *pressure* method is used, the brushes are omitted, and a resin strip or other means of maintaining pressure on the filling is prepared. In the pressure method, the mix is completed on the slab, the material is placed into the preparation with a stellite instrument, and pressure is applied by some means until the initial set of the material has been accomplished.

This type of filling is generally finished at a subsequent appointment. The instructions which accompany the material used in your office should be read carefully and the recommended procedure followed.

Finishing Plastic or Composite Fillings

Materials required:

1. Basic setup for nonoperative procedures
2. Fine sandpaper discs and mandrel
3. Right and left finishing burs for acrylic
4. Felt disc, moistened, on screw-mandrel
5. Dappen dish with moistened whiting
6. Gold-foil trimming knife

Preparation of Zinc Oxide-Eugenol Cement

Materials required:

1. Glass slab, parchment pad, or plastic pad
2. Steel spatula for mixing (one which is used only for this purpose)
3. Powder and liquid for zinc oxide-eugenol cement.
4. Plastic instrument for placing the mixed zinc oxide cement

When used, this material will usually be called for as part of an operative procedure, in which case no separate setup is required.

Preparation of Zinc Phosphate Cements

Materials required:

1. Glass slab, cooled to between 65° and 75° Fahrenheit
2. Stainless-steel cement spatula
3. Selected bottle of cement powder
4. Bottle of corresponding cement liquid

Zinc phosphate cements are used for bases under fillings and for cementing inlays, crowns, bridges, and jacket crowns. The consistency for bases is usually heavier than that used for cementation. For use as a base, this type of cement is usually mixed to a molasses-like consistency. For cementation the consistency is usually similar to thirty percent cream; if the spatula is quickly raised from the finished mix of cement on the slab, the cement will follow the spatula in a thin line without breaking momentarily. Zinc phosphate cements are *not* mixed like synthetic porcelain.

Gold-foil Filling Procedure

Materials required:

1. Basic setup for operative procedures

2. Rubber dam

3. Rubber-dam holder

4. Rubber-dam retainers

5. Rubber-dam retainer forceps

6. Rubber-dam punch

7. Petrolatum to lubricate punched holes in dam

8. Napkin face mask for rubber dam

9. Red stick compound (to stabilize retainer)

10. Alcohol lamp filled with alcohol (or electric annealer)

11. Leather-faced mallet, long handle (or automatic mallet, if used)

12. Prepared gold foil, pellets, cylinders, or ropes, as desired

13. Gold-foil pluggers, trimming knives, trimming files, and holders

14. Chisels and excavators as required for cavity preparation

15. Polishing strips, discs, rubber cups, and fine-polishing abrasives

Your assistance is usually needed for a rapid application of the rubber dam to the required area of the patient's mouth.

Your direct and constant assistance is required in *condensing* and in *annealing* the gold foil into the cavity preparation when ready. Some dentists require the assistant to wield a mallet, applying the strokes to the end of a gold-foil condenser manipulated by the dentist on the foil in the cavity preparation. Other methods include the use of automatic malleting devices.

If you are using cohesive gold foil, it must be annealed. If you are using noncohesive gold foil, it is not annealed. However, restorations in which noncohesive gold foil is used are usually completed by the use of cohesive gold foil. Thus the entire setup of materials required, as listed above, is necessary for either type of restoration.

Practice alone will help the dental assistant understand and become adept at assisting with gold-foil work. It is one of the most exacting, precise operative procedures used in the dental office.

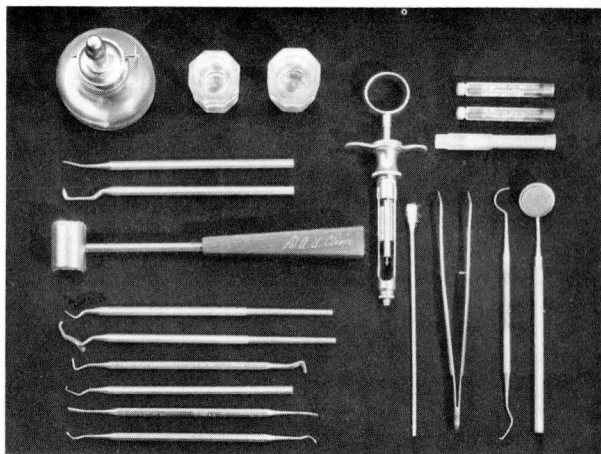

Fig. 45.12. Gold-foil tray

Temporary Crown Procedure

Materials required:

1. Basic setup for operative procedures
2. Diamond discs and mounted diamond wheels
3. Excavators, small, left and right
4. Zinc phosphate cement and liquid
5. Glass slab and stainless spatula for item 4
6. Plastic instrument
7. Set of contouring pliers for steel crowns
8. Crown and bridge scissors, curved

In cases involving extremely deep decay or pulp exposure, the following may be required by your dentist also.

9. Calcium hydroxide base material
10. Sterile glass slab for above items
11. Bottle of adrenalin
12. Sterile dappen dish for item 11
13. Sterile cotton pellets
14. Sterile No. 8 round burs for contra-angles
15. Other materials your dentist may use for pulp treatment
16. Rubber-dam setup

Temporary steel crowns are set at the same sitting that the preparation is made. No subsequent appointment for setting the crown is required.

The procedure involving treatment of the pulp requires extremely close assisting in the various steps, especially in the event that the patient is a very young child.

Orthodontic Procedures

Orthodontics is that specialty of dentistry which deals with the prevention and correction of irregularities of the teeth and malocclusion.

Study models are widely used in orthodontics as records of progress in treatment. Algi-nate materials are perhaps most commonly used as an impression material for these study models. A more detailed and specific method of shaping the model bases and of articulating the models is used, for which purposes several assisting devices are available.

Casts or models which are kept for reference purposes are often shown to patients and therefore should possess a neat and artistic appearance. White is the most common color for the artificial stone used in making these reference casts.

In order to keep such reference casts really white and clean, you should soak them or coat them with a surfacing material. Once the surface coating has dried, any dust or finger marks can be readily wiped off.

The construction of appliances involves the use of banding material, attachments of many kinds, arch wires of various types, and the use of soldering equipment or welding equipment. Instruments include contouring and bending pliers, crown shears, band drivers, cementing instruments, mirrors, and explorers.

Methods of radiographic cephalometry, which involve processing of extraoral film cassettes and intensifying screens, are used in many orthodontic offices.

Many orthodontists also use both intraoral and extraoral color photography as a means of recording case progress and results.

The latter procedures, X ray and photography, are usually so organized that their use is one of routine procedure, with positioning controlled for purposes of accurately repeating various views.

Records are maintained in a highly detailed manner, often involving the dictation of information relating to individual cases, with treatment planned for each.

Organization and control of the appointment schedules are extremely important because of the large number of short adjustment appointments involved in this specialty.

Endodontic Procedure for Routine Treatment (Pulpitis)

Intracanal Tray

Materials required:

1. Mirror
2. Explorer
3. Excavator
4. Cotton pliers
5. Irrigation syringe (2 or 3 cc.) with needle
6. Scissors
7. Hemostat
8. Plastic instrument
9. Spreader
10. Plugger
11. Measuring gauge
12. 2 dappen dishes
13. 3 2″ x 2″ gauze sponges
14. 2 1″ cotton rolls
15. 2 applicator sticks
16. Topical anesthetic
17. Syringes with cartridge of local anesthetic

Equipment and Supplies

18. Reamers and files (standardized A.A.E. sizes 10-140)
19. Gutta-percha points (standardized A.A.E. sizes 25-140)
20. Silver points (standardized A.A.E. sizes 10-60)
21. Broaches, smooth and barbed
22. Paper points
23. Rubber or silicone stops
24. Glass bead or salt sterilizer
25. Electric pulp tester
26. Culture tubes
27. Endodontic cement (sealer)
28. Mixing slab and spatula
29. Cavit
30. Cements: zinc oxide-eugenol, zinc phosphate, and silicate

Medicaments

31. Zonite (1% sodium hypochlorite)
32. Eugenol
33. Camphorated paramonochlorophenol
34. Cresatin
35. Beechwood creosote
36. Alcohol
37. Tincture of Mercresin (untinted)
38. Eucalyptol
39. EDTAC

Also Available

40. Rubber-dam squares
41. Rubber-dam punch
42. Rubber-dam clamp forceps
43. Rubber-dam holder

The purpose of this procedure is devitalization of the tooth involved, without apical surgery. A series of such treatments may be required.

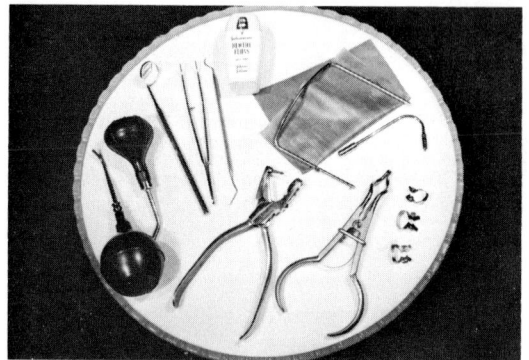

Fig. 45.13. Rubber-dam tray

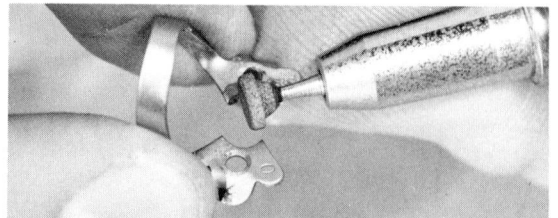

Fig. 45.14. Custom-contouring jaws of rubber-dam clamp when necessary.

Minimum Endodontic Setup for Apicoectomy (or Apical Curettage)

All materials and instruments needed to perform the work should be arranged in an orderly fashion. For efficiency in operating, there must be no delay to search for instruments or prepare materials once the work is begun.

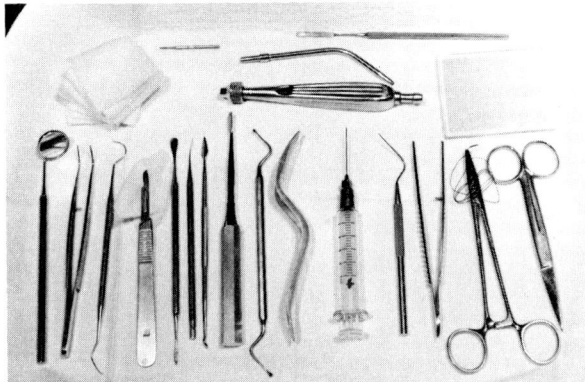

Fig. 45.15. Endodontic tray: apicoectomy or apical curettage.

Periapical Surgery Tray

Materials required:

1. Gilmore probe
2. Vehe carver
3. Scalpel (no. 15 blade)
4. Periosteotome
5. Burs (nos. 557 and 560 carbide)
6. Needle holder
7. Scissors
8. Bone chisel
9. 3 periapical curettes
10. Tissue retractor
11. Needle (with silk suture)
12. 5 2″ x 2″ gauze sponges
13. 2 applicator sticks
14. Sterile water of saline
15. Topical anesthetic
16. Syringes with cartridges of local anesthetic

The purpose of this procedure is devitalization of the tooth, together with removal of a portion of the root tip and the surrounding bony structure.

Care and Medication Preliminary to Surgery Under Local or General Anesthesia

Medical history: The dental office usually attempts to determine the present history of the patient, his sensitivity to drugs, and any medication being taken. Three questions commonly serve this purpose: Are you sensitive to any drugs? Are you taking any drugs? Are you under the care of a physician?

Preoperative medication is valuable in bringing the patient to a condition of quietness and complacency which eliminates, so far as possible, the apprehension, fear, and resistance to anesthesia.

Posture, the proper position of the patient, is most important. The upright position for dental surgery is the usual position advocated for surgery in the dental office. Trendelenburg's position is advisable for surgery in the hospital.

Clothing should be adjusted so that the patient can *ventilate* properly—that is, breathe easily through the air passages.

Your dentist will have recognized and questioned the patient about any pulmonary or respiratory disease before administering an anesthetic which is inhaled.

If a patient enters the office and shows blueness of the lips (cyanosis) or shortness of breath, it should be called to your dentist's attention in order that he may question the patient about his health factors which indicate that he should not be given an anesthetic. Blueness at the base of the fingernails and/or varicosities in the veins under the tongue can be checked by your dentist.

If general anesthesia is being used, the complete absence of liquids or solids in the stomach is essential; also, the bladder should be emptied just prior to induction. All removable dental appliances should be removed from the mouth.

The jaw should be supported to insure an adequate airway.

Clearing of the nasopharynx and maintenance of adequate breathing are required. Eliminate the accumulation of fluids and secretions in the lungs by medications and by aspiration.

Foreign bodies—dislodged teeth, dental materials, etc.—must be promptly removed.

Surgical Procedures

Materials required:

1. Basic setup for nonoperative procedures
2. Cotton swabs and exodontia sponges, sterile
3. Rubber gloves, if used
4. Topical antiseptic or anesthetic, as pre-preferred
5. Syringes with cartridges of local anesthetic
6. Surgical burs and sterile handpiece sheath, or turbine equipment
7. Bone chisels and mallet; impactors, automatic chisels, if used
8. Elevators and forceps as required
9. Bone rongeurs and bone files
10. Tissue scissors
11. Sutures, prepared with needles
12. Hemostats, for handling suture needles
13. Antibiotics, if used in the wound
14. Emesis basin (sometimes called a *kidney dish*), if used

15. Aspirator equipment, if used
16. Glass of cold water to clear aspirator tips when necessary
17. Glass of saline (water) and water syringe for flushing or irrigating
18. Throw-apron placed over patient
19. Towel over patient's eyes, if used
20. Towel at the chair
21. One or two sponges clipped to right bib-holder clip
22. Vaseline, for coating lightly over patient's lips
23. Tissue holders (similar to cotton pliers, except for notched beaks)

Both dentist and assistant should scrub thoroughly. While maintenance of a truly sterile field in oral surgery is not always possible, every attempt should be made to do so.

The assistant should keep the field free from blood and debris during the operation by swabbing or aspirating as frequently as necessary. Should the dentist change the position of the patient, the assistant should quickly adjust the position of the spotlight accordingly. Maintain a reassuring manner toward the patient at all times. Watch for the patient's comfort.

In suturing in the mouth, the assistant can be of help by holding loose tissue for penetration by the suture needle, using tissue forceps or cotton pliers.

At conclusion of the operation, see that the patient's face is cleaned of any debris or blood.

Any postoperative instructions are preferably given in writing, together with an envelope containing postoperative medications, if used. Orally given instructions will not usually be remembered with accuracy or detail.

Procedure for Removal of Teeth

Materials required:

1. Premedication, if required, given to patient

2. Basic setup for nonoperative procedures

3. Syringe and local anesthetic cartridges

4. Postoperative medication prepared in envelope, if required

5. Forceps as required

6. X rays on view-box

7. The dentist will inform you of the need for other instruments

If the premedication is desired, and has not been given to the patient to take at home prior to the appointment, it should be given immediately upon his arrival at the office.

No one considers the removal of a tooth a pleasant matter. It is not necessary, of course, to be at all morbid. Remain calm and poised at all times. Make no remarks which would indicate surprise at anything you may observe. Always conduct yourself so as to indicate to the patient that the appointment is proceeding in a perfectly customary manner. Should either the assistant or the dentist inadvertently indicate surprise at some state of the proceedings, the patient will very quickly become alarmed. While the removal of teeth usually proceeds as expected, the only dentist who does not experience difficulty at times is the dentist who does not remove teeth.

Upon completion of the operation, make sure that the patient is presentable by assisting in wiping any debris from his face.

Present the patient with the postoperative medication, if used. Any instructions are preferably given in written form. These commonly include the following (others may be used in your office):

The mouth should not be rinsed for twelve hours after the extraction; then a rinse consisting of one-half teaspoonful salt in a glass of tepid water may be used, gently, after eating and as frequently as necessary.

A certain amount of bleeding is normal following the removal of a tooth. However, if bleeding fails to stop within a reasonable time, place a roll of sterile gauze, about the size of the index finger, over the wound and hold it firmly for thirty minutes. A tea bag dipped in cold water may be used if bleeding persists, rolled and used as was the gauze. Avoid hot liquids.

A certain amount of swelling is to be expected. This may be held to a minimum by applying cold packs outside the face, over the area of the removal only, for one-half hour; no cold pack the second half hour; then cold pack again the third half-hour period. Should any unusual degree of swelling occur, an unusual degree of pain, or persistent bleeding, do not hesitate to call Dr. Raywin. The office telephone is 926-1414, the residence 920-1234.

If the removal has been quite difficult, the patient may be asked to return in twenty-four hours for examination of the wound. If the removal has been quite routine, it is highly recommended that you call the patient by telephone the next day and merely indicate that your office is interested in his comfort, therefore your call to inquire. Any negative comments should be referred to your dentist.

Cast-gold Restoration Procedure (Inlay, Three-quarter Crown, or Full Crown)

Materials required:

1. Basic setup for operative procedures

2. Block of diamond or carbide cutting instruments and handpieces

3. Double-ended Wedelstaedt chisels

4. Double-ended hatchets, one pair, right and left

5. Double-ended gingival margin trimmers, one pair, right and left

6. Excavators, one pair, right and left

7. Fine sandpaper discs and mandrels, straight and angle

8. Impression materials of choice

9. Impression trays or bands as indicated

10. Crown and bridge scissors

11. Dark red sheet wax to check clearance

12. Matrix holder, Tofflemire

13. Matrix bands, molar medium and bicuspid medium

14. Wedges

15. Stick of inlay wax

16. Plugger (Black No. 5)

17. Plastic instrument

18. Amalgam carver (Walls)

19. Sprue pins

20. Sprue base

21. Lighted gas burner or alcohol torch

22. Squares of hard gutta-percha for posterior temporary fillings; crown forms or resin forms with zinc oxide-eugenol paste for anterior teeth

23. Zinc oxide-eugenol cement

24. Cement slab and spatula

25. Peso pliers

26. Box of aluminum shells for temporary crowns (posterior only)

27. Box of crown forms or resin forms for temporary crowns (anterior only)

Cast-gold inlays are set at a subsequent appointment. Provide sufficient time between appointments for completion of the required laboratory work. For cementing inlays, see "Setting Gold Inlays, Crowns, Bridges, and Jacket Crowns."

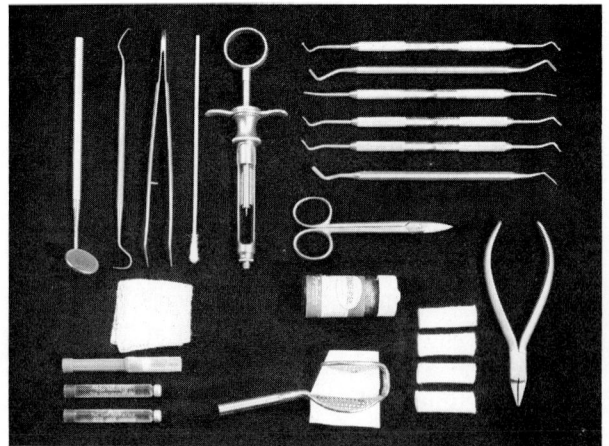

Fig. 45.16. Inlay tray

Fixed Prostheses or Bridge Procedure

Materials required:

1. Basic setup for operative procedures
2. Bridges may be supported entirely on full crowns, on three-quarter crowns, on jacket crowns, inlays, or any combination of these These are *abutments*. Instruments and materials should be prepared according to the types of support required for the particular bridge under construction.

In the Laboratory

3. Impression trays as your dentist designates
4. Impression material as your dentist designates
5. Equipment for preparation of the impression material

A bridge replacing one missing tooth is called a *three-tooth bridge*. It consists of two abutments, or supports, and a *pontic*, or replacement for the missing tooth. The abutments, of course, are placed on the natural teeth which are nearest the space left by the missing tooth in the mouth. The total length of a bridge is designated as the number of abutments plus the number of pontics.

Upper posterior bridges generally have a different type of pontic than a lower posterior bridge. Since a smile lifts the corners of the mouth upward, usually a porcelain or acrylic portion is made, called a *facing*, on the pontics of an upper posterior bridge. In the lower arch, food is passed between the tongue, cheeks, and lips during mastication. To provide for better mouth hygiene, lower posterior pontics

are often made without facings and with some opening between the chewing surface and the ridge below it—somewhat as though the pontic is a hammock suspended between the abutment teeth. This type is referred to as a *hygienic* pontic.

When preparation of the teeth for support of a bridge has been completed, it is necessary to construct by some means an accurate model of the abutments, the ridge area between the abutments, the relationship of these two items to each other, and the relationship of the opposing arch to the area involved in the bridge.

Many different techniques are used to secure these impressions. A dentist may take individual impressions of the abutments, construct the abutment crowns, and have an appointment with the patient at which these abutments are placed in the mouth and a relationship impression taken in plaster. The bridge is then finished from this impression.

A dentist may make a direct wax pattern of each abutment crown in the mouth, cast these patterns in gold, and then proceed as above.

A dentist may take a hydrocolloid impression over the entire bridge area and completely finish the bridge on the model made from this impression. The same procedure may be followed using one of the rubber-base materials or silicone materials available for this purpose. These procedures are entirely indirect.

The various methods of arriving at a wax pattern are discussed more fully under that title.

For cementing bridges, see "Setting Gold Inlays, Crowns, Bridges, and Jacket Crowns."

Jacket Crown Procedure

Materials required:

1. Basic setup for operative procedure
2. Diamond instrument block
3. Zinc oxide
4. Eugenol-thymol bottle with dropper
5. Glass slab
6. Steel spatula
7. Peso pliers
8. Crown and bridge scissors
9. Box of copper bands, or impression trays
10. Stick of inlay wax
11. Dark red sheet wax
12. Box of crown forms
13. Shade guides

In the Laboratory

14. Impression plaster
15. Trays for relationship impression
16. Tray for opposing arch impression
17. Sticky wax
18. Bunsen burner, matches

Shade guides used may consist of individually processed "chips" of material prepared from contents of the stock bottles of material to be used in the final crown itself; or shade guides provided by the various manufacturers of teeth for artificial dentures are sometimes used. Generally, a drawing of the tooth crown with the distribution of the various shades over various parts of the tooth is made as a guide.

Jacket crowns are set at a subsequent appointment. Provide sufficient time between appointments for the required laboratory work. For cementing, see "Setting Gold Inlays, Crowns, Bridges, and Jacket Crowns."

Hydrocolloid Impression Procedure Multiple Inlay or Bridge

Materials required:

1. Basic setup for nonoperative procedures
2. Impression trays (the dentist will select)
3. Rubber hoses for connecting trays with cold-water outlet for cooling impression
4. Cold water for cooling. During the winter months, the water supply at the unit may be cold enough for this purpose, and in some areas the same may be true in summer. If the water at the unit is not sufficiently cold, at least two quarts of ice water for each impression should be made available at the chair.
5. Hydrocolloid conditioner for preparing the hydrocolloid and for storage of the prepared hydrocolloid
6. Two tubes or containers of hydrocolloid for one impression; three or four tubes or containers to be prepared for two impressions
7. (a) Hydrocolloid syringes, small, loaded with hydrocolloid material, or

    (b) Jar of hydrocolloid material diluted with an equal amount of water (60% hydrocolloid and 40% water may be preferred in your office); brushes to apply (prepared sticks for syringes are available)
8. Glass of tepid salt water for rinsing (or a rinse such as Lavoris) to remove debris and saliva from the patient's mouth, used before your dentist prepares the mouth for the impression
9. Gum retraction kit
10. Wax (a high-melting-point variety) to build up trays as required

In the Laboratory

11. Materials required to pour artificial stone casts

12. Materials required to pour die stone

13. A device for positioning brass dowel pins directly in the center of each die

14. Separating medium

The main point of difference between this procedure and that for a partial denture is the necessity to apply a thinner form of hydrocolloid in and around all recesses of the prepared teeth to eliminate trapping fine air bubbles in the impression. The small hydrocolloid syringe material can be used for this purpose, since the fine syringe needle permits squirting a thin, controlled layer of hydrocolloid material where the dentist desires.

Another method is called the *paint-on* method. The thinned mix of hydrocolloid is prepared by measuring, for example, 100 cc. of water into a Pyrex jar which has an airtight stopper. Heat to a boil. Add 100 cc. of hydrocolloid material. Stir until smoothly combined with the water. The jar is then closed and placed in the storage bath of the hydrocolloid conditioner ready for use. It is applied in the mouth by brushes. Some dentists prefer this method to the syringe method when it is necessary to cover a larger number of prepared teeth, such as four or five teeth on each side of the same arch.

The balance of the procedure is the same as for partial denture impressions. Timing is important in that the tray must be ready for insertion into the mouth at precisely the same instant that the dentist has completed applying the preliminary thinner mix of hydrocolloid.

Casts are best poured immediately in your office, especially the first half which is poured in die stone and has the brass dowel pins placed. If two such impressions are to be prepared for the same patient at the same sitting, it is generally best that the first half (die stone portion) of the first impression be poured before proceeding to take the second impression in the patient's mouth.

Chloroform will wipe off hydrocolloid stains from equipment, such as the hydrocolloid conditioner chambers.

Silicone Elastic and Synthetic Rubber Impression Procedures

These materials are the more recently developed types which can be used for a wide variety of impression work. The silicone elastic impression materials, especially, can be used as part of the procedure in taking a full-denture impression, for rebasing impressions using the denture as the tray, as a correction material in the saddle areas of partial dentures, as the material for multiple inlay or bridge impressions, and also as a material for a single-tooth impression.

Each of these materials is supplied in two basic types—a heavier-bodied material for tray or band use and a lighter-bodied material for use in a syringe (or other mechanism) for placement around the preparations in the mouth before the loaded tray is seated. The general procedure is much the same as that used for hydrocolloid in taking impressions in multiple inlay or bridge procedures, with several notable exceptions: the material does not have to be heated or otherwise treated before use; impressions do not need to be poured as promptly as do those taken in hydrocolloid; the impressions are not as subject to error through mishandling as are those taken in a hydrocolloid.

Silicone elastic materials and synthetic rubber materials do require good timing and teamwork between you and your dentist in achieving good results. This is necessary whenever the tray material and the syringe material are to be used to take a single impression. Your dentist will prepare the first material to be used, generally the syringe material, and you will prepare the tray material—usually with a small delay in time. While the dentist is placing the syringe material in the mouth, you will be loading the tray or band, ready to take the used syringe from the dentist and hand him the prepared tray or band. This is referred to as a *double-mix technique.*

Constant improvement and change in these materials require that you study all directions for their use very carefully. Be sure that you understand each step of the instructions before you attempt to work with the material. Know where you keep the instruction sheet for future reference and replace it with the instruction sheet from each new package you open.

Compound Impression Procedure

Materials required:

1. Basic setup for nonoperative procedures
2. Trays selected by the dentist
3. Two cakes of impression compound for each arch to be taken
4. Compound heater filled with water and set at the correct temperature to properly soften the impression compound used in your office (see the instructions for temperature packed with each box of compound)
5. Lighted gas burner or alcohol torch

This method of taking an impression is sometimes used in making study models of both arches, whether with or without teeth.

The compound should be placed in the compound heater, resting on a gauze or heavy glazed paper to prevent sticking to the interior of the compound heater. Preparation of the compound is begun about ten minutes before appointment time. Check the material in the compound heater periodically to be sure that it is not overflowing the gauze or paper upon which it has been placed.

After the impression has been taken, it should be thoroughly chilled in cold water. Either plaster or artificial stone may be used in pouring the model, as is required. Since the compound will not change shape unless heated, the impressions may be left on the laboratory bench until a convenient time is available to pour the casts.

When the casts have thoroughly set, they are easily removed from the impression compound by immersing the tray, compound, and cast in water in the compound heater set at five degrees less than the temperature used to prepare the material originally. After eight to ten minutes at this temperature, remove from the compound heater and carefully separate the casts from the impression compound.

Compound which sticks to the cast at this moment is easily "picked off" by using a larger wad of soft compound in your fingers.

To clean the trays it may be necessary to hold them in a flame momentarily to soften any remaining compound. The compound can then be wiped off the tray, using disposable tissue or cloth. Trays are then sterilized and returned to their storage place.

Individual Tooth Impressions for Dies

Impressions for larger restorations than individual inlays and crowns are discussed in previous sections. The same general procedure is used in taking an impression of an individual tooth preparation except for a difference in the device for holding the impression and the fact that there are a greater number of impression materials to choose from for this purpose.

Since an individual tooth is small, a copper or aluminum cap or band or very small tray is substituted for the tray used in the larger types of impressions. A copper band is a thin tube of copper, available in lengths of 1/2 inch, 5/16 inch, and 1 inch. Various "gauges," or thicknesses, of the metal are available. Copper bands are also supplied in diameters from the very small to those large enough to go around the largest molars. The size is designated by number, beginning with the smallest band as No. 1. The grading system for sizes is not always the same for the various manufacturers, so when reordering copper bands, it is best to order the same brand as used previously to be sure of getting the size you wish.

Modeling Compound Method

A copper band of the dentist's choice is fitted over the tooth in which the preparation has been completed. The band is trimmed at the lower edge to correspond to the curvature of the preparation at the gingival. It is then filled with the impression material.

Modeling compound may at times be used for such an impression. For this purpose, a stick of the material is used, rather than a cake form. The dentist warms the stick in a burner until the compound is soft and very moldable, fills the copper band with it, then slips the band with its modeling compound over the tooth. A finger is placed over the open top end of the band to help force the material around the tooth and into the preparation. With a saliva ejector in place, the band is chilled while in position on the tooth, using cold water in a hand syringe. The band is carefully removed from the tooth. The modeling compound within the band will have a negative impression of the preparation in the tooth which, when it has been packed with amalgam to form a die, will form the amalgam into a positive, or duplicate, of the tooth with its preparation.

Silicone Material and Rubber Material Method

The *base* material is sometimes used for single-tooth impressions without using *syringe* material. If the preparation of which the impression is to be made is a complicated one, the syringe method might well be used; on the other hand, if the preparation is more simple in line—such as a full-crown preparation—the base material may be used alone.

The band used for the impression must be coated with an *adhesive* supplied for the specific material being used. This is applied in a thin, uniform coat over the entire area which will be in contact with the impression material. Heavy layers will not give the good adhesion given by a thin coat. The adhesive must dry thoroughly before it is ready for use.

Benzene on a gauze will remove the synthetic rubber materials from spatulas or fingers. If permitted to set thoroughly before attempting removal, you may sometimes find a slight stain remains. Benzene can also be used to remove this stain. By using a napkin or tissue, the elastic silicones can usually be wiped clean from most surfaces in the unset state. After setting, it will completely strip from surfaces.

It is usually much easier to clean up after either type of material when it has thoroughly set. The only time it is necessary to clean up the unset material might be when reusing the equipment to prepare more material before the first mixing has set.

According to the manufacturers, these materials will not shrink or distort if left exposed to the air for some hours before making the die. It is always preferable, however, to pour all casts and to make all models and dies as soon as possible, if for no other reason than to keep up-to-date with the work which must be accomplished in the dental office.

Setting Gold Inlays, Crowns, Bridges, and Jacket Crowns

Materials required:

1. Basic setup for operative procedure
2. Orangewood stick
3. Leather-faced mallet
4. Glass slab for cement preparation
5. Spatula for cement preparation
6. Silver cement for full gold crowns; regular zinc phosphate cement for three-quarter or veneer crowns, for inlays or jacket crowns
7. Finishing burs
8. Straight handpiece burs for carving
9. Roll of articulating paper (carbon paper)
10. Mounted stone, small, green Carborundum
11. Burlew disc on mandrel
12. Fine sandpaper discs and mandrels, straight and angle
13. Dappen dish with whiting-tin oxide mixture
14. Prophylactic contra-angle with rubber cup
15. Cotton-roll holder for lower arch

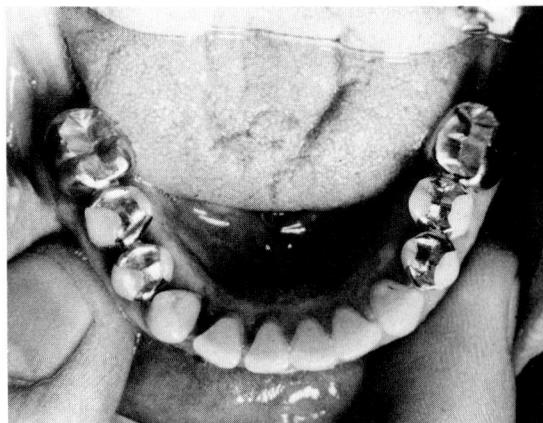

Fig. 45.17. Clinical picture of cast-gold restorations

Alginate Impression Technique

Materials required:

1. Basic setup for nonoperative procedures
2. Paper cup or glass containing tepid salt water for mouth rinse
3. Stick of red boxing or carding wax for building up trays

In the Laboratory

4. Alginate impression material
5. Measuring devices, if required. Some material is packaged in single units; some is available in bulk cans.
6. Plastic mixing bowl and plastic spatula
7. Sufficient water at the recommended temperature for the mix. If no temperature is specified, 70° may be satisfactory. Higher temperatures hasten setting. When the correct temperature has been decided upon, always use it exactly so that the material will react consistently.
8. The required trays (the dentist will usually select these)
9. Fixing solution prepared, if required, for immersion of the finished impressions prior to pouring the casts

Read the instructions for the alginate material used in your office. Comply with the manufacturer's recommendations exactly.

Mix the alginate as instructed. Usually the dentist prefers to place the material into the tray. At this time the patient is instructed to rinse his mouth thoroughly. The dentist will proceed with one impression, usually taking the upper impression first if both upper and lower are to be taken.

Upon completion of impressions, they are rinsed thoroughly in cool running water to remove all saliva and are placed in the fixing solution for the required period of time. Alginate impressions should be poured as soon as possible to reduce the possibility of inaccurate casts.

Hand the patient a disposable tissue and a hand mirror to clean up any material which may remain on his face. When he has finished, take these items from him.

When the alginate impressions have been poured, completely immerse in cool water. Do not remove casts and impressions from this bath in less than the time specified for the cast material to attain a hard set. Then gently separate the casts from the impressions. Write the patient's name on the back surface of each cast, immediately, with an indelible pencil (if the casts are too wet, a wipe with a towel will remove the excess water). Set the casts to dry.

Clean trays thoroughly. The type used for the alginate material usually has some means of locking the material into the tray, which necessitates careful cleaning. Trays are then sterilized and replaced in their proper storage area.

Hydrocolloid Impression Procedure
Partial Denture

Materials required:

1. Basic setup for nonoperative procedures

2. Impression trays (the dentist will select)

3. Rubber hoses for connecting trays with cold-water outlet for cooling impression

4. Cold water for cooling. During the winter months, the water supply at the unit may be cold enough for this purpose, and in some areas the same may be true in summer. If the water at the unit is not sufficiently cold, at least two quarts of ice water for each impression should be made available.

5. Hyrocolloid conditioner for preparing the hydrocolloid and for storing the prepared hydrocolloid

6. Prepare 2 tubes for 1 impression, 3 or 4 tubes for 2 impressions.

7. Glass of tepid salt water for rinsing (or a mouthwash) to remove debris and saliva from the patient's mouth; used immediately before impression is taken

8. Wax (a high-melting-point variety) to build up trays as required

In the Laboratory

9. Materials required to pour artificial stone casts

10. Fixative for hydrocolloid, if required, or storage facilities

The hydrocolloid must be prepared in advance of the appointment time. If a hydrocolloid conditioner is available for the purpose, preparation may be completed as far in advance of the appointment as you wish, since a mechanism designed for the purpose will keep the hydrocolloid ready for use for an indefinite period. Hydrocolloid should be prepared exactly according to the directions for the specific brand used in your office.

For example, Surgident impression material, a hydrocolloid, is supplied in a plastic jacket, much like the skin on a wiener. This material is used in the original jacket when a hydrocolloid conditioner is used in its preparation. Surgident is completely submerged in water of 208°F. to 212°F. until fluid, which takes approximately eight to twelve minutes. The material in its jacket is then placed in a storage bath at a temperature of 142°F. to 155°F., which will keep it in a liquid state for ten hours or more. The warmed tray is filled when the material is taken directly from the storage bath, and the filled tray is immersed for ten to fifteen minutes in a final tempering bath at 115°F. before placing it in the patient's mouth. Surgident instructions state that the impression should be rinsed with water upon its removal from the patient's mouth and should be immediately poured. If a delay in pouring is necessary, the impression should be submerged in Surgident control solution, *not* in plain or distilled water, and should be poured as soon as possible.

Your dentist will prepare the trays by building up with wax or other material, where necessary, to prevent loss of the hydrocolloid material when the tray is placed in the mouth (an upper tray, for example, is often built up across the back edge to prevent the flow of material in the direction of the throat). When the trays have been prepared, you will fill each with hydrocolloid material. An upper tray is filled by opening the tube or container of hydrocolloid to its greatest possible size by cutting across the tube with a scissors. A lower tray is filled through a smaller opening such as that formed by removing a cap from the tube if it has one or by cutting off a small corner if no cap is present. Air must not be trapped in this process; therefore each tray is completely filled in one movement across the length of the tray.

The trays are then placed in the tempering bath for the required period of time. If the upper impression is to be taken first, this tray is removed from the tempering bath, is connected to the water hoses, and a sharp-edged knife is used to scrape away just the surface hydrocolloid which has been somewhat diluted by contact with water. The prepared tray is then handed to the dentist for placement in the patient's mouth. The dentist, in the meantime, has taken care of preparation of the mouth for the impression material by rinsing, and drying with gauze, or whatever method he prefers.

When the tray has been seated properly, the dentist will signal. You will then start the water flowing through the tray, being careful to control the pressure so that the hoses will not be forced off the tray.

While the first tray is being chilled, prepare the second tray for the tempering bath, if not already prepared, keeping in mind that the cooling process for the tray now in the patient's mouth will take about six minutes. Upon completion of the cooling process, the dentist will usually prefer to have the water turned off while he removes the tray from the patient's mouth.

After the dentist has examined the impression, you will take it to the laboratory for storage until you have both impressions ready to pour. Be prepared to handle the material

properly. Some hydrocolloid may be safely stored for a few minutes by draping a thoroughly wetted facial tissue over the complete tray as it lies on the laboratory bench. Other hydrocolloid materials may require immersion in a specially prepared solution for a limited period of time. The accuracy of the material is very definitely affected by the manner in which you handle a completed impression; therefore you should know exactly and in detail just how the hydrocolloid used in your office is to be handled.

When the first impression has been properly protected, remove the second tray from the hydrocolloid conditioner tempering bath, connect it to the water hoses, scrape the surface material away, and hand it to your dentist. When your dentist has indicated that the tray is seated, start the water circulating.

Return to the laboratory and immediately proceed to pour the cast in the first impression taken, according to the recommended procedure for the material used in your office. If you have been prepared in advance to pour this impression, you will have sufficient time to complete the job and return to the chair within the five or six minutes it takes to chill the second impression.

When the second impression is removed and the dentist has examined it, you again pour it immediately, according to the recommended procedure for the material used in your office. Do this before dismissing the patient, unless there are other employees present to assist. The object of the appointment is to prepare accurate casts. If it is necessary to choose between handling the hydrocolloid properly in order to secure accurate casts or leaving the patient unattended for a short period of time, it is better to leave the patient unattended until you have properly cared for the casts.

Partial Denture Procedure

Primary Impressions

Materials required

1. Basic setup for nonoperative procedures

2. Alginate impression or other material of choice

The purpose of this appointment is to make impressions for study models. These study models are usually mounted in a simple articulator for preliminary study and are later placed on a "surveying" instrument to design the clasps which will hold the partial in the mouth.

If individualized impression trays are to be made, allow sufficient time for the laboratory procedures to be completed prior to the next appointment. If two partials, an upper and a lower, are to be constructed, both study models are poured in plaster. If but one partial is to be constructed, the *opposing* model is poured in artificial stone, not in plaster, since it may be used opposite the finished model of the arch which will have the partial.

Partial Dental Procedure (Continued)

Final Impressions

Materials required:

1. Basic setup for operative procedures
2. Hydrocolloid impression materials, or material of choice

The object of this appointment is to make an accurate impression to be used as the working model in constructing the partial or partials. The operative setup is listed because it is frequently necessary to prepare room for occlusal rests as determined in designing the case on the study models. If operative work is required in the mouth, it is usually completed before proceeding with the construction of partial dentures.

If but one partial is to be constructed, only this arch needs retaking for the final working impression. The previously made opposing cast poured in artificial stone is used.

Prior to the next appointment, time must be reserved for the construction of bite rims on the working models. In some cases, the partial dentures may be constructed at this point without making bite rims, etc., eliminating the next sitting. If so, the facebow transfer is accomplished at this sitting, and selection of mold of teeth and selection of shade are completed as well. The third sitting is thus combined with the second.

Partial Dental Procedure (Continued)

Interocclusal Records and Tooth Selection

Materials required:

1. Basic setup for nonoperative procedures
2. Gas burner or alcohol torch
3. Heavy wax spatula
4. Tooth mold and shade-selecting equipment
5. Facebow and its auxiliary equipment, if used, or equipment of choice

The object of this appointment is to register the correct relationship of the upper and lower arches and to duplicate this relationship in mounting the casts in the articulator. The desired shape (mold) and color (shade) of the replacement teeth must also be selected at this time.

Try-in

Materials required:

1. Disclosing paste
2. Mounted green stones
3. Articulating paper

The object of this appointment is to verify all preceding steps before final insertion. The cast framework is tried in and adjusted to fit accurately. The occlusion is checked to be sure the interocclusal records were accurate and the mounting correct. The mold and shade selection is checked to be certain no error was made in tooth selection.

Partial Dental Procedure (Continued)

Insertion

Materials required:

1. Basic setup for operative procedures
2. Vulcanite burs for any necessary trimming of the partial denture base
3. Small mounted stones (S. S. White No. 48) for adjusting occlusion
4. Articulating paper or sections of typewriter ribbon

At this appointment the partial or partials are inserted in the patient's mouth. Any obvious adjustments are made at this time. The patient is usually given another appointment within 1 to 3 days for follow-up and as often as needed thereafter.

Adjustments

Materials required (Same as for previous appointment):

1. Basic setup for operative procedures
2. Vulcanite burs for any necessary trimming of the partial denture base
3. Small mounted stone (S. S. White No. 48) for adjusting articulation
4. Articulating paper or sections of typewriter ribbon

These appointments are for the purpose of checking the progress and comfort of the patient. Since patients who wear partial dentures must have natural teeth present, their recall control cards are marked for the usual recall period.

Complete Denture Procedure

Primary Impression

Materials required:

1. Basic setup for nonoperative procedures

2. For full upper and lower dentures: impression material of choice

3. For single full denture: in addition, impression material of choice for impression of opposing arch

The object of this appointment is to make impressions for study models of the mouth for complete denture construction. If only one denture is to be constructed, an impression of the opposing arch or denture is made and poured in artificial stone. It then becomes the final opposing model.

Sufficient time will be required for the construction of a tray or trays for the final impression(s) between appointments.

Complete Denture Procedure (Continued)

Final Impressions

Materials required:

1. Basic setup for nonoperative procedures
2. Previously prepared tray(s) for final impression(s)
3. Final impression material, with appropriate mixing pad and spatula
4. Cleansing agent for removing material from skin surfaces

The object of this appointment is to make final impressions of the complete denture area. Various materials are used for final impressions, many of which are varieties of zinc oxide paste. To separate a cast from the zinc oxide type of material, the cast and impression are immersed in water in the compound heater at a temperature of 160° for five minutes. Separation is then easily accomplished.

Time will be needed for the construction of bite rim(s) before the next appointment of the patient.

Complete Denture Procedure (Continued)

Intermaxillary Records and Tooth Selection

Materials required:

1. Basic setup for nonoperative procedures

2. Previously prepared bite rim(s)

3. Facebow and auxiliary equipment

4. Mold and shade guides

The object of this appointment is to register the relationship of the upper and lower arches, to duplicate this relationship in mounting the casts in the articulator, and to select the correct mold and shade of teeth to be used in the denture(s).

Sufficient laboratory time will be needed for setting up the teeth in the trial denture before the next appointment.

Complete Denture Procedure (Continued)

Try-in

Materials required:

1. Basic setup for nonoperative procedures
2. Previously prepared trial denture setup(s)
3. Compound heater, all trays removed, set at 120° to soften wax
4. Bite registration wax, if desired
5. Cold water for chilling bite registrations
6. Large scissors for cutting registration wax into strips
7. Large hand mirror
8. Husband or wife of the patient

The object of this sitting is to register the *condylar inclinations* of the patient; also, and by no means incidentally, to verify the appearance of the teeth by having a close relative of the patient express an opinion, in addition to the patient's personal reaction.

Time will be needed for the final processing of the denture(s) before the next appointment.

Complete Denture Procedure (Continued)

Insertion

Materials required:

1. Basic setup for nonoperative procedures
2. Previously processed denture(s)
3. Articulating paper or piece of typewriter ribbon to check articulation of teeth
4. Disclosing wax, if desired
5. Mounting records retained from previous work
6. Compound heater, all trays removed, water at 120° for wax softening
7. Bite-registration wax
8. Scissors, large
9. Cold water for chilling registrations

The object of this appointment is to insert the denture(s) and to instruct the patient in their care. Sometimes a *checkbite* is taken at this time, and the dentures are remounted in the articulator to further refine the occlusion and to look for premature occlusal contacts.

Be sure to retain the mounting records to facilitate remounting the dentures at the next sitting. In some offices, these records are kept permanently.

The patient's recall control card is dated for recall one year from this appointment, unless natural teeth are present.

Denture Adjustment Procedure or Denture Patient Recall Procedure

Materials required:

1. Basic setup for nonoperative procedures

2. Vulcanite burs for trimming denture bases

3. Articulating paper or typewriter ribbon

4. Small mounted stones for adjusting articulation

5. Disclosing wax, if desired

The purpose of these appointments is to relieve denture soreness or improper function when it occurs

Denture recall appointments require the same materials as listed above under denture adjustment procedures. Should the dentures require it, they are cleaned and polished on the laboratory lathe. If calculus has collected on the dentures, it is removed by soaking them for a few minutes in a fifty percent solution of hydrochloric acid and then brushing them thoroughly with soap and water. Be careful of acid. It can burn! Ultrasonic cleaning mechanisms are also available.

Recall Prophylaxis and Examination Appointment

Materials required:

1. Basic setup for nonoperative procedures
2. Scalers
3. Dental tape
4. Bitewing films and tabs
5. Full-mouth films, if desired
6. Paper cup and mouth rinse
7. Dappen dish with prophylaxis paste
8. Prophylaxis right angle for handpiece, with rubber cup
9. Prophylaxis brush mounted in contra-angle, if desired
10. For the young child, the dappen dish with paste, the prophylaxis right angle with rubber cup, and child's size bitewing films with tabs

Seat the patient and place the bib or napkin. Place the patient's last films, if any, on the view-box, his records convenient to the dentist.

When the oral examination is made upon completion of the prophylaxis, be prepared to note information required.

Before dismissing the patient, be sure that his face is clean. If it is not, offer a disposable tissue. If a powder corner is not available, offer a hand mirror.

If dental work has been found necessary, see that the patient has an appointment for its completion. Some dental offices develop the X-ray films while the patient is still present to complete the examination. Otherwise, if no dental work is found to be necessary, inform the patient that he will be notified if any work is found on examination of the X rays. If none is found, he will be notified when it is time for his next prophylaxis and examination.

The patient's recall control card is dated at this time for the month and year of his next recall and is placed properly in the recall file.

In many dental offices, full-denture patients are recalled once each year for examination. Adjustment of articulation is made if required or appointments are arranged for relining, rebasing, or new dentures if necessary. Material required for this type of recall will depend upon the dentist but may include carbon paper or a section of typewriter ribbon for occlusal marking, or disclosing wax for the same purpose, plus small mounted stones for adjustment of individual areas on the artificial teeth, and vulcanite burs for adjustment of the denture base, if required.

Summary

Four-handed dentistry has become necessary because the assistant becomes a second pair of hands for the dentist, relieving him of eyestrain and saving his time. Six-handed dentistry increases the time-saving factor, as the chairside assistant never leaves the dentist and patient. She is served any materials which are not at her worktable.

Learn to anticipate the dentist's needs and have material or instruments ready *in advance of his request.*

This chapter is devoted to a listing of materials for each dental operation. They are *suggested* lists based on most frequent reported usage. This chapter should be marked up by the dentist or assistant to include the materials which the dentist prefers and eliminate those he does not use.

Eventually the dental assistant should have memorized the materials necessary for any specific operation.

Study Questions

1. Describe four-handed dentistry.
2. Describe six-handed dentistry.
3. What is the advantage of each?
4. What is a basic setup for nonoperative dentistry?
5. What is meant by nonoperative dentistry?
6. What is a basic setup for operative dentistry.
7. What is meant by operative dentistry?
8. Pick two or three setups and list the materials required for each.

APPENDIX

TABLES OF WEIGHTS AND MEASURES

Avoirdupois Weight

1 pound = 1.2153 pounds troy

Grains gr.		Drachms dr.		Ounces oz.		Pound lb.
27.34375	=	1				
437.5	=	16	=	1		
7000	=	256	=	16	=	1

Apothecaries' Weight

Grains gr.		Scruples Э		Drachms ʒ		Ounces ℥		Pound lb.
20	=	1						
60	=	3	=	1				
480	=	24	=	8	=	1		
5760	=	288	=	96	=	12	=	1

Apothecaries' Measure

Minims ♏		Fluidrachms fʒ		Fluidounces f℥		Pints O.		Gallon C.
60	=	1						
480	=	8	=	1				
7,680	=	128	=	16	=	1		
61,440	=	1024	=	128	=	8	=	1

Comparative Values of Standard and Metric Measures of Length

Inches	Centimeters	Inches	Millimeters
1	2.54	1/25	1.00
2	5.08	1/12	2.12
3	7.62	1/8	3.18
4	10.16	1/4	6.35
5	12.70	1/3	8.47
6	15.24	1/2	12.70
7	17.78	5/8	15.88
8	20.32	2/3	16.93
9	22.86	3/4	19.05
10	25.40	5/6	21.16
11	27.94	7/8	22.22
12	30.48	11/12	23.28

Metric Weights

1 gram = 1 cubic centimeter of distilled water at 4° C.

		Grams		Grains		Av. Ounces
Milligram	=	0.001	=	0.01543		
Centigram	=	0.01	=	0.15432		
Decigram	=	0.1	=	1.54324		
Gram	=	1.	=	15.43248	=	.03528
Decagram	=	10.	=		=	.3528
Hectogram	=	100.	=		=	3.52758
Kilogram	=	1,000.	=		=	35.2758

Comparative Values of Apothecaries' and Metric Liquid Measures

Minims	Cubic Centimeters	Flui-drachms	Cubic Centimeters	Fluid-ounces	Cubic Centimeters
1	0.06	1	3.70	1	29.57
2	0.12	2	7.39	2	59.15
3	0.19	3	11.09	3	88.72
4	0.25	4	14.79	4	118.29
5	0.31	5	18.48	5	147.87
6	0.37	6	22.18	6	177.44
7	0.43	7	25.88	7	207.01
8	0.49			8	236.58
9	0.55			9	266.16
10	0.62			10	295.73
11	0.68			11	325.30
12	0.74			12	354.88
13	0.80			13	384.45
14	0.86			14	414.02
15	0.92			15	443.59
16	0.99			16	473.17
17	1.05			17	502.74
18	1.11			18	532.31
19	1.17			19	561.89
20	1.23			20	591.46
25	1.54			21	621.03
30	1.85			22	650.60
35	2.16			23	680.18
40	2.46			24	709.75
45	2.77			25	739.32
50	3.08			26	768.90
55	3.39			27	798.47
				28	828.04
				29	857.61
				30	887.19
				31	916.76
				32	946.33

Metric Linear Measure

		Meter		U. S. Inches		Feet		Yards		Miles
Millimeter	=	.001	=	.03937	=	.00328				
Centimeter	=	.01	=	.3937	=	.03280				
Decimeter	=	.1	=	3.937	=	.32808	=	.10936		
Meter	=	1.	=	39.37	=	3.2808	=	1.0936		
Decameter	=	10.	=		=	32.808	=	10.936		
Hectometer	=	100.	=		=	328.08	=	109.36	=	.062137
Kilometer	=	1,000.	=		=	3,280.8	=	1,093.6	=	.62137

TABLES OF WEIGHTS AND MEASURES—(Continued)

Table for Converting Metric Weights into Apothecaries' Weights

Grams	Exact Equivalents in Grains	Grams	Exact Equivalents in Grains
0.01	0.1543	12.0	185.189
0.02	0.3086	13.0	200.621
0.03	0.4630	14.0	216.054
0.04	0.6173	15.0	231.486
0.05	0.7716	16.0	246.918
0.06	0.9259	17.0	262.351
0.07	1.0803	18.0	277.783
0.08	1.2346	19.0	293.216
0.09	1.3889	20.0	308.648
0.1	1.543	21.0	324.080
0.2	3.086	22.0	339.513
0.3	4.630	23.0	354.945
0.4	6.173	24.0	370.378
0.5	7.716	25.0	385.810
0.6	9.259	26.0	401.242
0.7	10.803	27.0	416.674
0.8	12.346	28.0	432.107
0.9	13.889	29.0	447.538
1.0	15.432	30.0	462.971
2.0	30.865	31.0	478.403
3.0	46.297	32.0	493.835
4.0	61.730	40.0	617.294
5.0	77.162	45.0	694.456
6.0	92.594	50.0	771.618
7.0	108.027	60.0	925.942
8.0	123.459	70.0	1080.265
9.0	138.892	80.0	1234.589
10.0	154.324	90.0	1388.912
11.0	169.756	100.0	1543.236

Table for Converting Apothecaries' Weights into Metric Weights

Grains	Grams	Grains	Grams
1/250	0.00130	50	3.240
1/32	0.00202	51	3.305
1/20	0.00324	52	3.370
1/18	0.00360	53	3.434
1/16	0.00405	54	3.499
1/15	0.00432	55	3.564
1/12	0.00540	56	3.629
1/10	0.00648	57	3.694
1/8	0.00810	58	3.758
1/6	0.01080	59	3.823
1/5	0.01296	60	3.888
1/4	0.01620	61	3.953
1/3	0.02160	62	4.018
1/2	0.03240	63	4.082
3/4	0.04860	64	4.147
1	0.0648	65	4.212
2	0.1296	66	4.277
3	0.1944	67	4.342
4	0.2592	68	4.406
5	0.3240	69	4.471
6	0.3888	70	4.536
7	0.4536	71	4.601
8	0.5184	72	4.666
9	0.5832	73	4.730
10	0.6480	74	4.795
11	0.7128	75	4.860
12	0.7776	76	4.925
13	0.8424	77	4.990
14	0.9072	78	5.054
15	0.9720	79	5.119
16	1.037	80	5.184
17	1.102	81	5.249
18	1.166	82	5.314
19	1.231	83	5.378
20	1.296	84	5.443
21	1.361	85	5.508
22	1.426	86	5.573
23	1.490	87	5.638
24	1.555	88	5.702
25	1.620	89	5.767
26	1.685	90	5.832
27	1.749	91	5.897
28	1.814	92	5.962
29	1.879	93	6.026
30	1.944	94	6.091
31	2.009	95	6.156
32	2.074	96	6.221
33	2.138	97	6.286
34	2.203	98	6.350
35	2.268	99	6.415
36	2.333	100	6.480
37	2.398	120	7.776
38	2.462	150	9.720
39	2.527	180	11.664
40	2.592	200	12.958
41	2.657	480	31.103
42	2.722	500	32.396
43	2.786	600	38.875
44	2.851	700	45.354
45	2.916	800	51.833
46	2.981	900	58.313
47	3.046	960	62.207
48	3.110	1000	64.799
49	3.175		

TABLES OF WEIGHTS AND MEASURES—(Continued)

Metric Doses with Approximate Apothecary Equivalents

The approximate dose equivalents in the following table represent the quantities that would be prescribed, under identical conditions, by physicians trained, respectively, in the metric or in the apothecary system of weights and measures.

When prepared dosage forms such as tablets, capsules, pills, etc., are prescribed in the metric system, the pharmacist may dispense the corresponding approximate equivalent in the apothecary system, and vice versa. However, this does not authorize the alternative use of the approximate dose equivalents given below for specific quantities on a prescription that requires compounding, nor in converting a pharmaceutical formula from one system of weights or measures to the other system; for such purposes exact equivalents must be used.

LIQUID MEASURES		WEIGHTS	
Metric	Approximate Apothecary Equivalents	Metric	Approximate Apothecary Equivalents
1000 cc.	1 quart	30 Gm.	1 ounce
750 cc.	$1\frac{1}{2}$ pints	15 Gm.	4 drachms
500 cc.	1 pint	10 Gm.	$2\frac{1}{2}$ drachms
250 cc.	8 fluidounces	7.5 Gm.	2 drachms
200 cc.	7 fluidounces	6 Gm.	90 grains
100 cc.	$3\frac{1}{2}$ fluidounces	5 Gm.	75 grains
50 cc.	$1\frac{3}{4}$ fluidounces	4 Gm.	60 grains (1 drachm)
30 cc.	1 fluidounce	3 Gm.	45 grains
15 cc.	$\frac{1}{2}$ fluidounce (4 fluidrachms)	2 Gm.	30 grains ($\frac{1}{2}$ drachm)
10 cc.	$2\frac{1}{2}$ fluidrachms	1.5 Gm.	22 grains
8 cc.	2 fluidrachms	1 Gm.	15 grains
5 cc.	75 minims ($1\frac{1}{4}$ fluidrachms)	0.75 Gm.	12 grains
4 cc.	1 fluidrachm	0.6 Gm.	10 grains
3 cc.	45 minims	0.5 Gm.	$7\frac{1}{2}$ grains
2 cc.	30 minims	0.45 Gm.	7 grains
1 cc.	15 minims	0.4 Gm.	6 grains
0.75 cc.	12 minims	0.3 Gm.	5 grains
0.6 cc.	10 minims	0.25 Gm.	4 grains
0.5 cc.	8 minims	0.2 Gm.	3 grains
0.3 cc.	5 minims	0.15 Gm.	$2\frac{1}{2}$ grains
0.25 cc.	4 minims	0.12 Gm.	2 grains
0.2 cc.	3 minims	0.1 Gm.	$1\frac{1}{2}$ grains
0.1 cc.	$1\frac{1}{2}$ minims	75 mg.	$1\frac{1}{4}$ grains
0.06 cc.	1 minim	60 mg.	1 grain
		50 mg.	$\frac{3}{4}$ grain
		40 mg.	$\frac{2}{3}$ grain
		30 mg.	$\frac{1}{2}$ grain
		25 mg.	$\frac{3}{8}$ grain
		20 mg.	$\frac{1}{3}$ grain
		15 mg.	$\frac{1}{4}$ grain
		12 mg.	$\frac{1}{5}$ grain
		10 mg.	$\frac{1}{6}$ grain
		8 mg.	$\frac{1}{8}$ grain
		6 mg.	$\frac{1}{10}$ grain
		5 mg.	$\frac{1}{12}$ grain
		4 mg.	$\frac{1}{15}$ grain
		3 mg.	$\frac{1}{20}$ grain
		2 mg.	$\frac{1}{30}$ grain
		1.5 mg.	$\frac{1}{40}$ grain
		1.2 mg.	$\frac{1}{50}$ grain
		1 mg.	$\frac{1}{60}$ grain
		0.8 mg.	$\frac{1}{80}$ grain
		0.6 mg.	$\frac{1}{100}$ grain
		0.5 mg.	$\frac{1}{120}$ grain
		0.4 mg.	$\frac{1}{150}$ grain
		0.3 mg.	$\frac{1}{200}$ grain
		0.25 mg.	$\frac{1}{250}$ grain
		0.2 mg.	$\frac{1}{300}$ grain
		0.15 mg.	$\frac{1}{400}$ grain
		0.1 mg.	$\frac{1}{600}$ grain

NOTE: A cubic centimeter (cc.) is the approximate equivalent of a milliliter (ml.).

Source: "Blakiston's New Gould Medical Dictionary," 2d ed., McGraw-Hill Book Company, Inc., Blakiston Division, New York, 1956.

TABLE OF THE MORE COMMON LATIN OR GREEK TERMS AND ABBREVIATIONS
USED IN PRESCRIPTION WRITING

Term or Abbreviation	Latin or Greek	Translation
a.c.	ante cibum	before meals
ad	ad	to, up to
ad lib.	ad libitum	at pleasure
alternis horis	alternis horis	every other hour
ante	ante	before
aq.	aqua	water
b.i.d.	bis in die, bis in dies	twice daily
bis	bis	twice
caps.	capsula	a capsule
d.t.d. No. iv	dentur tales doses No. iv	let 4 such doses be given
et	et	and
H.	hora	an hour
hor. som., H.S.	hora somni	at bedtime
in d.	in dies	from day to day, daily
m.	minimum	a minim
min.	minimum	a minim
no.	numero, numerus	number
noctis	noctis	of the night
non	non	not
non rep.	non repetatur	do not repeat
omn. hor.	omni hora	every hour
omni nocte	omni nocte	every night
p.c.	post cibos; post cibum	after eating; after food
p.r.n.	pro re nata	as occasion arises, occasionally
q.h.	quaque hora	each hour, every hour
q.i.d.	quater in die	4 times a day
q.s.	quantum sufficit; quantum sufficiat; quantum satis	a sufficient quantity; as much as is sufficient
sig.	signa; signetur	write (thou); let it be written; label (thou)
sine	sine	without
ss, ss̄	semis	a half
tabel.	tabella (dim. of *tabula,* a table)	a lozenge
t.i.d.	ter in die	3 times a day

Source: "Blakiston's Illustrated Pocket Medical Dictionary," 2d ed., McGraw-Hill Book Company. Inc., Blakiston Division, New York, 1960.

TABLE OF THERMOMETRIC EQUIVALENTS*

Centigrade to Fahrenheit Scales

$$\frac{9}{5} \text{ C.}° + 32 = \text{F.}°$$

C. °	F. °	C. °	F. °	C. °	F. °	C. °	F. °	C. °	F. °
−20	−4.0	21	69.8	61	141.8	101	213.8	141	285.8
−19	−2.2	22	71.6	62	143.6	102	215.6	142	287.6
−18	−0.4	23	73.4	63	145.4	103	217.4	143	289.4
−17	1.4	24	75.2	64	147.2	104	219.2	144	291.2
−16	3.2	25	77.	65	149.	105	221.	145	293.
−15	5.	26	78.8	66	150.8	106	222.8	146	294.8
−14	6.8	27	80.6	67	152.6	107	224.6	147	296.6
−13	8.6	28	82.4	68	154.4	108	226.4	148	298.4
−12	10.4	29	84.2	69	156.2	109	228.2	149	300.2
−11	12.2	30	86.	70	158.	110	230.	150	302.
−10	14.	31	87.8	71	159.8	111	231.8	151	303.8
− 9	15.8	32	89.6	72	161.6	112	233.6	152	305.6
− 8	17.6	33	91.4	73	163.4	113	235.4	153	307.4
− 7	19.4	34	93.2	74	165.2	114	237.2	154	309.2
− 6	21.2	35	95.	75	167.	115	239.	155	311.
− 5	23.	36	96.8	76	168.8	116	240.8	156	312.8
− 4	24.8	37	98.6	77	170.6	117	242.6	157	314.6
− 3	26.6	38	100.4	78	172.4	118	244.4	158	316.4
− 2	28.4	39	102.2	79	174.2	119	246.2	159	318.2
− 1	30.2	40	104.	80	176.	120	248.	160	320.
0	32.	41	105.8	81	177.8	121	249.8	161	321.8
1	33.8	42	107.6	82	179.6	122	251.6	162	323.6
2	35.6	43	109.4	83	181.4	123	253.4	163	325.4
3	37.4	44	111.2	84	183.2	124	255.2	104	327.2
4	39.2	45	113.	85	185.	125	257.	165	329.
5	41.	46	114.8	86	186.8	126	258.8	166	330.8
6	42.8	47	116.6	87	188.6	127	260.6	167	332.6
7	44.6	48	118.4	88	190.4	128	262.4	168	334.4
8	46.4	49	120.2	89	192.2	129	264.2	169	336.2
9	48.2	50	122.	90	194.	130	266.	170	338.
10	50.	51	123.8	91	195.8	131	267.8	171	339.8
11	51.8	52	125.6	92	197.6	132	269.6	172	341.6
12	53.6	53	127.4	93	199.4	133	271.4	173	343.4
13	55.4	54	129.2	94	201.2	134	273.2	174	345.2
14	57.2	55	131.	95	203.	135	275.	175	347.
15	59.	56	132.8	96	204.8	136	276.8	176	348.8
16	60.8	57	134.6	97	206.6	137	278.6	177	350.6
17	62.6	58	136.4	98	208.4	138	280.4	178	352.4
18	64.4	59	138.2	99	210.2	139	282.2	179	354.2
19	66.2	60	140.	100	212.	140	284.	180	356.
20	68.								

* Courtesy, *The Pharmacopeia of the United States of America.*

From THE DENTAL ASSISTANT edited by John C. Brauer & R. E. Richardson. 3rd Ed., Copyright © 1964 by McGraw-Hill, Inc. Used by permission of McGraw-Hill Book Company.

TABLE OF THERMOMETRIC EQUIVALENTS - (Continued)

Fahrenheit to Centigrade Scales

$$(\text{F.}^\circ - 32) \times \tfrac{5}{9} = \text{C.}^\circ$$

F. °	C. °	F. °	C. °	F. °	C. °	F. °	C. °	F. °	C. °
0	−17.78	51	10.56	101	38.33	151	66.11	201	93.89
1	−17.22	52	11.11	102	38.89	152	66.67	202	94.44
2	−16.67	53	11.67	103	39.44	153	67.22	203	95.
3	−16.11	54	12.22	104	40.	154	67.78	204	95.56
4	−15.56	55	12.78	105	40.56	155	68.33	205	96.11
5	−15.	56	13.33	106	41.11	156	68.89	206	96.67
6	−14.44	57	13.89	107	41.67	157	69.44	207	97.22
7	−13.89	58	14.44	108	42.22	158	70.	208	97.78
8	−13.33	59	15.	109	42.78	159	70.56	209	98.33
9	−12.78	60	15.56	110	43.33	160	71.11	210	98.89
10	−12.22	61	16.11	111	43.89	161	71.67	211	99.44
11	−11.67	62	16.67	112	44.44	162	72.22	212	100.
12	−11.11	63	17.22	113	45.	163	72.78	213	100.56
13	−10.56	64	17.78	114	45.56	164	73.33	214	101.11
14	−10.	65	18.33	115	46.11	165	73.89	215	101.67
15	−9.44	66	18.89	116	46.67	166	74.44	216	102.22
16	−8.89	67	19.44	117	47.22	167	75.	217	102.78
17	−8.33	68	20.	118	47.78	168	75.56	218	103.33
18	−7.78	69	20.56	119	48.33	169	76.11	219	103.89
19	−7.22	70	21.11	120	48.89	170	76.67	220	104.44
20	−6.67	71	21.67	121	49.44	171	77.22	221	105.
21	−6.11	72	22.22	122	50.	172	77.78	222	105.56
22	−5.56	73	22.78	123	50.56	173	78.33	223	106.11
23	−5.	74	23.33	124	51.11	174	78.89	224	106.67
24	−4.44	75	23.89	125	51.67	175	79.44	225	107.22
25	−3.89	76	24.44	126	52.22	176	80.	226	107.78
26	−3.33	77	25.	127	52.78	177	80.56	227	108.33
27	−2.78	78	25.56	128	53.33	178	81.11	228	108.89
28	−2.22	79	26.11	129	53.89	179	81.67	229	109.44
29	−1.67	80	26.67	130	54.44	180	82.22	230	110.
30	−1.11	81	27.22	131	55.	181	82.78	231	110.56
31	−0.56	82	27.78	132	55.56	182	83.33	232	111.11
32	0.	83	28.33	133	56.11	183	83.89	233	111.67
33	0.56	84	28.89	134	56.67	184	84.44	234	112.22
34	1.11	85	29.44	135	57.22	185	85.	235	112.78
35	1.67	86	30.	136	57.78	186	85.56	236	113.33
36	2.22	87	30.56	137	58.33	187	86.11	237	113.89
37	2.78	88	31.11	138	58.89	188	86.67	238	114.44
38	3.33	89	31.67	139	59.44	189	87.22	239	115.
39	3.89	90	32.22	140	60.	190	87.78	240	115.56
40	4.44	91	32.78	141	60.56	191	88.33	241	116.11
41	5.	92	33.33	142	61.11	192	88.89	242	116.67
42	5.56	93	33.89	143	61.67	193	89.44	243	117.22
43	6.11	94	34.44	144	62.22	194	90.	244	117.78
44	6.67	95	35.	145	62.78	195	90.56	245	118.33
45	7.22	96	35.56	146	63.33	196	91.11	246	118.89
46	7.78	97	36.11	147	63.89	197	91.67	247	119.44
47	8.33	98	36.67	148	64.44	198	92.22	248	120.
48	8.89	99	37.22	149	65.	199	92.78	249	120.56
49	9.44	100	37.78	150	65.56	200	93.33	250	121.11
50	10.								

From THE DENTAL ASSISTANT edited by John C. Brauer & R. E. Richardson. 3rd Ed., Copyright © 1964 by McGraw-Hill, Inc. Used by permission of McGraw-Hill Book Company.

TABLE OF CERTAIN DISEASES

Disease	Age	Transmission	Incubation
Bacterial Meningitis	Any age, but younger more susceptible.	Direct or indirect contact with patient.	Variable.
Chickenpox	2 to 8 years.	Air-borne spread, contact with discharges from skin lesions or nose or throat of patient.	10 to 21 days. More commonly 14 to 16 days.
Diarrheal Diseases	Birth to 5 years most common.	Direct contact fecal contamination.	Variable. 2 to 4 days.
Diphtheria	1 to 14 years.	Direct contact with nose or throat discharges of carrier or patient.	1 to 6 days.
German Measles	2 to 15 years.	Air-borne spread, and direct contact with nose or throat discharges of patient.	10 to 28 days. More commonly 14 to 21 days.
Impetigo	Any age.	Contact with lesions or infected articles, especially found on face.	2-5 days.
Infectious Hepatitis	Any age.	Contact with patient, or contaminated water or food or fecal contamination.	Usually 3 to 4 weeks, but can be 2 to 7 weeks.
Infectious Mononucleosis	2 to 20 years.	Believed to be direct contact with nose and throat discharges of infected patient. Also air-borne spread.	Believed to be 2 to 6 weeks. Really unknown.
Influenza	Any age.	Air-borne spread possible. Direct or indirect contact with nose or throat discharges of patient.	1 to 2 days.
Measles	2 to 8 years.	Air-borne spread. Direct and indirect contact with nose and throat discharges of patient.	10 to 12 days usually, but 7 to 14 days possible.
Mumps	Usually 2 to 14 years.	Nose and throat discharges of patient.	Usually 16 to 20 days, but 12 to 28 days possible.
Poliomyelitis	Any age; more common among infants and children.	Focal contamination. Direct or indirect contact with nose and throat discharges of patient.	Usually 7 to 12 days, but 3 to 28 days possible.

Early Symptoms	Length of Illness	Length of Contagion	Permanent Aftereffects
Headache, irritability, fever, nausea, muscular rigidity.	Variable, usually 1 to 3 weeks.	Variable. Probably less than one day after beginning of treatment.	Brain damage is frequent. Death occurs in about 10% of the cases.
Characteristic eruption, with slight fever.	9 to 14 days.	One day before ill until skin lesions scab.	Rare.
Nausea, vomiting, fever, abdominal pain, prostration.	Variable. Usually 2 to 5 days, but sometimes longer.	Shortly before onset until 5 days after onset usually.	Variable.
Sore throat, running nose, mild fever.	Variable. Possibly several weeks.	Usually 3 days before to 10 days after onset.	Possible heart or nervous system damage. Up to 10% of the cases may die.
Rash, swelling of lymph glands, slight fever.	1 to 4 days.	One week before to disappearance of rash.	Rare. However, damage to fetus early in pregnancy if a pregnant woman contracts the disease.
Circular raised lesion, usually on face, becomes crusted.	Varies.	Until sores heal.	None.
Mild headache, chilliness, jaundice, fever.	Variable. 2 to 4 weeks.	Unknown.	Rarely. Death and chronic liver disease do occur.
Sore throat, fatigue, enlarged lymph nodes, fever, possibly rash.	1 week to several months. Highly variable.	Unknown.	Rare.
Muscular pain, dry cough, sudden fever, marked prostration.	3 to 10 days.	1 day before to 4 days after onset.	Very rare.
Cold, severe cough, gradually increasing fever, running nose, conjunctivitis.	6 to 12 days.	4 days before to end of rash.	Occasionally death or brain damage.
Fever, swelling of salivary glands.	4 to 10 days.	1 week before onset to end of swelling.	Very rarely there is brain damage.
Fever, sore throat, headache, nausea, vomiting, muscle pain, and weakness.	Highly variable. Some possibility of several months.	Usually 3 days before to 10 days after onset.	Death in 5% to 10% of paralytic cases. Some paralysis may be permanent.

TABLE OF CERTAIN DISEASES—(Continued)

Disease	Age	Transmission	Incubation
Roseola	6 months to 3 years.	Unknown, probably air-borne spread, or contact with nose and throat discharges of infected patient.	Unknown. Believed to be 10 to 15 days.
Scarlet Fever or Scarlatina	1 to 9 years.	Direct or indirect contact with a carrier or a patient.	1 to 5 days.
Smallpox	Any age.	Air-borne spread. Contact with throat or skin discharges of patient.	7 to 16 days.
"Strep Throat," (acute pharyngitis)	Any age.	Droplet infection, infected milk.	Varies.
Syphilis	Usually post-puberty.	Contact with lesion.	Usually 21 days.
Tetanus (lockjaw)	Any age.	Puncture wound.	4-21 days.
Vincent's Disease (Trench mouth)	Any age.	Direct contact and contaminated articles.	Undetermined.
Whooping Cough	Birth to 8 years.	Direct contact with discharges of nose or throat from a carrier or patient.	Usually 7 to 10 days, but 5 to 16 days possible.

Early Symptoms	Length of Illness	Length of Contagion	Permanent Aftereffects
High fever for 3 to 5 days. Rash appears after temperature returns to normal.	4 to 6 days.	Unknown.	Rare.
Vomiting, sore throat, fever, nausea.	4 to 10 days.	Highly variable. Usually 1 to 2 weeks, but can be several months.	Kidney disease. Rheumatic heart disease.
High fever, characteristic eruption, prostration.	1 to 7 weeks.	4 to 5 days before rash until scabs disappear.	Blindness, brain damage, pox scars. 1% to 40% cases may die.
Severe sore throat, high fever, general aches.	Varies.	Until antibiotics take effect.	Not dangerous unless complications occur, such as rheumatic fever.
Running sore is usually a primary sore.	Varies.	Until antibiotics take effect.	Varies, depending on when treatment is begun. Early treatment can leave no aftereffects.
Muscle spasms, first local, then general paralysis.	Varies.		Highly fatal.
Painful ulcers of gums and mouth tissues, sore throat, slight fever.	Varies, depending on care.	As long as disease is present.	None if properly cared for.
Cold, with a gradually increasing intermittent dry cough.	Usually 4 to 6 weeks, but 2 to 10 possible.	Variable. Usually first 2 weeks.	In infants death and brain damage.

GLOSSARY

This glossary is not intended to be a technical dictionary. It is an attempt to explain commonly used words in language which can be understood by the beginner. This guide has been compiled as an aid to pronunciation without conforming to standard dictionary methods. The long sound of vowels is indicated by the symbol (⁻) above the vowel. We suggest that after becoming familiar with the words in this section, the dental assistant consult *Current Clinical Dental Terminology*, edited by Carl O. Boucher and published by the C. V. Mosby Company, St. Louis, Missouri, in 1963. In addition, it may be helpful to use *The American Illustrated Medical Dictionary* by W. A. Newman Dorland, published by Saunders Company, Philadelphia, or the *New Gould Medical Dictionary*, published by the Blakiston Company, Toronto and Philadelphia. These medical dictionaries give technical definitions of these words in language commonly used by dentists and physicians.

A

abnormal (ab-nor′-mal) Markedly irregular. Deviating from the normal; not conforming with the general rule.

abrasion (uh-brā′-zhun) The wearing away of a tooth by mechanical means. Example: A person who chews tobacco markedly wears away his teeth over many years.

abscess (ab′-ses) Pus formation which is localized and limited in extent in any part of the body.

absorption (ab-sorp′-shun) 1. A substance passes into the interior of another by penetration or by solution. This process is called absorption. (Definition for Anesthesiology) 2. Skin, mucous surfaces, dental materials, etc., take up fluids or other substances. The process is called absorption. (Definition for Prosthodontology) 3. Radiation imparts energy to any material through which it passes by absorption. (Definition for Radiography)

abutment (a-but'-ment) Support. The natural tooth which is nearest the space left by a missing tooth when it has been crowned (or fitted with an inlay) and becomes one end of a bridge. An abutment is also a natural tooth to which the clasp of a partial denture is fitted.

accelerator (ak-sel'-er-ā-ter) In dentistry it is a chemical which causes a reaction to happen faster than it would happen without the chemical.

account (a-kount) A formal record of the charges, payments, and balance of the patient whose name is at the top of the card or sheet.

aciculae (ā-sik'-ū-lī) Needle-form crystals found in general-purpose artificial-stone preparations.

acrylic (uh-kril'-ik) One of a group of synthetic thermoplastic substances resembling clear glass but lighter in weight. It can be colored as desired. It is used in making both partial and full dentures and is colored pink to resemble natural gum color. It is also used for individual tooth restorations and colored the desired shade for the individual tooth. Methyl methacrylate resin is most commonly used in dentures at present.

acute (uh'-kūt) Severe, coming quickly to a crisis. It is therefore different from a chronic ailment which lasts over a long period of time.

adaptation (ad-ap-tā'-shun) Modification to fit the conditions of the environment.

adhesion (ad-hē'-zhun) Molecular binding.

aerobe (ay-ur-ōb) A microorganism that must have oxygen to live.

aerobic (ay-ur-ō-bik) Growing in free oxygen.

aesthetic (es-the'-tik) Appreciation of the beautiful in nature and art.

aesthetic dentistry Pleasing and beautiful dental operations aside from the purely practical function of replacement.

aesthetic try-ins A trial fitting of artificial teeth to check appearance before final processing.

aesthetics The study of those components which make up beauty—color, form, etc. Applied to dentistry, it refers to the qualities involved in the appearance of a restoration—whether it is pleasing to the viewer.

alcohol (al'-kuh-hol) A transparent, colorless, volatile, mobile liquid which is most effectively used as a disinfectant at 70% strength. It can precipitate a protective coat around bacteria contained in blood, pus, mucus, and should be used only after the instruments are thoroughly cleaned. Any residue of blood, etc., left on the instrument can cause infection on the next use even if alcohol has been used to disinfect it.

alkali (al'-kuh-lī) A strong, water-soluble chemical base, obtained from the ashes of plants. It is largely potassium or sodium carbonate. When in solution, it dissociates, forming hydroxyl (OH) ions. The term is used in Anesthesiology.

alkaline (al'-kuh-līn) Having the properties of an alkali, commonly having a pH of more than 7.

alkaloid (al'-kuh'loid) A bitter, alkaline, organic derivative of plants which is highly active physiologically.

　synthetic alkaloid A synthetically prepared compound which has the chemical characteristics of alkaloids. (These terms are used in Oral Medicine and Pharmacology.)

allergy (al'-er-jē) A hypersensitive (exaggerated) reaction of the body to a substance which is harmless in most other persons. In the affected individual it produces asthma, hay fever and other respiratory disturbances, eczema, dermatitis, stomatitis, migraine headaches, edema, erythema, and other reactions. Some of the common allergies are allergies to dust, weeds, pollen, and certain foods and drugs.

alloy (a'-loi) Two or more metals are "fused" (melted together) to form a new metal called an "alloy." In dentistry the amalgam used for filling cavities is made of a silver alloy combined with mercury.

alveolar process (al-vē'-ō-lar prah'-ses) *Process* in anatomy means an outgrowth or projecting part. The alveolar process is the part of the bone which projects from the maxilla (upper jaw) and mandible (lower jaw) and supports the roots of the teeth. It forms their sockets (alveoli).

alveolus (al-vē'-ō-lus) (pl., alveoli) The tooth socket in the alveolar process.

amalgam (uh-mal'-gam) A mixture of mercury with any other metal or metals.

　dental amalgam A compound of mercury, silver, tin, and other metals for filling teeth. A.D.A. Specification No. 1 for dental amalgam alloys requires the chemical composition to be within these limits: silver, 65% minimum; copper, 6% maximum; zinc, 2% maximum; and tin, 25% minimum.

ameloblast (am-el'-ō-blast) A dental-enamel-forming cell. One of a group of cells from which the enamel on teeth is formed.

ammeter (am'-ēt-er) A contraction of the word *amperemeter*. It is an electrical device which measures the flow of electricity. An ammeter is used on dental X-ray machines to measure the current flowing through the X-ray tube. The higher the ammeter reading, the greater the amount of current flowing through the tube and the less time needed to record a satisfactory image on the film.

amorphous (uh-mor'-fus) Shapeless. A substance having no specific form in space. The molecules are distributed at random.

ampere (am'-peer) A unit of electrical current. It is the amount of electrical current produced by one volt acting through a resistance of one ohm. The measurement in dental X ray is usually in milliamperes, which is 1/1000 of one ampere.

ampul, ampule (am'-pūl) A small container, usually glass, which can be perfectly sealed (hermetically sealed). It is used to keep its contents sterile until needed. Local anesthetic comes in ampules in the dental office. Ampules are used for many types of hypodermic solutions.

anaerobe (an-ay-ur-ōb) A microorganism which grows where there is no oxygen. If these microorganisms are exposed to air for any length of time, they are usually destroyed.

analgesic (an"-al-jēs'-ik) A mild remedy for relieving pain, such as aspirin, Anacin, Bufferin, A.S.A.

anaphylaxis (an"-uh-fuh-lak'-sus) A dangerous, violent reaction characterized by respiratory and circulatory failure or a sudden collapse or shock. It can occur following an injection. It is an allergic reaction following the injection of an allergen. A patient so reacting requires *immediate,* prompt treatment to prevent death.

anatomy (ah-nat'-ō-mē) The science that studies the way the parts of the body are formed and how the parts are related to each other. Anatomy applies to all plant and animal life, but we are interested in it only as it refers to human anatomy.

anemia (uh-nē'-mē-uh) A decrease in the number of red blood cells or in the amount of hemoglobin they contain. Anemia is referred to as a quantitative or qualitative deficiency of the blood. The result is that the blood is unable to carry oxygen in sufficient amount for use by the body.

anesthesia (an"-es-thē'-sē-a) Loss of bodily feeling due to receiving an anesthetic or to disease. Thus, you do not feel pain when you are given an anesthetic.

anesthetic (an"-es-thet'-ik) A drug or gas which takes away the sense of feeling.

> **general** A drug or gas which produces unconsciousness (and, thus, the loss of feeling) either by inhalation (ether, chloroform, vinathene) or by injection (sodium pentothal).
>
> **local** A drug which when injected into the tissues and absorbed into a nerve will temporarily cause loss of feeling in the area supplied by that nerve. It is called local (to differentiate from general) because the area so anesthetized is only a part of the patient's body.
>
> **topical** A drug which is applied to the surface of tissues and produces the loss of feeling in that tissue area. It is used prior to the insertion of a hypodermic needle, preparatory to injection, to prevent pain.

angina (an-jī'-nuh) Derived from the Latin *angere* which means "to strangle"; thus any disease accompanied by a spasmodic, choking pain or suffocation is called angina. There are other words added to differentiate the kind of angina, such as angina pectoris.

anneal (uh-nēl') To toughen, temper, or make glass or metal more lasting. This is accomplished by heating the metal or glass and slowly cooling it so that it is less brittle, relieving internal strain.

anode (an'-ōd) The target of the roentgen-ray tube. It is a tungsten block set at an angle of either 20° or 45° to the cathode. The electronic stream from the cathode strikes the target; and since the anode is the positive terminal, it emits roentgen rays at this point which are then directed through the opening in the tube head and are used for oral radiography.

anodontia (an"-ō-don'-shē-ah) Without teeth. Teeth may not have erupted. Teeth may be missing from lack of care or old age, or may never have formed.

anomaly (uh-nom'-uh-lē) Any noticeable change from the normal form, abnormal or irregular.

anoxia (an-oks'-ē-ah) An insufficient supply of oxygen in the body. The disturbance of bodily functions due to insufficient oxygen.

anterior (an-tē'-rē-or) Front or in the front or forward part of. Anterior teeth are the six front teeth in both the upper and lower arches.

antibody (an'-ti-bah-dē)   A specific substance produced by an animal as a reaction to the presence of an antigen (a toxin or enzyme). It reacts specifically with the antigen. It neutralizes the toxins, precipitates the antigen invaders, or gathers the bacteria cells into a mass.

antibiotic (an"-te-bī-ot'-ik)   A medication made from certain microorganisms and given a patient either orally or by injection to prevent or fight an infection.

antidote (an'-te-dōt)   Medicine given to counteract a poison.

antigen (ant'-i-jen)   A substance which, when introduced into an individual to which it is foreign, stimulates the formation of antibodies which react with it. It is usually a protein or carbohydrate (as a toxin or enzyme).

antipyretic (an-te-pi-ret'-ik)   A medicine used to reduce a fever.

antiseptic (an-te-sep'-tik)   A substance that is used to arrest the growth of disease germs (bacteria) or prevent putrefaction. It does not necessarily kill the bacteria.

anti-sialagogue, antisialagog (an-te-sī-al'-a-gog) A medication which reduces the flow of saliva.

apex (ā'-peks)   (pl., apices)   Tip. In dentistry it refers to the tip of the root of a tooth.

aphthous ulcer, aphtha stomatitis (af'-thoos-ul-sir)   Commonly called the canker sore. An ulcer of unknown origin which appears on the mucous membrane, similar to herpes simplex lesion which appears on skin, but not of viral origin as is herpes lesion.

apical (āp'-i-kal)   At or pertaining to the tip or apex.

apical foramen (āp'-i-kal for-ā'-men)   The tiny opening of the pulp canal at the tip end of the root of the tooth. The vessels and nerves of the dental pulp pass through the apical foramen.

apoplexy (ap'-up-plek-sē)   Sudden loss of consciousness, voluntary motion, and sensation caused by rupturing or obstruction of an artery of the brain. Commonly called a stroke.

arch, dental   (See dental arch)

armamentarium (ar"-mah-men-tā'-rē-um)   All the materials, equipment, books, journals, and supplies owned by a dentist to help him practice dentistry. (It also applies to a physician or hospital.) Also, the materials, equipment, supplies, etc., required to complete a specific operation.

aromatic (ar-ō-mat'-ik)   Fragrant, spicy smelling.

articulate (ar-tik'-ū-lāt) 1. To adjust the relationship of natural or artificial teeth so that they work properly for the mastication of food and for proper distribution of stresses. 2. To form sound into words.

articulator (ar-tik'-ū-lā-tor) 1.   An instrument which holds models or casts of a patient's dental arches in a given relative position while work is done on occlusion and articulation for either natural or artificial teeth. The patient's mandibular movements (lower jaw) may or may not be duplicated depending on the complexity of the articulator. 2. The articulators of the speech mechanism are the lips, teeth, jaw, tongue, soft palate, uvula, and pharyngeal wall.

artifact (ar'-te-fakt)   An apparently diseased area visible in dental X ray which is caused by faulty manipulation of film developer or foreign matter.

artificial teeth (ar-ti-fish'-al)   A full or partial denture, or bridgework. The teeth are either porcelain or acrylic.

artificial stone.   (See stone, artificial)

asepsis (ah-sep'-sis)   Freedom from living germs of disease and decay (without decay).

aseptic (ah-sep'-tik)   Surgically clean; free of all microorganisms.

asphyxia (as-fiks'-ē-ah)   Suspension of breathing and animation because the body is deprived of oxygen, as in drowning or suffocation.

aspirate (as'-pi-rāt)   To withdraw by suction.

aspiration (as-pir-ā'-shun)   Using the aspirator or low-pressure evacuator to suck fluids and gases from the oral cavity (patient's mouth).

aspirator (as'-pir-ā-tor)   A piece of equipment which has a hose and nozzle which the dental assistant holds at the patient's mouth during the preparation of a tooth. The aspirator is a vacuum, and all debris and water from the patient's mouth are sucked up by the aspirator nozzle and carried away.

aspirin (as'-pir-in)   A mild pain-relieving drug; also reduces above-normal body temperature.

astringent (as-trin'-jent)   A medication which tends to contract body tissue.

atom (at'-um)   The smallest unit of an element that can exist either alone or in combination.

atrofe, atrophy (at'-rō-fē)   The wasting away of tissue or parts through lack of use or disease.

attrition (ah-trish'-un)   Normal wearing away by friction. In dentistry it refers to wearing down the surfaces of the teeth by mastication of food.

autoclave (aw'-tō-klāv)   A device for sterilizing instruments by steam under pressure.

auxiliary personnel.   (See personnel)

axial (ak′-sē-al)   The axis of a tooth is an imaginary line passing through the center of the tooth the long way (from apex to occlusal or incisal surface). *Axial* refers to all lines, angles, and surfaces of a tooth which are parallel to this line.

B

bacillus (bah-sil′-us)   (pl., bacilli) A group of bacteria that are shaped like rods and frequently appear in chains.

backing (bak′-ing)   The metal back of a bridge or pontic to which the tooth or facing is attached.

bacteremia (bak-ter-ē′-mē-ah)   Bacteria in the blood.

bacterial plaque (bak-tē′-rē-al plak)   A filmlike covering on the teeth which is often very difficult to see in a well-kept mouth.

bacterial spore (bak-tē′-rē-al spor)   The rough, resistant reproductive cell enabling some bacteria to remain alive under adverse conditions. A spore has a thick cell wall and the spore can remain dormant until conditions are favorable for bacteria to reproduce. This dormant stage of bacterial life is highly resistant to sterilizing procedures.

bactericide (bak-ter′-i-sīd)   A substance (usually in liquid form) which kills bacteria.

bacteriostatic (bak-ter′-ē-ō-stat′-ik)   Inhibits or arrests the growth of bacteria.

bacterium (bak-tē′-rē-um)   Singular of bacteria. Any one of an important group of microscopic one-celled vegetable organisms some of which are harmless, some of which produce disease. They were discovered by L. Pasteur who found that they were responsible for producing disease. They are spherical, rod-shaped, or spiral. They live on organic matter, dead or alive.

band, orthodontic.   A thin strip of metal used to encircle the crown of a tooth closely. It wraps around the tooth horizontally. A band is used in orthodontic treatment to bodily move a tooth to its new position.

barbiturate (bar-bich′-a-rit)   Any of the derivatives of barbituric acid. Its use is as a sedative.

base for filling.   A cement or other protective material placed over the pulpal area of the tooth to reduce thermal shock and irritation when a restoration is large.

benign (bē-nīn′)   Usually refers to a tumor which is not malignant and will not kill.

bicuspid (bī-kus′-pid)   *Bi* means "two," *cusp* means "a prominent shape of a tooth"; so a bicuspid is a tooth with two cusps, or rounded parts.

bifurcate (bī-fur′-kāt)   Divided into two branches or forks.

bile (bīl′)   A viscid, alkaline fluid secreted by the liver which aids in the digestion and absorption of fats. It is yellow or greenish.

biology (bī-ahl′-uh-jē)   The science of living matter in all its forms.

biopsy (bī-ahp′-sē)   The removal of tissue from a living person and examination of this tissue by microscope for diagnosis. There are several methods of securing the tissue. When possible, part of a lesion and some of the normal tissue beside it are removed so that a comparison can be made.

bite fork   Part of the mechanism used in face-bow transfer.

bite rims   A temporary wax shape to hold an initial setup of artificial teeth for checking.

boxing of an impression   The process of enclosing an impression with wax, clay, or wet asbestos to shape the base of the cast while it hardens.

bridgework (brij-work)   A missing tooth is replaced by a *bridge*. Sometimes 2 or 3 teeth may be replaced by a bridge. The bridge consists of a pontic (name of artificial tooth replacing the missing natural tooth) and two crowns or inlays which are cemented to the teeth on either side of the missing tooth. These crowns are called abutments. The entire bridge (pontics and abutment crowns) is a one-piece appliance, either cast as a whole unit or soldered together. It is usually "fixed" or cemented in place. Some bridges are removable fixed bridges (removable by the dentist only), and occasionally there are removable bridges which the patient can remove as he would a partial or full denture.

bruxism (bruk′-sizm)   Gnashing the teeth. Usually a person does this unconsciously in his sleep or when he is under nervous strain.

buccal (buk′-al)   *Bucca* is the Latin word for "cheek." Buccal in dentistry means the side of the tooth which is next to the cheek.

bur   A cutting instrument used by the dentist in preparing a tooth for a restoration. Burs come in many shapes and sizes and of various materials. See illustrations of burs, chapter 33.

C

calcification (kal″-si-fi-kā′-shun)   The deposit of calcium in the tissues of the body.

calcarious deposit   *See* calculus.

calcining (kal-sīn′-ing)   Removing water by heat in the manufacture of artificial stone and plaster from gypsum.

calculus (kal'-kū-lus) The technical name for tartar. It is a hard calcium deposit on the tooth—usually near the gum line or where teeth overlap—places which are hard to brush clean. The dentist or dental hygienist removes this deposit with a scaler during prophylaxis.

canal (ka-nal') A narrow channel between two larger spaces (as Panama Canal). In dentistry it refers to tiny tubes or ducts as the salivary ducts which permit the flow of saliva to the mouth from the salivary glands or the root canal of the tooth through which the nerves and blood supply pass.

cancer (kan'-ser) A malignant tumor. Malignant means capable of causing death.

canine eminence (kā'-nīn em'-i-nens) A noticeable bulge over the cuspid tooth on the upper jaw, just below and to the outside of the nose.

capsule (kap'-sūl) 1. A shell found around certain bacteria which protects the bacteria from destruction. 2. A tiny container of gelatin which holds disagreeable medicine and may be swallowed. The capsule is made of gelatin which is dry and hard at room temperature but melts when wet. Capsules are often cylindrical in shape and are usually made in two pieces which slip together.

carbolic acid (kar-bol'-ik a'-sid) More properly called phenol.

Carborundum (kar-bō-run'-dum) An abrasive which is extremely hard (harder than emery). It is a registered trade name for silicon carbide.

Carborundum stones and wheels are used in dentistry to polish restorations and teeth. They mount in the handpiece, and the unit motor makes them spin as a bur spins.

carcinoma (kar"-si-nō'-mah) From the Greek *karkinoma* which means "cancer." A malignant tumor. It originates in the epithelium.

cardiac (kar'-dē-ak) Refers to the heart. A patient with cardiac disease frequently requires special attention in the dental office.

cardiovascular (kar"-dē-ō-vas'-kū-lar) *Cardio* comes from the Greek, meaning "heart." *Vascular* comes from the Latin meaning "vessel." Thus, cardiovascular refers to the heart and blood systems; the carrying of the blood throughout the body.

caries (kār'-ēz) (dental caries) Decay. A disease process which attacks the hard tissues of the teeth, demineralizing and eventually destroying these hard tissues through loss of both organic and inorganic elements.

interproximal caries The interproximal surface of the tooth is that surface which touches another tooth. Thus, interproximal caries is decay found on the surfaces of the teeth which are in contact with other teeth.

carious (kār'-ē-us) Refers to caries or decay.

carotene (kār'-ō-tēn) An orange pigment which may be converted to vitamin A by digestive process within the body. It is found in leafy vegetables, carrots, and other vegetables. Our bodies need both carotene which can be *converted* to vitamin A and vitamin A which does not have to be converted.

carpule (kar'-pūl) The name given by the Novol Chemical Company to the glass cartridge containing Novocaine ready for use.

carrier (care'-ē-er) One who harbors or carries a disease and transmits it to other people but does not necessarily have the disease himself. A typhoid "carrier" can infect anyone with whom he has contact, but he does not have typhoid himself.

case history All the information your dentist is able to gather about a patient which will help in diagnosing and treating that patient. This information is strictly confidential.

cassette (kah-set') A holder for extraoral X-ray film or plates.

cast A positive reproduction made from an impression (or negative), usually of a dental arch.

casting Noun: A metallic object formed by using a wax replica, melting out the wax, and replacing it with molten metal which then hardens in the mold. Verb: The process of making the casting in the mold.

catalyst (kat'-ah-list) A chemical which accelerates a chemical reaction between two other chemicals but does not combine with either of these chemicals and does not permanently change itself.

cathode (kath'-ōd) The negative terminal of the roentgen-ray tube. It is a spiral of tungsten wire which focuses the electron stream at the anode.

caustic (kaws'-tik) A chemical which eats away tissue. It is very irritating, and it can burn.

cavity (kav'-i-tē) The hollow space in a tooth made by dental caries.

incipient interproximal cavity Decay which is just beginning in the area where two teeth are in contact with each other.

cavity liner Material used to line the preparation in a tooth before the tooth is fitted or crowned or has an inlay placed, usually a varnish.

cc   Abbreviation for cubic centimeter.

cement (se-ment′)   A substance which is used to seal inlays, crowns, bridges, and acrylic fillings in place. It may be used as a temporary filling also.

  zinc acid phosphate cement (zink as′-id fos′-fāt se-ment′)   Used as a base under metallic fillings and for placing gold inlays and crowns.

  zinc oxide-eugenol cement (zink ox′-īd ū-jen-ōl se-ment′)   When a tooth needs to be soothed, this "sedative" cement is used. It may be used as a temporary filling or as a base when sedation is required.

cementum (se-men′-tum)   A thin, bonelike tissue covering the root of a tooth.

centigrade (sen′-ti-grād)   Having one hundred equal grades or gradients. The freezing point is 0° and the boiling point is 100°. To change centigrade to Fahrenheit: $F = 9/5C + 32$.

centimeter (sen′-ti-mē″-ter)   The 100th part of a meter. It equals about 2/5 of an inch or 0.3937. The abbreviation is cm.

  cubic centimeter (cc)   1/1000 part of a liter.

centric relation   Objectionable as a noun. *See* occlusion, centric.

cephalometry (sef-ah-lōm′-eh-trē)   Measurement of bone structure of the head by use of lateral and anteroposterior radiographs which can be reproduced.

cervix (ser′-viks)   Latin for *neck*. Neck of a tooth. The neck of the tooth is located where the root of the tooth and the crown of the tooth join.

cervical (ser′-vi-kal)   Pertaining to the neck or cervix.

cervical line   The line at which the cementum meets the enamel on a tooth.

cheilitis (kī-lī′-tis)   Inflammation of the lip or lips.

cheilosis (kī-lō′-sis)   Fissuring at the corners of the mouth caused by vitamin B complex deficiency, drooling, decreased vertical measurements, or infection. The lips do not show inflammation but can be chapped.

chemotherapy (ke-mō-ther′-uh-pē)   The use of chemicals to cure or arrest the process of diseases.

chronic (kron′-ik)   Continuing for a long time and the opposite of acute; habitual. A chronic ailment is one which is not acute and is long established.

chronological (krahn-uh-lahg′-i-kal)   An arrangement of events in the order in which they occur.

cingulum (sin′-gū-lum)   The lump on the lingual of the anterior teeth in the gingival third.

cleft palate (kleft pal′-at)   The dictionary defines cleft as a crack or split. The palate is the roof of the mouth. A cleft palate is one which has a crack or split in it because the two sides of the palate did not grow together along the midline of the roof of the mouth prior to birth. It may be a partial cleft with a small split only in the soft palate, or it may be a complete cleft and extend from the uvula through the soft and hard palates, the nose and upper lip. *See* oral pathology, p. 328 for a nontechnical explanation.

coccus (kok′-us) (pl., cocci)   One of the three forms of bacteria (see bacterium). Cocci are spherical in shape.

codeine (ko′-dēn)   One of the stronger pain relievers. It is made from opium, hence is a narcotic and may only be prescribed by a dentist or physician holding a narcotic license.

colloid (kuh′-loid)   A suspension of particles in a dispersion medium. The particles are somewhat larger than the molecules of material found in a solution. Dental examples: hydrocolloids and silicate cements.

colloidal (kuh-loi′-dal)   Pertaining to colloid.

coma (kō′-ma)   Prolonged loss of consciousness which does not reverse by itself.

composite filling material   A material composed of two distinct phases (plastic and filler) which are bonded together. The dispersed phase (or filler) complements the physical properties of the continuous phase (plastic) matrix material.

compound (kom′-pound)   A material used in dentistry which can be shaped when warm. It is often used for preliminary impressions in prosthetics.

conductivity (kon-duk-tiv′-i-tē)   Ability to convey or carry. In electricity or radiography, the ability to carry electric current.

conductor (kon-duk′-tor)   Certain substances transmit electricity, heat, cold, or sound. That is, they pass the heat or electricity along. Copper is a good conductor of electricity so it is used as a wire to pass electricity from the power station to your light. Gold is a good conductor of heat and cold so crowned teeth may allow the person to notice more temperature change when he masticates food.

condyle (kon′-dīl)   A knoblike part on the end of a bone. In dentistry it refers to that part of the mandible which *articulates* with the rest of the skull.

congenital (kon-jen′-i-tal)   Any condition which was present when the person was born is referred to as congenital.

connector (kuh-nek′-tor)   There are several types of connectors used in dentistry. A connector is usually a device to unite two parts of a dental prosthesis. Sometimes it is removable, sometimes it is fixed. A connector is found on a bridge, uniting the pontic with the abutments, and on partials and splints.

consultation (kon-sul-tā'-shun) If two or more dentists, or a dentist and a physician, examine a patient and together decide on a diagnosis and treatment, it is called a consultation.

contact area (kon'-takt a'-rē-ah) Refers to the part of a tooth which touches or contacts the tooth next to it.

contact point Refers to the point of a tooth which touches the next tooth (in contrast to a larger part called an area).

contaminate (kon-tam'-i-nāt) To soil, dirty, or make impure by touching. A sterile instrument is no longer sterile when you have touched it with your bare hands. It has been contaminated with microorganisms.

contour, height of (kon'-tour) A contour is an outline of a curve. The height of contour is the point where the curve has "bulged" the farthest.

contra-angle (kon'-trah-ang'-l) An attachment for a straight handpiece. With it the dentist can use burs, diamond stones, and discs at a right angle to the shaft, thus enabling him to reach areas not readily accessible to the straight handpiece.

convulsion (kon-vul'-shun) An involuntary, irregular, intermittent, and variable muscular contraction, often accompanied by loss of consciousness.

coronal (kor-ō'-nal) Referring to the crown or visible portion of a tooth as seen in the mouth.

coronoid (kor'-ō-noid) The protuberance (swelling out) of the upper forward portion of the ramus of the mandible to which a large part of the temporal muscle is attached. (*See* anatomy).

corrode (kuh-rōd) A chemical or electrolytic action which wears away the surface of metal, such as rusting or tarnishing.

corrosion (kuh-rō'-zhun) A disintegration of a metallic surface by attack of electrolytic or chemical process.

C.P. Chemically pure. This abbreviation is used for chemicals which meet the U.S. Government standards for chemical purity.

crown (krown) The part of the tooth which is visible in the mouth, under normal circumstances. It is covered with enamel.

　anatomical crown (an-uh-tom'-i-kal) That portion of a tooth which is covered with enamel, whether visible or not.

　artificial crown (ar-ti-fish'-al) A dental substitute for the natural crown.

clinical crown (klin'-i-kal) That portion of the tooth which is visible upon examination.

　full veneer crown A complete shell replacement of the outer portion of the natural crown.

　three-quarter crown A shell replacement, except for labial or buccal surface, of the outer portion of the natural crown.

crucible (kroo'-si-bl) A container which withstands high heat. It is used for melting or holding material.

　crucible former (sprue base) A stand into which a sprued pattern is placed. It controls the shape or form of the hollowed-out end of the investment in the casting ring, which receives molten metal through the sprue hole.

crystal (kris'-tal) A solid which is produced by nature. The final units of the substance from which it is formed are arranged systematically.

cubic centimeter (ku-bik sen'-ti-mē-ter) 1/1000 part of a liter. Abbreviation: cc. Used to measure liquids.

culture (kul'-chur) Microorganisms are grown in the laboratory in a special environment.

　culture medium Some liquid or solid in which the bacteria grow well.

　pure culture A bacterial colony which contains only one kind of bacteria.

cusp (kusp) A pointed or rounded part of a tooth, usually on the occlusal surface.

cuspid (kus'-pid) A tooth having one cusp (the canine tooth, the eye tooth, the stomach tooth).

cutaneous (kū-tā'-nē-us) Refers to the skin. The skin is an external, limiting layer of an animal.

cyclopropane (sī"-klō-prō'-pān) A colorless, inflammable gas used for general anesthesia.

cyst (sist) A sac with a distinct wall containing fluid and at times other material such as hair, serum, or blood, or abnormally developed teeth, found in the body tissues.

D

D.D.S. Abbreviation for Doctor of Dental Surgery, the degree from dental college which a dentist receives.

debris (de-brē') Fragments, rubbish, loosely attached to a tooth.

decalcification (dē"-kal-si-fi-kā'-shun) The removal of calcium from the tooth surface by acid. Beginning of formation of cavity.

delirium (di-lir'-ē-um) A state of mental excitement, usually including hallucinations, illusions, delusions, or confusions. The delirium is usually brought on by toxicity produced by disease or drugs.

dental hygienist *See* hygienist, dental.

density (den'-si'-tē) The ratio of mass to volume; such as the less air remaining in investment after mixing, the more solid is the finished material; its density has been increased.

dental arch The horseshoe-shaped curve made by the bony projection, gums, and teeth of either the upper or lower jaw.

dentifrice (den'-ti-fris) A cleanser used for brushing the teeth. It may be a powder or paste. It is usually flavored and may contain medicaments for specific purposes in mouth care. (For example, caries preventives, oxygenating agents, antiseptics, etc.)

dentin, dentine (den'-tin) Calcified hard tissue forming the main body of the tooth. The dentin has innumerable tiny canals, many fibers which make the junction of the enamel with the dentin a very sensitive area. Dentin is slightly elastic, although not visibly so, and is very strong.

dentinocemental junction (den'-ti-nō-se-men'-tal) That junction of the inner surface of the cementum with the dentin.

dentition (den-ti'-shun) 1. The natural teeth in their normal position in the dental arches. 2. The process of eruption of the teeth through the alveolar ridge and gum.

  dentition, deciduous (*also* primary dentition) (dē-sid'-ū-us) The twenty teeth of childhood which are normally replaced by permanent teeth (second dentition). Syn: deciduous teeth, primary teeth, milk teeth, baby teeth.

  dentition, mixed 1. The teeth found in the dental arch after some of the permanent teeth have erupted but while some of the deciduous teeth are still present. 2. The teeth found in the dental arch when some are natural teeth and some are artificial.

  dentition, permanent (Secondary dentition, permanent teeth) The teeth of adulthood which erupt as the primary teeth are shed and which replace or add to the dentition. (There are 32 teeth in a complete set.)

dentoenamel junction That junction of the inner surface of the enamel crown with the dentin. Syn: amelodentinal junction.

denture (den'-tūr) An entire set of teeth—either natural or artificial, deciduous or permanent.

  artificial denture Substitute for natural teeth.

  immediate denture Substitute for natural teeth inserted at time of extraction of remaining natural teeth.

partial denture Substitute for part of natural dentition of either arch.

dermatitis (der-ma-tī'-tis) Inflammation of the skin.

dermatosis (der-ma-tō'-sis) (pl. dermatoses [sēz]) A disease, any disease, of the skin can be called dermatosis.

detergent (dē-ter'-gent) A cleanser. There are several types of detergents, with some differences in their actions, but all are cleansers.

diabetes (dī-uh-bē'-tēz) An inheritable disease, the cause of which is unknown. The islet cells of the pancreas fail to produce insulin. The body tissues fail to oxidize carbohydrate at a normal rate. There is excess sugar in the blood, sugar in the urine, excessive passage of urine, excessive thirst, deficiency in insulin, weakness, increased susceptibility to infection, and in advanced states, coma.

  A diabetic is likely to have multiple periodontal abscesses.

diagnose (dī'-ag-nōs) To recognize the nature of a disease, to make a diagnosis of.

diagnosis (dī'-ag-nō-sis) 1. The art of determining one disease from another. 2. The conclusions arrived at.

diaphoretic (dī"-uh-for-ret'-ik) A drug or medicine which increases perspiration.

diastema (dī"-uh-stē'-mah) A spacing between the teeth. This word usually is used in speaking about deciduous anterior teeth. Occasionally the condition is present in the permanent dentition.

die An exact reproduction regardless of material used, of an original object. In dentistry it commonly refers to the reproduction of an individual tooth (die) on which a restoration may be constructed (such as a wax pattern).

diet (dī'-et) The food and drink consumed by a person during a day. It is not the same as nutrition. Some of the diet may not be utilized by the body.

diplococcus (dip"-lō-kok'-us) Gram positive, elongated bacteria cells growing in pairs or short chains. They are usually parasitic.

direct technique *See* technique, direct.

disease (di'-zēz) Illness or sickness; any state other than that of good health.

  acute disease Illness which appears suddenly and lasts a short time.

  chronic disease Illness which progresses slowly and continues over a long period of time.

disinfectant (dis"-in-fek'-tant) An agent, usually a chemical substance, which destroys or inhibits the microorganisms causing disease.

dislocation (dis-lō-kā′-shun) The displacement of any part of the body (especially bones) from the normal position. (Out of location.)

distal (dis′-tal) Away from the median line or center—thus, the distal side of a tooth is that which is away from the median line of the face or the back surface of a posterior tooth.

diuretic (dī″-ū-ret′-ik) An agent which increases the secretion of urine.

D.M.D. Abbreviation for Doctor of Dental Medicine, a degree granted by some dental colleges, similar to Doctor of Dental Surgery.

dram, drachm (dram) A unit of weight. It equals 1/8 part of an apothecaries′ ounce, or 60 grains. Symbol 3.

drug Any crude medicinal substance; a medicine.

duct (dukt) A passage with well-defined walls such as a tube for saliva to flow from the salivary gland to the mouth.

ductile (duk′-tal) Capable of being drawn out thinly into a wire, such as copper or gold.

dysfunction (dis-funk′-shun) Malfunction. Any impairment or abnormality of the normal working of a part of the body.

dyspnea (disp′-nē-ah) Difficult breathing, labored breathing.

E

ecchymosis (ek-i-mō′-sis) Bleeding into the tissues under the skin. The skin is discolored to purple, which gradually changes to brown, green, and yellow—such as a "black" eye or "black and blue" mark.

edema (i-dē′-mah) When tissue fluid collects in a large amount in one place in the body there is a swelling known as edema. It is commonly noticed around the ankles of some pregnant women, some people with cardiac conditions, and persons having dropsy.

edematous (i-dem′-ah-tus) Affected by edema.

edentulous (ē-den′-tū-lus) Without teeth.

elastic (ē-las′-tik) Adjective: Capable of being stretched and then returning to its original shape.

elastic limit. When any material is stretched beyond the point where it will return to its original shape, that point is known as the elastic limit.

elastic memory Capacity of a material to return to its original shape. The material is warmed, shaped, cooled, and then rewarmed. Upon rewarming, it returns to its original shape.

elastics (orthodontics) A rubber band used to apply force to teeth for orthodontic purposes.

electron (ē-lek′-tron) More frequently it is a unit of negatively charged electricity called a nega-

tron. It is a necessary part of all atoms. It is sometimes a positively charged unit of electricity called a positron.

embolus (em′-buh-lus) A blood clot or other foreign matter which travels in a bloodstream, lodges in some blood vessel, and obstructs the flow of blood.

embrasure (em-brā′-zhur) The opening with sloping sides formed by the adjacent surfaces of teeth.

empyema (em″-pī-ē′-ma) The presence of pus in a cavity, space, or hollow organ.

emulsion (e-mul′-zhun) Two liquids are mixed, but they will not blend. For example, oil and milk will not blend when poured in the same container. The oil remains in small particles.

emulsion, photographic A suspension of silver halide salts impregnated in gelatin and used to make radiographic film.

enamel (ē-nam′-l) The surface of the crown, which you see, is enamel, the hardest material in the body. The enamel forms a shell, covering the crown or coronal portion of the tooth. It varies in thickness, being heaviest on the chewing or biting surface of the tooth, and becoming thin toward that part of the crown which is farthest from the chewing or biting surface. The enamel consists of microscopic "rods." Calcium and phosphorus make up approximately ninety percent of the enamel. The rest is made up of other materials, plus a small amount of organic matter.

endocrine glands (en′-du-krin) Glands inside the body which do not have ducts. They are often called the *ductless glands*. They secrete hormones directly into the bloodstream. The endocrine glands which are known are pituitary, adrenals, parathyroids, thyroid, islet cells of the pancreas, and certain cells of the gonads. There are two glands which are not as well documented. They are the thymus and the pineal. They may be discovered to belong to the endocrine family.

endodontics (en″-dō-don′-tiks) Branch of dentistry which cares for teeth no longer vital or with severely damaged pulps.

enzyme (en′-zīm) An organic compound, frequently a protein, which can by catalytic action promote a chemical change.

epilepsy (ep′-i′-lep″-sē) A chronic disease in which the patient has convulsive seizures with loss of consciousness. A seizure may last from 5 to 20 minutes. A patient who gives a history of taking Dilantin sodium is subject to epilepsy.

epithelium (ep″-i-thē′-lē-um) The covering of the skin and mucous membranes.

epulis (ep-ū′-lis) Any benign neoplasm of the gingiva, usually pedunculated and raised, like a small toadstool.

erosion (ē-rō′-zhun) In dentistry the destruction of superficial layers of the tooth at the neck beginning with the enamel and working inward. It is probably due to a combination of chemical action and abrasion. The cavities have dense and polished surfaces.

eruption (ē-rup′-shun) The process of a new tooth entering the mouth from its place of formation.

erythema (er-uh-thē′-ma) Abnormal redness of the skin. An acute inflammatory reaction seen in the skin and sometimes in mucous membranes. Cause is unknown, although hypersensitivity and virus infection have been suggested as possibilities.

   E. multiforme complex An acute inflammation characterized by various lesions of the skin and mucosa.

ether (ē-ther) An inhalation anesthetic used for general anesthesia.

ethical (eth′-i-kal) In accordance with the rules governing the conduct of a specific group. Ethical conduct for dental assistants would mean observing the correct standards of conduct set for the profession. One example would be keeping as confidential all information learned about a patient.

ethics (eth′-iks) The science of right conduct.

ethyl chloride (eth′-il klō′-rīd) A colorless, inflammable liquid used as a local anesthetic. It is applied in a spray and its effect is of short duration. (CH_3CH_2Cl)

ethylene (eth′-i-lēn) A colorless gas used as a general anesthetic. It is inhaled.

etiology (ē-tē-ol′-ō-gē) The study or science related to the cause of any disease.

examination (eks-am-i-nā′-shun) In dentistry, a careful inspection to determine (or diagnose) the conditions which exist in a patient's mouth.

exfoliation (eks′-fō-lē-ā-shun) Shedding. Thus, in dentistry, the shedding of a tooth.

exfoliation time Refers to the proper age at which the shedding of primary dentition should occur.

exodontics, exodontia (eks″-ō-don′-tiks, eks″-ō-don′-she-ah) The art and science of the removal of teeth.

exodontia sponge A folded square of sterile gauze used to remove debris, blood, and mucus in oral surgery, usually 2″ x 2″.

exostosis (eks-os-tō′-sis) Overgrowth of bone projecting outward from the usual surface; the most common are the tori, bony protuberances occurring along the midline of the hard palate in about twenty percent of the population (this protuberance is called a torus palatinus), and the bilateral or unilateral protuberances occurring on the lingual surface of the mandible in the premolar region in about seven percent of the population (torus mandibularis).

expectorate (eks-pek′-tō-rāt) To spit.

expiration (eks′-pir-ā-shun) The act of expelling air from the lungs.

expire (eks-pīr) Cessation. A person is said to expire when he dies.

explorer (eks-plor′-er) An instrument with a sharp point, in various shapes, used to test the surface of the tooth for cavity formation.

eye tooth The cuspid tooth of the upper arch.

F

facebow A mechanism used together with an articulator to construct dentures that will work together in the same relationship as do the patient's dental arches.

facial (fā′-shal) Referring to the face. Refers to those surfaces of the upper and lower teeth toward the lips and cheeks.

facial surface See surface.

facing (fā-sing) A piece of plastic or porcelain shaped to replace the outer surface of a tooth. It may be reinforced by gold and restores the full form of the natural tooth.

Fahrenheit scale (fah′-ren-hīt) Another method of scaling temperatures. The scale has 180° between the freezing and boiling points of water. Freezing is 32° and boiling 212°. To change F to C: $C = (F-32) \times 5/9$.

faint See syncopé.

false teeth Correctly called dentures.

febrile (feb′-ril) Relating to fever or feverish. A synonym for fever.

fibroma (fī-brō′-mah) A benign neoplasm of fibrous connective tissue.

filled plastic Filling material is composed of two phases (plastic and filler) like the composite, but they are not bonded together and hence do not complement each other's physical properties.

fissure (fish′-ūr) A long, narrow fault in the surface of a tooth caused by imperfect joining of the enamel of different lobes.

fistula (fis′-tū-lah) A deep, sinuous ulcer or canal-like tube into the cavity of an alveolar abscess.

flora (flō'-ruh) Bacteria living in various parts of the digestive tract.

floss (dental) Heavy nylon or silk cord, waxed or unwaxed. It is used to clean between the teeth. Some dentists also use it to hold a rubber dam in position at the neck of a tooth. Dental tape is the same as floss except that tape is wider and more ribbonlike.

flow Continuous movement. The change in shape of a material when placed under a given load, such as wax or amalgam.

fluorescence (flur-es'-ens) When some objects are exposed to X rays, they emit light. They emit light only as long as they are being irradiated. The ability to emit this light is referred to as fluorescence.

fluoridation (flur″-i-dā'-shun) Adding fluorides to the water supply of any community to aid in control of dental caries. The recommended concentration is one part fluoride per million parts of water.

fluoroscope (flur'-uh-skōp) An apparatus used in a darkened room with X ray to see on the fluorescent screen that which would be visible on a radiograph. No film is used, but the radiologist reads the results on the fluorescent screen. When he wishes, he has a radiograph made. Most commonly used to diagnose the conditions in the digestive system.

fluorosis (flur-ō'-sus) When an individual consumes excessive fluorides in drinking water during the development of teeth, pitting occurs on the enamel surface which is easily stained by foods. This pitting is called mottling of the enamel. This condition is called fluorosis and is chronic fluoride poisoning.

focus (fō'-kus) of infection. The center of a disease from which the infection and its products are spread throughout the body through the circulatory system.

follicle (fol'-li-kl) A small sac enclosing a developing tooth.

foramen (for-ā'-men) A hole in bone.

  mental foramen A foramen in the lower jaw for the mental nerve and vessels.

forceps (for'-seps) An instrument with 2 blades and 2 handles, like pliers, used to take out teeth.

fordyce's spots (for'-dīs-es) Harmless, brownish, slightly raised spots on the oral mucosa or lips, found in more than seventy percent of the population. Erroneously called Fordyce's disease.

formaldehyde (for-mal'-duh-hīd) A liquid which is colorless and volatile. It is used as a preservative and a general antiseptic.

fossa (fos'-sah) A round or angular depression, pit, or hollow on the surface of a tooth, usually in the lingual surfaces of the anterior teeth and in the occlusal surfaces of the bicuspids and molars.

fracture (frak'-chur) The breaking of a part, especially with reference to bone.

free gum margin That portion of the unattached gum encircling the neck of a tooth. Somewhat like a short cuff, usually not more than 1/16 inch in height. Also called free gingiva.

frenum (fre'-num) (pl., frena) A weblike fold of the integument or mucous membrane that limits the movements of an organ or part. There are frenii inside the middle of each lip connecting the lips to the gum and one under the tongue connecting the tongue to the floor of the mouth. It is called lingual frenum. Frena contain no muscle tissue.

fulcrum (ful'-krum) A point at which an action of balance or movement occurs. Therefore, the jaw pivot is a fulcrum.

fusion (fū'-zhun) The act of melting; uniting as by melting together.

G

gastrointestinal (gas'-trō-in-tes'-ti-nal) *Gastro* means "stomach," and thus gastrointestinal refers to both the stomach and the intestines.

germicidal Destructive to germs.

germicide An agent that destroys germs. Same as bactericide.

gingiva (jin'-ji-vah) (pl., gingivae) The part of the oral mucous membrane which is located nearest the neck of the tooth and covers the alveolar process; pale pink color when healthy; and when wiped dry, appears to be finely stippled, somewhat like a very fine sandpaper.

gingival line (jin'-ji-val) The line which marks the limit of the gingival crest around the tooth. It gradually moves from a position above the cervical line of the tooth crownwise toward the root of the tooth as age advances.

gingival crevice The space between the cervical enamel of a tooth and the free gum margin (or the overlying unattached gingiva). Also called subgingival space.

gingival papillae Projections of gum tissue that fill or nearly fill the interproximal spaces.

gingivitis Any inflammation of the gingiva (gum).

gingivitis, necrotizing ulcerative Also known as fusospirochetal gingivitis, trench mouth, ulcerative gingivitis, ulceromembranous gingivitis,

Vincent's gingivitis, Vincent's infection. An inflammation of the gingivae characterized by death of the interdental papillae (the pointed area of the gum which rises between teeth), ulceration of the gingival margins, and in cases of more severe infection by the appearance of a false or pseudomembrane, the entire mouth painful and tender, with a foul odor.

gland An organ which manufactures and secretes a specific product—as salivary glands manufacture and secrete saliva or a sweat gland manufactures and secretes sweat.

glossitis (glos-ī'-tis) Inflammation of the tongue.

gold foil Gold foil is basically in the same physical form as you associate with aluminum foil except that it is the thinnest sheet of metal made, about 1/10 the thickness of the average human hair.

gram A unit of weight in the metric system. One pound contains 454 grams. One kilogram is 1,000 grams.

granulation tissue (gran-ū-lā'-shun) New tissue found in the early stages of healing.

granuloma (gran-ū-lō'-mah) A dental granuloma may be found on the root of a tooth as a small mass of granulation tissue containing bacterial deposits.

groove A shallow, elongated depression in a tooth or bone. (Also called a sulcus.)

   developmental g A fine depressed line in the enamel of the tooth. When the tooth was developing, the lobes developed separately and joined when they had grown large enough. This fine line marks the union of the lobes of the crown.

H

halide (hal'-īd) A chemical element of the halogen group combined with a more electropositive element or radical.

hard palate An area forming the roof of the mouth which has a hard, bony support. It also forms the floor of the nasal passages.

harelip A split or cleft in the upper lip. An individual may have one or may have two. The cleft is congenital (present at birth).

hemihydrate (hem-i-hī'-drāt) The chemical form of plaster or artificial stone before being mixed with water.

hemoglobin (hē'-muh-glō-bin) The oxygen-carrying red pigment of the red blood cells. It is an iron-containing protein.

hemorrhage (hem'-or-āj) In Greek: *blood* plus *to burst forth*. Bleeding.

hemostat (hē-mō-stat) An instrument used to check hemorrhage. The instrument somewhat resembles a scissors, with flat serrated beaks, and can be locked in closed position over a cut or bleeding capillary, artery, or vein.

hemostatic agent Any drug used to arrest hemorrhage.

hepatitis, infectious (hep-uh-tī'-tus, in-fek'-shus) Hepatitis is inflammation of the liver. Infectious hepatitis is a viral hepatitis which can be epidemic, has an incubation period of 7-28 days, and even 50 days. It may be transmitted by human serum through transfusions and hypodermic injections. Autoclaving is the only safe method of sterilizing instruments to guard against transmitting this disease.

herpes simplex (her-pēz sim-plex) An infection caused by the virus of the same name. When it occurs on the lips, it is a cold sore; when it occurs on the mucosa, it is called herpetic gingivostomatitis, which may become acute.

histology (hiss-tahl'-uh-gē) A branch of anatomy which studies the minute structure and composition of plant and animal tissues which are discernible with the microscope.

homogeneity (hō-mō-gi-nē'-i-tē) The quality or state of being uniform in structure or composition throughout.

homogeneous (hō-mō-jē'-nē-us) Greek: *Same kind*. Uniform, similar in makeup throughout.

hormone (hor'-mōn) A biochemical secretion of the endocrine glands which partially regulates the functional activity of organs, tissues, other glands, or the nervous system. The blood carries the hormones from the gland which produces them to the parts of the body which need them.

horn, pulpal A small projection of pulp tissue which lies directly under a cusp or lobe of a tooth.

hydrated (hī-drā-ted) Combined with water, forming a hydrate or a hydroxide.

hydrocal (hī-drō-kal) A trade name for artificial stone made from gypsum and used for making casts.

hydrocolloid A material used in dentistry for making an accurate impression (negative) for certain types of dental restorations such as partial dentures, inlays, crowns, or bridgework. It is liquefied by heating to the temperature of boiling water and is solidified by cooling the tray which holds it while taking the impression (water-cooled trays).

hygiene (hī'-jēn) The science of health and how to preserve it.

hygienist, dental (hī-jēn'-ist) A person trained and licensed by the state in which he lives to practice dental prophylaxis under the direction of a licensed dentist.

hygroscopic (hī-gruh-skahp'-ik) Able to absorb moisture. Such a material has so strong an affinity for water that it absorbs moisture from the air to an unusual degree.

hypercementosis (hī"-per-cē"-mēn-tō'-sis) An excessive formation of cementum usually at the apical portion of the root of a tooth, giving a bulbous appearance to the root tip.

hyperplasia (hī-per-plā'-zhē-uh) An abnormal increase in the *number* of cells in normal arrangement in tissue. The tissue thickens or enlarges. One of the possible reactions of tissue to irritation, injury, or drugs; for example, continued long-term intake of Dilantin to control epileptic seizure may cause the formation of hyperplastic gingival tissue (Dilantin enlargement).

hypersecretion (hī-per-sē-krē'-shun) Hyper means increase, thus increased secretion or excessive secretion. Excessive discharge of the liquid which the gland manufactures or stores.

hypersensitive (hī-per-sen-si-tiv) Abnormally sensitive, i.e., more sensitive than average.

hypertrophy (hī'-per-trō-fē) Greek: *overnutrition.* The abnormal increase in the *size* of the cells of a tissue, resulting in an enlargement or thickening of the tissue. True or physiologic hypertrophy results from excessive activity of muscle: for example, exercise makes a muscle larger.

hypnosis (hip-nō'-sis) The science of artificially induced sleep, or a trance induced by drugs, psychology, or both.

hypnotic (hip-not-ik) 1. Inducing sleep. 2. Pertaining to hypnotism. 3. Sleep may be induced by certain drugs which produce normal sleep.

hypo- (hī'-pō) Beneath, under, insufficient.

hypoplasia (hī-pō-plā'-zē-ah) Greek: *hypo* means "under" and *plasia* means "formation." Incomplete or defective development of any tissue. In dentistry, mostly associated with enamel hypoplasia: pits or ringlike grooves left in enamel due to interference with the function of the ameloblasts (enamel-forming cells) at the particular time this area was being formed. Hypoplasia is often associated with a highly infectious illness with high temperature. The age at which this occurred can be estimated quite accurately by the position of the defect.

hypothyroidism (hī-pō-thī'-roid-izm) Insufficient secretion from the thyroid gland. It lowers the basal metabolism rate, reduces growth, produces lethargy and a tendency to obesity. In children it may produce cretinism. Teeth may erupt late. In adults it may produce myxedema.

I

idiosyncrasy (id-ē-ō-sin'-krah-sē) A characteristic which is peculiar to an individual. An abnormal response to a drug, food, or cosmetic. This reaction may be quite violent.

immune (im-ūn) Latin: *safe.* Protected against a specific disease. It may be "natural" immunity or produced by vaccination or inoculation.

impaction (im-pak-shun) Confinement of a tooth in the jaw so that its eruption is prevented. May be complete or partial.

impression (im-presh'-un) A metal band for a single tooth, or a tray full of "impression material" is placed over the teeth and ridges of either dental arch and allowed to "set." The hollows and grooves so formed (a negative) are called an impression or mold, and this may be filled with a stone mixture to form a cast, or positive.

impulse (im'-puls) An uncontrollable wave of excitation transmitted through tissues, especially nerve fibers and muscles following a stimulus. The result is physiological activity or inhibition of an activity.

incisal (in-sī-zal) Cutting.

incisal edge The cutting edge of an anterior tooth formed where the labial and lingual enamel plates join.

incisal papilla or palatine papilla The hump in the median line behind the two central incisors forming the front part of the hard palate which forms a pad protecting the anterior palatine foramen.

incisor A tooth with an incisal (cutting) edge. Man has four incisors in each dental arch. They are "anterior" teeth.

inclination (in-kli-nā'-shun) Tilting. To say "A tooth is mesially inclined" means it is tilted to the mesial.

infection (in-fek'-shun) Invasion of tissues by pathogenic microorganisms followed by a typical reaction in the area of invasion.

inferior (in-fē'-rē-or) Below or lower.

infiltration (in-fil-trā'-shun) To pass through or into by filtering or permeating. To permeate by penetrating.

inlay (in'-lay) A filling made outside the mouth in the shape of the preparation cut in the tooth. When it has been finished, it is cemented into the tooth. Inlaid as in woodworking.

insulator (in-sah-lā-tor)   Any material which will prevent the transfer of heat, electricity, or sound. In dentistry, cements may be used as insulators against extreme changes in temperature.

interdental space   The space between two neighboring approximating teeth.

internal   Within or inside.

interproximal space (in-ter-proks'-i″-mul)   Situated between the proximal surfaces of adjoining teeth of the same arch. Same as interdental space.

intramuscular (in-trah-mus'-kū-lar)   Latin: *within muscle*. Inside the substance of a muscle.

intravenous (in-trah-ve'-nus)   Into the vein, in the vein, or from within the vein.

investing   The process of placing investment material, of covering or enveloping an object to be cast, cured, or soldered.

investment   1. Material enclosing the wax pattern for crowns, inlays, and dentures while they are being cast or processed. 2. Material enclosing parts to be soldered. It is usually some form of plaster.

ion (ī'-on)   An atom which carries a positive or negative electrical charge because it has lost or gained one or more electrons.

ionization (ī″-un-ī-zā'-shun)   This refers to the process of being ionized.

ionize (ī'-un-īz)   To convert partly or wholly into ions.

K

kilovolt (kil'-uh-volt)   A thousand volts. Refers to the quality of penetration of the X-radiation.

Koplik's spots (Kop'-liks)   The oral lesions of measles (Rubeola). Small white or bluish-white spots surrounded by a red area, occurring on the mucous membrane of the lips and buccal mucosa before the actual outbreak of the usual skin symptoms.

L

labial (lā'-bē-al)   Pertaining to the lips.

labial commissure   The thin connecting fold at the corners of the lips. It is quite tender. Protect during dental operations with a very light coating of vaseline to prevent soreness.

labial surface   That surface of an anterior **tooth** which is next to the lips.

labiomental groove (lā-bē-ō-men'-tal)   A groove running parallel to the lower lip and slightly below it.

laboratory stone   *See* artificial stone.

lactobacillus (lak-tō-buh-sil'-us)   Bacteria which forms lactic acid.

lancet (lan'-set)   A small, two-edged, pointed surgical knife.

lesion (lē-zhun)   Latin: *to hurt*. Any change in continuity of a tissue due to disease or injury, or the loss of function of a part.

leukemia (lū-kē'-mē-ah)   Greek: *white blood*. A fatal disease of the blood-forming organs, showing as a severe increase in the number of white blood cells and an increase in size or activity of the blood-forming organs.

leukoplakia (lū-kō-plā'-kē-ah)   A white, opaque, leathery plaque formed on the oral mucous membrane. Considered premalignant. Resembles lichen planus in appearance; differentiated by biopsy.

lichen planus (lī'-ken plan-us)   A disease of unknown etiology affecting either skin or oral mucous membranes, sometimes both together. The oral lesion appears on the buccal mucous membrane most commonly, a lacy pattern of raised bluish-white or white porcelain-like fine lines or dots. Painless and harmless. Distinguished from leukoplakia by biopsy (the removal of a small tissue sample from the suspect area for the purpose of microscopic examination).

ligature (lig'-uh-chur)   A cord, thread, or wire used to tie off or bind. One type is used to hold rubber dam in place. Another type is used in an orthodontic appliance.

ligature wire (ortho)   Steel filaments of several diameters are used to bind teeth together. The size of the filament is determined by the orthodontist for the particular work he wishes to accomplish. The purpose of binding the teeth together is to stabilize and immobilize or to produce minor movements.

linear (lin'-ē-er)   Straight, or involving a single dimension. Thus a straight line is linear.

lingual (lin'-gual)   Refers to the tongue.

lingual frenum   A weblike fold of mucosa from the under surface of the tongue to the floor of the mouth near the lower front teeth, along the midline, restricting extension of the tongue.

lingual surface   The surface of any tooth which is next to the tongue. All teeth have a lingual surface.

lobe (lōb)   A somewhat rounded projection or division of an organ of the body or a gland.

local   Restricted to one spot or area. Not general.

local anesthetic   *See* anesthetic.

M

malaise (ma-lāz')   This is the French word for *illness*. Any indisposition, discomfort, or distress.

malar (mā'-lar)   Referring to the cheek or cheek bone.

malignant (mah-lig′-nant) A term used to describe a neoplasm in the human body which will kill the human. Most people use the term as "a malignant tumor"—meaning a cancer which must be completely removed if the individual is to continue living.

malleable (mal′-ē-ah-bl) Latin: *to hammer.* Susceptible to being beaten or hammered out into a thin plate or sheet. Gold is extremely malleable.

malocclusion (mal″-ō-klū′-shun) *Mal* in Latin means "ill." Poor positioning of the teeth so that they interfere with best efficiency during mastication. Malocclusion can usually be corrected by correcting the articulation of the teeth through orthodontic procedures.

malpractice Latin: *bad* plus *practice.* Unskillful or faulty medical or dental treatment.

mamelon, mammelon (mam′-e-lon) One of the three rounded prominences on the incisal edge of a newly erupted incisor.

mandible The horseshoe-shaped bone forming the lower jaw. It provides support for lower teeth and provides places for attachment of various muscles which make it possible to chew. Also called the inferior maxilla.

mandrel A shaft which holds a tool for rotation.

margin The bounding line or border of a surface of a tooth or a cavity.

marginal ridge An elevation of enamel known as the margin of a surface of a tooth.

masticate Chew.

mastication The act of chewing food.

materia alba Soft white matter often found on the necks of teeth when not properly cleansed.

materia medica Latin: *medical material.* A branch of medical study dealing with the sources, uses, and preparation of drugs.

matrix (mā′-tricks) In *biomaterials:* the matrix refers to the continuous phase of the material which holds, and in amalgam, silicate, or composites, bonds to the dispersed phase (unreacted particles or filler). In *restorative dentistry:* a matrix is an instrument or device used to replace the missing walls of the cavity, provide form and contour, and retain the restorative material as it is being placed and allowed to harden in the cavity.

maturation (mach-uh-rā′-shun) The time or point at which something is fully developed—or fully grown.

maxilla One of a pair of bones forming the upper jaw (superior maxilla).

median (mē′-dē-an) In the middle—dividing into two equal halves.

median line An imaginary line dividing the body into right and left halves.

medication (med-i-kā′-shun) A drug or substance used to treat a disease. Also, the process of medicating.

medicine 1. Any drug or substance used to treat disease. 2. The art of healing.

medicine, oral The specialty in dentistry which concerns itself with the significance and relationship of oral and systemic diseases.

mental Latin: *mind* and *chin.* 1. Refers to the chin. 2. Refers to the mind.

mental foramen (men-tal fo-rā′-men) *See* foramen.

mercury (mer′-kur-ē) (quicksilver) A liquid metallic element. It is combined with silver alloy to make silver amalgam for filling teeth.

mesial (mē′-zē-al) Greek: *middle.* Toward the median line following the curve of the dental arch.

mesial surface Surface of the tooth following the dental arch nearest the median line.

metabolism (me-tab′-ō-lizm) Greek: *change.* The process by which the body changes food into material which can be used by the body to rebuild tissue or to provide energy.

metal A chemical element which is opaque, fusible, malleable, ductile, typically lustrous, and possesses the ability to conduct electricity and heat.

metastasis (meh-tas′-tuh-sis) The transfer of disease from one organ or one place in the body to another organ or another place by diseased cells or pathogenic organisms via the blood or lymph streams.

method, indirect The formation of a wax pattern by taking an impression in the patient's mouth and working up the wax pattern *outside* the mouth (indirect) as opposed to direct method when the pattern is made in the mouth on the patient's tooth.

microorganisms (mī-krō-or′-ga-nizms) Tiny (or minute) living organisms, including bacteria, viruses, rickettsiae, yeasts, and fungi. They may be part of the normal flora without producing disease, but they may also overgrow and produce disease. It is possible that organisms which are foreign to the individual may produce disease.

microscope (mī′-krō-skōp) An instrument through which objects too small to be seen with the naked eye can be viewed.

microscopic (mī-krō-skop′-ik) Something so small that it can be seen only by assisting normal vision is said to be microscopic. Very tiny in size.

milleroentgen (mil-ē-rahnt'-gen) One one-thousandth of a roentgen.

milliammeter (mil-ē-am'-i-ter) A meter which indicates the milliamperes flowing in an X-ray tube.

milliampere (mil-ē-am'-per) One one-thousandth of an ampere. In X ray it is used to indicate the amount of current flowing in the X-ray circuit. When combined with seconds (time measurement), it is an indication of the quantity of roentgen ray.

mineral (min'-er'al) A substance not derived from plant or animal life, usually a solid.

model (mah'-del) A positive reproduction of any part of a tooth or dental arch made by filling an impression with a molding material. *See* cast and impression.

molar (mō'-lar) One of the grinding teeth found in the back of the mouth. They have three or more cusps. There are twelve molars in the upper and lower dental arches—first, second, and third molars in each quadrant. The first molar refers to the six-year molar. The second molar is the twelve-year molar. The third molar is the wisdom tooth. The terms first, second, and third molar are preferred terminology.

mold guide A group of porcelain or plastic teeth supplied by a manufacturer of artificial teeth. There is a tooth in each size and shape variation made by that firm. The dentist (and his patient) can select the correct tooth size and shape for the appliance or replacements to be made.

molecule (mahl'-i-kyul) The smallest part of an element or compound which is capable of keeping its chemical identity with the substance in mass.

morphology (mor-fol'-ō-jē) The science which deals with structure and form of organic beings in all their variations and in all stages. (*See* microbiology.)

mottled enamel. Due to excessive intake of fluoride during tooth development. *See* fluorosis.

mucin (mū'-sin) From mucous membranes originate various proteins which are called mucin.

mucobuccal fold The space or troughlike area between the gums and cheek. The little trough between the gingivae and the inner surface of the cheek.

mucocele (mū'-kō-sēl) A dilated gland or duct filled with mucous secretion.

mucosa (mū-kō-sah) The mucous membrane.

mucus (mū'-kus) A viscid, watery secretion which covers all mucous membranes.

mucous gland Glands occurring in all mucous membrane.

mucous membrane Pink to red tissue lining the mouth and other areas. It contains many tiny glands which secrete mucus, a viscid, watery secretion.

N

narcotic (nar-kot'-ik) A drug which relieves pain while it tends to produce stupor or sleep at the same time, depending on the dosage.

nasal Refers to the nose.

nausea (naw'-sē-ah) Latin: *seasickness.* Sickness at the stomach, together with a tendency to vomit.

necrosis (nē-krō'-sis) Greek: *deadness of a certain portion of tissue,* not the entire body. Dental necrosis is decay of a tooth.

necrotic (nē-krot'-ik) Referring to (or affected with) necrosis.

neoplasm (nē'-ō-plasm) Greek: *new formation.* Any abnormal new growth, such as a tumor.

nevus (nē'-vus) A congenital malformation seen occasionally on the oral mucosa; can be vascular similar to a birthmark) or nonvascular with pigmentation. Some types can develop into malignancies.

nitrogen (nī'-trō-gen) An odorless, tasteless, colorless gaseous element which constitutes 78% of the atmosphere by volume. It is a constituent of all living tissues.

nitrous oxide (nī-trus ox'-īd) A colorless gas (N_2O) with a sweet taste and pleasant odor. It is used for minor surgery. It produces unconsciousness by temporary asphyxiation. It is also called laughing gas.

nomenclature (nō'-men-klā-tur) Latin: *name* plus *to call.* Terminology. A system of names in a particular science, art, or field of knowledge.

normal flora *See* flora.

notation (nō-tā'-shun) A system of designating teeth by figures, letters, and/or signs. (*See* notating teeth for the various systems of notation.)

O

occlude (ok-lūd') To fit close together. To shut.

occlusal (ok-lū'-sal) Refers to closing or shutting the masticating surfaces of the teeth (the occlusal surfaces).

occlusal surface The masticating surface of a bicuspid or molar tooth. This surface is in contact with the opposing dental arch when the jaws are closed.

occlusion The contact of the teeth of both jaws when closed or during the movements of the mandible in mastication.

balanced occlusion An ideal relationship of the teeth in both dental arches to each other during all the movements of the mandible as well as in centric closure.

centric occlusion Contact relationships of the teeth when the jaws are closed in normal position (subject to various interpretations).

malocclusion Any variation from the so-called normal relationships of the teeth (see malocclusion).

traumatic occlusion Malocclusion of the teeth which results in injury to the teeth, or the tissue either surrounding or underlying the teeth.

odontalgia (ō-don-tal'-jē-ah) Greek: *tooth* plus *pain*. Toothache.

odontoblast (ō-don'-tō-blast) Greek: *tooth* plus *germ*. A dentin-forming cell. Specialized connective tissue cells that develop the dentin and maintain its nutrition and translucency.

odontoma (ō-don-tō'-mah) Greek: *tooth* plus *tumor*. A tumor which is toothlike in structure. Some form at the time the tooth is developing. Some attack the tooth later. There are several types, each attacking a different part of the tooth.

opaque (ō-pāk') That which blocks light. Light rays cannot penetrate.

radiopaque That which blocks X ray (*See* radiolucent).

operation An act performed with the hands or instruments. In the dental office it usually refers to surgical procedures.

operatory A room in which dental treatment is performed.

optimum (op'-ti-mum) The most favorable conditions for any activity or function.

oral Refers to the mouth.

oral cavity The space which is enclosed by the lips in front, the cheeks on either side, the palate above, and the floor of the mouth below. Restricted sense: space enclosed by the teeth, when closed together, with the palate above, and the floor of the mouth below.

oral hygiene The science of health and its preservation, as related to the mouth.

oral medicine *See* medicine, oral.

oral pathology The study of diseases of the mouth.

oral surgery Surgery of the mouth (a special field of surgery or dentistry).

oral vestibule *See* mucobuccal fold.

organism (or'-gan-izm) An individual constituted to live by means of organs which are separate in function but mutually dependent.

orthodontics (or'-thō'-don-tiks) That branch of dentistry which deals with the causes, prevention, and treatment of the irregularities or malocclusion of the teeth and arches.

osmosis (ah-smō'-sis) When two solutions are separated by a membrane, the solvents from the lesser pass to the greater concentration. This movement of the solvent is called osmosis.

osteoblasts (os'-tē-ō-blasts) Greek: *bone* plus *germ*. Bone-forming cells. Any cell active in producing bone or any cell which develops into bone.

osteoclast (os'-tē-ō-klast) Greek: *bone* plus *break*. A large, multinuclei which absorbs and destroys bone.

osteology (ahs-tē-ahl'-uh-gē) Is the scientific study of bones and their structures.

oxidation (oxs-i-dā'-shun) The act of oxidizing or combining with oxygen.

oxidizing agent Anything which produces oxidation (such as the excess of oxygen in the flame of a blowtorch applied to casting gold).

oxygen A colorless, odorless, gaseous element which combines readily with most elements. It is necessary to all animal and vegetable life and for combustion. It makes up 20% by weight of the atmosphere and about 88% of water.

P

palatal (pal'-ah-tal) Refers to the roof of the mouth.

palate (pal'-at) Roof of the mouth.

hard palate The front and larger portion of the roof of the mouth is hard because it is formed by a bony arch.

soft palate That smaller portion toward the throat from which the uvula is suspended.

palatine (pal'-uh-tīn) Refers to the palate.

palliative treatment (pal'-ē-ā-tiv) Giving relief, but not curing a disease.

pallor Paleness, lack of color.

papilloma (pap-il-ō'-mah) An epithelial tumor, mushroom- or finger-like in appearance, found in other epithelial tissue (a wart is a papilloma).

parotid gland (pah-rot'-id) Greek: *near* plus *ear*. A gland in front and below the ear which produces saliva, entering the mouth through Stenson's duct in the cheek just across from the first or second molar of the upper arch.

parulis (pah-roo'-lis) Technical name for a gum boil.

pathogenic (path-ō-jen′-ik) Greek: *disease* plus *to produce*. Capable of causing disease.

pathology (pah-thol′-ō-jē) Greek: *disease* plus *discourse*. That science which studies the nature of disease, its causes, effects, and the changes produced by disease.

pedodontics (pē″-dō-don′-tiks) Greek: *child* plus *tooth*. That branch of dentistry which studies and cares for children's dental needs. (Syn. pedodontia)

pellagra (pel-lag′-rah) Latin: *skin* plus *seizure*. A disease caused by a diet deficient in nicotinic acid.

perforate (per′-fuh-rāt) Latin: *through* plus *to bore*. To puncture, bore, or pierce through.

periapical (per-ē-ā′-pi-kal) Surrounding the root or apex of the tooth.

pericoronitis (per″-ē-ko-ron-ī′-tis) Inflammation (*itis*) of the gingiva around the crown of a tooth, especially a newly erupting tooth.

periodontal (per″-ē-ō-don′-tal) Greek: *around* plus *tooth*. Around the tooth, especially refers to the periodontal membrane.

periodontal membrane The fibrous and connective tissue running from the cementum to the tooth socket, supporting the tooth in its socket.

periodontics Specialty of dentistry which deals with the treatment and prevention of diseases of the soft tissue and bone surrounding the teeth.

periodontitis (per-ē-ō-don-tī′-tis) Inflammation of the tissues that surround and support the teeth —the gingivae, the cementum of the tooth, the periodontal membrane, and the alveolar and supporting bone.

periodontosis (diffuse alveolar atrophy) (per-ē-ō-don-tō′-sis) A noninflammatory condition affecting the tissues listed under periodontitis, in which the fibers of the periodontal membranes degenerate, alveolar bone is resorbed, and the epithelial attachment is proliferated along the root surfaces. The end result of the process is the loosening and moving of teeth.

periosteum (per″-ē-os′-tē-um) Greek: *around* plus *bone*. Dental periosteum is another name for the periodontal membrane. It is also tough membrane around bones and adhering to their surfaces.

peripheral (per-if′-er-al) Situated near the periphery (external boundary of a surface or area).

permanent Lasting; intended to last indefinitely.

personnel, auxiliary The dental office staff hired by the dentist to assist him in his work. It includes dental assistants, dental hygienists, dental laboratory technicians, and any other classification the dentist deems essential in assistant personnel.

pH The concentration of hydrogen ions expressed as the negative logarithm of base 10. It is used in expressing both acidity and alkalinity on a scale whose values run from 0—14 with 7 representing neutrality, acid below 7 and alkalinity above 7.

phagocyte (fag′-ō-sīt) A cell that engulfs or devours microorganisms, cells, debris, and other substances.

phagocytosis (fag-ō-sī-tō′-sis) The engulfing and destruction of microorganisms, cells, or other substances by a cell called a phagocyte.

pharmacology (fahr-mah-kol′-ō-jē) Greek: *medicine* plus *discourse*. The science of drugs, their uses and actions.

phenol (fē-nol) Also called carbolic acid. A coal tar derivative used to cauterize in cavity preparation. It also may be used as a disinfectant and germicide.

phenol coefficient A formula showing how effective a given antisepetic is as compared with phenol. Not always a reliable indication of the ability of an antisepetic.

phonetics (fō-net′-iks) The study of the production and understanding of speech sounds including variations by individuals and groups. Phonetics also includes the classification of the sounds produced.

physician (fi-zish′-un) A person holding the degree of doctor of medicine (M.D.), legally qualified to practice medicine.

physiological (fi-zē-ō-loj′-i-kal) Refers to normal functions of an organism.

pit A small, sharp depression in the enamel surface of the tooth.

plaster A roasted (calcined) calcium sulfate powder which is mixed with water to make casts and impressions for dental use.

plastic (plas′-tik) Greek: *to mold*. Material which can be shaped or molded.

plasticizer (plas′-ti-sī′-zer) One of several substances added to a plastic material to give a soft, viscous property to the finished product.

pleomorphic (plē-ō-mor′-fik) More than one distinct form occurs in the life cycle of a plant.

plexus (pleks′-us) An interwoven combination of parts of a structure, thus, a network of nerves, veins, or lymphatics.

pneumatic (new-mat′-ik) Pertaining to air or gases in general; operated by air pressure.

pontic (pon'-tik) That part of a bridge or partial which replaces a missing tooth. Patients often refer to the pontic as the "false tooth."

porcelain, synthetic porcelain Terms used for silicate cement.

posterior (pos-tē'-rē-or) Situated behind; to the back.

premature (prē-ma-tūr') Latin: *before* plus *ripe*. Something which occurs too soon or before the proper time.

prescribe (prē-skrīb') To designate or indicate the directions for giving or using remedy or treatment.

prescription (prē-skrip'-shun) The written directions for the preparation and use of a drug, treatment, or remedy.

primary tooth *Primary* means first in order of time or any series, thus primary teeth means first teeth—those which are first seen in the child's mouth and are later replaced with permanent dentition. Synonyms: Deciduous dentition, baby tooth.

procedure (prō-sē'-dure) The manner of proceeding, a certain course of action.

process (pros'-es) A projecting part of bone.
  alveolar process A ridge in which the sockets of the teeth are found.

profession (prō-fesh'-un) A vocation for which specific study is necessary, usually requiring examination and licensing by the state in which the person wishes to practice his profession. (Examples: law, teaching, dentistry, medicine.)

professional Appropriate to a profession; in keeping with ethics.

prognosis (prahg-nō'-sis) A forecast as to the probable result of a disease or condition. Thus, in dentistry, an opinion about the probable success of a restoration.

proliferation (prō-lif"-er-ā'-shun) Latin: *offspring* plus *to bear*. To grow by reproduction or multiplication, referring especially to cells.

prophylactic (prō-fī-lak'-tik) A remedy which helps prevention of a disease.

prophylaxis (prō-fī-lax'-is) 1. The prevention of disease. 2. A procedure for removing substances from the surfaces of the teeth. Scaling and polishing techniques are used. The purpose of this procedure is the prevention of disease of the oral cavity.

prosthesis (pros'-thē-sis) Replacement of a natural part of the body with an artificial substitute.
  dental prosthesis Any replacement for natural dentition, as a bridge, denture, partial denture, etc.

prosthetic (pros-thet'-ik) Refers to prostheses.

prosthodontics (pros-thō-don'-tiks) The branch of dentistry concerned with making replacements for missing teeth.

protoplasm (prō'-tō-plazm) Greek: *first* plus *form*. A mixture of complex chemical compounds, mostly proteins and water, in a cell. The living matter of all vegetable and animal cells.

proximal (prok'-si-mal) Latin: *next*. Nearest to the chosen point or place.
  proximal surface One of the surfaces of a tooth, either mesial or distal, which is next to an adjacent tooth.
  interproximal The area between two adjacent teeth; bounded by the contact point above and extending gingivally between the two curving surfaces.

psychology (sī-kahl'-uh-gē) The science that studies the mental processes and the behavior of the individual. Modern psychology studies all the interactions between living organisms and their environment.

ptyalin (tī'-al-in) Greek: *spittle*. An enzyme found in the saliva of man and some of the lower animals which changes starch into dextrin, maltose, and glucose.

pulp The soft tissue found in the central cavity of a tooth (pulp chamber). It contains arteries, veins, lymphatic and nerve tissue—all of which connect to the rest of the body and supply the tooth its means of sensation and nutrition.

pulp canal The part of the pulp cavity found within the root or roots of the teeth.

pulp chamber That portion of the central cavity of the tooth which lies within the crown of the tooth. It has canals which form a passageway for blood vessels and nerve fibers to the tip of the root, the apex, and thence to the circulatory and nerve structures of the rest of the body.

pulpitis (pulp-ī'-tis) Inflammation of the dental pulp. Toothache.

pulpless tooth A tooth from which the pulp has been removed. A devitalized tooth, no longer alive.

pulpotomy (pulp-ot'-ō-mē) An operation in which part or all the pulp is removed from a tooth.

pumice (pum'-is) Spongy volcanic lava used in powdered form to clean and polish teeth and other dental materials such as dentures.

pus A liquid made up of white blood cells (leukocytes) and a thin fluid called liquor puris. It is the product of inflammation.

pyogenic (pī-ō-gen'-ik) Refers to the production of pus.

R

radiant energy The energy which travels as a wave motion; specifically, the energy of electromagnetic waves is called radiant energy. The waves are called roentgen rays.

radiation (rā-dē-ā′-shun) The processes of emission, transmission, and absorption of radiant energy combined.

radiation necrosis (rā-dē-ā′-shun ni-krō′-sis) Death of tissue caused by radiation. If treatment of carcinoma (cancer) of the throat, mouth, or lip is undertaken by means of X rays or cobalt, heavy destruction of bone and teeth with formation of a sequestrum (piece of dead bone, usually being expelled from the body) is generally one result. The destruction is apparently more easily controlled when teeth, if present in the area of treatment, are removed prior to exposure if possible.

radioactivity Some elements are capable of spontaneously emitting alpha, beta, or gamma rays by disintegration of the nuclei of atoms. This ability is called radioactivity.

radiodontics (rā′dē-ō-don-tiks) The specialty in dentistry which devotes itself to making and interpreting radiographs (X rays) of teeth and mouth.

radiograph (rā′-dē-ō-graf) X ray or roentgenogram.

radiography (rā-dē-ah′-graf-ē) Photography with X rays or roentgen rays.

radiology (rā-dē-ol′-uh-gē) A name for the branch of medical science which uses radiant energy in diagnosis and treatment. (Radiographs are made for diagnosis of conditions. Radioactive substances and roentgen rays are used to treat certain diseases.)

radiolucent (rā-dē-ō-lū′-sent) That which permits X rays to pass through, yet has some resistance to their passage.

ramus (rā-mus) Latin: *a branch*. In dentistry, especially that part of the lower jaw which articulates with the skull.

record (rek′-ord) Usually a written recounting of facts to be kept for future reference. The record may include X rays and study models as well as written history.

rehabilitation (rē-hab-il-i-tā′-shun) Restoring a person to useful activity who has been physically or emotionally injured.

    oral rehabilitation The restoration of the mouth to normal in all respects through dental work.

residual cyst (rē-zid′-ū-l sist) An odontogenic cyst that remains within the jaw after the tooth with which it was associated has been removed.

residual ridge (rē-zid′-ū-l) means *remainder*. The portion of the alveolar ridge which remains after the alveoli (sockets for the teeth) have disappeared from the alveolar process (the bone which surrounds and supports the teeth) following extraction of teeth.

resin (rez′-un) An organic substance, usually transparent or translucent which is not soluble in water but is soluble in ether, acetone, etc. They are nonconductors of electricity. They are used in medicine.

resorption (rē-sorp′-shun) Latin: *to suck up*. The removal or loss of tissue by absorption. The gradual disappearance of the root of a primary tooth is due to resorption.

rest position A position of the lower jaw, usually with the teeth slightly apart, though the lips remain closed.

restoration (res-tō-rā′-shun) A general term often used to designate the filling, crown, bridge, partial, or full denture used to restore part or all of the dentition to normal function.

resuscitate (rē-sus′-i-tāt) To restore to life or consciousness an individual who is apparently dead or unable to breathe.

retainer (rē-tān-er) An appliance designed to stabilize teeth after orthodontic treatment.

retarders (re-tard′-ers) *Retard*: to hold back, to slow down. A chemical is added to a substance to slow the chemical reaction. It prolongs the setting time of the material and provides more working time.

retraction (rē-trak′-shun) A shrinking of tissues, also a laying back of tissues to reveal or expose a given part.

rickets (rik′-its) A disease found in children and infants caused by vitamin D deficiency. It causes defective ossification of bone because the body is unable to properly utilize calcium and phosphorus without adequate vitamin D intake.

ridge Remainder of alveolar process (bone surrounding and supporting teeth) after teeth are removed.

roentgen (rent′-gen) The international unit of quantity or dose of roentgen (or X) ray and gamma rays. It shall be called the "roentgen" and be designated by the symbol *r*.

roentgenogram (rent-gen′-ō-gram) A photograph made with roentgen rays, or more technically, a shadow image of radiopaque anatomic structures which are recorded on film sensitized to roentgen rays.

roentgenology (rent-gen-ahl'-uh-gē) The study and use of roentgen ray in diagnostic and therapeutic areas in medicine and dentistry.

root That portion of the dentin which lies beyond the enamel-covered coronal part of each tooth. It is covered with cementum.

root canal A passageway for nerves and blood vessels to the pulp chamber of the tooth.

rouge An iron oxide in cake or stick form used for polishing gold on a muslin wheel. (Jeweler's rouge.)

rubber dam A thin sheet of very lively rubber which the dentist perforates in such a manner as to fit over a tooth or group of teeth preventing saliva from wetting that portion of the tooth exposed through the rubber.

S

saccharids (sak'-uh-rīds) A simple sugar, carbohydrate.

saddle That part of a partial denture which distributes stresses of mastication over the ridge area, usually carrying the replacement teeth, where natural teeth have been removed.

saliva (sah-lī'-vah) A clear liquid secreted by the salivary glands into the oral cavity through various ducts. Saliva aids in the digestion of foods. It contains ptyalin.

sanitary (san'-i-terry) Relating to health, hygienic. Relating to keeping something clean.

scurvy (skur'-vē) A disease which occurs as a result of vitamin C deficiency. Symptoms are weakness, anemia, hemhorrage under the skin and mucous membranes, poor healing of wounds and bone deformities, "spongy gums," and "loosening of the teeth."

secretion (si-krē'-shun) 1. The process of separating and releasing some material, 2. The material which is released. Thus, saliva is the secretion secreted by the salivary glands.

sedative (sed'-uh-tiv) A remedy that reduces activity or **excitement.**

senility (seh-nil'-i-tē) The physical and mental infirmity of old age.

sepsis (sep'-sus) A disease condition found in the mouth or adjacent areas which may affect the general health of the individual as well as the parts of the body adjacent to the diseased area because sepsis disseminates toxins. Sepsis may also be found in other areas of the body, but we are concerned with the term as it applies to dentistry.

septicemia (sep"-ti-cē'-mē-ah) Greek: *putrid* plus *blood.* A disease condition caused by the presence of microorganisms and their poisons in the blood.

septum (sep'-tum) A dividing wall or membrane. Interdental: the alveolar process (bone surrounding the teeth) extending between the roots of the teeth. Nasal: The membrane dividing the left and right nostrils.

shade guide A group of teeth furnished by a manufacturer of artificial teeth or filling material showing each color in which he manufactures his product. The dentist and patient are able to select the shades most suited to the patient's mouth for any artificial teeth or filling to be used.

shock A condition brought about by physical or emotional injury, consisting mainly of circulatory disturbances. Shock can lead to death if not successfully treated in time. An individual suffering from shock is pale, skin is clammy, pulse weak and rapid.

shoulder A term used in reference to a definite ledge or step in a dental preparation in the tooth structure.

sialolithiasis (si"-ah-lō-li-thi'-ah-sis) The formation of salivary calculi within the ducts of the salivary glands, or the condition or infection caused by such formation.

silicate cement (sil'-i'-kut se-ment') A filling material used in anterior teeth.

solder (sod'-er) An alloy which is used to join together other metal surfaces, requiring heat in its application.

soldering (sod'-er-ing) (ortho) The process of joining two pieces of metal by using an alloy which melts at a lower temperature than the metals to be joined. The alloy is melted and dripped on the joint, then allowed to harden.

solubility (sahl-ū-bil'-i-tē) Possible to dissolve.

solute (sahl-yūt') The dissolved member of a solution (usually the less abundant part) Thus, in sugary syrup, the sugar is the solute—it has been dissolved in the water.

solution (sō-lū'-shun) A liquid consisting of a mixture of two or more substances dispersed through one another uniformly.

solvent (sol'-vent) A chemical used to dissolve other substances.

spasm (spaa'-zm) A sudden, violent temporary, involuntary contraction of a muscle group when referring to physical spasms. There is also an emotional spasm which is a sudden, violent effort.

spatulation (spat-ū-lā'-shun) Mixing by use of a flat, blunt instrument.

specialist (spesh-ul-ist) In dentistry, a dentist who limits his practice to a certain type of treatment, such as orthodontics or pedodontics.

spirillum (spi-ril′-um) Spiral-shaped bacteria. Spirilla may have many forms—a single curve, coiled, many curves, or coiled and curved at the same time.

spirochete (spī-rō-kēt′) An organism which is elongated and flexible, twisted spirally around its long axis. It exhibits motility without possessing flagella.

spores A form of bacteria especially difficult to destroy.

spot welders (ortho) "Spot welding is a resistance-welding process in which the joining of two metals is done electrically without the application of flux and solder. High amperage current flowing through the metals creates an internal heat within the metals. The flow of electricity is concentrated so that the two metals melt at their point of contact between the electrodes. Because there is pressure between the electrodes of the welder, the two 'molten' spots are pushed together. When the 'molten' spot cools, the two metals become one at the point of the weld." Courtesy Rocky Mountain Dental Products Co., Denver, Colorado.

sprue In dentistry, the piece of metal or plastic attaching the wax pattern to the base; the hole through which the molten metal enters the mold; or the waste piece of the casting which filled this hole.

staphylococcus (staf″-i-lō-kok′-us) The bacteria most commonly found in abscesses and other pus-forming conditions.

sterilize The act of removing or destroying all microorganisms.

    hot-water sterilization Sanitizing.

    pasteurization Partial sterilization of a fluid at a temperature which destroys objectionable organisms without chemical alteration of the subject.

stomatitis (stō″-mah-tī′-tus) A general term for inflammation of the oral cavity which may occur from bacterial, viral, mechanical, chemical, electrical, thermal, or radiation injury, from allergens, and as secondary (in sequence of time or development) manifestation of a systemic disease. May also occur as a reaction to medications or irritants, or systemic changes such as pregnancy. In the case of pregnancy it is often referred to as *pregnancy stomatitis,* and at this time a patient may also exhibit a gingivitis with hypertrophy of the gums, and occasionally develop a *pregnancy tumor* on the gingiva. Such pregnancy tumors are easily removed.

stomatology (stō-ma-tahl′-uh-ge) A branch of medical science which studies structures, functions, and diseases of the mouth.

stone A tool or instrument used for abrading.

    Arkansas stone A fine-grained stone used in the final sharpening of instruments.

    Carborundum stone is made of silicon carbide. It is an abrasive, handpiece-mounted instrument. There are several sizes, shapes, and degrees of abrasiveness. They are used to shape (or contour) tooth structure.

stone, artificial A special calcined gypsum derivative similar to plaster. Its grains are nonporous, and therefore artificial stone is stronger than plaster.

streptococcus (strep″-tuh-kok′-us) A genus of microorganisms found in many pathologic conditions, occurring as chains of cells.

study model A duplication of the dental arch of a patient, used for treatment planning, as opposed to a "working" model on which a denture may be constructed, for example.

styptic (stip′-tik) An astringent agent used to stop bleeding.

sublingual (sub-ling′-gwal) Beneath the tongue.

submaxillary (sub-max′-i-lary) Beneath the mandible.

submucosa (sub-mew-kō′-sah) The layer of tissue beneath the mucous membrane.

succedaneous (suk-suh-dā′-nē-us) Substituted or serving as a substitute (or following after).

sulcus, gingival (sul-kus) Sulcus means groove. The gingival sulcus is the shallow groove between the gingiva and the surface of the tooth. It extends around the circumference of the tooth.

superior Above or upper.

surface, facial Surface means the external portion of an object, thus *facial surface* is the external side of a tooth which faces the lips and cheeks (the buccal and labial surfaces).

suture (sū′-chur) 1. A surgical stitch. 2. The line of junction of bones in the head. 3. The material used to sew up a wound.

syncopé (sin′-kō-pay) The act of fainting. It is directly caused by an insufficient supply of blood to the brain.

synthesis (sin′-thuh-sis) The combination of parts to form a whole.

synthetic (sin-thet′-ik) Produced artificially.

syringe An instrument for injecting liquids.

T

target In radiography the target is the tungsten button in the anode at which the electrons produced by the cathode are directed.

tartar A hard deposit on the surfaces of the teeth; more properly called "salivary calculus." Usually most heavily formed on those surfaces nearest the salivary ducts.

technique, direct Preparation of a crown wax pattern in the patient's mouth.

technique, indirect Preparation of the wax pattern outside the patient's mouth on a die.

temporary stopping A material containing gutta-percha, capable of being softened by low heat and immediately placed in a cavity preparation in the tooth.

temporomandibular joints The joints, just ahead of each ear, upon which the lower jaw swings open and shut and can also slide forward.

terminology (ter-mi-nol-ah-jē) The complete system of scientific or technical words applying to a science, art, or subject.

tincture (tink′-chur) An alcoholic solution of a medicinal substance.

therapeutics (ther-uh-pew′-tiks) Branch of medicine which deals with the treatment of disease. (*Therapeutic* is Greek for treatment.)

therapy Remedial treatment of disease or bodily disorder.

thermoplastic A material which is rigid at normal temperatures but becomes soft when heated. The material can be softened by applying heat any number of times.

thrush (moniliasis) A disease caused by the yeast-like *Candida albicans,* characterized by white, curdy, raised patches which can be scraped off leaving a base which bleeds.

thyroid The endocrine gland which lies at the base of the neck. It produces a hormone containing iodine.

tooth An organ of mastication. One of the hard bodies designed for the mastication of food. It is located in the oral cavity, attached to the alveolar process of the maxilla or mandible.

    deciduous tooth (dē-sid′-ū-us) A tooth which is shed; primary, baby, or milk tooth.

    impacted tooth (im-pak′-ted) A tooth which is in such a position within the jaws that it cannot erupt into complete visibility of the crown. A tooth may be partially or completely impacted.

    nonvital tooth (non-vī′-tal) A tooth which does not give a response to a stimulus because of a loss of "life."

    permanent tooth The tooth which replaces the primary tooth when it is shed.

    supernumerary tooth (sū-per-nū′-mer-ary) A tooth which is in excess of the usual or normally occurring number.

    unerupted tooth (un-ē-rup′-ted) A normal tooth before eruption into the mouth. Occasionally a tooth which lacks the physiologic impulse or erupting stimulus and therefore remains embedded. Not to be confused with "impacted."

    vital tooth (vī′-tal) A tooth which gives a response to an irritating stimulus, much as you would expect a person whose skin is pricked to say "ouch!"

topical (top′-i-kal) On the surface, locally.

toxicity (tox-is′-i-tē) Usually used as a measure of the kind and amount of toxin (poison) produced by a given microorganism.

toxin (tox′-in) A secretion of cells which is poisonous to animals or man, resulting in the formation of resisting substances called antibodies. Bacteria produce most of the toxins with which we are concerned.

trachea (trā′-kē-uh) The windpipe, extending from the lower part of the larynx to the point of division into two bronchi.

transformer A device used to convert variations of current in a primary circuit into variations of voltage and current in a secondary circuit. The principle of mutual induction is used for the conversion.

transfusion (trans-fū′-zhun) The process of passing from one to another, that is, transferring blood or saline solution into the vein or artery of a human.

transient (tran′-shent) Of short duration.

transilluminate (trans″-il-lū′-min-āt″) To pass through an area or organ in order to examine its condition.

trauma (trow′-ma) General: A hurt or wound to living tissue.

    dental An actual alteration of tissues produced by dental disharmony.

traumatic (trow-mat′-ik) Referring to that which has been caused by injury.

treatment (trēt-ment) The actual process of treating anything. The management of an illness by any means in an effort to bring relief or aid in a cure.

trituration (trit-ur-ā′-shun) To mix by grinding and rubbing.

tuberosity (tū-ber-os′-it-ē) A large, rough prominence on a bone. It is also used to refer in specific cases to a prominence made up of soft tissues (flesh).

tumor (tū′-mōr) A swollen or distended part of the body. However, usage has now made the word *tumor* synonymous with neoplasm, which means an abnormal mass of tissue with no physiologic function. It is an abnormal growth of a mass of cells in the body.

tungsten (tung′-sten) An element used especially for electrical purposes and in hardening alloys. It is gray-white, heavy, high-melting, ductile, hard, polyvalent, metallic, and resembles chromium and molybdenum.

U

ulcer (ul′-cer) An open sore, whether on an external or internal surface of the body.

U.S.P. An abbreviation for "United States Pharmacopeia," the authority for all drug standards.

V

varnish A solution of certain resins or gums in an evaporating base, used to form a shining, firm coating on a surface.

vascular (vas′-qū-lar) Relating to a channel for the conveyance of a body fluid, such as blood, or to a system of these channels, such as blood vessels.

vasoconstrictor (vas″-ō-kon-strik′-tor) A nerve or a drug which causes a blood vessel to become smaller in diameter, thus permitting less blood to flow through the blood vessel.

vasodilator (vas″-ō-dī-lā′-tor) A drug or nerve action which causes enlargement of a blood vessel, thus permitting more blood to flow through the blood vessel.

vestibule of the mouth (ves-ti-būl) The corridor or space between the alveolar gingiva and the lips and the cheeks.

virulent (vir′-yū-lent) Able to overcome bodily defenses, marked by a severe, extremely poisonous course.

virus (vī′-rus) The causative agent of a specific disease, smaller than bacteria. These agents are formed by various plants and animal forms, and are responsible for many common diseases in man.

vitamin (vī′-tah-min) A protein substance which is essential to the metabolic processes and closely associated with enzyme function. Vitamins are not produced by the human body but must come from plant sources and be injested in the diet.

volatilize (vol′-uh-til-īz) To cause to pass off as a vapor; evaporate.

volt The electromotive force necessary to cause one ampere of current to flow against one ohm of resistance.

voltmeter A meter which registers the volts being used in operating the machine to which the meter is attached.

W

wax A substance of complex chemical form, used in dentistry in many variations for various purposes. In general, waxes become soft and plastic when warmed, more resistant to molding when chilled or cold, are not soluble in water, are soluble in ether or chloroform.

weld To unite two or more pieces by the application of heat along the joint.

wire, separating Wires threaded interproximally between two adjacent teeth and tightened by twisting the ends together to wedge the teeth apart slightly. Used preparatory to adapting bands to teeth having tight contacts with adjacent teeth.

X

X ray (roentgen ray) Electromagnetic radiation when electrons strike a target in a vacuum tube. X ray is preferred when speaking with lay personnel. Roentgen ray is preferred in scientific communication.

Z

zoology The branch of biology concerned with the animal kingdom and its members as individuals as well as classes.

zygomatic arch (zī′-gō-mat-ik) An arch of bone commonly known as the "cheek bone." It begins just in front of the ear, arches slightly outward, forward, and then curves slightly inward to an area just below the outer corner of the eye. The *arch* portion of this bone is just above the ramus of the mandible. You can't get your finger under the arch because it is so blocked by muscles.

INDEX

(Numbers in bold type indicate pages on which illustrations occur.)

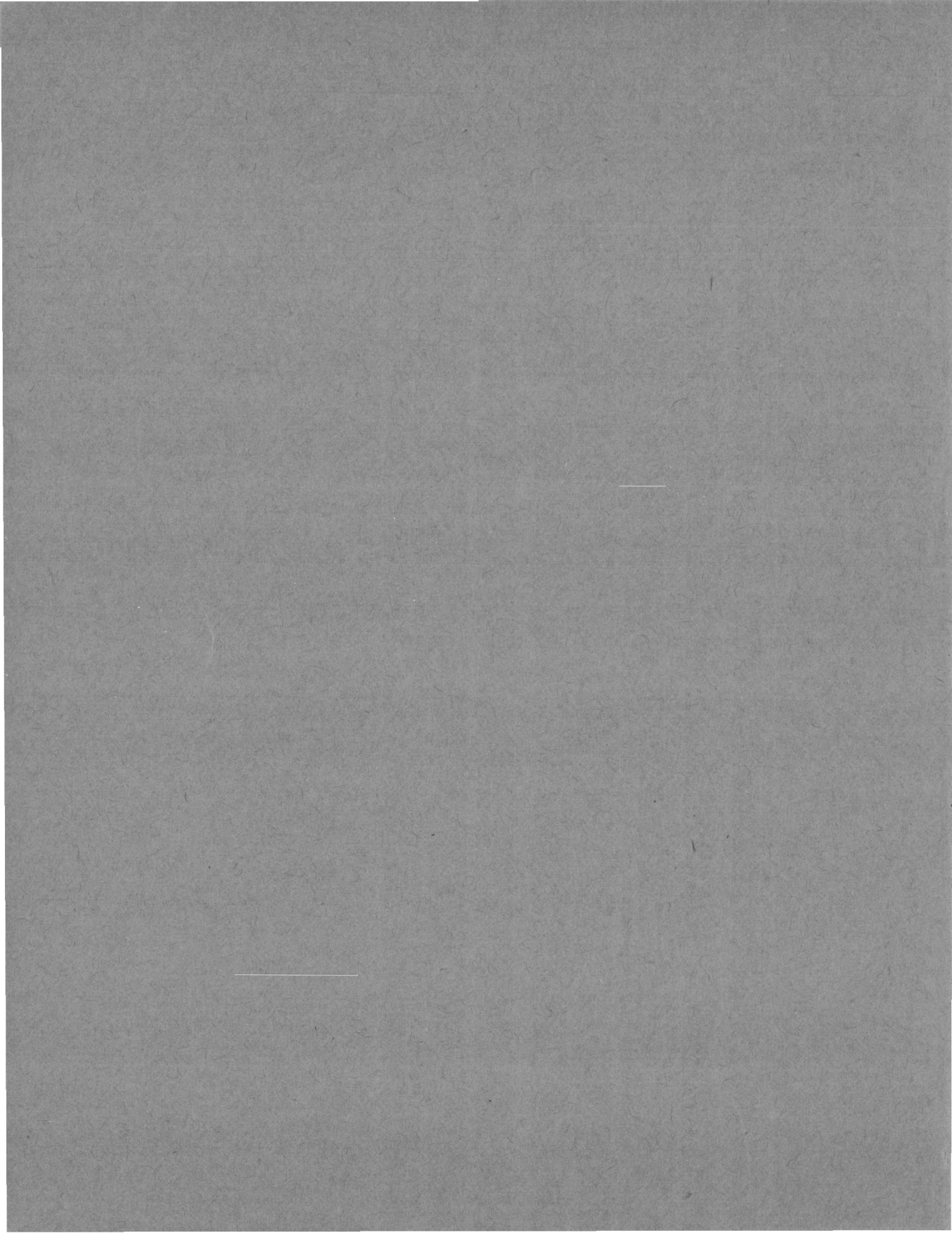